Anaesthesia for
Vascular Surgery

Anaesthesia for Vascular Surgery

Edited by

J Bannister
Department of Anaesthetics,
Ninewells Hospital and Medical School,
Dundee, UK

J A W Wildsmith
University Department of Anaesthesia,
Ninewells Hospital and Medical School,
Dundee, UK

A member of the Hodder Headline Group
LONDON
Co-published in the USA by Oxford University Press Inc., New York

First published in Great Britain in 2000 by
Arnold, a member of the Hodder Headline Group,
338 Euston Road, London NWI 3BH

http://www.arnoldpublishers.com

Co-published in the United States of America by
Oxford University Press, Inc.,
198 Madison Avenue, New York, NY 10016
Oxford is a registered trademark of Oxford University Press

British Library Cataloguing in Publication Data
A catalogue record for this book is available from the British
Library

Library of Congress Cataloging-in-Publication Data
A catalog record for this book is available from the Library of
Congress

ISBN 0 340 69204 9

1 2 3 4 5 6 7 8 9 10

Publisher: Joanna Koster
Project Editor: Melissa Morton
Production Editor: James Rabson
Production Controller: Priya Gohil
Cover design: Terry Griffiths

Typeset in 10/12 pt Minion by
Scribe Design, Gillingham, Kent
Printed and bound in Great Britain by the Bath Press, Avon

What do you think about this book? Or any other Arnold title?
Please send your comments to feedback.arnold@hodder.co.uk

Contents

Contributors

Jill J F Belch MB ChB FRCP MD
Section of Vascular Medicine and Biology, University Department of Medicine, Ninewells Hospital and Medical School, Dundee, UK

Margaret Bourke FFARCSI
Department of Anaesthesia, Beaumont Hospital, Dublin, Ireland

Andrew W Bradbury BSc MD FRCS Ed
Vascular Surgery Unit, University Department of Clinical and Surgical Sciences, Royal Infirmary, Edinburgh, UK

R Butler MB ChB MD MRCP
University Department of Clinical Pharmacology, Ninewells Hospital and Medical School, Dundee, UK

Michael J Cousins MBBS MD FANZCA FRCA
Department of Anaesthesia and Pain Management, Royal North Shore Hospital and University of Sydney, St Leonards, New South Wales, Australia

David M Coventry MB ChB FRCA
Department of Anaesthetics, Ninewells Hospital and Medical School, Dundee, UK

Anthony J Cunningham MD FRCPC
Department of Anaesthesia, Royal College of Surgeons in Ireland, Dublin, Ireland

Lesley A Duncan FRCA
Department of Anaesthetics, Ninewells Hospital and Medical School, Dundee, UK

Neal D Edwards FRCA
University Department of Surgical and Anaesthetic Sciences, Northern General Hospital, Sheffield, UK

Shirley J Fearn MB ChB PhD FRCS
Departments of Surgery and Anaesthesia, Withington Hospital, South Manchester University Hospitals NHS Trust, Manchester, UK

Pierre Foëx MA DPhil FRCA FANZCA F Med Sci
Nuffield Department of Anaesthetics, Radcliffe Infirmary, Oxford, UK

Megan Gray MBBS FANZCA
Department of Anaesthesia and Pain Management, Royal North Shore Hospital and University of Sydney, St Leonards, New South Wales, Australia

S J Howell MSc MRCP FRCA
Sir Humphrey Davy Department of Anaesthesia, Bristol Royal Infirmary, Bristol, UK

Gerard M A Keenan MB ChB FFARCSI FRCA
Department of Anaesthesia, The Royal Infirmary of Edinburgh, Edinburgh, UK

Andrew D Morris MSc MD FRCP
University Department of Medicine, Ninewells Hospital and Medical School, Dundee, UK

Andrew J Mortimer BSc MD FRCA
Department of Anaesthesia, Withington Hospital, South Manchester University Hospitals NHS Trust, Manchester, UK

Andrew Muir MB ChB
Section of Vascular Medicine and Biology, University Department of Medicine, Ninewells Hospital and Medical School, Dundee, UK

Alastair F Nimmo MB ChB FRCA
Department of Anaesthesia, The Royal Infirmary of Edinburgh, Edinburgh, UK

Christopher J O'Connor MD
Associate Professor, Department of Anesthesiology, Rush Medical College, Rush-Presbyterian-St Luke's Medical Center, Chicago, Illinois, USA

Charles S Reilly MD FRCA
Department of Surgical and Anaesthetic Sciences, University of Sheffield, Royal Hallamshire Hospital, Sheffield, UK

N B Scott FRCS FFARCS
Consultant Anaesthetist, Department of Anaesthesia,
HCI International Medical Centre, Clydebank, UK

J W Sear MA PhD FFARCS FANZCA
Honorary Consultant Anaesthetist, Nuffield Department
of Anaesthetics, University of Oxford, The John Radcliffe
Hospital, Oxford, UK

Graham Smith BSc MD FRCA
University Department of Anaesthesia, Leicester Royal
Infirmary, Leicester, UK

Peter A Stonebridge ChM FRCS
Department of Surgery, Ninewells Hospital and Medical
School, Dundee, UK

A D Struthers MD FRCP
Consultant Physician, University Department of Clinical
Pharmacology, Ninewells Hospital and Medical School,
Dundee, UK

Jonathan P Thompson BSc FRCA
University Department of Anaesthesia, Leicester Royal
Infirmary, Leicester, UK

Kenneth J Tuman MD
Department of Anesthesiology, Rush Medical College,
Rush-Presbyterian-St Luke's Medical Center, Chicago,
Illinois, USA

Malcolm O Wright MB ChB FRCS FDSRCS
Department of Biomedical Sciences, University of
Edinburgh, Edinburgh, UK

Preface

The performance of, and outcomes from, anaesthesia and surgery are inextricably linked. Vascular surgery is recognized and established as a subspecialty worldwide. The unique constellation of challenges which these patients present to their anaesthetist has given rise to the subspecialty of vascular anaesthesia.

Developments in surgical and anaesthetic technique and, along with them, increasing patient expectations, lead to ever older and frailer patients presenting for surgery. The patient who might have been refused major surgery fifteen years ago is now a fairly routine part of any vascular list. Patients undergoing emergency vascular surgery present the anaesthetist with an increasing spectrum of co-morbidities. A steadily increasing demand is placed on the knowledge and skills of the perioperative team.

As members of this perioperative team, anaesthetists find themselves more and more involved in all aspects including preoperative assessment and optimization, discussion of surgical options in terms of optimal risk benefit, and postoperative care in the Intensive Care or High Dependency Unit. Dialogue with colleagues now regularly includes not only surgeons, but radiologists, vascular physicians and cardiologists.

The expanding role of the anaesthetist has shaped the form of this book. It is written to reflect current best practice. Authors have been chosen for their individual knowledge, be they from anaesthetic, surgical or medical disciplines. The reader will find areas of overlapping subject matter in different chapters. In some aspects you will find opposing views from differing experts. Usually, however, there is simply a different emphasis placed, and the differing views complement each other. This diversity reflects the fact that there is no absolutely correct approach to these patients. This is not a recipe book for vascular anaesthesia – it is intended as an information and opinion resource for both the trainee and established practitioner.

ACKNOWLEDGEMENTS

We would like to thank Mrs Marie Thomson, Secretary to the University Department of Anaesthesia in Dundee, for her assistance, the publishers for their many contributions, and our families for their support, forbearing and tolerance of the editorial processes.

JB
JAWW

Epidemiology of peripheral vascular disease

PETER A STONEBRIDGE

LOWER LIMB OCCLUSIVE DISEASE

Atherosclerotic disease of the arteries of the lower limbs is a major cause of morbidity in the developed world with approximately 2 per cent of the populations of Western countries suffering from intermittent claudication. A recent modification of the World Health Organization questionnaire for diagnosing peripheral vascular disease, the Edinburgh Claudication Questionnaire, showed the prevalence to be 4.6 per cent in a population aged 55–74 years (Fowkes et al., 1991). The range is wide with a prevalence as high as 10 per cent in Eastern Finland (Heliovaara et al., 1978) and as low as 0.3 per cent in telephone employees in the USA (Holland et al., 1967).

Claudication increases with age (Hale et al., 1988) and is slightly more common in men than women (Hughson et al., 1978), although the Edinburgh Artery Study found an identical prevalence in the sexes (Table 1.1). This latter may have been because the group surveyed was older than in most cardiovascular studies. In a long-standing USA study (the 'Framingham' study) the biennial incidence rate was 7.1 per 1000 men and 3.6 per 1000 women (Kannel and McGee, 1984), with women having the incidence of men 10 years younger and this difference reducing with advancing age (Kannel et al., 1970).

The occupation of the patient also has an impact on incidence, if only by influencing whether a patient will complain of claudication or not, for example farmers having a higher incidence (Reuanen et al., 1982) than civil servants (Reid et al., 1974).

Asymptomatic disease follows a similar pattern to symptomatic. In a study from Basle the five-year cumulative incidence was 4 per cent in men aged 35–44 years and 18 per cent in those aged 65 or over (Widmer et al., 1985). In the Glostrup study from Denmark, a survey of 60-year-old patients found that 14 per cent had peripheral arterial disease manifest by an ankle–brachial pressure index (ABPI) < 0.9 (Reuanen et al., 1982). In a series of 293 unselected autopsies 15 per cent of men, and 5 per cent of women, had a common iliac artery stenosis >50 per cent (Mitchell and Schwartz, 1965). Finally, a

Table 1.1 *Prevalence of intermittent claudication in the Edinburgh Artery Study*

Age (years)	Intermittent claudication (%)	
	Men	Women
55–59	2.2	2.3
60–64	4.4	5.0
65–69	3.5	5.5
70–74	7.7	6.6

study in Malmö, Sweden (Sternby, 1968) of 1486 subjects aged 30–79 years produced similar findings, and also showed that the left common iliac artery was more commonly affected, even though the common femoral arteries were equally affected.

Outcome of lower limb ischaemia

The commonest concern of patients who consult a surgeon about leg ischaemia is of losing the limb, but only 10 per cent of such patients will require any form of local procedure. Silbert and Zazeela (1958) followed up 1115 patients with intermittent claudication for 3–25 years and found that 56 per cent remained the same and 44 per cent became worse. A similar study of 1476 patients revealed that 71 per cent remained stable or improved, and that 29 per cent became worse (Bloor, 1961). Poor prognostic indicators for limb survival include age over 65 years (Taylor and Calo, 1962), and distal vessel disease (Crawford et al., 1981). The amputation rate is related to the presenting symptom, being 3 per cent with claudication and 9 per cent with rest pain (Kannel et al., 1970). Within the group who present with claudication the amputation rate is three times greater in short- than long-distance claudicants (McAllister, 1976), but the most important predictor is smoking. Juergens and colleagues (1960) reported that claudicants who stopped smoking did not require amputation, whilst 11.4 per cent who did not stop smoking lost a limb. Diabetes increases the risk of amputation fivefold (Schadt et al., 1961).

If amputation is required only 20 per cent of patients maintain full mobility after major limb amputation (Jamieson and Ruckley, 1983). Furthermore, between 15 and 50 per cent of these patients will require a contralateral limb amputation within two years (Ecker and Jacobs, Kihn et al., 1972). Of even greater concern is the mortality rate of major amputees (Table 1.2). The reasons for this are not hard to find. In the Basle leg ischaemia study the combined prevalence of coronary and cere-

brovascular disease was 37 per cent, compared to 10 per cent in an age and sex matched population (Agner, 1981). The average prevalence of coronary disease derived from ten studies was 44 per cent. This was partly depending on the method of diagnosis, while the prevalence of cerebrovascular disease was between 4 and 52 per cent (De Weese and Rob, 1977; Turnipseed et al., 1980), again depending on whether it was diagnosed by clinical history or objective investigation. Such co-existing disease has a major impact on the mortality of patients with chronic leg ischaemia, with mean mortality being 30, 50 and 70 per cent at 5, 10 and 15 years after diagnosis. The most important risk factor is again smoking which may increase the mortality rate threefold (Biland et al., 1985). Diabetes is also a risk factor for death (Hertzer, 1981; Biland et al., 1985) as are hypertension and concomitant coronary or cerebrovascular disease (Malone et al., 1977; DeWeese and Rob, 1977). The site of the peripheral lesion also has an impact on mortality, with popliteal trifurcation disease being associated with a doubling of the five-year mortality rate (Kallero et al., 1985), although this may more reflect the pattern of diabetic vascular disease. In addition, the mean survival of patients with aorto-iliac disease has been shown to be longer (10.7 years) than those with femoropopliteal disease (7.2 years) (Reid et al., 1974).

Risk factors for lower limb arterial disease

TOBACCO

Cigarette smoking is probably the single most important risk factor for atherosclerotic peripheral artery disease. Between 80 and 100 per cent of individuals attending vascular outpatient clinics have been shown to be current or recent smokers (Lord, 1965; Lithel et al., 1975). The relative risk of smoking and developing peripheral arterial disease ranges from 1.4 (Gyntelberg, 1973) to more than 10.0 (Skalkidis et al., 1989), and it is thought to cause between 14 and 53 per cent of the disease in the community (Hughson et al., 1978; Heliovaara et al., 1978; De Backer et al., 1979). After 16 years of follow up, the Framingham study indicated that nearly 80 per cent of cases of intermittent claudication could be attributed to smoking (Kannel and Shurtleff, 1971). Autopsy studies suggest that cigarette smoking is a

Table 1.2 *Mortality after first amputation*

Hospital/one month	One year	Three years
14%	32%	61%

After Jamieson and Ruckley (1983), Myers et al. (1978), Rush et al. (1981).

more important risk factor for peripheral than coronary arterial disease (Strong and Richards, 1976). In a study of 1320 men aged 25–64 years, the extent of abdominal aortic atherosclerosis was more strongly associated with smoking than was that in the coronary arteries (Powell, 1991). Smoking is also associated with increases in haematocrit, fibrinogen and blood viscosity (Ernst and Matrai, 1987; Meade *et al.*, 1987).

LIPID METABOLISM

Serum triglycerides are elevated in patients with peripheral arterial disease (Leng and Fowkes, 1991). However, more recent studies have shown that this may be due to the correlation between triglycerides and high-density lipoprotein (HDL) and non-HDL cholesterol (Fowkes *et al.*, 1992). Triglyceride levels are also potential markers of the severity of disease (Fowkes *et al.*, 1992), although the relationship may not be with the absolute level of lipid, but rather its rate of removal. Patients with coronary and peripheral vascular disease have been shown to eliminate injected triglycerides slowly (Angquist *et al.*, 1982; Tollin *et al.*, 1984), but exercise has been shown to increase elimination (Ericcson *et al.*, 1982). The relationship between cholesterol and peripheral arterial disease has been examined most recently in the Edinburgh Artery Study. This showed that the relationship persisted after adjustment for other risk factors such as smoking (Fowkes *et al.*, 1992), although a similar study from Israel did not (Gofin *et al.*, 1987). Reduced levels of HDL cholesterol have been observed in hospital patients with arterial disease (Rohling *et al.*, 1989), although the Israeli study did not find this (Gofin *et al.*, 1987). However, the Edinburgh Artery Study did show a significant relationship between peripheral arterial disease, ABPI and HDL cholesterol (Fowkes *et al.*, 1992). Finally, although there is a link between lipoproteins A and B and coronary artery disease, this is less clear for peripheral vascular disease (Editorial, *Lancet*, 1988; Rosengren *et al.*, 1990).

DIABETES MELLITUS

Peripheral vascular, cerebrovascular and cardiovascular disease are all commoner in diabetics than in the normal population (Pyorala and Laasco, 1983). In the Framingham study, the age-adjusted incidence of intermittent claudication in diabetics was 12.6 per thousand men, and 8.4 for women; for non-diabetics the corresponding figures were 3.3 and 1.3 respectively (Kannel and McGhee, 1979). A prospective study using Doppler ABPI has shown that *occult* peripheral arterial disease is also much commoner in non-insulin-dependent diabetics than in controls: 22 versus 3 per cent (Beach *et al.*, 1988). Such patients, representing 90 per cent of diabetics, have a 7- to 20-fold increased risk of lower limb arterial occlusive disease (Beach *et al.*, 1982). Associated risk factors include raised plasma triglycerides, reduced plasma HDL, hypertension, and an elevated systolic blood pressure (Beach *et al.*, 1988). Such associations may make the role of diabetes spurious, but the Edinburgh Artery Study found that the relationship with altered ABPI was independent of other risk factors (Fowkes *et al.*, 1992). It is worthwhile noting that the progression of atherosclerotic occlusive disease is relatively rapid in diabetics, which suggests that those with symptomatic disease might benefit from aggressive early treatment (Bendick *et al.*, 1983).

Thirty-five to forty-five per cent of all lower limb amputations are in diabetics (although not solely for peripheral vascular disease), and standard of footcare, age and patient education are the most important factors (Lippmann and Farrar, 1979; Edmonds *et al.*, 1984). Diabetic foot problems are the commonest indication for hospital admission of these patients in the USA, where the amputation rate has been suggested as a marker of the adequacy of care. Diabetic patients may account for 50–70 per cent of all non-traumatic amputations, a figure well out of proportion to the number of diabetics (2 per cent) in the population (Ger, 1985; Stemmer, 1986). The risk of amputation for a diabetic is 15–70 times that for a non-diabetic (Waugh, 1988). Peripheral vascular disease is the costliest complication of diabetes mellitus in terms of inpatient bed usage, and in the USA it accounts for 1.2 per cent of all hospital costs (National Diabetes Advisory Board, 1980).

LoGerfo and Coffman (1984) conducted a literature review of macrovascular and microvascular disease in diabetes, highlighting the widespread misconception that arteriolar occlusive disease is an aetiological cause of lower limb ischaemic lesions. This belief stems from a report which described, in diabetic arterioles, periodic acid–Schiff-positive material which was interpreted as specific arteriosclerosis associated with diabetes mellitus (Goldenberg *et al.*, 1959). LoGerfo and Coffman (1984) pointed out that subsequent studies using Goldenberg's technique, arterial microcasting down to 10 μm, plethysmographically derived pressure–flow relationships, and blood-flow response to papavarine have all failed to confirm this. Barner and colleagues (1971) concluded that 'vascular reactivity is not impaired and arterial reconstruction should not be withheld on the basis of arteriolar–capillary involvement [in subjects with diabetes]'.

The distribution of macrovascular occlusion in diabetes does differ from that of the non-diabetic population. Amputation specimens from diabetics have revealed that their occlusive atherosclerosis tends to involve the infrageniculate arteries between the knee and ankle, sparing the foot. This has been confirmed in a more recent angiographic study which showed that the dorsalis pedis was spared in two-thirds of patients (Menzoian *et al.*, 1989).

OTHER FACTORS

The Framingham study has shown after 26 years follow up that hypertension increases the risk of claudication by a factor of three (Ruckley, 1991). The Glostrup study showed something similar (Reuanen *et al.*, 1982), although the Basle study did not (da Silva *et al.*, 1979).

Blood viscosity (Ernst and Matrai, 1987; Hell *et al.*, 1989; Lowe *et al.*, 1993) and plasma fibrinogen (Christie *et al.*, 1984; Ernst and Matrai, 1987; Hell *et al.*, 1989) have consistently been found to be higher in patients with intermittent claudication than in control subjects. Increased haematocrit has also been shown to be related to peripheral arterial disease (Lowe *et al.*, 1986), although the Framingham study did not find any relationship with the development of intermittent claudication (Ruckley, 1991). It may be that these factors are co-incidental because they are all also related to smoking (Lowe *et al.*, 1986). Other factors such as fibrinolysis time, decreased fibrinolytic activity and raised factor VIII, factor XIII, plasminogen and platelet function have also been implicated. On the positive side, both exercise (Hell *et al.*, 1989; Housley, 1991) and drinking small quantities of alcohol have a beneficial effect.

Natural history of lower limb ischaemia

Over a five-year period, 75 per cent of claudicants will stabilize (Imperato *et al.*, 1975; McAllister, 1976),

Bloor (1961) reporting that 7 per cent had an amputation within five years and 12 per cent within 10 years. In the unselected populations in the Basle and Framingham studies only 2 per cent proceeded to amputation (Kannel *et al.*, 1970; Widmer *et al.*, 1985). About one-third of claudicants present with bilateral symptoms (Taylor and Calo, 1962), and approximately 15 per cent of patients with critical limb ischaemia have both legs equally effected (Bloor, 1961). Smoking in excess of 40 pack-years (number of packs of cigarettes per day multiplied by the number of years smoked) triples the likelihood of surgery (Cronenwett *et al.*, 1984), and diabetic claudicants have a 21 per cent risk of amputation (McDaniel and Cronenwett, 1989). An ABPI of <0.5 is also a strong predictor of local deterioration (Jelnes *et al.*, 1986).

Critical limb ischaemia has no clear definition, the usual one being a clinical state that will inevitably lead to amputation if not improved. More precise definitions, not open to individual interpretation, have been attempted and found difficult to define. The latest attempt involves the use of toe pressures. It is either persistently recurring ischaemic rest pain requiring regular analgesics for more than 2 weeks, or ulceration or gangrene of the toe or foot, and associated with an ankle systolic pressure <50 mmHg and/or a toe systolic pressure <30 mmHg (European Working Group, 1991). The incidence of critical limb ischaemia is approximately 500–1000 patients per million per year (Wolfe, 1986; DHSS, 1986). Progression to amputation is not inevitable with 30–75 per cent of patients with rest pain improving spontaneously (Bloor, 1961; Taylor and Calo, 1962). Assessment of the true natural history of this condition is no longer possible because 50–60 per cent undergo some sort of limb salvage procedure, although 20 per cent still require an amputation (Wolfe, 1986). Randomized placebo-controlled trials have provided data on patients with unreconstructable critical limb ischaemia. Thirty-five per cent will lose the leg within 6 months and 15 per cent will die (Lowe *et al.*, 1982; Belch *et al.*, 1983). Not unexpectedly, ulceration and gangrene carry a greater risk of amputation (Wolfe, 1986).

Claudicants have mortality rates two to three times that of matched controls (Davey Smith *et al.*, 1990; O'Riordain and O'Donnell, 1991), and the outlook for patients with critical limb ischaemia is as grim as for Dukes 'B' carcinoma of the colon, with 20 per cent dying in one year (Myers *et al.*, 1978; Wolfe, 1986). The five-year mortality rate of patients with rest pain is 50 per cent (Bolin *et al.*, 1988) and 95 per cent of patients with gangrene are dead within ten years (DeWeese and Rob, 1977). An ischaemic electrocardiogram (ECG) in a claudicant confers a life expectancy similar to that of one who has survived a myocardial infarction (Juergens *et al.*, 1960), but if the ECG is normal, life expectancy is similar to controls (Vecht *et al.*, 1982). The ABPI also relates to prognosis, with a figure >0.5 being associated with normal life expectancy (O'Riordain and O'Donnell, 1991).

Relationship to generalized disease

The risk factors for peripheral arterial disease are also those for vascular disease at other sites. Clinical history and ECG reveal that ischaemic heart disease is present in 40–60 per cent of patients with leg ischaemia (Crawford *et al.*, 1981; Dormandy and Murray, 1991). Coronary angiography shows that 90 per cent of patients have disease there, it being severe in 28 per cent (Hertzer *et al.*, 1984). Both the prevalence of cardiac disease and the frequency of cardiac events are related to the severity of the peripheral disease (Kallero *et al.*, 1985; Dormandy and Murray, 1991). Furthermore, the severity of coronary artery disease has been shown to be related to the resting ABPI (Hertzer *et al.*, 1984).

Carotid artery disease, as measured by duplex scanning, is present in 25–50 per cent of claudicants (Turnipseed *et al.*, 1980; Klop *et al.*, 1991). It has been reported that symptomatic disease is not associated with a higher risk of stroke in patients with peripheral arterial occlusive disease (Ellis *et al.*, 1992) and that the relative stroke risk of patients with claudication is approximately three (Smith *et al.*, 1990).

Renal artery disease is also associated with peripheral arterial occlusive disease, with 15 per cent of patients having a stenosis >50 per cent (Choudhri *et al.*, 1990; Missouris *et al.*, 1994). Patients with both peripheral arterial occlusive disease and hypertension are three times more likely to have renal artery stenosis (Choudhri *et al.*, 1990).

CEREBROVASCULAR DISEASE

Cerebrovascular diseases include all those of the vascular system which cause ischaemia or infarction of

the brain. There are four groups of clinical manifestations:

- *Transient ischaemic attack* (TIA) is an acute loss of focal cerebral or monocular function, but with symptoms lasting less than 24 hours, which, after adequate investigation, is presumed to be embolic or thrombotic in origin.
- *Stroke* is a rapidly developing clinical condition with signs of focal, and at times global, loss of cerebral function. Symptoms persist for longer than 24 hours and there should be no cause apparent other than a vascular one. The condition may last for a few days, be permanent and disabling, or cause death.
- *Reversible ischaemic neurological deficit* (RIND) is a term used for a condition similar to stroke but with symptoms lasting between 1 and 7 days.
- *Multi-infarct dementia* is a deterioration in previously normal cerebral function (intellect and memory) due to multiple, individually 'silent' infarcts.

Stroke is the third most common cause of death after coronary heart disease and cancer in Western countries. It causes 12 per cent of deaths in England and Wales, and accounts for about 7 per cent of all hospital bed days, and 6 per cent of hospital running costs in Scotland. Eighty per cent of first-time strokes are due to cerebral infarction, 10 per cent to primary intracerebral haemorrhage and 5 per cent to subarachnoid haemorrhage. The incidence in the UK is about 2 per thousand population per year, rising rapidly with age (Table 1.3). In UK patients under the age of 65 years, stroke mortality is greater in deprived than in affluent areas (Carstairs and Morris, 1990), and amongst the unemployed (Franks *et al.*, 1991). There is also evidence that poor maternal and infant health is associated with stroke many decades later (Barker and Osmond, 1987). Finally, stroke mortality is greater in winter than summer. One explanation may be that the complications of stroke

Table 1.3 *Incidence of stroke (per thousand population) related to age*

Year of study	Age (years)		
	55–64	65–74	75–84
1983	2.9	6.9	14.3
1988	2.8	5.4	14.6

(e.g. pneumonia) are more likely to be fatal in the colder winter months, but the same phenomenon has been observed in the warmer climate of Israel (Berginer et al., 1989).

Risk factors for stroke

Age is the strongest risk factor, being 0.57 per thousand per year in patients aged 45–54 years, and 25 times greater (14.3 per thousand per year) at ages 75–84 years. Men are only marginally more susceptible to stroke than women, contrary to the situation with coronary and peripheral vascular diseases. Hypertension may increase stroke risk by increasing the severity and extent of atheroma (Lusiani et al., 1987), and producing intracerebral microvascular disease (Russell, 1963). The risk is related to both diastolic and systolic blood pressures (Sharper et al., 1991), doubling with each 7.5 mmHg increase in diastolic pressure (MacMahon et al., 1990). Treating hypertension reduces the risk (Collins et al., 1990). Autopsy (Flegel et al., 1987), cohort (Kannel et al., 1983) and case-controlled (Herman et al., 1983) studies have shown a clear association with coronary disease. This may be a causal relationship and due to emboli of cardiac origin, or due to co-incidental atheroma. Atrial fibrillation is a potential source of such emboli and although it is present in only 20 per cent of cerebral infarct patients (Sandercock et al., 1992), 2.5 per cent of patients with atrial fibrillation will suffer a stroke. From this it is not surprising that ECG abnormalities reflecting hypertension and coronary artery disease are also risk factors, as is cardiac failure (Kannel et al., 1983; Sharper et al., 1991).

Smoking increases stroke risk in a dose-related manner equally in both sexes (Shinton and Beevers, 1989), but lipids have not been shown to be related to stroke risk despite the causal relationship with coronary disease (Quizilbash et al., 1992). The reasons are complex, relating to the age at which strokes occur and a negative association with intracerebral haemorrhage (Iso et al., 1989). Diabetes doubles the risk (Kannel and McGhee, 1979), probably independently of other factors (Rosengren et al., 1989). Plasma fibrinogen levels have a consistent relationship with stroke (Meade et al., 1987), but platelet coagulation and fibrinolytic parameters have not.

AORTIC ANEURYSM

Prevalence and risk factors

The prevalence of aortic aneurysm is not easy to establish because the definition is based on the maximum aortic diameter, and this varies quite significantly. For example, in men aged 65–74 years, it ranges from 1.5 to 2.4 cm (Liddington and Heather, 1992). A ratio of 'normal' to 'abnormal' aortic diameters has been used, but this still depends on the definition of 'normal'. The most practical method of assessing the abdominal aorta is ultrasound screening because clinical examination is unreliable (Robicsek, 1981), but even ultrasound has a margin of error of 0.5 cm (Ellis et al., 1991). Thus identifying both prevalence and risk factors is difficult.

Most screening studies have been restricted to potentially high-risk groups, patients with either peripheral vascular disease (prevalence 10–14 per cent) (Allardice et al., 1988; Galland et al., 1991) or hypertension (prevalence 10.7 per cent) (Twomey et al., 1984). Because aneurysms may be familial, siblings can be considered at risk. A Swedish study showed that 29 per cent of brothers, and 6 per cent of sisters, of aneurysm patients were affected (Bengtsson et al., 1989). However, the aneurysms appeared no different in type to the sporadic ones (Darling et al., 1989). Similarly, an Oxford screening study found that 25 per cent of brothers of aneurysm patients also had aneurysms (Collin and Walton, 1989).

Collin and colleagues (1988), in a large community-based study of 426 men aged between 65 and 74 years of age invited for screening (with a 52 per cent response rate), found that 2.3 per cent had aneurysms greater than 4 cm in diameter. The same study confirmed the increased prevalence in patients who had evidence of peripheral arterial disease (17.9 per cent), but did not find a higher rate in hypertensive men. A study of 1800 patients over 50 years of age undergoing abdominal ultrasound for other reasons found an aneurysm greater than 3 cm in anteroposterior diameter in 8.8 per cent of men and 2.1 per cent of women (Akkersdijk et al., 1991).

Age has a strong effect, increasing the prevalence of aortic aneurysms in both sexes. The mortality from aortic aneurysm is ten times greater in men over 85 years than in those between 55 and 64 years, and 100 times greater than in those younger than 55 years. The increase in aneurysm prevalence with age is steeper in women, reducing the male to female ratio from 3.5 at 55–64 years to 2.1 at over 85 years (HMSO, 1984). Aneurysms in younger people (under 40 years) are usually associated with tissue disorders such as Marfan's syndrome and Ehlers–Danlos type IV. Racial differences have been studied in the United States where an autopsy and computed tomography study showed aneurysms to be twice as common in whites as blacks (Johnson et al., 1986). Smoking is associated with abdominal aortic aneurysm (Hammond et al., 1967) and with death due to the condition (Strachan, 1991).

In Scotland, the rate of diagnosis of abdominal aortic aneurysm was 25.8 per 100 000 population in 1971, but 63.6 in 1984 (Naylor et al., 1988), and similar trends have been noted in both the United States and Australia (Melton et al., 1984; Castleden, 1986). The age standardized mortality from aneurysm rose 20-fold in men, and 11-fold in women, between 1950 and 1984 (Fowkes et al., 1989), and this is thought to reflect a true increase in the prevalence of the condition. This has also been manifested by an increase in the incidence of ruptured aortic aneurysms (Jenkins et al., 1986; Mealy and Salman, 1988), the majority of such patients dying unless operated upon (Armour, 1977).

Natural history of aortic aneurysm

An early study of 102 patients with an aortic aneurysm showed that the five-year survival rate was 19 per cent, 63 per cent dying of rupture (Estes, 1950). The annual growth rate of an aortic aneurysm, as recorded by serial ultrasound or computed tomography, is 0.4–0.52 cm, although aneurysms vary in both average growth rates and the rate of expansion at different times (Draper et al., 1996). However, these figures for growth rate have been challenged by a population based study of 103 patients who received more than one ultrasound scan. The median annual growth rate was 0.21 cm per year with only 24 per cent showing an expansion rate of 0.4 cm or more per year (Nevitt et al., 1989). Although it is not possible to predict the growth rate of an individual aneurysm, large aneurysms tend to expand more quickly than small ones (Draper et al., 1996; Sterpetti et al., 1987).

The risk of rupture increases with size (Darling, 1970), as can be predicted from Laplace's law (tension = pressure × radius). An autopsy study of 473

patients with untreated aneurysms showed the rate of rupture to be 60 per cent at a diameter of greater than 10 cm, 45 per cent between 7 and 10 cm, 25 per cent per cent between 4 and 7 cm, and 9.5 per cent for those less than 4 cm in diameter (Darling et al., 1977). It has been calculated that small aneurysms are associated with a risk of death from rupture of 5 per cent per year, with rupture being associated with diastolic hypertension and chronic obstructive airways disease (Cronenwett et al., 1985). Collin (1987) estimated that the presence of a small aneurysm raises the annual death rate by 230 per cent in 60–64-year-old men. A much more favourable prognosis was suggested by a follow-up study of 176 patients with aortic aneurysms in Rochester, Maine, in which the overall risk of rupture was 6 per cent and 8 per cent at five and ten years, respectively. The risk was zero if the aneurysm was less than 5 cm in diameter and 25 per cent if it was over 5 cm (Nevitt et al., 1989). Recently, however, estimates of the risk of rupture have been increased, although not to previous levels, by a follow-up study of 300 patients with aortic aneurysms which showed a 1 per cent cumulative incidence of rupture at six years for aneurysms smaller than 4 cm, and 2 per cent for those between 4·0 and 4.9 cm. The median annual growth rate was 0.3 cm a year (Guirguis and Barber, 1991). The actual site of rupture is thought to be a localized weakness or 'bleb' on a more diffusely weakened aneurysm wall (Hunter et al., 1989). Most rupture posterolaterally into the retroperitoneal space and occasionally a patient may survive for weeks or months with a contained rupture (Rosenthal et al., 1986). There has been some debate as to whether aneurysms are more likely to rupture in colder weather, but this has not been confirmed by the largest study to date (Castleden, 1986; John and Stonebridge, ·1993).

It should be noted that life expectancy is the same after successful repair of a ruptured aortic aneurysm as it is after elective repair and this is, in turn, virtually the same as in an age- and sex-matched population (Stonebridge et al., 1993).

A review of the deaths reported to the Scottish Audit of Surgical Mortality (a national audit, which includes all hospital and immediately post-hospital deaths in Scotland) revealed that the commonest vascular case involving significant delay is ruptured aortic aneurysm. Delay in these cases was ascribed to two main causes: failure to make an early diagnosis, and simple lack of urgency once the diagnosis has been made. Despite the well-documented increase in the incidence of aortic aneurysm, the diagnosis of rupture in a collapsed or hypotensive elderly patient appears often not to be considered, producing a consequent delay in referral (9.5 per cent incidence). The subsequent lack of urgency is possibly due to the misleading impression of stability in some of these patients. A stable patient with a ruptured aortic aneurysm is in a very transient and precarious state (Scottish Audit of Surgical Mortality, 1994).

VARICOSE VEINS

Epidemiology

The most widely accepted classification of varicose veins is that used by Widmer (1978), who defined three categories (Table 1.4), but it is not universally

Table 1.4 *Basle study venous classification*

- No venous disease
- Varicosities
    Hyphenwebs; reticular varices; trunk varices
- Chronic venous insufficiency
    I. Dilated subcutaneous veins
    II. Hyperpigmented or depigmented areas
    III. Open or healed ulcer

accepted. Therefore the prevalence of varicose veins is difficult to assess. It depends on the nature of the population investigated (age, occupation, race) and the definition used. A recent review (Callam, 1994) showed that in an unselected Western adult population, the prevalence may be 15 per cent in men and 25 per cent in women, with an apparent association with pregnancy. There is a common belief that varicose veins run in families and studies seem to confirm this (Widmer, 1978; Belcaro, 1986), but it is not possible to say that there is an association with occupations that involve prolonged standing (Callam, 1994).

INTERCURRENT DISEASE AND DECISION MAKING

There are two key facts that must be in the forefront of the clinician's mind when dealing with patients with peripheral arterial disease. The first is that it should be assumed that all patients with peripheral arterial disease are very likely to have coronary artery and/or cerebrovascular disease. In fact it is misleading to refer to peripheral arterial disease as a separate entity because it rarely, if ever, exists in isolation and simply indicates the peripheral arterial element of a widespread condition – the tip of an iceberg so to speak. Other manifestations may not be clinically apparent, but they must be assumed to exist. The second fact is that the risk factors which predispose the patient to arterial disease (e.g. smoking, hypertension and diabetes) also predispose the patient to other conditions. The patient presenting with claudication may also suffer from chronic obstructive airways disease, cancer (especially of lung and stomach), hypertension and diabetes, to say nothing of their complications such as cardiac failure, renal failure, neuropathy and blindness.

These two key facts influence decision making by affecting the risk–benefit ratio. As an obvious example, a patient who suffers from angina and presents with claudication is at increased risk of peri-operative myocardial infarction and therefore death. Furthermore, an operation which increases the blood supply to the leg may increase walking distance beyond 100 m, but there is little point if angina develops at 150 m. The patient is exposed to a significant peri-operative risk for a limited post-operative benefit. The same analysis may be true of exertional dyspnoea of either respiratory or cardiac origin. It would therefore appear unreasonable to perform an operative procedure for claudication on a patient who also has significant other exercise-induced symptoms.

The case is slightly different with aortic aneurysm repair. The operation is prophylactic, but there is increasing risk of premature death as the diameter of the aneurysm increases. In 'normal' circumstances the recommended aneurysm diameter for operative intervention is 5.5–6 cm. However, as the peri-operative risk increases because of concomitant disease, so the aneurysm diameter at which intervention is advised will also increase. The risk of the condition must remain significantly greater than the risk of the procedure. This may mean that the threshold for intervention continues to increase as the patient becomes older and peri-operative risk factors escalate. In addition, and because the operation is prophylactic, the patient must have an anticipated survival of greater than two to three years so that statistical benefits clearly accrue from the procedure. This may lead to a situation where the operation is never performed because the risk of the procedure never becomes significantly less than the risk of the aneurysm rupturing, and the patient's anticipated survival gradually decreases to less than two years. The same argument also holds true for carotid endarterectomy. The patient must survive this long for the risks of the procedure to be outweighed by the risks doing nothing.

With respect to carotid endarterectomy, the European and North American carotid trials demonstrated a benefit for surgery in symptomatic severe carotid stenosis (European Carotid Surgery Trialists' Collaborative Group, 1991; North American Symptomatic Carotid Endarterectomy Trial Collaborators, 1991). A key factor in this risk–benefit analysis is the peri-operative stroke rate and, for this reason, it has been strongly suggested that only surgeons and anaesthetists with regular commitments and interest in carotid artery surgery should perform the procedure (Brown and Humphrey, 1992). A recent systematic review of the morbidity and mortality of carotid endarterectomy revealed that female sex, symptomatic disease, cerebral symptoms, systolic blood pressure greater than 180 mmHg and contralateral carotid artery occlusion increased the risk of surgery. If no risk factors were present, then the risk of death or stroke was 2 per cent, but if there were more than three the risk was 18.5 per cent (Rothwell and Warlow, 1996). The question therefore arises as to what one does with a woman with transient hemiplegia and a contralateral occluded carotid. The simple approach would be that the risks of peri-operative death or stroke are too great and that the operation should be refused, but what if the risk factors for a non-operative stroke are the same? There is no answer available for such questions because the numbers involved prohibit study. However, a broader view shows that the risk profile of patients now undergoing carotid endarterectomy may be different to that of the patient population studied in the two major trials (da Silva and Harris, 1995). It may not be valid to apply the findings of those trials to patients in much higher risk groups. This is complicated even further with the development of new antiplatelet drugs and combinations of drugs which invalidate the previous non-intervention statistics.

The question becomes even more complex when one asks how low a bypass success rate is acceptable for critical limb ischaemia – 75, 50, or even (as has been suggested) as low as 25 per cent? At what level is it better to go straight to primary amputation rather than attempt a bypass procedure? The combined risk of a failed bypass and an amputation is greater than that of a primary amputation, but the mortality rate of a successful bypass is less than that of a primary amputation. Quite where the point is reached when a bypass is more of a risk is almost a matter of personal belief.

Despite the speciality of vascular surgery/anaesthesia being the subject of more than the usual number of prospective studies, much of the decision making revolves around the skill, experience and philosophy of individual clinicians. There is a lot of guidance in the literature, but unfortunately it does not cover all of the problems encountered. The best philosophy remains the oldest – *'first do no harm'*.

REFERENCES

Agner, E. 1981. Natural history of angina pectoris, possible previous myocardial infarction and intermittent claudication during the eighth decade. *Acta Medica Scandinavica* **210**, 271–276.

Akkersdijk, G.J.M., Puylaert, J.B.C.M. and de Vries, A.C. 1991. Abdominal aortic aneurysm as an incidental finding in abdominal ultrasonography. *British Journal of Surgery* **78**, 1261–1263.

Allardice, J.T., Allwright, G.J., Wafula, J.M.C. and Wyatt, A.P. 1988. High prevalence of abdominal aortic aneurysm in men with peripheral vascular disease: screening by ultrasonography. *British Journal of Surgery* **75**, 240–242.

Angquist, K.A., Johnson, O., Ericsson, M. and Tollin, C. 1982. Serum lipoproteins and apolipoproteins AI and AII in male patients with peripheral arterial insufficiency. *Acta Chirurgica Scandinavica* **148**, 675–678.

Armour, R.H. 1977. Survivors of ruptured abdominal aortic aneurysms: the iceberg's tip. *British Medical Journal* **ii**, 1055–1057.

Barker, D.J. and Osmond, C. 1987. Death rates from stroke in England and Wales predicted from past maternal mortality. *British Medical Journal* **295**, 83–86.

Barner, H.B., Kaiser, G.C. and Willman, V.L. 1971. Blood flow in the diabetic leg. *Circulation* **43**, 391–394.

Beach, K.W., Brunzell, J.D. and Strandness, D.E. 1982. Prevelence of severe arteriosclerosis obliterans in patients with diabetes mellitus. *Arteriosclerosis* **2**, 275–280.

Beach, K.W., Bedford, G.R., Berglin, R.O. *et al.*. 1988. Progression of lower-extremity arterial occlusive disease in Type 2 diabetes mellitus. *Diabetic Care* **11**; 464–472.

Belcaro, G.V. 1986. Sapheno-femoral incompetence in young asymptomatic subjects with a family history of varices of the lower limbs. In Negus, D. and Jantet, G. (eds), *Phlebology '85*. London: John Libbey, 30–32.

Belch, J.J.F., McArdle, B., Pollock, J.G. *et al.* 1983. Epoprostenol (prostacyclin) and severe arterial disease. A double-blind trial. *Lancet* **i**, 315–317.

Bendick, P.J., Glover, J.L., Kuebler, T.W. and Dilley, R.S. 1983. Progression of atherosclerosis in diabetics. *Surgery* **93**, 834–838.

Bengtsson, H., Norrgård, O., Angquist, K.A. *et al.* 1989. Ultrasonographic screening of the abdominal aorta among siblings of patients with abdominal aortic aneurysms. *British Journal of Surgery* **76**, 589–591.

Berginer, V.M., Goldsmith, J., Batz, U. *et al.*. 1989. Clustering of strokes in association with meteorological factors in the Negev Desert of Israel: 1981–1983. *Stroke* **20**, 65–69.

Biland, L., daSilva, A., Zemp, E. and Widmer, L.K. 1985. Occlusive peripheral artery disease (OPAD). Mortality and risk profile. In *Proceedings of the 13th International Congress of Angiology, Athens, 9–14 June 1985*.

Bloor, K. 1961. Natural history of arteriosclerosis of the lower extremities. *Annals of the Royal College of Surgeons (England)* **28**, 36–52.

Bolin, T., Aldman, A., Gustavsson, P-O. *et al.*. 1988. Hur gar det for patienter med viloischemi som ej operaras? *Läkartidningen* **85**, 2398–2399.

Brown, M.M. and Humphrey, P.R.D. 1992. Carotid endarterectomy: recommendations for management of transient ischaemic attack and ischaemic stroke. *British Medical Journal* **305**, 1071–1074.

Callam, M.J. 1994. Epidemiology of varicose veins. *British Journal of Surgery* **81**, 167–173.

Carstairs, V. and Morris, R. 1990. Deprivation and health in Scotland. *Health Bulletin* **48**, 162–175.

Castleden, C.M. 1986. Abdominal aortic aneurysms in Western Australia: descriptive epidemiology and patterns of rupture. *British Journal of Surgery* **73**, 551–553.

Choudhri, A.H., Cleland, J.G.F., Rowlands, P.C. *et al.* 1990. Unsuspected renal artery stenosis in peripheral vascular disease. *British Medical Journal* **301**, 1197–1198.

Christie, M., Delley, A., Marbet, G.A. *et al.* 1984. Fibrinogen, factor VIII related antigen, anti-thrombin III and alpha 2–antiplasmin in peripheral arterial disease. *Thrombosis and Haemostasis* **52**, 240–242.

Collin, J. 1987. Elective surgery for small abdominal aortic aneurysms. *Lancet* **i**, 909.

Collin, J. and Walton, J. 1989. Is abdominal aortic aneurysm familial? *British Medical Journal* **299**, 493.

Collin, J., Araujo, H., Sutton, G.L.J. and Lindsell, D. 1988. Oxford screening programme for abdominal aortic aneurysm in men aged 65 to 74 years. *Lancet* **ii**, 1431–1432.

Collins, R., Pet, R., MacMahon, S. *et al.*. 1990. Blood pressure, stroke and coronary heart disease. Part 2. Short-term reductions in blood pressure: overview of randomised drug trials in their epidemiological context. *Lancet* **335**, 827–838.

Crawford, E.S., Bomberger, R.A., Glaeser, D.H. *et al.*. 1981. Aortoiliac occlusive disease: factors influencing survival and function following reconstructive operation over twenty-five year period. *Surgery* **90**, 1055–1067.

Cronenwett, J.L., Warner, K.G., Zelenock, G.B. *et al.*. 1984. Intermittent claudication. *Archives of Surgery* **119**, 430–436.

Cronenwett, J.L., Murphy, T.F., Zelenock, G.B. *et al.*. 1985. Actuarial analysis of variables associated with rupture of small abdominal aortic aneurysms. *Surgery* **98**, 472–482.

da Silva, A. and Harris, P.L. 1995. Changing risk factors in patients referred for carotid endarterectomy. *British Journal of Surgery* **82**, 548.

da Silva, A., Widmer, L.K., Ziegler, H.W. *et al.*. 1979. The Basle longitudinal study: report on the relation of initial glucose level to baseline ECG abnormalities, peripheral artery disease, and subsequent mortality. *Journal of Chronic Diseases* **32**, 797–803.

Darling, R.C. 1970. Ruptured arteriosclerotic abdominal aortic aneurysms. A pathologic and clinical study. *American Journal of Surgery* **119**, 397–340.

Darling, R.C., Massina, C.R., Brewster, D.C. and Ottinger, L.W. 1977. Autopsy study of unoperated abdominal aortic aneurysms. The case for early resection. *Circulation* **56** (Suppl. 2), 161–164.

Darling, R.C., Brewster, D.C., Darling, R.C. *et al.* 1989. Are familial abdominal aortic aneurysms different? *Journal of Vascular Surgery* **10**, 39–40.

Davey Smith, G., Shipley, M.J. and Rose, G. 1990. Intermittent claudication, heart disease risk factors and mortality (The Whitehall Study). *Circulation* **82**, 1925–1931.

De Backer, I.G., Kornitzer, M., Sobolski, J. and Denolin, H. 1979. Intermittent claudication – epidemiology and natural history. *Acta Cardiologica* **34**, 115–124.

Department of Health and Social Security, 1986. *DHSS Amputation Statistics for England, Wales and Northern Ireland.* London: DHSS.

DeWeese, J.A. and Rob, C.G. 1977. Autogenous venous grafts ten years later. *Surgery* **82**, 775–784.

Dormandy, J.A. and Murray, G.D. 1991. The fate of the claudicant – a prospective study of 1969 claudicants. *European Journal of Vascular Surgery* **5**, 131–133.

Draper, T.D., Stonebridge, P.A., Kelmen, G. *et al.* 1996. Growth rate of infrarenal aortic aneurysms. *European Journal of Vascular and Endovascular Surgery* **11**, 70–73.

Ecker, M.L. and Jacobs, B.S. 1970. Lower extremity amputation in diabetic patients. *Diabetes* **19**, 189–195.

Editorial. 1988. Apolipoprotein-B and atherogenesis. *Lancet* **i**, 1141–1142

Edmonds, M.E., Blundell, M.P., Morris, M. and Watkins, P.J. 1984. Reduction in the number of major and minor limb amputations, impact of a new combined diabetic foot clinic. *Diabetologia* **27**, 272A.

Ellis, M., Powel, J.T. and Greenhalgh, R.M. 1991. Limitations of ultrasonography in surveillance of small abdominal aortic aneurysms. *British Journal of Surgery* **78**, 614–616.

Ellis, M.R., Franks, P.J., Cuming, R. *et al.* 1992. Prevalence, progression and natural history of asymptomatic carotid stenosis: is there a place for carotid endarterectomy? *European Journal of Vascular Surgery* **6**, 172–177.

Ericsson, M., Johnson, O., Tollin, C. *et al.* 1982. Serum lipoprotein, apolipoprotein and intravenous fat tolerance in young athletes. *Scandinavian Journal of Rehabilitation Medicine* **14**, 209–212.

Ernst, E.E. and Matrai, A. 1987. Intermittent claudication, exercise and blood rheology. *Circulation* **76**, 1110–1114.

Estes, E. 1950. Abdominal aortic aneurysms: a study of 102 cases. *Circulation* **2**, 258–264.

European Carotid Surgery Trialists' Collaborative Group. 1991. MRC European carotid surgery trial: interim results for symptomatic patients with severe (70–99 per cent) or with mild (0–29 per cent) carotid stenosis. *Lancet* **337**, 1235–1243.

European Working Group on Critical Leg Ischaemia. 1991. Consensus Document. *Circulation* **84**, 1–26.

Executive Committee for ACAS Study. 1995. Endarterectomy for asymptomatic carotid artery stenosis. *Journal of the American Medical Association* **273**, 1421–1428.

Flegel, K.M., Shipley, M.J. and Rose, G. 1987. Risk of stroke in non-rheumatic atrial fibrillation. *Lancet* **i**, 526–529.

Fowkes, F.G.R., Macintyre, C.C.A. and Ruckley, C.V. 1989. Increasing incidence of aortic aneurysms in England and Wales. *British Medical Journal* **298**, 33–35.

Fowkes, F.G.R., Housley, E., Cawood, E.H.H. *et al.* 1991. Edinburgh Artery Study: Prevalence of Asymptomatic and Symptomatic Peripheral Arterial Disease in the General Population. *International Journal of Epidemiology* **20**, 384–392.

Fowkes, F.G.R., Housley, E., Riemersma, R.A. *et al.* 1992. Smoking, lipids, glucose intolerance and blood pressure as risk factors for peripheral atherosclerosis compared with ischaemic heart disease in the Edinburgh Artery Study. *American Journal of Epidemiology* **135**, 331–340.

Franks, P.J., Adamson, C., Bulpitt, P.F. and Bulpitt, C.J. 1991. Stroke death and unemployment in London. *Journal of Epidemiology and Community Health* **45**, 16–18.

Galland, R.B., Simmons, M.J. and Torrie, E.P.H. 1991. Prevalence of abdominal aortic aneurysm in patients with occlusive peripheral vascular disease. *British Journal of Surgery* **78**, 1259–1260.

Ger, R. 1985. Prevention of major limb amputations in the diabetic patient. *Archives of Surgery* **120**, 1317–1320.

Gofin, R., Karic, J.K., Friedlander, Y. *et al.* 1987. Peripheral vascular disease in a middle-aged population sample. The Jerusalem Lipid Research Clinic Prevalence Study. *International Journal of Medical Science* **23**, 157–167.

Goldenberg, S.G., Alex, M., Joshi, R.A. and Blumenthal, H.T. 1959. Nonatheromatous peripheral vascular disease of the lower extremity in diabetes mellitus. *Diabetes* **8**, 261–273.

Guirguis, E.M. and Barber, G.G. 1991. The natural history of abdominal aortic aneurysms. *American Journal of Surgery* **162**, 481–483.

Gyntelberg, F. 1973. Physical fitness and coronary heart disease in male residents in Copenhagen aged 40–59. *Danish Medical Bulletin* **20**, 105–112.

Hale, W.E., Marks, R.G., May, F.E. *et al.* 1988. Epidemiology of intermittent claudication: Evaluation of risk factors. *Age and Ageing* **17**, 57–60.

Hammond, E. and Garfinkel, L. 1967. Coronary heart disease, stroke and abdominal aortic aneurysm. Factors in the etiology. *Archives of Environmental Health* **19**, 167–182.

Heliovaara, M., Karvoren, M.J., Vilhaven, R. and Punsar, S. 1978. Smoking carbon monoxide and atherosclerosis. *British Medical Journal* **i**, 268–270.

Hell, K.M., Balzereit, A., Diebold, U. and Bruhn, H.D. 1989. Importance of blood viscoelasticity in arteriosclerosis. *Angiology* **40**, 539–546.

Herman, B., Schmitz, P.I.M., Leyten, A.C.M. *et al.* 1983. Multivariate logistic analysis of risk factors for stroke in Tilburg, The Netherlands. *American Journal of Epidemiology* **118**, 514–525.

Hertzer, N.R. 1981. Fatal myocardial infarction following lower extremity revascularisation – Two hundred and seventy three patients followed six to eleven post-operative years. *Annals of Surgery* **193**, 492–498.

Hertzer, N.R., Beven, E.G., Young, J.R. *et al.* 1984. Coronary artery disease in peripheral vascular patients – a classification of 1000 coronary angiograms and results of surgical management. *Annals of Surgery* **199**, 223–233.

HMSO. 1984. *Population mortality statistics. England and Wales*. London: HMSO.

Holland, W.W., Raftery, E.B., McPearson, P. and Stone, R.W. 1967. A cardiovascular survey of American East Coast telephone workers. *American Journal of Epidemiology* **85**, 61–71.

Housley, E. 1991. Exercise. In Fowkes, F.G.R. (ed.), *Epidemiology of peripheral vascular disease*. London: Springer-Verlag, 227–234.

Hughson, W.G., Mann, J.I. and Garrod, A. 1978. Intermittent claudication: prevalence and risk factors. *British Medical Journal* **I**, 1379–1381.

Hunter, G.C., Leong, S.C., Yu, G.S.M. *et al.* 1989. Aortic blebs: possible site of aneurysm rupture. *Journal of Vascular Surgery* **10**, 93–99.

Imperato, A.M., Kim, G., Davidson, T. and Crowley, J.G. 1975. Intermittent claudication: its natural course. *Surgery* **78**, 795–799.

Iso, H., Jacobs, D.R., Wentworth, D. *et al.* 1989. Serum cholesterol levels and six-year mortality from stroke in 350 977 men screened for the multiple risk factor intervention trial. *New England Journal of Medicine* **320**, 904–910.

Jamieson, M.G. and Ruckley, C.V. 1983. Amputation for peripheral vascular disease in a general surgical unit. *Journal of the Royal College of Surgeons (Edinburgh)* **28**, 46–50.

Jelnes, R., Gaardsting, O., Hougaard Jensen, K. *et al.* 1986. Fate in intermittent claudication; outcome and risk factors. *British Medical Journal* **293**, 1137–1140.

Jenkins, A.M.L., Ruckley, C.V. and Nolan, B. 1986. Ruptured aortic aneurysm. *British Journal of Surgery* **73**, 395–398.

John, T.G. and Stonebridge, P.A. 1993. Seasonal variation in operations for ruptured aortic aneurysm and acute lower limb ischaemia. *Journal of the Royal College of Surgeons (Edinburgh)* **38**, 161–162.

Johnson, W.C., Gale, M.E., Gerzof, S.G. *et al.* 1986. The role of computer tomography in symptomatic aortic aneurysms. *Surgery, Gynecology and Obstetrics* **162**, 49–53.

Juergens, J.L., Barker, N.W. and Hines, E.A. 1960. Arteriosclerosis obliterans: review of 520 cases with special reference to pathogenic and prognostic factors. *Circulation* **21**, 188–195.

Kallero, K.S., Bergqvist, D., Cederholm, C. *et al.* 1985. Late mortality and morbidity after arterial reconstruction: the influence of arteriosclerosis in popliteal artery trifurcation. *Journal of Vascular Surgery* **2**, 541–546.

Kannel, W.B. and McGhee, D.L. 1979. Diabetes and cardiovascular disease. The Framingham Study. *Journal of the American Medical Association* **41**, 2035–2038.

Kannel, W.B. and McGee, D.L. 1984. Update on some epidemiological features of intermittent claudication. *Journal of the American Geriatrics Society* **33**, 13–18.

Kannel, W.B. and Shurtleff, D. 1971. The natural history of atherosclerosis obliterans. *Cardiovascular Clinics* **3**, 37–52.

Kannel, W.B., Skinner, J.J., Schwartz, M.J. and Shurtleff, D. 1970. Intermittent claudication: Incidence in the Framingham Study. *Circulation* **41**, 875–883.

Kannel, W.B., Wolf, P.A. and Verter, J. 1983. Manifestations of coronary disease predisposing to stroke. The Framingham Study, *Journal of the American Medical Association* 250, 2942–2946.

Kihn, R.B., Warren, R. and Beebe, G.W. 1972. The 'geriatric' amputee. *Annals of Surgery* **176**, 305–314.

Klop, R.B.J., Eikelboom, B.C. and Taks, A.C.J.M. 1991. Screening of the internal carotid arteries in patients with peripheral vascular disease by colour-flow Duplex scanning. *European Journal of Vascular Surgery* **5**, 41–45.

Leng, G.C. and Fowkes, F.G.R. 1991. Lipids: epidemiology. In Fowkes, F.G.R. (ed.), *Epidemiology of peripheral vascular disease*. London: Springer-Verlag, 165–179.

Liddington, M.I. and Heather, B.P. 1992. The relationship between aortic diameter and body habitus. *European Journal of Vascular Surgery* **6**, 89–92.

Lippmann, H.I. and Farrar, R. 1979. Prevention of amputation in diabetics. *Angiology* **30**, 649–658.

Lithel, H., Hedstrand, H. and Karlsson, R. 1975. The smoking habits of men with intermittent claudication. *Acta Medica Scandinavica* **197**, 473–476.

LoGerfo, F.W. and Coffman, J.D. 1984. Vascular and microvascular disease of the foot in diabetes. *New England Journal of Medicine* **311**, 1615–1619.

Lord, J.W. 1965. Cigarette smoking and peripheral atherosclerotic occlusive disease. *Journal of the American Medical Association* **191**, 249–251.

Lowe, G.D.O., Dunlop, D.J., Lawson, D.H. *et al.* 1982. Double-blind controlled clinical trial of Ancrod for ischaemic rest pain of the leg. *Angiology* **33**, 46–50.

Lowe, G.D.O., Sanibadi, A. and Turner, A. 1986. Studies on haematocrit in peripheral arterial disease. *Klinische Wochenschrift* **64**, 969–674.

Lowe, G.D.O., Fowkes, F.G.R., Dawes, J. *et al.* 1993. Blood viscosity, fibrinogen, and activation of coagulation and leukocytes in peripheral arterial disease and the normal population in the Edinburgh Artery Study. *Circulation* **87**, 1915–1920.

Lusiani, L., Visona, A. and Castellani, V. 1987. Prevalence of atherosclerotic involvement of the internal carotid artery in hypertensive patients. *International Journal of Cardiology* **17**, 51–56.

MacMahon, S., Peto, R., Cutler, J. *et al.* 1990. Blood pressure, stroke and coronary heart disease. Part 1. Prolonged differences in blood pressure: prospective observational studies corrected for the regression dilution bias. *Lancet* **335**, 765–764.

Malone, J.M., Moore, W.R. and Goldstone, J. 1977. Life expectancy following aortofemoral arterial grafting. *Surgery* **81**, 551–555.

McAllister, F.F. 1976. The fate of patients with intermittent claudication managed nonoperatively. *American Journal of Surgery* **132**, 593–595.

McDaniel, M.D. and Cronenwett, J.L. 1989. Basic data related to the natural history of intermittent claudication. *Annals of Vascular Surgery* **3**, 273–277.

Meade, T.W., Mellow, S. and Brozovic, M. 1986. Haemostatic function and ischaemic heart disease: principal results of the Northwick Park Heart Study. *Lancet* **ii**, 533–537.

Meade, T.W., Imeson, J. and Stirling, Y. 1987. Effects of changes in smoking and other characteristics on clotting factors and the risk of ischaemic heart disease. *Lancet* **ii**, 986–988.

Mealy, K. and Salman, A. 1988. The true incidence of ruptured abdominal aortic aneurysms. *European Journal of Vascular Surgery* **2**, 405–408.

Melton, L.J., Bickerstaff, L.K., Hollier, L.H., *et al.* 1984. Changing incidence of abdominal aortic aneurysms: a population based study. *American Journal of Epidemiology* **120**, 379–386.

Menzoian, J.O., LaMorte, W.W., Paniszyn, C.C. *et al.* 1989. Symptomatology and anatomic patterns of peripheral vascular disease: differing impact of smoking and diabetes. *Annals of Vascular Surgery* **3**, 224–228.

Missouris, C.G., Buckenham, T., Cappucio, F.P. and MacGregor, G.A. 1994. Renal artery stenosis: a common and important problem in patients with peripheral vascular disease. *American Journal of Medicine* **96**, 10–14.

Mitchell, J.R.A. and Schwartz, C.J. 1965. *Arterial disease.* Oxford: Blackwell.

Myers, K.A., King, R.B., Scott, D.F., Johnson, N. and Morris, P.J. 1978. Surgical treatment of the severely ischaemic leg: survival rates. *British Journal of Surgery* **65**, 460–464.

National Diabetes Advisory Board. 1980. *The treatment and control of diabetes.* Publication No. 82–224. United States Department of Health, Education and Welfare. Public Health Service. Bethesda, MD: National Institutes of Health.

Naylor, A.R., Webb, J., Fowkes, F.G.R. and Ruckley, C.V. 1988. Trends in abdominal aortic aneurysm surgery in Scotland (1971–1984). *European Journal of Vascular Surgery* **2**, 217–221.

Nevitt, M.P., Ballard, D.J. and Hallett, J.W. 1989. Prognosis of abdominal aortic aneurysms. A population based study. *New England Journal of Medicine* **321**, 1009–1014.

North American Symptomatic Carotid Endarterectomy Trial Collaborators. 1991. Beneficial effect of carotid endarterectomy in symptomatic patients with high grade carotid stenosis. *New England Journal of Medicine* **325**, 445–453.

O'Riordain, D.S. and O'Donnell, J.A. 1991. Realistic expectations for the patient with intermittent claudication. *British Journal of Surgery* **78**, 861–863.

Powell, J.T. 1991. Smoking. In Fowkes, F.G.R. (ed.), *Epidemiology of peripheral vascular disease.* London: Springer-Verlag, 141–153.

Pyorala, K. and Laasko, M. 1983. Diabetes in epidemiological perspective. In Mann, J.I., Pyorala, K. and Teuscher, A. (eds), *Macrovascular disease in diabetes mellitus.* Edinburgh: Churchill Livingstone, 183–186.

Quizilbash, N., Duffy, S.W. and Warlow, C. 1992. Lipids are risk factors for ischaemic stroke: overview and review, *Cerebrovascular Disease* **2**, 127.

Reid, D.D., Brett, G.J., Hamilton, P.J.R. *et al.* 1974. Cardiorespiratory disease and diabetes among middle aged male civil servants. *Lancet* **i**, 469–473.

Reunanen, A., Takkunen, H. and Aromaa, A. 1982. Prevalence of intermittent claudication and its effect on mortality. *Acta Medica Scandinavica* **211**, 249–256.

Robicsek, F. 1981. The diagnosis of abdominal aneurysms. *Surgery* **89**, 275–276.

Rohling, K., Zabel-Langhenning, R., Till, U. and Thielmann, K. 1989. Enhanced net mass transfer of HDL cholesterylesters to apo B containing lipoproteins in patients with peripheral vascular disease. *Clinica Chimica Acta* **184**, 289–296.

Rosengren, A., Welin, L., Tsipogianni, A. and Wilhelmsen, L. 1989. Impact of cardiovascular risk factors on coronary heart disease and mortality among middle aged diabetic men: a general population study. *British Medical Journal* **299**, 1127–1131.

Rosengren, A., Wilhelmsen, L., Eriksson, E. *et al.* 1990. Lipoprotein (a) and coronary heart disease: a prospective case-control study in a general population sample of middle-aged men. *British Medical Journal* **301**, 1248–1251.

Rosenthal, D., Clark, M.D., Stanton, P.E. and Lamis, P.A. 1986. 'Chronic-contained' ruptured abdominal aortic aneurysm: is it real? *Journal of Cardiovascular Surgery* **27**, 723–724.

Rothwell, P.M. and Warlow, C.P. 1996. Systematic review of the morbidity and mortality of carotid endarterectomy. *British Journal of Surgery* **83**, 564.

Ruckley, C.V. 1991. Symptomatic and asymptomatic disease. In Fowkes, F.G.R. (ed.), *Epidemiology of peripheral vascular disease*. London: Springer-Verlag, 97–108.

Rush, D.S., Juston, C.C., Bivins, B.A. and Hyde, G.L. 1981. Operative and late mortality rates of above-knee and below-knee amputations. *American Surgeon* **47**, 36–39.

Russell, R.W.R. 1963. Observations on intracerebral aneurysms. *Brain* **86**, 425–442.

Sandercock, P.A.G., Bamford, J., Dennis, M. *et al.* 1992. Atrial fibrillation and stroke: prevalence in different types of stroke and influence on early and long term prognosis. (Oxfordshire Community Stroke Project). *British Medical Journal* **305**, 1460–1465.

Schadt, D.C., Hines, E.A., Juergens, J.L. and Barker, N.W. 1961. Chronic atherosclerotic occlusion of the femoral artery. *Journal of the American Medical Association* **175**, 937–940.

Sharper, A.G., Phillips, A.N., Pocock, S.J. *et al.* 1991. Risk factors for stroke in middle aged British men. *British Medical Journal* **302**, 1111–1115.

Shinton, R. and Beevers, G. 1989. Meta-analysis of relation between cigarette smoking and stroke. *British Medical Journal* **298**, 789–794.

Silbert, S. and Zazeela, H. 1958. Prognosis in atherosclerotic peripheral vascular disease. *Journal of the American Medical Association* **166**, 1816–1821.

Skalkidis, Y., Katsouyanni, K., Petridou, E. *et al.* 1989. Risk factors of peripheral arterial occlusive disease: a case control study in Greece. *International Journal of Epidemiology* **18**, 614–618.

Smith, G.D., Shipley, M.J. and Rose, G. 1990. Intermittent claudication, heart disease, risk factors, and mortality. The Whitehall Study. *Circulation* **82**, 1925–1931.

Stemmer, E.A. 1986. Influence of diabetes mellitus on the patterns of vascular occlusive disease. In Moore, W.S. (ed.), *Vascular Surgery – a comprehensive review*, 2nd edn. Orlando, FL: Grune and Stratton, 543–560.

Sternby, N.H. 1968. Atherosclerosis in a defined population. An autopsy study in Malmö, Sweden. *Acta Pathologica Microbiologica Scandinavica*, Suppl. 194, 5.

Sterpetti, A.V., Schultz, R.D., Feldhaus, R.J. *et al.* 1987. Factors influencing enlargement rate of small abdominal aortic aneurysms. *Journal of Surgical Research* **43**, 211–219.

Stonebridge, P.A., Callam, M.J., Bradbury, A.W. *et al.* 1993. Comparison of long-term survival after successful repair of ruptured and nonruptured abdominal aortic aneurysm. *British Journal of Surgery* **80**, 585–586.

Strachan, D.P. 1991. Predictors of death from aortic aneurysm among middle aged men: the Whitehall study. *British Journal of Surgery* **78**, 401–404.

Strong, J.P. and Richards, M.L. 1976. Cigarette smoking and atherosclerosis in autopsied men. *Atherosclerosis* **23**, 451–476.

Taylor, M.S. and Calo, M.R. 1962. Atherosclerosis of arteries of lower limbs. *British Medical Journal* **24**, 507–519.

Tollin, C., Ericsson, M., Johnson, O. *et al.* 1984. Decreased removal of triglycerides from blood – a mechanism for the hypertriglyceridaemia in male patients with coronary artery disease. *International Journal of Cardiology* **5**, 185–192.

Turnipseed, W..D, Berkoff, H.A. and Belzer, F.O. 1980. Postoperative stroke in cardiac and peripheral vascular disease. *Annals of Surgery* **192**, 365–368.

Twomey, A., Twomey, E.M., Wilkins, R.A. and Lewis, J.D. 1984. Unrecognised aneurysmal disease in male hypertensive patients. *British Journal of Surgery* **71**, 307–308.

Vecht, R.J., Nicolaides, A.N., Brandao, E. *et al.* 1982. Resting and treadmill electrocardiographic findings in patients with intermittent claudication. *International Angiography* **1**, 119–121.

Waugh, N.R. 1988. Amputations in diabetic patients – a review of rates, relative risks and resource use. *Community Medicine* **10**, 279–288.

Widmer, L.K. 1978. *Peripheral venous disorders.* Bern: Hans Huber.

Widmer, L.K., Greensher, A. and Kannel, W.B. 1964. Occlusion of peripheral arteries. A study of 6400 working subjects. *Circulation* **30**, 836–842.

Widmer, L.K., Biland, L. and Da Silva, A. 1985. Risk profile and occlusive peripheral artery disease (OPAD). In *Proceedings of 13th International Congress of Angiology. Athens, 9–14 June, 1985.*

Wolfe, J.N. 1986. Defining the outcome of critical ischaemia; a one year prospective study. *British Journal of Surgery* **73**, 321.

2

The scope of vascular surgery

ANDREW W BRADBURY

INTRODUCTION

Vascular surgery can be defined as surgery of extracranial and extrapericardial arteries and veins. It is arguably the fastest growing surgical subspeciality in the UK with over one-third of general surgeons expressing a vascular interest. Vascular surgery overlaps with a large number of other surgical and medical subspecialities. For example, in addition to anaesthetists, the vascular surgeon will liaise with neurologists in the management of patients with carotid disease, with renal physicians in the care of patients with renal artery disease and those requiring access for haemodialysis, with gastrointestinal surgeons in the management of mesenteric ischaemia, and with cardiologists and respiratory physicians during pre-operative assessment for major arterial surgery. The surgeon will also develop close links with the laboratories, particularly those providing coagulation and the transfusion services, and with his or her radiological colleagues who provide both diagnostic imaging and an increasingly wide range of percutaneous endoluminal interventions.

The vascular surgeon and anaesthetist must be constantly aware of the fact that they are dealing with an incurable multisystem disorder – vascular

disease somewhere, vascular disease everywhere. Unlike the gastrointestinal surgeon who can usually cut back to normal bowel to perform the anastomosis, the vascular surgeon is always operating on the arterial equivalent of Crohn's disease – there is no normal bowel. But unlike the Crohn's patient, the typical vascular patient is elderly and has limited cardiorespiratory reserve. For all these reasons it is absolutely imperative that the vascular surgeon develops a close working relationship with his or her anaesthetic colleagues to assess the patient's fitness for surgery, take them through the surgical insult and look after them post-operatively in the high-dependency and intensive therapy units.

There can be no other subspeciality where such major surgery is carried out prophylactically; that is, to prevent catastrophe in the future. Repair of abdominal aortic aneurysm to prevent rupture and carotid endarterectomy to prevent stroke are the two most obvious examples. Because both operations are associated with a major morbidity and mortality rate of the order of 5 per cent, the balance of risks between surgery and best medical therapy can be a fine one. The vascular surgeon and anaesthetist must liaise constantly if correct judgements about whether, when and how to intervene surgically are to be reached. To quote a senior UK vascular surgeon, 'it is a poor bargain to exchange possible death at an uncertain date in the future for a high probability of death within hours of prophylactic surgery' (Collins, 1994).

The aim of this chapter is examine the current scope of vascular surgery and to give the reader a clearer idea of why his or her surgical colleague wants to undertake a particular operation, how to set about it, what particular problems may arise as a result, and how management of that condition might change in the foreseeable future as the result of new knowledge and technical innovation.

ANEURYSMAL DISEASE

Abdominal aortic aneurysm

Abdominal aortic aneurysm (AAA) is present in 5 per cent, and responsible for the death of 1 per cent, of men over the age of 60 years. The primary cause of death is rupture. Other complications include distal embolism from thrombus lying within the aneurysm sac (Fig. 2.1), inflammation of the wall leading to abdominal and back pain, compression of surrounding structures and rarely thrombotic occlusion. The annual risk of rupture varies quite widely between different reports but is probably of the region of: 4 cm, 1–2 per cent; 5 cm, 5–10 per cent; 6 cm, 10–15 per cent; and 7 cm, 20 per cent or more. Only one-third of patients with ruptured AAA survive to reach hospital and of those that are operated, only half survive, giving a community mortality of 80–90 per cent. Until rupture occurs, most AAA are completely asymptomatic and those operated upon electively before rupture are usually identified by chance. The mortality of elective AAA repair is 5–10 per cent in many UK centres and may be rising as older and less fit patients are accepted for surgical repair.

Ultrasound-based screening (Fig. 2.2) has been used in some centres to increase the number of asymptomatic aneurysms being detected and operated. The inference is that this will, in time, reduce the number of patients operated for rupture and, thus, overall mortality from the condition. However, the resource implications and cost–benefit ratio of population screening have not been adequately addressed and no national programme is imminent or likely. Most vascular surgeons therefore undertake 'opportunist' screening; that is, they actively search for AAA either by means of clinical examination or by performing an ultrasound in patients who consult them for other reasons. Some extend this to screening first-degree relatives of AAA patients and to other high-risk groups such as those patients attending hypertension and cardiology outpatient clinics.

Although most AAA gradually increase in size, the rate of growth is highly variable both between patients and within an individual patient over time. Thus, in general, the lifetime threat posed by a 5-cm AAA is considerably higher in a 50-year-old man than it is in

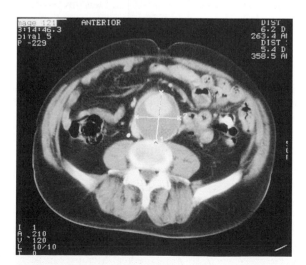

Figure 2.1 *Computed tomogram showing a large abdominal aortic aneurysm containing a large amount of laminated thrombus that may dislodge and embolize distally.*

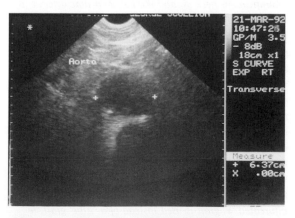

Figure 2.2 *Ultrasound scan demonstrating an abdominal aortic aneurysm in transverse section.*

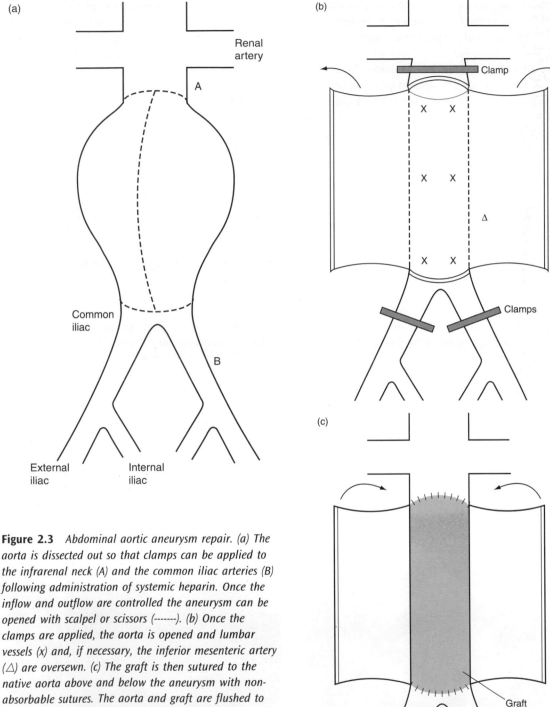

(a)

Renal
artery

A

Common
iliac

B

External
iliac

Internal
iliac

(b)

Clamp

x   x

x   x

Δ

x   x

Clamps

(c)

Graft

Figure 2.3 *Abdominal aortic aneurysm repair. (a) The
aorta is dissected out so that clamps can be applied to
the infrarenal neck (A) and the common iliac arteries (B)
following administration of systemic heparin. Once the
inflow and outflow are controlled the aneurysm can be
opened with scalpel or scissors (-------). (b) Once the
clamps are applied, the aorta is opened and lumbar
vessels (x) and, if necessary, the inferior mesenteric artery
(△) are oversewn. (c) The graft is then sutured to the
native aorta above and below the aneurysm with non-
absorbable sutures. The aorta and graft are flushed to
expel any thrombus and then clamps are removed to
reperfuse the lower limbs. The aneurysm sac is then
wrapped around the graft to exclude it from the
peritoneal cavity. (d) If iliacs are also aneurysmal then a
bifurcated 'Y' graft is used instead of a 'tube' graft. (e)
The Y-graft in position. At least one internal iliac artery
must be 'plumbed in' to prevent pelvic ischaemia.*

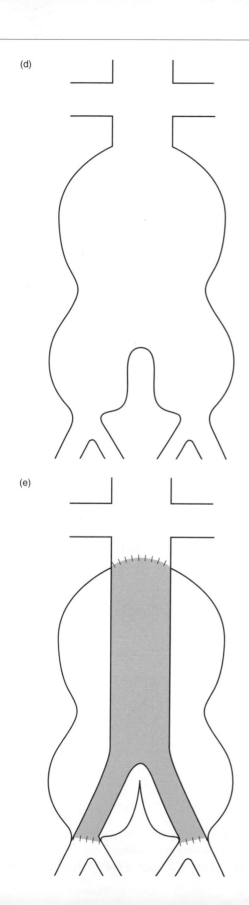

(d)

(e)

a man in his late seventies. The unpredictable nature of AAA expansion means that vascular surgeons will usually organize repeated ultrasound examinations at three- to six-monthly intervals to assess the AAA in those patients initially managed conservatively.

The decision to operate (Fig. 2.3) upon an asymptomatic AAA requires the surgeon to balance the risk of leaving the AAA in place versus the risks of surgery. The risk of the former depends primarily upon size, the presence of symptoms, and to some extent the age of the patient. The risk of surgery depends primarily upon the cardiorespiratory status of the patient. The anaesthetist and other colleagues such as cardiologists can help the surgeon assess the risk of surgery more precisely, as well as any limitation of life expectancy from co-morbid conditions. Clearly, there is no advantage to be gained in repairing a small aneurysm at low risk of rupture in an elderly gentleman with severe myocardial disease whose cardiac prognosis is very poor.

Thoraco-abdominal aneurysm

Standard teaching states that 90 per cent of all AAA arise below the renal arteries. However, with increased awareness of the condition and better imaging techniques, particularly computed tomography (CT), it has become apparent that perhaps 15–20 per cent involve the abdominal aorta above the level of the renal arteries and/or the thoracic aorta (Fig. 2.4). The risk of rupture from thoraco-abdominal aortic aneurysm (TAAA) appears to be

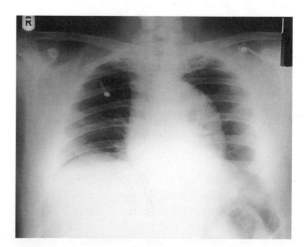

Figure 2.4 *Thoracic aneurysm causing mediastinal widening on a chest radiograph.*

the same as for infra-renal aneurysm. TAAA may also lead to aortic dissection and compress surrounding structures such as the oesophagus leading to dysphagia, or a main bronchus leading to lobar

collapse and recurrent pneumonia. TAAA may also cause severe chest and back pain, especially if large and eroding in to the vertebral column. TAAA are usually repaired for the symptoms or complications outlined above. The operation is performed in only a few specialist centres in the UK, with the details of the techniques involved being beyond the scope of this chapter. Suffice it to say, however, that the complexity and thus the risks of TAAA repair are considerably higher than for infra-renal AAA repair. As a result, for patients without symptoms, the risk–benefit equation outlined above with regard to infra-renal aortic aneurysms must be modified considerably.

Popliteal aneurysm

One in ten patients with AAA has a popliteal artery aneurysm (PAA) and 50 per cent of patients with PAA have an AAA (Fig. 2.5). The main complication of PAA is thrombosis with or without distal embolization. Again, because the aneurysm is usually asymptomatic until this point, most patients with PAA present as emergencies with acute limb ischaemia or are identified incidentally on examination. Acute thrombosis of a PAA is associated with a high rate of limb loss because the distal calf vessels often thrombose at the same time. In some cases, small thrombi from within the PAA have been chronically embolizing downstream leading to obliteration of the distal calf and foot vessels. This makes

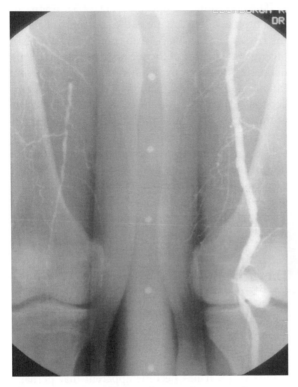

Figure 2.5   *Lower limb angiogram demonstrating a large left popliteal artery aneurysm.*

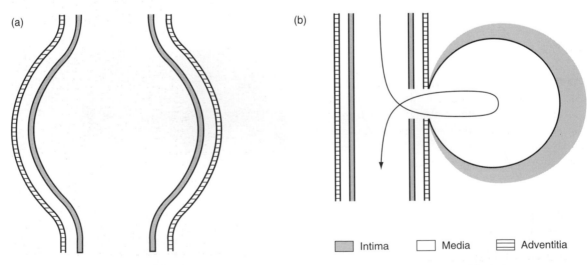

Figure 2.6   *Schematic diagram indicating the difference between a true and false aneurysm. (a) The true aneurysm has all three layers of the normal arterial wall in its wall. (b) The false aneurysm wall is formed only by a fibrous capsule and is kept open by flowing blood which enters and leaves the aneurysm through a hole in the arterial wall.*

surgery technically difficult because there is no distal 'run-off' for the surgeon to use for a bypass graft. Thrombosed PAA is one accepted indication for thrombolysis which can be used to dissolve clot in the calf vessels. This can be done either pre-operatively by the radiologist through a femoral catheter or by the surgeon directly in the operating theatre. Despite these techniques, half of all patients presenting acutely with thrombosed PAA lose the limb.

The indications for elective repair of asymptomatic PAA are controversial although many surgeons would operate when they exceed 2 cm in diameter or when they contain a significant amount of thrombus. About 20 per cent of patients with PAA have bilateral disease so the other limb should be carefully examined and if a PAA found it should be repaired. The standard operation for PAA is reversed vein bypass together with ligation of the aneurysm immediately above and below the sac.

False aneurysm

Most false aneurysms (Fig. 2.6) are iatrogenic and follow arterial puncture of the common femoral artery for the purposes of arteriography. If a false aneurysm is small then it may close spontaneously if the patient is not anticoagulated. It is possible to induce thrombosis in small aneurysms by compressing them under ultrasound guidance. However, if the aneurysm is large, too tender to compress or continuing to expand then surgical repair is necessary. This is usually a straightforward procedure which entails suturing the hole in the artery and obliterating the aneurysm sac to prevent refilling.

False aneurysms can also develop at the site of an anastomosis between prosthetic material and native artery after vascular reconstruction. In these circumstances the surgeon should always consider the possibility of graft infection. Such anastomotic aneurysms may require operative repair to prevent rapid expansion and haemorrhage.

LOWER LIMB ISCHAEMIA

Intermittent claudication

Intermittent claudication is the mildest form of lower limb ischaemia and affects approximately 5 per cent of men aged over 60 years. In the majority of cases claudication is due to atherosclerosis of the superficial femoral artery in the thigh (Fig. 2.7). At rest, the leg's oxygen requirements are met by

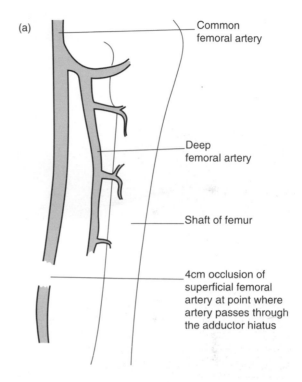

(a)

Common femoral artery

Deep femoral artery

Shaft of femur

4cm occlusion of superficial femoral artery at point where artery passes through the adductor hiatus

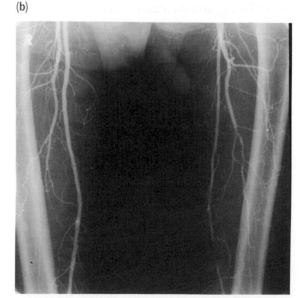

(b)

Figure 2.7 *(a) Intermittent claudication due to left superficial femoral artery occlusion. (b) Angiogram showing left superficial femoral artery occlusion.*

(a)

(b)

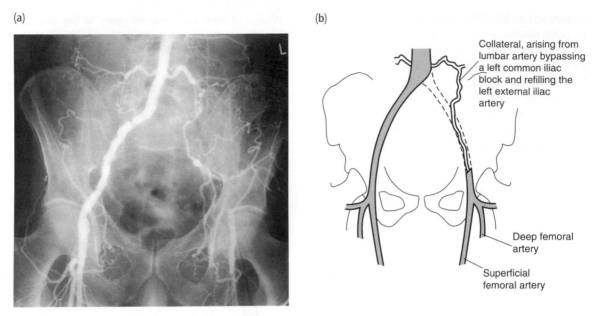

Figure 2.8   *(a) Angiogram showing left common iliac occlusion. (b) Intermittent claudication due to left common iliac occlusion.*

collateral circulation through the profunda system which joins the popliteal artery below the occlusion, usually just above the knee. As the thigh muscles have a normal blood supply, the pain is usually felt in the calf only. If the stenosis is more proximal, for example in the iliac system, the pain will be felt in the whole leg, and even the buttock, if internal iliac flow is compromised (Fig. 2.8). Such patients may also complain of inability to sustain an erection. The combination of bilateral lower limb and buttock claudication with vasculogenic impotence is termed Leriche's syndrome.

It is important to reassure the anxious claudicant that the risk of requiring surgical intervention and/or amputation is small, less than 1–2 per cent per year. For this reason, the standard treatment for the majority of patients with claudication has been to 'stop smoking and keep walking'. The patient should be warned about the hazards of continued smoking, screened and treated for correctable risk factors (diabetes and hyperlipidaemia) and told to exercise to the point of pain regularly in order to build up the collateral circulation. Fortunately, the majority of patients will accept the wisdom of this advice and attempt to alter their lifestyle. However, a proportion will not comply and/or will not accept their level of disability and in these patients the surgeon may have to consider intervention.

The role of percutaneous transluminal angioplasty (PTA) is controversial. There have been few direct comparisons, but where patients have been randomly allocated to either conservative therapy or PTA, PTA has not been shown to confer any additional long-term benefit. In the first six months, PTA might provide quicker symptomatic improvement, but in the long-term medical therapy will not only ameliorate the symptoms of claudication bilaterally but will also increase longevity by reducing the risk of death from ischaemic heart disease, stroke and bronchial carcinoma – by far the most frequent causes of death in this group of patients. Moreover, PTA costs £500–1000 per procedure and, although arguably safer than open surgery, is associated with a 1–2 per cent major morbidity and mortality rate.

The role of surgery in the management of claudication is also contentious. The natural history of the condition is benign in terms of limb loss in the great majority of cases. Thus, any excess mortality or limb loss arising as a consequence of surgery is a disaster for the patient. There is a morbidity and mortality rate of at least 1 per cent associated with femoro-popliteal bypass, and for major aorto-iliac reconstruction that figure may rise to 5 per cent.

Despite the increased risk, most surgeons will have a lower threshold for reconstructing aorto-iliac disease for the following reasons: the body's ability to compensate for aorto-iliac occlusion by developing collateral vessels is not as good as it is in the case of infra-inguinal disease; the long-term results of aorto-iliac reconstruction are considerably better than those of infra-inguinal bypass (more than 80% of aorto-bifemoral grafts placed for claudication will be patent at ten years); bilateral claudication can be corrected by a single operation; patients affected by aorto-iliac disease are generally younger and more likely to have their livelihood threatened by their disability.

By contrast, surgeons are much less enthusiastic about performing infra-inguinal bypass for femoropopliteal disease because: at five years, only about 70 per cent of grafts are still patent; bilateral claudication is common, requires two operations, and so doubles the risk; patients with claudication due to infra-inguinal disease compensate well by developing collaterals; and insertion of a bypass graft leads to involution of collateral pathways. If the graft subsequently occludes, the patient is often returned to a worse level of ischaemia than that which was present pre-operatively. A proportion of these patients will develop rest pain and, in these circumstances, the surgeon is forced to re-operate. The long-term results of repeat surgery are less impressive than those of primary reconstruction.

In summary, there can be few experienced vascular surgeons who have not seen a patient die or lose a limb as a result of vascular surgery that was initially performed for claudication. In the UK, most surgeons adopt an extremely conservative approach, and in general, less than 5–10 per cent of infra-inguinal grafts are performed for claudication.

Critical limb ischaemia

Critical limb ischaemia (CLI) can be defined as rest pain requiring strong (opiate) analgesia for a period of two weeks or more, or tissue loss, in association with an ankle pressure of less than 50 mmHg (European Consensus Document on Critical Leg Ischaemia, 1992). The inference is that without intervention, a patient with CLI will come to major limb amputation within weeks or at most months.

Although the treatment of CLI is primarily surgical, medical treatment serves two important roles. Firstly, treatment of heart failure, intercurrent infection, anaemia and diabetes, administration of intravenous antibiotics, good pain control, and use of

heparin, warfarin, and perhaps some of the newer prostacyclin based drugs, can lead to symptomatic improvement in patients with early rest pain and very limited tissue loss. Secondly, medical therapy is vital to ensure that the patient is in optimum condition prior to embarking upon major surgery.

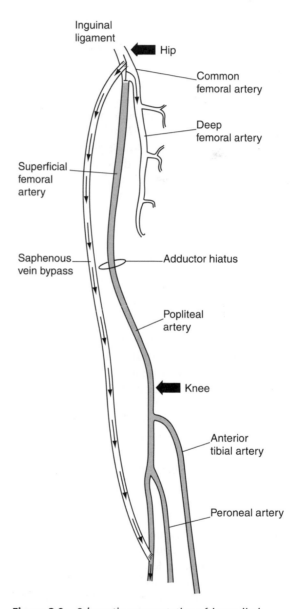

Figure 2.9 *Schematic representation of lower limb arterial anatomy and femorodistal bypass. Patients with CLI usually have extensive multi-level arterial occlusion. The mainstay of treatment is bypass, preferably using saphenous vein. The bypass usually begins at the common femoral artery and ends as far distally as is necessary; in this case, the posterior tibial artery.*

The role of PTA has not been adequately defined in this group of patients and remains contentious. The majority view is that, in patients with early rest pain and/or minimal tissue loss, sometimes called 'sub-critical ischaemia', PTA may tip the balance just enough to salvage the limb of a patient who is either not suitable or not fit for surgical reconstruction. However, some experts believe that all patients with CLI should be managed in the first instance with PTA and that surgery should be reserved for those who do not respond.

Sympathectomy has little role to play in patients with CLI although patients with early rest pain may experience some relief. Amputation is a last resort and every patient with CLI should first be assessed by a vascular surgeon. Although primary amputation is increasingly indicated in the elderly frail patient with extensive tissue loss, there are situations where the interests of patients and their families are best served by providing tender loving care only.

Bypass surgery, and to a far lesser extent local endarterectomy, are the mainstay of treatment for CLI (Fig. 2.9). These are generally unfit patients with multisystem medical and vascular problems and for this reason the mortality of so-called 'limb salvage surgery' may be as high as 10–20 per cent.

In CLI, aorto-iliac disease usually presents in conjunction with infra-inguinal disease. In patients with limited disease, the treatment of choice may be PTA, often supported with a stent. In patients who are deemed unsuitable for PTA the standard operation is aorto-bifemoral bypass grafting. In patients who are not fit for aortic surgery, then extra-anatomical bypass is frequently performed. If a patient has iliac occlusion on one side, and a relatively disease-free iliac on the other, a femoro-femoral crossover graft can be performed; an alternative is the axillo-bifemoral graft (Fig. 2.10).

The term femorodistal bypass is used to describe any arterial reconstruction which originates below the inguinal ligament and terminates at a more distal point on the same leg. The requirements for a successful distal bypass include good inflow, a reliable conduit and good outflow. Inflow is usually provided by the ipsilateral iliac system and iliac disease should be corrected where possible by PTA with or without placement of a stent. With regard to conduit, there is no doubt that autogenous vein provides the best long-term results, especially if the distal anastomosis is below the knee. The patency of long prosthetic bypasses (PTFE or Dacron) can be

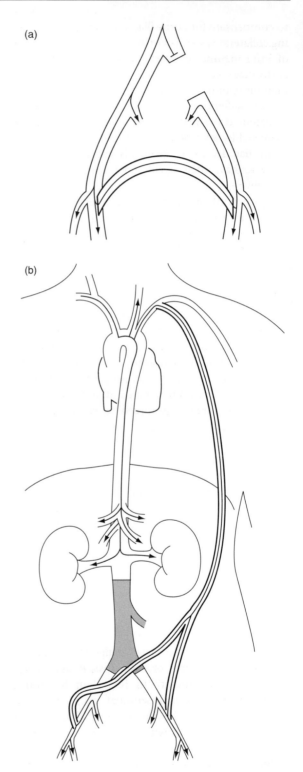

(a)

(b)

Figure 2.10 *Extra-anatomic bypass. (a) Femoro-femoral cross-over graft for unilateral iliac occlusion. (b) Axillo-bifemoral graft for aortic occlusion in a patient unfit for aortic surgery.*

improved by using a vein interposition cuff at the distal anastomosis (Stonebridge *et al.*, 1997). Vein grafts may be placed in a reversed manner or *in situ*. In the former, the vein is reversed to remove any obstruction to flow that may occur due to intact valves. In the latter, the vein is not reversed and the valves are cut. Although no significant difference in patency between these two techniques has ever been demonstrated, there are considerable advantages from a technical point of view in the *in situ* technique when long bypasses to calf and foot vessels are being constructed. Outflow (or 'run-off') refers to the vessels into which the graft is going to deliver blood and these are of great importance. If the graft is essentially delivering blood to a dead end, then it will block.

Because graft patency depends on so many different factors, most of which cannot be defined with precision, it is difficult to predict how long a particular graft will remain open. However, as at least 50 per cent of patients with CLI will be dead at five years, the graft need not remain open for a prolonged period in order to allow patients to live out the rest of their lives with two legs. Thus, many surgeons believe that if there is at least a 70 per cent chance of the graft remaining patent at two years, then it should be performed.

The great majority of patients with bypass grafts are prescribed aspirin because it both increases graft patency and reduces the risk of future myocardial infarction and stroke. Certain surgeons prescribe warfarin to some or all of their patients with femorodistal grafts although there is no definite evidence that this enhances patency, and anticoagulation in an elderly population is not without hazard.

The diabetic foot

Patients with diabetes have a propensity to develop, often quite suddenly, severe ischaemia and infection in their feet leading to rapid tissue necrosis and the requirement for amputation – the so-called 'diabetic foot'. This is due to vascular disease and neuropathy. In diabetes, peripheral vascular disease develops earlier in life, and tends to be more extensive and distal. This makes intervention, either by means of angioplasty or surgery, more difficult and technically demanding. Sensory neuropathy means that they do not respond to minor trauma, such as a stone in the shoe, and that they tend to ignore ischaemia and

infection in their feet which would be intolerably painful for someone without neuropathy. Autonomic neuropathy leads to a lack of sweating and the development of dry, fissured skin which permits entry of bacteria. Motor neuropathy leads to wasting and weakness of the small muscles of the feet, loss of the longitudinal and transverse arch structure of the foot, and development of abnormal pressure areas such as over the metatarsal heads. The principles of management are best medical care (control of diabetes, antibiotics etc.), wide debridement of devitalized tissue and drainage of pus, and revascularization of the foot when necessary.

Acute limb ischaemia

The vast majority of acute limb ischaemia is caused by either embolism or thrombosis *in situ*. By far the commonest source of embolus is the left atrium due to atrial fibrillation. Embolic occlusion usually leads to sudden and profound ischaemia with early loss of motor and sensory function. The need to act quickly is usually obvious and embolectomy is usually successful. In patients with thrombosis *in situ* the presentation is often less clear cut and the treatment more difficult because of pre-existing arterial disease. Simple surgical thrombectomy will rarely succeed and arterial bypass or thrombolysis is usually required.

The surgeon faced with the acutely ischaemic limb must primarily address two questions. Is the limb salvageable and, if so, is the limb threatened? If the limb is beyond salvage, the surgeon must decide whether it is appropriate to offer amputation or whether conservative treatment is the best option. Increasingly, however, acute-on-chronic limb ischaemia is simply the external manifestation of another terminal illness such as cardiac failure or malignancy. Subjecting such patients to amputation just before they die of underlying pathology is not good practice. The threatened limb can be defined as an ischaemic limb that is likely to become non-viable within 6 hours in the absence of revascularization. Features of the threatened limb include loss of sensation and active movement, pain on passive movement and when calf muscles are squeezed, and absent capillary return. If embolism cannot be diagnosed with certainty, then many surgeons would arrange urgent angiography to avoid operating 'blind'. An alternative is to perform 'on-table' angiography in the operating theatre. The type of surgical revascularization required will depend on the images obtained. In a patient whose limb is threatened, but whose general condition precludes long and complicated arterial surgery, amputation may be the only option. If the limb is not threatened, a period of medical optimization and heparin therapy may lead to spontaneous improvement due to collateralization. Angiography and reconstruction can then be performed on a semi-elective basis if required. An alternative is to commence thrombolysis which will lyse thrombus *in situ* over a 12–24-hour period.

Amputation

Arterial reconstruction, where possible, is a far better option than amputation for several reasons. Amputation is associated with a 10–20 per cent mortality. Stump infection and ischaemia are common and in up to 10 per cent of cases lead to major wound revision or amputation at a higher level. Less than two-thirds of below-knee, and less than one-third of above-knee, unilateral amputees are independently mobile two years after operation. And lastly, although a distal bypass for limb salvage may cost £5000, a major limb amputation frequently costs ten times that amount once the costs of rehabilitation, artificial limbs and long-term care are taken into consideration. Because rehabilitation after amputation is directly related to level of amputation, every effort should be made to preserve the knee if it is mobile and there is a prospect of the patient being fitted with, and using, a prosthesis. Although numerous investigations have been proposed, there is no single test which will reliably predict which amputation level will heal. Level of amputation remains, therefore, largely a matter of clinical judgement on the part of the surgeon.

Many patients requiring amputation for ischaemia have considerable pre-operative pain. Adequate analgesia around the time of surgery is vital for both humane reasons and because it hastens recovery and rehabilitation. The anaesthetist is usually closely involved in this aspect of care. Phantom pain, a continuation or worsening of the pain experienced in the limb prior to amputation, often with a distressing sensation that the limb is still present, is a common post-operative phenomenon. Various treatments have been advocated including transcutaneous electrical nerve stimulation, anticonvulsants

and tricyclic antidepressants. There is some evidence that, if the patient goes to theatre absolutely pain free, then the incidence of phantom pain is reduced. For this reason some surgeons request that the anaesthetists insert an epidural catheter prior to operation (Katz, 1997).

VISCERAL ISCHAEMIA

Renal artery disease

Renal artery stenosis (RAS) is usually asymptomatic and an incidental finding at post-mortem or on angiography performed for another indication (Fig. 2.11). RAS leads to decreased renal perfusion and the release of renin from the juxtaglomerular apparatus. Renin converts angiotensinogen to angiotensin I which is converted to angiotensin II in the lung. Angiotensin II causes vasoconstriction and the release of aldosterone from the adrenal cortex. The effect is salt and water retention and an increase in blood pressure. This may normalize renal perfusion in the short term, but progressive stenosis will lead to worsening ischaemia, hypertension, loss of nephrons, atrophy and irreversible renal failure. The two main causes of RAS are atheroma (60 per cent) and fibromuscular dysplasia (up to 40 per cent).

Renovascular hypertension affects a large number of people. For example, approximately 10 per cent of the adult population in the UK is hypertensive and in perhaps 10 per cent of cases, RAS is responsible.

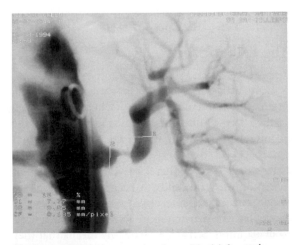

Figure 2.11 *Angiogram showing critical left renal artery stenosis.*

Renal failure due to RAS is much less common, but should always be considered in the differential diagnosis of renal failure, particularly in patients with peripheral vascular disease.

Successful surgical and/or radiological correction of RAS reduces the long-term complications of hypertension such as: stroke and heart failure; the requirement to continue on life-long antihypertensive medication; and the risk of dialysis. However, the diagnosis can be difficult to make and clinically suspected RAS is usually confirmed by means of angiography.

Balloon angioplasty is now considered the first-line treatment of most RAS, particularly that due to fibromuscular dysplasia. Surgery provides better long-term results than PTA, but is associated with greater morbidity and mortality. Most patients are therefore only operated on if medical therapy and PTA have failed. The commonest operation performed is aorto-renal bypass using long saphenous vein. Extra-anatomic renal revascularization can be achieved through hepaticorenal and splenorenal bypasses. In expert hands, these operations can be expected to provide long-term blood pressure control in 85–90 per cent of patients with a mortality of less than 5 per cent and a major morbidity of less than 10 per cent. In patients with a small non-functioning kidney, nephrectomy may be the only option.

Mesenteric ischaemia

It is important to distinguish chronic from acute mesenteric ischaemia because their presentation, investigation, management and prognosis are quite different. Due to the impressive ability of the gastrointestinal circulation to develop collaterals, the great majority of patients with chronic mesenteric arterial disease are asymptomatic. Symptomatic patients typically complain of severe abdominal pain after eating, and of weight loss. This presentation mimics many other abdominal pathologies and it is frequently the case that the patient has had numerous inconclusive investigations before the diagnosis is finally made almost as one of exclusion. The diagnosis can only be made with certainty on angiography. Surgical revascularization is the mainstay of treatment. The commonest operation is to take a graft from the aorta to the superior mesenteric artery and the coeliac axis. Although this is a major surgical undertaking, and associated with significant risk, the long-term results are good and the alternative is a slow and painful death from progressive cachexia.

Acute occlusion of a previously healthy mesenteric artery by embolus, most often arising from the left atrium due to fibrillation, leads to rapid gut infarction and a dramatic clinical presentation with sudden onset of severe abdominal pain, peritonitis and collapse which rapidly results in death. Sudden occlusion of a previously diseased mesenteric artery due to thrombosis *in situ* leads to a more insidious onset of symptoms due to the presence of collaterals. If the diagnosis is in doubt, and the patient's condition permits, angiography will confirm the diagnosis in the majority of cases. The standard operation for embolus is embolectomy and resection of any non-viable intestine. The surgical options for thrombosis are resection of ischaemic bowel if enough healthy bowel remains, or, if not, construction of a surgical bypass. A second look laparotomy to assess the viability of the remaining bowel at 24 hours is usually recommended. The mortality associated with embolus is 50 per cent and with thrombosis *in situ* as high as 90 per cent.

UPPER LIMB ISCHAEMIA

The leg is affected by ischaemia eight times more commonly than the arm because atherosclerosis affects the leg more frequently, the arterial supply of the leg (in terms of muscle bulk) is much poorer than that of the arm, and the ability of the arm vessels to develop a collateral supply appears superior. Unlike the leg, the commonest cause of upper limb ischaemia remains embolism and the standard treatment is embolectomy. Upper limb ischaemia can progress rapidly and clearly loss of any part of the upper limb has a devastating functional result.

Thoracic outlet syndrome (TOS)

Thoracic outlet syndrome occurs when the lower trunk of the brachial plexus and/or the subclavian artery are compressed as they pass over the first rib, or a cervical rib or band. The majority of patients complain of neurological symptoms. Only 5 per cent present with arterial symptoms, most commonly claudication or Raynaud's phenomenon. Turbulent flow caused by the stenosis may lead to a post-stenotic dilatation of the subclavian artery and this may in turn develop into an aneurysm. This may become lined with thrombus and give rise to distal emboli. In the absence of objective neurological damage and arterial ischaemia, the patient should be treated symptomatically with physiotherapy in an attempt to improve posture and strengthen muscles of the neck and shoulder girdle. Failure of these measures requires consideration of operative decompression. Much controversy surrounds the surgical approach to this complex area. If a cervical rib or fibrous band is present then it can be excised through a supraclavicular approach. If not, many advocate excision of the first rib through a transaxillary approach. A subclavian aneurysm requires excision and grafting. When the symptoms are clear-cut and the diagnosis certain then the results of surgery are good. In other circumstances, when the symptoms, signs and investigations are unconvincing, the surgeon and the neurologist are at a loss, and surgery is performed almost as a diagnostic test or desperate last resort, the results are poor.

Raynaud's phenomenon

In most cases, patients with Raynaud's phenomenon can be reassured about the usually benign nature of their condition, advised to stop smoking, and to avoid cold. Numerous drugs have been used to treat Raynaud's phenomenon, the best of which appears to be the calcium-channel blocker, nifedipine. Vasodilators may also be useful. In patients with severe disease, admission to hospital for a five-day infusion of prostacyclin may provide symptomatic relief. Sympathectomy is associated with poor long-term results in the hand, especially in secondary Raynaud's phenomenon, but appears more useful in the feet. Digits affected by severe ulceration, or calcium deposits in the CREST (calcinosis, Raynaud's, (o)esophagitis, sclerodactyly, telangectasia) syndrome, may require amputation although every attempt should be made to preserve as much tissue as possible.

CAROTID ARTERY

Carotid endarterectomy

Approximately 80 per cent of all strokes are ischaemic as opposed to haemorrhagic, and, of

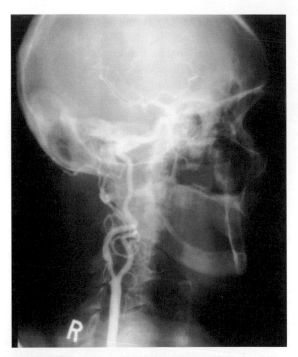

Figure 2.12 *Angiogram showing 80 per cent stenosis at the origin of the internal carotid artery.*

these, as many as half are due to distal embolization from, or thrombotic occlusion of, the carotid artery bifurcation consequent upon atherosclerotic narrowing (Fig. 2.12). Cholesterol embolization to the eye leads to a transient loss of vision, called 'amaurosis fugax', in the ipsilateral eye. Embolization to the middle cerebral artery leads to hemispheric symptoms, usually a contralateral hemiparesis. If symptoms last less than 24 hours, the event is termed a 'transient ischaemic attack' (TIA).

Two large randomized controlled trials have indicated that in patients presenting with amaurosis fugax, TIA, or stroke with good recovery, and an internal carotid artery stenosis of 70 per cent or greater, the risk of future stroke is significantly reduced by carotid endarterectomy (Fig. 2.13) in addition to best medical therapy when compared to best medical therapy alone (European Carotid Surgery Trialists' Collaborative Group, 1991; North American Symptomatic Carotid Endarterectomy Trial Collaborators, 1991). Stenoses less than 70 per cent should be treated medically in most circumstances. The risks of surgery in patients with acute stroke, and in those with completed stroke with poor recovery, outweigh the benefits. There is also mounting evidence that patients with high-grade asymptomatic stenoses may benefit from surgery, but

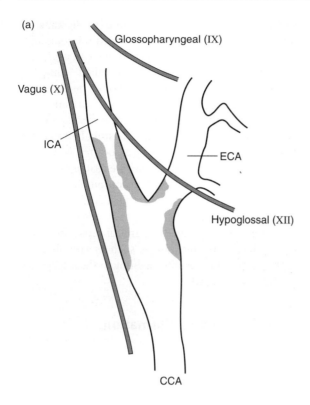

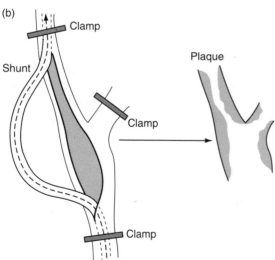

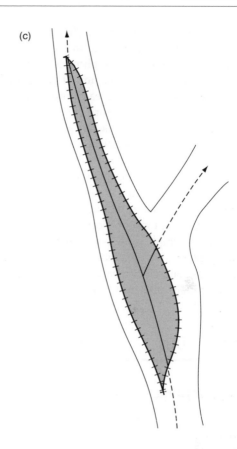

Figure 2.13 *Carotid endarterectomy. (a) The carotid bifurcation is dissected out, being careful not to dislodge plaque or damage adjacent nerves. Heparin is given, the clamps applied and the artery opened. (b) The plaque is removed. If the brain is hypoxic with the clamps on, a shunt can be put in to maintain cerebral blood flow. (c) The artery is then closed, sometimes with a patch of vein or prosthetic material to prevent narrowing. Normal flow is then restored.*

most UK surgeons are awaiting the results of further trials before they start operating on this potentially very large group of patients. The benefits of the operation depend crucially upon a low peri-operative stroke rate which should be less than 7.5 per cent in patients with previous stroke, less than 5 per cent in patients with TIA and amaurosis fugax, and less than 3 per cent in asymptomatic patients

Trials are underway comparing carotid endarterectomy with angioplasty and stenting. Early data indicate that the immediate complication rate from endovascular treatment is higher than that associated with carotid endarterectomy, and at present there is no evidence that angioplasty reduces the risk of future stroke to the same extent as surgery. However, with the development of new technology, at least a proportion of these patients may be treated non-operatively in the future.

Carotid body tumours

Carotid body tumours are paragangliomas that arise in the carotid body or less commonly in one of the adjacent nerves such as the vagus. They are rare and usually present as a painless lump in the neck. They are frequently mistaken for lymph nodes or parotid lesions and a significant proportion of patients presenting to vascular surgeons already have scar in the neck due to previous exploratory surgery. Very few carotid body tumours secrete active substances and, in the absence of symptoms, there is no requirement to routinely check circulating catecholamines. Carotid body tumours should be excised because they grow and the larger the tumour, the more difficult will the surgery be in the future. In addition, a small but significant proportion of tumours may metastasize to lymph nodes. Radiotherapy might provide an alternative to surgery, but as recurrence is high, it is generally reserved for symptomatic treatment of inoperable tumours.

MISCELLANEOUS

Vascular trauma

The commonest causes of injury to blood vessels in the UK are road traffic accidents (usually blunt injuries), penetrating injuries due to knife (and far less commonly gunshot) wounds and medical intervention (so-called 'iatrogenic injury'). Injury to the brachial and common femoral arteries at angiography and angioplasty are by far the commonest examples of the latter.

Bleeding may be external and obvious, or internal and thus clinically inapparent. Blood loss is greater if there is only partial transection because the laceration is held open. In complete transection the artery goes into spasm and thromboses, so limiting the volume of blood lost. Ischaemia may be severe because the patient has not normally had an opportunity to establish collaterals. The diagnosis is made on clinical examination with the aid of hand-held Doppler ultrasound and angiography.

As in any acutely ill patient, management begins with resuscitation. Urgent control of haemorrhage by direct pressure and restoration of normal flow is essential. This can be achieved either by directly repairing the artery, and accompanying large veins if possible, or by means of bypass grafting. Prosthetic materials should be avoided wherever possible because of the risk of infection. Upon reperfusion,

tissues become oedematous due to leakage of intravascular fluid from the damaged microcirculation. Such swelling of the calf muscles can aggravate ischaemia and, to prevent the so-called 'compartment syndrome', the surgeon will often perform fasciotomy at the time of surgical revascularization.

If, as a result of trauma, there is damage to an adjacent artery and vein, then a fistula between the two may develop. This may be associated with pain, swelling, distal ischaemia, venous engorgement, and (if the connection is large) high-output cardiac failure. On examination there is a thrill and a 'machinery murmur' throughout the cardiac cycle. Treatment usually involves surgical repair but various endovascular techniques such as embolization and covering the fistulous opening in the artery with a stent may be used.

Arteriovenous malformations

Arteriovenous malformations (AVM) are congenital abnormalities. They are almost invariably present at birth, but may not present until much later in life. AVMs arise when there are abnormal communications between arteries and veins. The more proximal in the circulation, the greater the transmitted flow. A proportion of malformations appear to be entirely venous. Patients usually present with swelling, discoloration and bleeding. Pain, high-output cardiac failure, limb hypertrophy and ulceration are less common. Apart from biopsy to exclude malignancy in cases of doubt, the diagnosis is usually clinical. Magnetic resonance imaging (MRI), which is now the investigation of choice, will give valuable information about the deep extent of the lesions in cases where excision is being contemplated. The principles of treatment are control of symptoms and prevention of complications whilst, at the same time, minimizing intervention. Excision, where possible and safe, provides good long-term control, but is rarely possible. Amputation is sometimes required as a last resort. Therapeutic embolization is usually the mainstay of treatment, but is highly skilled, requires careful planning, and is not without risk of rendering surrounding or distal vital tissues ischaemic. Angiography and embolization in children (and some adults) is usually carried out under general anaesthesia to reduce the stress on the patient, and also to prevent the patient from moving unexpectedly.

CHRONIC VENOUS INSUFFICIENCY

Up to 20 per cent of the adult population have varicose veins and some 50 000 patients undergo surgery for this condition each year in the UK, the great majority for cosmetic reasons or for minor leg symptoms which are often not related to venous pathology. It is likely that this activity will be drastically reduced as part of healthcare rationing. Although varicose vein surgery is usually considered minor and straightforward there are many traps for the unwary and there is no doubt that it is often performed extremely badly by unsupervised junior surgeons. This is perhaps one reason why varicose vein surgery is one rapidly growing area for medico-legal complaint.

A more important health problem is posed by chronic venous insufficiency and ulceration which affects up to 5 per cent of the elderly population and costs the health service at least £500 million per annum. There is increasing evidence that timely superficial venous surgery, interruption of perforating veins and skin grafting can augment ulcer healing and reduce ulcer recurrence. However, it has to be appreciated that this is a very different group of patients from those undergoing typical varicose vein surgery. They are old, they often have significant medical co-morbidity, have often suffered previous deep venous thrombosis, and are much more akin to the 'arterial' patient. The surgery is also more complex and extensive, and particular care has to be taken with antibiotic and thromboembolic prophylaxis.

THE FUTURE

Many of the techniques, and much of the knowledge, outlined in this chapter have only become available and apparent in the last twenty to thirty years. This rapid pace of technological advance continues, particularly with regard to minimally invasive and endovascular techniques. For example, several centres in the UK are now repairing certain abdominal aortic aneurysms by means of a stent–graft combination placed percutaneously through the femoral artery without the need for an abdominal incision. Laparoscopic intra-abdominal arterial surgery, although still in its infancy, shows promise for the future. Equally impressive have been the advances in non-invasive imaging. Many radiologists believe that within the next ten years, MRI will have largely replaced conventional angiography and computed tomography in the assessment of the central and peripheral vascular systems. High-quality real-time colour flow duplex ultrasound imaging has revolutionized the imaging of arteries and veins. New ultrasound contrast media may allow certain vessels such as the renal and mesenteric arteries, previously often inaccessible to ultrasound diagnosis, to be imaged with increasing ease and accuracy. It is likely that there will also be major advances in the development of prosthetic grafts that can match the long-term performance of autologous vein. In addition, there is much basic science work directed towards allowing human cadaver and animal arteries to be used as arterial conduits in man.

In summary, vascular surgery is a young subspeciality, but growing fast. With the ageing population, and no evidence of a decline in tobacco consumption or in the prevalence of diabetes, there is undoubtedly going to be an ever growing need for arterial surgery for many years. Increasing surgical and anaesthetic specialization and expertise, together with the technological advances outlined above, mean that the profession is well placed to meet these future demands.

REFERENCES

Collins, J. 1994. Aneurysms. In Galland, R.B. and Clyne, C.A.C. (eds) *Clinical problems in vascular surgery.* London: Edward Arnold, 89–96.

European Consensus Document on Critical Leg Ischaemia. 1992. *European Journal of Vascular Surgery* **6** (Suppl. A), 1–28.

Stonebridge, P.A., Prescott, R.P. and Ruckley, C.V. 1997. Randomised trial comparing infrainguinal PTFE bypass grafts with and without a vein interposition cuff at the distal anastomosis. *Journal of Vascular Surgery* **26**, 543–550.

Katz, J. 1997. Prevention of phantom limb pain by regional anaesthesia. *Lancet* **349**, 519–520.

European Carotid Surgery Trialists' Collaborative Group. 1991. MRC European Carotid Surgery trial: interim results for symptomatic patients with severe (70–99 per cent) or with mild (0–29 per cent) carotid stenosis. *Lancet* **337**, 1235–1243.

North American Symptomatic Carotid Endarterectomy Trial Collaborators. 1991. Beneficial effect of carotid endarterectomy in symptomatic patients with high-grade carotid stenosis. *New England Journal of Medicine* **325**, 335–351.

3

Vascular risk, prophylaxis of thromboembolism and the vasculitides: the physician's approach

JILL J F BELCH AND ANDREW MUIR

INTRODUCTION

The medical management of peripheral vascular disease is complex, involving strategies for vascular risk reduction and lifestyle modification, as well as drug therapy. Target areas for the vascular team are outlined in Table 3.1, but a number relate to outpatient or non-surgical provision of care. This review will concentrate on the aspects relevant to the patient undergoing vascular surgery.

MODIFYING VASCULAR RISK

'I say that this [angina pectoris] exactly corresponds to the sense of weakness and want of muscular power which exists in persons who have the arteries of the legs obstructed or ossified.'

(B.C. Brodie, 1841)

This statement from the mid-nineteenth century demonstrates that clinicians have long recognized that peripheral arterial occlusive disease (PAOD) of the lower limb is a marker for potentially lethal coronary atherosclerosis (Brodie, 1841; McKenna *et al.*, 1991). However, the strength of this link has only been appreciated recently. Intermittent claudication is the prime symptom of lower limb ischaemia and the natural history of leg disease in claudicating patients is usually benign. Fewer than 5 per cent of patients ever require amputation, and spontaneous remission of symptoms is common. However, their mortality is two to three times higher than that of non-claudicating patients of a similar age (Leng and Fowkes, 1993). This increased death rate is mainly due to cardiovascular disease: 50 per cent die from ischaemic heart disease (IHD), 15 per cent from cerebral vascular events, 10 per cent from abdominal vascular pathology and only 25 per cent of patients from non-vascular events. Such is the strength of the association between PAOD and cardiac mortality that even in asymptomatic disease detected by a decreased lower limb blood pressure, the relative risk of a cardiac event is greatly enhanced (Table 3.2). Thus medical management goals are directed not only at reducing or preventing progression of leg ischaemia, but also at reducing the risk of IHD and thrombotic stroke.

Table 3.1 *Medical management of peripheral arterial disease*

- **Modify vascular risk**
  Antiplatelet therapy
  Cigarette smoking
  Diabetes
  Hypertension
  Hyperlipidaemia
  Thrombophilia

- **Intermittent claudication**
  Exercise
  ? Drug therapy

- **Acute critical limb ischaemia (CLI)**
  Thrombolysis
  Anticoagulation

- **Chronic critical limb ischaemia**
  Control oedema
  Control infection
  Improve cardiac output
  ? Prostanoids

- **Embolism**
  Detect and treat arrhythmia and cardiac thrombus

- **Deep-vein thrombosis (DVT)**
  Prophylaxis
  Treatment

- **Vasculitides**
  Connective-tissue disease
  Raynaud's phenomenon
  Vasculitis
  Antiphospholipid syndrome

- **Perioperative**
  Modify risk
  Optimize cardiac function
  DVT prophylaxis
  Detect arrhythmias and cardiac thrombus in acute CLI

Table 3.2 *The ankle–brachial pressure index (ABPI) as a marker for increased cardiovascular risk*

ABPI	Subjects	Relative risk (95% CI)	Measure
< 0.85	Population study	2.36 (1.60–3.48)	Total mortality[1]
< 0.40	Population study	4.49 (3.52–5.64)	Total mortality[1]
< 0.90	Elderly men (≥ 50 years)	2.0 (1.4–2.9)	Ischaemic heart disease mortality[2]
< 0.90	Elderly women	2.1 (1.4–3.1)	Ischaemic heart disease mortality[2]
≤ 0.90	Hypertensives	4.1 (2.0–8.3)	Total mortality[3]

1, McKenna *et al.* (1991). 2, Vogt *et al.* (1993). 3, Newman *et al.* (1993).

Over the past decade, modification of risk factors has been a major remit for cardiologists who have set important targets to be achieved in vascular event reduction in coronary disease by the year 2000. In the UK government's White Paper *The Health of the Nation*, targets include a reduction in death rate from IHD and stroke by at least 40 per cent in people under 65 years of age, and 30 per cent in those aged 65–74 years. Similar goals have been set in the USA with the *Healthy People 2000* objectives. Despite major public health campaigns and doctor education programmes combined with these government directives, doctors have failed to significantly increase risk factor modification after myocardial infarction (MI) until fairly recently. The Action on

Secondary Prevention through Intervention to Reduce Events study (ASPIRE, 1996) indicated that 50 per cent of those diagnosed as glucose intolerant at the time of MI had received no treatment after six months, 25 per cent remained hypertensive and over 75 per cent had a cholesterol above the recommended level. It is likely that the rate of take-up for risk factor modification is even lower in patients with PAOD because the importance of these (apart from cigarette smoking) is not widely recognized, and historically (in the UK at least) vascular physicians who would manage them are in short supply. Thus the hospital admission of a patient for vascular surgery offers a golden opportunity for assessment of risk profile. This has two advantages: firstly, modification of risk

Table 3.3 *The predictive value of some risk factors for total mortality and for progression of PAOD in 1969 patients with claudication. Relative risk with 95% confidence intervals. (After Dormandy and Murray, 1991)*

Parameter	Total mortality	Progression of PAOD
ABPI ≤ 0.5	2.0 (1.3–3.2)	2.3 (1.6–3.4)
Age (per 10 years)	2.1 (1.6–2.7)	1.2 (1.0–1.4)
Male sex	1.3 (0.7–2.3)	1.7 (1.0–2.8)
Recent smoking (within 6 months)	0.8 (0.5–1.3)	1.4 (0.9–2.2)
Hypertension	1.8 (1.1–2.8)	1.0 (0.7–1.4)
Diabetes mellitus	1.7 (1.0–2.8)	1.3 (0.8–2.1)
Previous vascular surgery	0.6 (0.3–0.9)	1.7 (1.2–2.4)

will decrease the likelihood of coronary artery events and stroke in the future; and secondly, such risk factor modification may attenuate the disease process in the peripheral vessels, thus maximizing the potential benefits of surgery. It is a careless plumber who repairs a blocked pipe, but does not seek out the cause (e.g. rubbish in the outlet).

Risk factors in PAOD

The factors associated with the development of PAOD have been identified in numerous cross-sectional studies (Table 3.3). Unfortunately, there have been relatively few cohort studies performed to date, but the evidence suggests that cigarette smoking (Levy, 1989), hyperlipidaemia (Fowkes *et al.*, 1995), hypertension (Strano *et al.*, 1993) and diabetes mellitus (Beks *et al.*, 1995) are of particular importance. Each will be addressed in turn. Haemorheological and coagulation abnormalities (Fig. 3.1) are also involved, including one of the best recognized risk factors – increased platelet aggregation (Belch *et al.*, 1983) – and also the activated white blood cell (WBC) (Hickman *et al.*, 1994), free-radical generation (Belch *et al.*, 1995), increased plasma fibrinogen (Lowe *et al.*, 1991) and decreased fibrinolysis (Smith *et al.*, 1993). Of these, platelet activation has been best studied, and the use of antiplatelet agents in PAOD should, by now, be established practice.

Antiplatelet therapy

PERIPHERAL ARTERIAL OBSTRUCTIVE DISEASE (PAOD)

The role of platelet aggregation in arterial thrombosis has been well documented. Other relevant aspects include the role of platelet-release products. Thromboxane A_2 (TXA$_2$) and serotonin (5-hydroxytryptamine, 5-HT) cause vasoconstriction, and increased

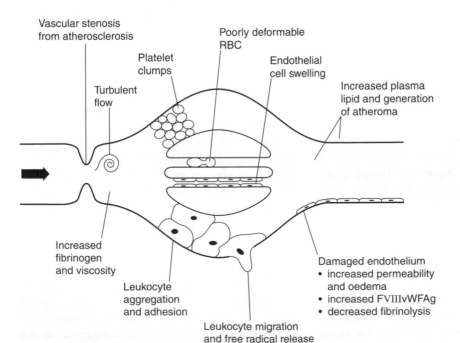

Vascular stenosis from atherosclerosis

Platelet clumps

Turbulent flow

Poorly deformable RBC

Endothelial cell swelling

Increased plasma lipid and generation of atheroma

Increased fibrinogen and viscosity

Leukocyte aggregation and adhesion

Leukocyte migration and free radical release

Damaged endothelium
• increased permeability and oedema
• increased FVIIIvWFAg
• decreased fibrinolysis

Figure 3.1 *Abnormalities of blood and vessel wall contributing to PAOD. FVIIIvWFAg is factor VIII von Willebrand factor antigen.*

levels of TXB_2 (the stable metabolite of TXA_2) have been detected in PAOD (FitzGerald *et al.*, 1984). TXA_2 formation is inhibited by aspirin and this may be relevant to its use in peripheral arterial disease (Lau *et al.*, 1991a). Serotonin (released from activated platelets) is a weaker vasoconstrictor, but it still induces platelet aggregation. Patients with PAOD have lower intraplatelet 5-HT levels than controls suggesting increased release into the plasma (Barradas *et al.*, 1988), and thus increased platelet activation.

Beta-thromboglobulin (βTG) is another marker of platelet activation *in vivo* and plasma levels are elevated in patients with PAOD (Zahavi and Zahavi, 1985). Whilst the biological function of βTG is not fully defined, it may include a contribution to WBC activation through neutrophil-activating peptide formation. Platelet factor 4 (PF4), which neutralizes the body's natural anticoagulant, heparin, and platelet-derived growth factor (PDGF), which stimulates proliferation of vascular smooth muscle cells, are also released from activated platelets and may play a role in atherosclerosis. Platelet release of plasminogen activator inhibitor-1 (PAI-1), which inhibits the activation of plasminogen activator and thus decreases fibrinolysis, may also contribute to this process.

CLINICAL TRIALS OF ANTIPLATELET AGENTS

Pharmacotherapy for PAOD has been difficult to study because of the disease's variable natural history. Some small trials have evaluated antiplatelet therapy for claudication, but there have been very few randomized trials of sufficient size to clearly define the efficacy of such drug therapy (Cameron *et al.*, 1988). With the realization that platelets may be involved in other manifestations of arterial disease in the claudicating patient (such as MI and stroke) interest has grown in the use of antiplatelet agents as prophylaxis for other arterial events and disease progression. Table 3.4 summarizes the clinical approaches to antiplatelet treatment which have been studied in PAOD.

Aspirin

Aspirin is the most commonly used antiplatelet agent because it is the best studied in clinical trials and is currently the cheapest agent available. It irreversibly inhibits the cyclooxygenase enzyme by acetylating the serine residue number 529 near the

Table 3.4 *Antiplatelet agents and peripheral arterial disease*

Clinical situation	Antiplatelet agents providing benefit
Primary prevention of PAOD	Not yet studied
Primary prevention of PAOD surgery	Aspirin
Secondary prevention of PAOD progression	Aspirin and dipyridamole
Prevention of re-occlusion after re-vascularization	Aspirin Aspirin and dipyridamole Ticlopidine
Prevention of coronary and cerebrovascular events in PAOD	Aspirin Ticlopidine Clopidogrel

active site of the enzyme (Patrono, 1994). The synthesis of TXA_2 is therefore decreased and platelet aggregation attenuated. Platelets are unable to synthesize new enzyme and are therefore inactive for their 8–10-day lifetime. Aspirin has been used in patients with PAOD to prevent progression of arterial disease and to prevent MI and stroke. The Physicians' Health Study carried out in the USA (Goldhaber *et al.*, 1992) provided data on the primary prevention of peripheral vascular surgery. Healthy doctors received placebo or 325 mg of aspirin every other day. The risk of undergoing peripheral vascular surgery was decreased by 46 per cent in the aspirin group compared to placebo. In a subgroup analysis, those with claudication were also found to require less vascular surgery than equivalent control patients. However, aspirin did not affect the likelihood of developing claudication *de novo* in the study period.

Only a few small studies have examined aspirin's ability to prevent progression of PAOD. Hess and colleagues (1985) did evaluate 240 patients, and they were able to show that aspirin and dipyridamole inhibited angiographic progression of the disease, and that the combination of aspirin and dipyridamole was superior to aspirin alone. However, it should be noted that pre-existing vascular stenoses were found more frequently in the aspirin group and this may explain the failure to obtain a statistically significant difference from placebo with aspirin alone. The most convincing data in support of the use of aspirin in these patients come from the

Antiplatelet Trialists Collaboration (1994a). In this meta-analysis of 174 randomized trials of antiplatelet therapy (mainly aspirin in doses of 75–325 mg per day), the data showed antiplatelet agents to decrease non-fatal MI, non-fatal stroke and vascular death in patients with cardiovascular disease (Antiplatelet Trialists Collaboration, 1994b). In a subgroup analysis of high-risk patients, which included those with a history of vascular surgery, peripheral angioplasty or PAOD, the percentage odds reductions were: 32 per cent from the risk of vascular death, MI or stroke; 32 per cent also for non-fatal MI; 46 per cent for non-fatal stroke; and 20 per cent for death from vascular causes. There was no evidence that the higher doses were more effective than the lower ones.

Occlusion of vascular grafts has also been studied. There is a significant failure rate after infra-inguinal bypass surgery (Taylor et al., 1990) and this is more likely with artificial materials (49 per cent) than with vein grafts (12 per cent). The underlying mechanisms of occlusion are likely to be related to platelet behaviour because early thrombosis can occur by activation of platelets on exposed artificial surfaces. Stenosis at anastomoses may take place because of smooth muscle cell proliferation which may be related, in part, to PDGF release from the platelet (Reidy et al., 1992). Early randomized controlled studies evaluated aspirin alone or in combination with dipyridamole for infra-inguinal prosthetic grafts. Both treatments decreased re-occlusion rates (Green et al., 1982; Goldman et al., 1983; Clyne et al., 1987) and these data are supported by a meta-analysis (Antiplatelet Trialists Collaboration, 1994c). In this overview (n = 3000 PAOD patients), antiplatelet agents were given for a mean of 19 months and decreased the risk of occlusion from 25 per cent in control patients to 16 per cent in those treated. Thus the addition of aspirin to the regime will prevent nine out of every 100 patients from developinging a vascular occlusion (Lualdi et al., 1995). As with the trials of secondary prevention of vascular events, a variety of aspirin doses were used and larger ones were not significantly more effective than 75 mg per day. Most patients should be on aspirin before pre-operative assessment, but if it has not been started, it appears from these studies that it may be introduced post-operatively without loss of efficacy. In contrast, smaller studies appear to support the introduction of aspirin pre-operatively (Kohler et al., 1984). Those clinicians concerned about antiplatelet drug effects on haemostasis or during spinal anaesthesia may prefer to consider post-operative administration, although the evidence that this is acceptable is not yet conclusive.

It is of interest that while aspirin appears to prevent secondary vascular events in patients receiving prosthetic grafts, it does not increase vein graft patency rates. McCollom and colleagues (1991), in one of the largest studies (n = 549), found no statistically significant difference between re-occlusion rates in the active (aspirin) or placebo groups. Nevertheless, it should still be given to these patients because of the proven benefits of aspirin in MI and stroke prevention. A compound affecting other mechanisms of the coagulation cascade may be of use in improving graft patency and clinical studies in this area are currently underway.

Aspirin is contraindicated in patients with active peptic ulceration and gastrointestinal haemorrhage, but previous peptic ulceration is not a contraindication if ulcer prophylaxis (e.g. an H_2-receptor antagonist) is given. Aspirin intolerance is mainly secondary to gastrointestinal effects, which may be minimized by administration on alternate days. Efficacy does not appear to be lost with this regime (Goldhaber et al., 1992). If true aspirin intolerance does occur, dipyridamole alone or ticlopidine (see below) may be used. Recent work with clopidogrel makes it an attractive alternative for the aspirin-intolerant patient (CAPRIE Steering Committee, 1996).

Dipyridamole

Dipyridamole's antiplatelet effect is thought to be due to three actions. Firstly it may increase and potentiate the effects of prostacyclin (PGI_2). Secondly, it may inhibit platelet phosphodiesterase, the enzyme which breaks down cyclic AMP, and finally it may inhibit cellular uptake of adenosine, thereby increasing the plasma concentration of this autologous antiplatelet vasodilator agent (FitzGerald, 1987). Clinical studies of dipyridamole have used doses between 75 and 400 mg per day, usually in three divided doses. There has been much controversy over the use of dipyridamole in combination with aspirin. Early work appeared to show benefit from combined therapy, but this fell into disrepute in the 1980s when aspirin alone was favoured. More recently, the large stroke studies have convincingly demonstrated the benefit of the combination, and Hess *et al.* (1985) found it more effective in the prevention of peripheral graft failure. With the current evidence of possible tachyphylaxis occurring in patients developing stroke on aspirin, it is our current practice to add in dipyridamole if thrombosis has already occurred on aspirin. Large comparative clinical studies are urgently required in this area. In PAOD, dipyridamole is at present mainly reserved for the aspirin-intolerant patient.

Ticlopidine

Ticlopidine appears to inhibit platelet aggregation by interfering with the binding of macromolecules such as fibrinogen to the group IIb–IIIa complex (McTavish *et al.*, 1990). The dose is 250 mg twice a day. It causes leukopenia in 1–2 per cent of patients. In patients with PAOD, ticlopidine decreases the rate of cardiac events. Boissel *et al.* (1989) performed a meta-analysis of a number of claudication studies to show a statistically significant reduction in the rate of fatal and non-fatal cardiovascular events following ticlopidine: 3 per cent in the active group compared to 9 per cent in the placebo group. In addition, the Swedish Ticlodipine Multicenter Study (STIMS) has shown a reduction in the rate of primary cardiovascular events such as transient ischaemic attacks (TIAs), strokes and MI in patients with claudication (Janzon *et al.*, 1990). This was an 'on treatment' analysis. Mortality was decreased when the analysis was carried out on an intention-to-treat basis. Further evaluation of STIMS (Bergqvist *et al.*, 1995) also showed a reduction in the requirement for lower limb vascular surgery during treatment with ticlopidine. This supports earlier work by the EMATAP Group (Blanchard *et al.*, 1993) where ticlopidine significantly reduced the need for vascular surgery.

Clopidogrel

Clopidogrel is chemically related to ticlopidine, but has a potentially greater antithrombotic effect (Herbert *et al.*, 1993a). It blocks activation of platelets, selectively and irreversibly inhibiting the binding of ADP to its receptors, thereby affecting ADP-dependent activation of the group IIb–IIIa complex (Herbert *et al.*, 1993b). Clopidogrel 75 mg per day appears to be equipotent to ticlopidine 250 mg b.d. and is not associated with the same degree of leukopenia. The Clopidogrel versus Aspirin in

Patients at Risk of Ischaemic Events (CAPRIE) study compared the two agents, potential benefits in reducing the risk of stroke, MI, or vascular death in 19 185 patients with recent stroke, MI or PAOD. There were 1960 'first' events. Clopidogrel produced a 'risk of event' rate of 5.32 per cent per annum compared to 5.83 per cent with aspirin, reflecting a relative risk reduction of 8.7 per cent in favour of clopidogrel. There were no major differences in safety between clopidogrel and aspirin, with neutropenia occurring in 0.1 per cent of clopidogrel patients and 0.17 per cent of those taking aspirin. Subgroup analysis demonstrated that patients with PAOD benefited to a greater extent from clopidogrel than other groups, the annual event rate being 3.71 compared to 4.86 in patients taking aspirin, a relative risk reduction of 23.8 per cent in favour of clopidogrel. Because approximately 30 per cent of all patients given aspirin develop gastrointestinal side effects, it is likely that clopidogrel will be reserved for them, at least until the prices of the two are comparable.

Other agents

Ketanserin is a selective $5-HT_2$-receptor antagonist that inhibits serotonin-induced platelet aggregation (Brogden and Sorkin, 1990). The Prevention of Atherosclerotic Complications with Ketanserin (PACK) (1989) trial group evaluated its role in the prevention of vascular events and vascular death. Unlike aspirin, ticlopidine and clopidogrel, ketanserin did not prevent such primary endpoints and cannot be recommended for prophylaxis of vascular events in PAOD.

Iloprost, a synthetic prostacyclin analogue with potent antiplatelet and vasodilator effects (Belch *et al.*, 1984a), has been evaluated in a number of multicentre studies as a treatment for critical limb ischaemia (CLI). The meta-analysis of these studies showed a statistically significant decrease in amputation and death in the iloprost group (Loosemore *et al.*, 1994). It is not known whether the combined endpoint suggests cardiovascular protection from iloprost over and above the effects it has on the CLI itself. Further work is required.

Of interest is the recent work by Mangano and colleagues (1996) on atenolol given intravenously immediately before and after operation (and orally thereafter) in patients at risk of IHD events. The operations were all non-cardiac, with 81 patients out of 200 undergoing major peripheral vascular surgery. It was considered that atenolol might have a number of beneficial effects in this patient group, including an antiplatelet action. All cause mortality was significantly decreased in the atenolol group compared to placebo at six months (0 per cent versus 8 per cent), at one year (3 per cent versus 14 per cent) and at two years (10 per cent versus 21 per cent). The principal effect was a reduction in death from cardiac causes. Further work is needed, perhaps with assessment of the newer, non-vasoconstrictor beta-blockers.

CONCLUSION

There is growing evidence that antiplatelet agents such as aspirin are effective in preventing cardiac and stroke events in patients with PAOD. Additionally, they will decrease occlusion rates after vascular grafting. Antiplatelet drugs should be prescribed unless there is a clear contraindication in an individual patient. Peri-operative admission is the ideal setting for starting such therapy should it not already be prescribed.

Cigarette smoking

Smoking has long been known to increase the risk, and contribute to the progression, of peripheral arterial disease (Krupski, 1991). In 1904, Read observed that cigarette smokers had a significantly higher incidence of peripheral atherosclerosis than non-smokers, and in 1908, Buerger described another peripheral vascular complication, thromboangiitis obliterans (Buerger's disease). Of all the risk factors, the use of tobacco correlates most strongly with the development of occlusive arterial disease. The mechanisms whereby cigarette smoking produces vascular morbidity and mortality are multiple. Cigarette smoke contains more than 4000 substances, of which carbon monoxide and nicotine have been best studied (Krupski, 1991). Nicotine raises the systolic blood pressure and increases heart rate. Carbon monoxide directly reduces oxygen availability and is atherogenic. Cigarette smoking induces platelet aggregation and decreases fibrinolysis (Belch et al., 1984b), damages the vascular endothelium and also appears to have a detrimental effect on lipid profile (McGill, 1988). Total cholesterol levels average 3 per cent more in smokers than in non-smokers. According to the Framingham

study (Kannel and McGee, 1985), smokers are twice as likely to develop intermittent claudication as their non-smoking counterparts, and indeed 70–90 per cent of patients with intermittent claudication smoke.

Atherosclerosis is more likely to progress to CLI in subjects who smoke, and amputation is more common than in non-smokers (Hughson et al., 1978; Jonason and Ringqvist, 1985). Crucially, vascular grafts are far more likely to fail if smoking continues. In one study, the five-year cumulative patency rates of femoropopliteal and aortofemoral bypass grafts were 80 per cent and 90 per cent respectively, in non-smokers, but in patients smoking more than five cigarettes per day, the corresponding rates were 45 per cent and 30 per cent (Myers et al., 1978). Because this recurrence of ischaemia is both frequent and rapid in smokers, it is crucial that stopping smoking is given a firm priority at the time of surgery. This is, however, difficult because 90 per cent are addicted to nicotine (Jarvis and Russel, 1989). Although 60–70 per cent of smokers would like to give up, the majority have tried more than once (Russel, 1990) and almost three-quarters of those who do stop are smoking again within three months (Benowitz, 1988).

There are two aspects to nicotine addiction: psychological and physiological dependence. The former relates to the rapid, pleasurable, mood-enhancing effect of nicotine, with smokers using cigarettes as a reward mechanism, and to alleviate anxiety and boredom. The physiological dependence is due to the action on acetylcholine receptors increasing arousal and concentration (US Department of Health and Human Services, 1988). Higher levels of nicotine inhibit the receptors, producing sedative and stress-relieving effects. Thus, when smokers try to stop, they experience both behavioural and physical withdrawal symptoms. Although the withdrawal symptoms are often short-lived, they can exert a strong influence on a smoker's will to stop, so it makes sense to offer support in overcoming both aspects of the addiction. About 5 per cent of smokers stop after receiving only medical advice (Fiore et al., 1990), but provision of increased support and counselling improves this rate (Abelin, 1989). Whilst in hospital for vascular grafting, patients should be given the opportunity to be referred to the smoking clinic, which may be either a primary care or hospital-based facility. Nicotine-replacement therapy is an effective aid (Silagy et al., 1994), overcoming the early problems of physical addiction and allowing the smoker to concentrate on combatting the psychological addition.

The first type of nicotine replacement therapy (NRT) to become widely available was nicotine-containing chewing gum (Lam et al., 1987). Other forms include transdermal patches, intranasal sprays and inhalers, but the latter two are not yet licensed for clinical use. These forms of therapy may attenuate some of the problems seen with the gum, such as transfer of dependency (Hughes et al., 1986) and gastrointestinal side effects (Henningfield et al., 1990). A recent meta-analysis of 53 trials of NRT (42 gum, 9 patch, 1 spray, 1 inhaler) with data on 17703 subjects was carried out (Silagy et al., 1994). NRT increased the odds ratio for abstinence to 1.61 for gum, 2.07 for patch, 2.92 for nasal spray and 3.05 for inhaled nicotine. The authors concluded that the currently available forms of NRT are effective aids to stopping smoking, but they are contraindicated in acute MI, unstable angina and cardiac arrhythmias, so its introduction should take account of this.

Diabetes mellitus

The association between diabetes mellitus and PAOD has been recognized for some time. Brandman and Redisch (1953) estimated that 50 per cent of patients with diabetes have evidence of PAOD ten to fifteen years after the onset of their disease. Furthermore, the arteriographic extent of disease has been correlated with glucose intolerance (Kingsbury, 1996). The scale of the clinical problem is such that 29 per cent of below-knee amputations are performed on diabetic patients, a figure that rises to 45 per cent when distal amputations are included (Connor, 1987). When the risk profiles of diabetics who died were compared with those who did not, the incidence of PAOD was the most significant predictor of death: 92 per cent versus 39 per cent (Stiegler et al., 1992). Vascular disease is the major cause of morbidity and mortality in patients with both non-insulin- and insulin-dependent diabetes mellitus (NIDDM, IDDM). They have an overall mortality of 50 per cent within four years of diagnosis compared with only 10 per cent of a control population (Deckert et al., 1978). Some of this enhanced mortality results from diabetic microvascular disease (Wilson et al., 1992) and some from the macrovascular disease which occurs at an earlier age, probably

with its roots in childhood (Belch et al., 1996b). This premature macrovascular disease affects coronary, cerebral, carotid and peripheral vessels.

Asymptomatic peripheral arterial disease, as detected by a decrease in ankle brachial systolic blood pressure index (ABPI), occurs approximately 20 times more frequently in diabetic patients (Fabris et al., 1994). The mechanism of development of premature vascular disease in a diabetic patient is complex and multifactorial, and includes contributions from hypertension, hyperlipidaemia (Jones et al., 1989), abnormalities of free-radical activity (Jennings et al., 1991) and abnormalities of haemostasis (Lowe et al., 1986). There is an enhanced oxidative stress in diabetes mellitus compared to both control and to non-diabetic PAOD patients (Belch et al., 1996a).

Defence against free-radical attack is provided in part by the body's antioxidants. Plasma vitamin E and ascorbic acid levels are lower in diabetics (Karpen et al., 1985) and, interestingly, some of the capillary basement membrane changes are similar to those occurring in scurvy. Other free-radical scavengers have also been reported to be decreased in diabetic PAOD patients compared to non-diabetics (Belch et al., 1996a). A number of haemostatic and fibrinolytic abnormalities have been detected in diabetes (McLaren et al., 1990), but the most compelling and reproducible abnormalities have been those of platelet behaviour with enhanced release of platelet products and platelet aggregation (Lagarde et al., 1980; Oswald et al., 1988). Links between platelet aggregation and the increase in free-radical generation have been studied. Free radicals have been shown to increase platelet aggregation, with antioxidants decreasing aggregation (Salonen, 1989). Antiplatelet therapy has been used in the secondary prevention of arterial disease in general, as described earlier, but also specifically in diabetic patients (Sivenius et al., 1992; ETDRS Investigators, 1992). The Early Treatment of Diabetic Retinopathy Study (ETDRS) showed aspirin to provide cardiovascular protection equal to that seen in non-diabetic groups when given for primary prevention of diabetic retinopathy. Additionally, aspirin had no greater side effects in the diabetic population than in non-diabetics.

Diabetes mellitus presents three problems perioperatively. First, there is care of the previously diagnosed patient at a time of metabolic stress, and second the introduction of antiplatelet treatment such

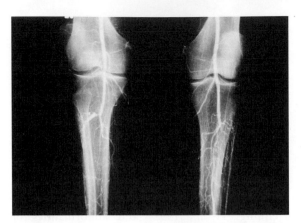

Figure 3.2   *Angiographic pattern of 'distal' disease seen in diabetes mellitus.*

as aspirin. The third aspect is diagnosis of 'occult' diabetes. Of 100 consecutive diabetic patients presenting to a group of vascular surgeons, 72 had been diagnosed by finding a random or fasting blood sugar in the diabetic range; 28 had normal random or fasting blood sugar levels (Muir *et al.*, 1997), but had an abnormal glucose tolerance test. The difficulty is knowing which patients require this test if the fasting or random glucose is normal, but our current practice is to do it in two groups of patients. First, those in whom the distal distribution of arterial disease arouses the suspicion of diabetes (Fig. 3.2); 12 of the 100 consecutive patients were diagnosed in this way. Another clue is a 'diabetic' lipid profile in which both total plasma cholesterol and fasting triglyceride levels are increased, and HDL levels are decreased. This group comprised the other 16 subjects in the study. Diabetes mellitus is consistently underdiagnosed (Gerstein and Yusuf, 1996) and this can have serious consequences in the vascular patient, either acutely in the post-operative period or over the longer term with uncontrolled disease progression. A high index of suspicion is required because all risk factors are synergistic not merely additive in terms of vascular disease production (Muhlhauser, 1990). Failure to diagnose underlying diabetes in a smoking claudicant will have serious consequences for that patient.

Hypertension

An elevated blood pressure (BP) has been associated with the development of PAOD in both cross-sectional and case–control surveys. Some studies suggest that a raised systolic BP may be the most important component (Schroll and Munck, 1981), although others suggest an association with both diastolic and systolic BP (Reid *et al.*, 1966). However, results from prospective studies are less convincing (Da Silva *et al.*, 1979; Kannel and McGee, 1985). Nevertheless, an elevated BP can have serious consequences for a patient with vascular disease and it is well recognized that it contributes to aneurysm formation. Those patients with substantial hypertension (particularly with higher nocturnal pressures) have higher mortality, a greater prevalence of cerebral lacunar infarcts and more left ventricular hypertrophy (Shimada *et al.*, 1992).

Epidemiological studies show a predominance of cardiovascular events in the early hours of the morning: sudden cardiac death, non-fatal MI and stroke occurring most commonly at this time (Muller *et al.*, 1985). Clinical impressions suggest acute critical limb ischaemia may then present also. A rapid increase in BP is evident in these early hours and this suggests a role in the acute presentation of the disease. Interestingly, other factors such as platelet aggregation and WBC activation, also peak at this crucial time (Bridges *et al.*, 1992). The management of hypertension is outwith the remit of this chapter, but is mentioned to remind the clinician of its importance as a potential risk factor for cardiovascular disease (Fig. 3.3). While 'white coat' hypertension may usually have little detrimental effect (White *et al.*, 1989), it has, if sustained, synergistic effects with other risk factors on progression of disease. A note of caution is needed for patients with CLI because it may be that limb perfusion is only maintained by an elevated BP. Too rapid a reduction may significantly worsen the CLI and particular care must be taken with these patients, as with those with severe carotid disease. Nevertheless, pre-operative admission is an ideal time to detect hypertension and institute treatment.

Hyperlipidaemia

Most patients undergoing vascular surgery do so as a result of atherosclerosis. The characteristic lesion is the fat-rich fibrous plaque, composed of a central cholesterol core with an overlying cap of smooth muscle cells and collagen covered by endothelium. The plaque can bulge into the media of the vessel,

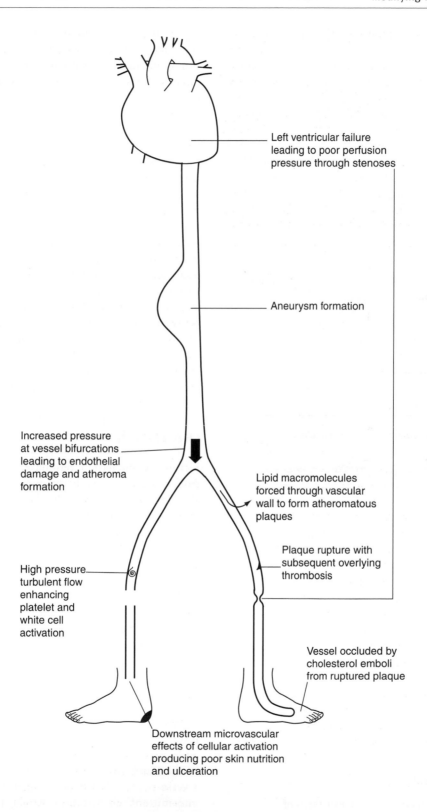

Left ventricular failure
leading to poor perfusion
pressure through stenoses

Aneurysm formation

Increased pressure
at vessel bifurcations
leading to endothelial
damage and atheroma
formation

Lipid macromolecules
forced through vascular
wall to form atheromatous
plaques

Plaque rupture with
subsequent overlying
thrombosis

High pressure
turbulent flow
enhancing
platelet and
white cell
activation

Vessel occluded by
cholesterol emboli
from ruptured plaque

Downstream microvascular
effects of cellular activation
producing poor skin nutrition
and ulceration

Figure 3.3   *Potential deleterious effects of hypertension in a patient with PAOD.*

thus retaining the circular vascular lumen, but reducing its diameter. The composition varies widely from solid hard plaques of mainly smooth muscle cells to those containing large pools of cholesterol covered only by a thin fibrous cap. These are the more dangerous, tending to fissure and ulcerate. The initiating event in atherosclerosis is thought to be a 'response-to-injury' by the endothelium. Low-density lipoprotein (LDL) accumulates at the site of injury. This attracts WBCs which adhere to the endothelium and penetrate the intima where they engulf the lipid-containing fatty streaks. With time, the endothelium over the streaks breaks and is repaired by smooth muscle cell proliferation, probably stimulated by

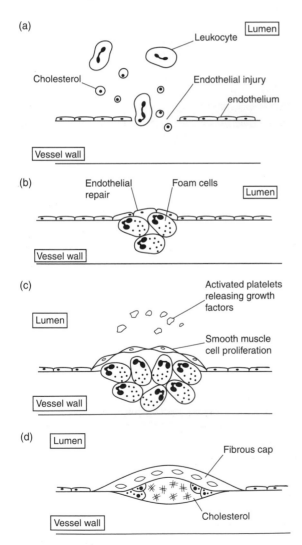

(a)

Leukocyte

Lumen

Cholesterol

Endothelial injury

endothelium

Vessel wall

(b)

Endothelial repair   Foam cells

Lumen

Vessel wall

(c)

Activated platelets releasing growth factors

Lumen

Smooth muscle cell proliferation

Vessel wall

(d)   Lumen

Fibrous cap

Cholesterol

Vessel wall

Figure 3.4 *Response-to-injury hypothesis of atherosclerosis. (a) Endothelial injury; (b) fatty streak; (c) early plaque; (d) cholesterol with plaque.*

PDGF from adherent platelets attracted by the endothelial breakdown (Fig. 3.4).

Hyperlipidaemia contributes in three ways to the vascular disease. First, elevated levels of lipids are available for the formation of the fatty streaks. Second, the cholesterol-rich plaques are unstable and may rupture to stimulate *in situ* thrombosis with increased risk of thrombus and cholesterol embolization. Finally, endothelial function is perturbed. Patients with intermittent claudication and hyperlipidaemia have decreased endothelial vasodilatory responses which can be normalized by lipid lowering (Khan *et al.*, 1995). Elevation in cholesterol without triglyceride elevation is called 'hypercholesterolaemia', whereas an elevated triglyceride level is 'hypertriglyceridaemia'. When both occur together the combined term mixed hyperlipidaemia is used. The relationship between cholesterol level and IHD risk is continuous, with no cut-off point between 'safe' and 'unsafe' levels. It is likely to be the same for patients with PAOD. Dyslipidaemia has been evaluated in patients with PAOD. In general, high lipid levels occur most commonly in the elderly, in patients with diabetes (Laakso *et al.*, 1988) and in obese subjects (Van Gaal *et al.*, 1988).

CHOLESTEROL

Elevated cholesterol levels have been detected in patients with peripheral arterial disease (Cardia *et al.*, 1990) and positive associations between serum cholesterol and the development of PAOD have been detected in two longitudinal studies. After 26 years, the Framingham study found cholesterol to be a weak, but significant risk factor for claudication (Kannel and McGee, 1985). The Danish study found, over a ten-year period, that cholesterol levels correlated with ABPI at the age of 50 years and this was independent of other risk factors (Schroll and Munck, 1981).

It is likely that the LDL subfraction is of prime importance in PAOD. LDL carries cholesterol from the liver to the periphery, from where it is returned to the liver by high-density lipoprotein (HDL). An imbalance, with excess LDL, encourages peripheral atherosclerosis. Reduced HDL has been detected in PAOD (Angquist *et al.*, 1982) and is associated with an increased disease severity (Jacobson *et al.*, 1984). In the Edinburgh Artery Study, there was a strong inverse relationship between HDL cholesterol and intermittent claudication which persisted after adjustment for other lipids, obesity and diabetes (Fowkes *et al.*, 1992).

TRIGLYCERIDE

The majority of studies of PAOD have found elevated serum triglyceride levels in this group of patients (Fowkes *et al.*, 1992). Longitudinal studies evaluating future development of PAOD include the Basle Study (Da Silva and Widmer, 1980) and the Glostrup Study (Schroll and Munck, 1981). Of the 2759 men in the Basle Study, 174 developed disease during five years and, of these, 59 per cent had elevated triglyceride levels. Interestingly, the strong apparent relationship with triglycerides and PAOD may be explained by the correlation of triglyceride level with LDL and it may be the increase in LDL, or the decrease in HDL, which provides the vascular risk (Fowkes *et al.*, 1992).

CLINICAL STUDIES

There have been no clinical studies of lipid-lowering agents in PAOD using a vascular event as an endpoint. Attempts to establish such a study have met with lack of enthusiasm from the pharmaceutical industry which perceives coronary disease as the larger market. Studies in PAOD have looked at progression of disease rather than vascular risk and, although some regression has been seen, many workers remain unconvinced (Zelis *et al.*, 1970; Blankenhorn *et al.*, 1978) due in part to short-term follow up and the use of less-powerful lipid-lowering agents.

There have been three major clinical studies of lipid lowering in recent years. These are the Scandinavian Simvastatin Survival Study (4S) (4S Study Group, 1994), the West of Scotland Coronary Prevention Study (WOSCOPS) (Shepherd *et al.*, 1995) and the Cholesterol and Recurrent Events (CARE) trial (Sacks *et al.*, 1996). The 4S evaluated 4444 subjects with a past history of MI or angina and cholesterol levels between 5.5 and 8.0 mmol/L, but triglycerides <2.6 mmol/L. Median duration of treatment was 5.4 years at which point the study was terminated because of a 30 per cent decrease in overall mortality with simvastatin treatment. This was due to a 42 per cent decrease in IHD mortality. Additionally, major coronary events were decreased as was the need for coronary revascularization. Stroke was also less common in the treated group. These data suggest that four out of nine deaths occurring in a group of subjects with cholesterol >5.5 mmol/L would be prevented by treatment.

WOSCOPS was a primary prevention trial where 6595 asymptomatic men with cholesterol levels of >6.5 mmol/L were allocated to pravastatin or placebo for about five years. There was a 31 per cent reduction of non-fatal MI and IHD death, and a 30 per cent decreased requirement for revascularization procedures. The CARE trial was a secondary prevention study in which 4195 patients with a past history of MI were enrolled. After five years there were 24 per cent fewer coronary deaths and non-fatal MIs if pravastatin was taken, with a 27 per cent decrease in the need for coronary revascularization and angioplasty. The importance of this trial is that the drug appeared to be beneficial in secondary prevention even when cholesterol levels were 'normal'.

How do these major trials impact on PAOD? It may be that subset analysis might provide data on patients and subjects with PAOD, both relating to vascular events in claudication and the development of disease in a normal population. If the pattern reflects that seen in the antiplatelet trials then this subgroup of PAOD subjects should do very well on active treatment. Until these and other data are available, it is our current practice to intervene if total cholesterol is >5.2 mmol/L or LDL cholesterol is >3.2 mmol/L. Furthermore, the majority of our patients have IHD, often silent, and admission for peripheral vascular surgery is an ideal time to assess lipid profiles and manage elevated levels. A fasting sample on the morning of the operation is ideal. Spurious 'low' levels can be found in times of physical stress and samples should not be taken until six weeks after the operation.

LIPID-LOWERING THERAPY

Adherence to a lipid-lowering diet can reduce levels by a modest 10–15 per cent (Cooke and Creager, 1991). Our own, somewhat pragmatic, approach is to concentrate the patient's mind on stopping smoking whilst we improve the lipid profile with diet if possible, but more often pharmacologically. A number of drugs can be used for reducing LDL cholesterol, but the statins (HMG-CoA reductase inhibitors) are preferred for patients with multiple-risk factors. This will be the majority of PAOD patients who exercise poorly, smoke and may be obese. Furthermore, these compounds have been shown to conclusively decrease vascular events. In diabetics, where mixed hyperlipidaemia is found (i.e. triglycerides are also increased), fibrates may be selected because of their stronger effects on triglycerides and HDL cholesterol. Nevertheless, statins are well-tolerated alternatives because patients with diabetes and mixed hyperlipidaemia did well on statin therapy in both secondary prevention studies described earlier.

Thrombophilia

Prothrombotic or hypercoagulable states occur when deficiencies in natural anticoagulants exist, imbalance occurs in the fibrinolytic system, coagulation or platelet activation is accelerated or there is endothelial cell dysfunction. Hypercoagulable states can be classified into two broad categories, hereditary and acquired (Table 3.5), with the former often referred to as inherited thrombophilic disorders. Whilst some of the risk factors for PAOD such as increased platelet aggregation may contribute to an acquired hypercoagulable state, the term 'acquired thrombophilia' is usually reserved for well-defined syndromes such as the antiphospholipid syndrome (APS) formally called 'lupus anticoagulant'.

Table 3.5 *Acquired and hereditary thrombophilia. Clinical markers for thrombophilia*

Acquired
  Antiphospholipid syndrome (previously 'lupus anticoagulant')
  Heparin-induced thrombocytopenia
  Malignancy
  Post-operative state
  Pregnancy
  Oral contraceptives
  Nephrotic syndrome

Inherited
  Protein C deficiency
  Resistance to activated protein C
  Protein S deficiency
  Antithrombin III deficiency
  Homocysteinaemia

Clinical markers for thrombophilia
  Young patients (< 50 years old)
  Systemic lupus erythematosus
  History of unexplained arterial or venous thrombotic events
  Previous unexplained failed vascular reconstruction
  Unexplained prolonged APPT
  Strong family history of thrombosis

Inherited thrombophilia disorders are frequently characterized by venous thrombosis (especially in an unusual site), whereas hypercoagulable states tend to present with both venous and arterial thrombi. More recently, a number of reports of patients with hereditary thrombophilias experiencing arterial thrombosis have been published, and many groups have reported a significant incidence of these syndromes in patients undergoing vascular surgery. In prospective studies, the overall incidence of hypercoagulability varies from 10 to 25 per cent, and increases to about 50 per cent in patients with clinical markers for thrombophilia (Table 3.5) (Eldrup-Jorgensen et al., 1989; Donaldson et al., 1990; De Frang et al., 1994). It is very important to identify these patients pre-operatively because the immediate and medium term failure of the vascular reconstruction is reported to be as high as 50 per cent (Ahn et al., 1988; Donaldson et al., 1990). Additionally they are at risk of developing deep-vein thrombosis (DVT). This infrequent occurrence does not justify screening all potential vascular surgery patients, but a more selective approach, reserving screening for those patients with multiple bypass failures, is appropriate (De Frang et al., 1994).

PROTEIN C AND PROTEIN S DEFICIENCY

Protein C, and its cofactor protein S, are physiological inhibitors of coagulation. Protein C is activated by thrombin and, with protein S, will inhibit factors Va and VIIIa. Protein S deficiency appears to represent a particular risk for arterial thrombosis (Schafer and Kroll, 1993). In a study of protein S-deficient subjects who had no other vascular risk factors, the incidence of IHD and cerebrovascular disease was 14 per cent (Vianna et al., 1994). There have also been many reports of patients with protein C deficiency who have developed atrial thrombus manifest by TIA, stroke, MI and acute CLI (Conard and Samama, 1986; Coller et al., 1987; De Stafano et al., 1991). These deficiencies are detected in only 20–40 per cent of patients who develop unexplained thrombosis, but recent studies have shown that a newly described inherited defect (resistance to activated protein C) may be important. This factor V Leiden mutation (Dahlback and Hildebrand, 1994) has not been evaluated in PAOD, although it may be of some relevance.

ANTITHROMBIN III DEFICIENCY

As with protein C and S deficiencies, this defect is more commonly associated with venous thrombosis. Antithrombin III, as its name suggests, inhibits thrombin and also other factors such as factor Xa and IXa. It is inherited as an autosomal dominant trait and occurs in between 1 in 1000 and 2000 individuals. It may occur more frequently in subjects with arterial disease, particularly in thromboembolism secondary to atrial clot formation (Conard and Samama, 1986; Hirsh *et al.*, 1989). Anticoagulation of these patients, as well as those with protein S and C deficiency, may be required post-operatively. Because of the potential for skin necrosis, heparinization should be instituted initially. These abnormalities can be detected by asking the haematology department for a thrombophilia check on a clotting screen blood sample (citrate anticoagulant).

HOMOCYSTEINAEMIA

Premature atherosclerosis, and arterial and venous thromboses, are all clinical features of homocysteinaemia (Rees and Rodgers, 1993). It causes endothelial cell dysfunction and damage, and particular inhibits fibrinolysis (Rodgers and Conn, 1990). Although patients with homozygous disease are diagnosed early because of the severity of symptoms, patients with heterozygous disease may merely appear to have premature atherosclerosis. It has been estimated that 20–40 per cent of patients presenting with premature PAOD or stroke have heterozygous homocysteinaemia (Taylor and Porter, 1993). Pyridoxine reduces the incidence of thrombotic events in homozygous patients, but it is not known if it, or other vitamins affect the course of the condition in heterozygous subjects. Nevertheless, other risk-factor management should be more actively pursued if homocysteinaemia is detected.

ANTIPHOSPHOLIPID SYNDROME

Of all the hypercoagulable states occurring in patients undergoing vascular surgery, antiphospholipid syndrome (APS) is the most frequently detected (Eldrup-Jorgensen *et al.*, 1989). It was initially described in patients with systemic lupus erythematosus (SLE), hence its original name of 'lupus anticoagulant'. However, it can occur in isolation or in association with a number of other diseases. The paradoxical nature of the old term (anticoagulant) in a disease which produces thrombosis led to it being renamed APS. Evidence indicates that APS, as defined by prolonged Activated Partial Thromboplastin Time (APTT) and elevated anticardiolipin antibody titres in blood, defines two distinct, but related patient populations, each with an increased risk of arterial and venous thrombosis (Bick and Baker, 1992). Both its true incidence and the risk of thrombosis are unknown, and the clinical manifestations are diverse, including DVT and pulmonary embolus, stroke, MI, thrombosis of arterial reconstructions and obstetric complications (Rosove and Brewer, 1992). APS is one of the most common causes of TIA and stroke in young individuals (Ginsburg *et al.*, 1992). Treatment is with anticoagulants when there is evidence of thrombosis, but they may not always protect against recurrent thrombosis (Vianna *et al.*, 1994). Aspirin is being used if APS is detected as an incidental finding in an otherwise normal individual or the diagnosis is secondary to fetal loss.

Vascular risk: conclusion

When a patient is admitted for elective vascular surgery there is an ideal opportunity for the critical assessment of vascular risk factors. Active intervention at this time will not only decrease the risk of coronary and cerebral events, but also improve graft patency rates and limit progression of the arterial disease. This approach is important now, and is likely to become even more important in the future when management strategies for the more recently described risk factors become available. The recent emphasis on the importance of oxidative stress (Lau *et al.*, 1991b) in PAOD as a contributor to direct vascular damage and as a mechanism for oxidizing lipids (Hickman *et al.*, 1994) has opened up a number of potential therapeutic avenues. CHAOS evaluated the role of antioxidant vitamin E after myocardial infarction in 2002 subjects and the risk of non-fatal MI was significantly decreased in the treatment group (Stephens *et al.*, 1996). Antioxidant treatment has not been evaluated in PAOD, but the Prevention of Progression of Asymptomatic Diabetic Arterial Disease study will evaluate the effect of antioxidant and aspirin therapy on four-year cardiovascular mortality in patients with low ABPI and diabetes mellitus.

Another area of current study is the relationship between endothelium and WBC cell adhesion molecules because there is a link between re-stenosis after peripheral angioplasty and E-selectin levels (Belch *et al.*, 1997). E-selectin is a cell-adhesion molecule specific to activated endothelium and antibodies are now being developed which may provide for interesting therapeutic interventions in the future.

PROPHYLAXIS OF DEEP-VEIN THROMBOSIS

Pulmonary thromboembolism remains one of the commonest causes of death in the hospital patient (Rubenstein *et al.*, 1988; Hauch *et al.*, 1990). It is most likely to occur after major trauma, orthopaedic surgery and major abdominal surgery, but it also occurs in medical patients (Belch *et al.*, 1981) and was the commonest cause of death in the Maternal Perinatal Mortality study (Turnbull *et al.*, 1989). In the absence of prophylaxis, the frequency of fatal pulmonary embolism ranges from 0.1 per cent to 0.8 per cent in patients undergoing general surgery (International Multicenter Trial, 1975). In 1993, the Scottish Audit of Surgical Mortality, and the National Confidential Enquiry into Perioperative Death (NCEPOD) in England, both highlighted the major contribution of pulmonary embolism to perioperative death. It is surprising therefore that physicians and surgeons still do not comply with the recommendations for prophylaxis of venous thromboembolism despite the fact that there is convincing evidence of the efficacy and safety of a number of agents (Colditz *et al.*, 1986; Clagett and Reisch, 1988). There is now a consensus of expert opinion that routine prophylaxis should be used in patients at moderate or high risk of venous thromboembolism. In 1992, separate groups each published recommendations for prophylaxis of venous thromboembolism in the UK (THRIFT, 1992), mainland Europe (European Consensus Statement, 1992) and the USA (Clagett *et al.*, 1992). These measures are relevant to most operations discussed in this book.

Risk factors for deep-vein thrombosis

Many clinicians recognize that the risk of venous thromboembolism increases with both background

Table 3.6 *Risk factors for venous thromboembolism*

Background	'Acute'
Advancing age	Immobility
Obesity (bodyweight ≥ 80 kg)	Surgery
Pregnancy	Malignancy
Puerperium	Heart failure
Thrombophilia	Recent MI*
Previous DVT/PTE*	Infection
High-dose oestrogens	

*DVT = deep-vein thrombosis; PTE = pulmonary thromboembolism; MI = myocardial infarction.

and acute precipitating factors (Table 3.6). Low-risk (Table 3.7) hospital patients have a risk of DVT of <10 per cent, and should be encouraged to mobilize early, but they do not merit the risks and costs of specific prophylaxis (THRIFT, 1992). Moderate-risk groups have an incidence of DVT of between 10 and 40 per cent, and an average risk of pulmonary embolism of 1 per cent, so they should also receive

Table 3.7 *Risk 'groups' for hospital patients for deep-vein thrombosis (DVT) and pulmonary thromboembolism (PTE)*

- *Low risk* (< 10% chance of DVT, 0.01% fatal PTE)
  Minor surgery (< 30 min); no other risk factors
  Major surgery (> 30 min); age < 40 years; no other risk factors
  Minor trauma or medical illness; no DVT, PTE or thrombophilia

- *Moderate risk* (10–40% chance of DVT, 0.1–1% fatal PTE)
  Major general, urological, gynaecological, cardiothoracic, vascular or neurological surgery; age ≥ 40 years or other risk factors.
  Major medical illness: heart or lung disease, cancer or inflammatory bowel disease
  Major trauma, burns
  Low-risk group but previous DVT, PTE or thrombophilia

- *High risk* (40–80% chance of DVT, 1–10% fatal PTE)
  Critical lower limb ischaemia
  Major lower limb ischaemia
  Fracture or major surgery of pelvis, hip or lower limb
  Major pelvic or abdominal surgery for cancer
  Moderate risk with previous DVT, PTE or thrombophilia
  Lower limb paralysis

specific prophylaxis. High-risk patients have a higher incidence of DVT (40–80 per cent) and an above average risk of fatal pulmonary embolism (1–10 per cent). In addition to mobilization, they should receive intensive specific prophylaxis.

Prophylactic agents used in vascular surgery

These include standard heparin (usually in low dosage), low-molecular-weight heparins, heparinoids, oral anticoagulants, Dextran 70 and aspirin.

LOW-DOSE STANDARD HEPARIN

Low-dose standard heparin (5000 IU 8–12 hourly) given subcutaneously is effective in preventing DVT and pulmonary embolism in medical patients, and in moderate-risk surgical patients. There is an increased risk of wound haematoma, but monitoring of clotting times is not routinely required.

LOW-MOLECULAR-WEIGHT HEPARINS AND HEPARINOIDS

Low-molecular-weight heparins and heparinoids are also given subcutaneously for prophylaxis of venous thromboembolism, but some are given once daily with obvious benefit. They are significantly more effective in orthopaedic surgery and slightly more effective in general surgery without increasing the risk of bleeding (Nurmohamed et al., 1992). Contraindications are as for standard heparin and monitoring of the anticoagulant effect is not required.

ORAL ANTICOAGULANTS, DEXTRAN 70 AND ASPIRIN

Oral anticoagulants such as warfarin are effective in the prophylaxis of venous thromboembolism and have been used peri-operatively, especially for hip surgery, but they require daily monitoring of the International Normalized Ratio (INR). Contraindications include bleeding disorders and, particularly, spinal or epidural analgesia. Although effective, warfarin therapy is more complicated to manage and thus rarely used (British Society of Haematology, 1990).

The peri-operative intravenous infusion of Dextran 70 has limited efficacy in prevention of DVT after general surgery, but appears more effective in preventing thrombosis after hip surgery. Complications include increased risk of bleeding, fluid overload and allergic reactions. DVT prophylaxis is not a licensed indication for use in the UK.

Aspirin also shows limited efficacy in preventing DVT (Antiplatelet Trialists Collaboration, 1994a), but appears less effective in preventing pulmonary embolism than heparin, oral anticoagulants or dextran. It is not recommended as an alternative routine prophylactic method in vascular surgery patients.

Duration of prophylaxis

Prophylaxis should continue at least until hospital discharge because patients continue to be at risk (Arcelus and Caprini, 1993) and there is increasing evidence that the risk continues for several weeks after hospital discharge. Patients with continuing risk factors (e.g. immobility secondary to amputation or healing ulcers) should be considered for prophylaxis after hospital discharge and good communication with the primary care team prior is obviously essential.

Recommendations for vascular surgery

The specific recommendation for vascular surgery is either subcutaneous low-dose traditional heparin (5000 IU 8–12 hourly) or subcutaneous low-molecular-weight heparin (Nurmohamed et al., 1992; Leizorovicz et al., 1992; SIGN, 1996). Ideally prophylaxis should be started before the operation and continued until the patient is fully mobile (Pineo et al., 1995). Some surgeons consider that pre-operative administration should be avoided in patients who are to receive heparin during the operative procedure because excess bleeding has been reported (Belch et al., 1980). Some anaesthetists consider that pre-operative heparin should also be avoided in patients who are to receive regional anaesthesia because of the perceived risk of spinal haematoma (Wildsmith and McClure, 1991). Thus local protocols should be established after discussions between all interested parties.

Routine monitoring of coagulation is not required, but a little remembered screening test for those receiving subcutaneous heparin prophylaxis

Table 3.8 *Size of vessel and type of vasculitis*

Disorder	Aorta and branches	Large and medium-sized arteries	Medium-sized arteries	Small arteries	Arterioles, capillaries and vessels
Takayasu's arteritis	X				
Thromboangiitis obliterans (Buerger's disease)	X	X			
Giant cell arteritis (temporal arteritis)	X	X			
Polyarteritis nodosa		X	X		
Wegener's granulomatosis		X	X		
Connective-tissue disorders			X	X	
Rheumatoid vasculitis			X	X	
Cutaneous vasculitis (leukocytoclastic vasculitis)				X	

for over five days is a platelet count. Heparin-induced thrombocytopenia occurs in about 3–4 per cent of patients given prophylactic heparin and the Committee on Safety and Medicines in the UK recommends that the platelet count should be checked every five days, up to 20 days. Because arterial or venous thrombosis occurs in 1 per cent of patients with heparin-induced thrombocytopenia, this is crucial for the vascular graft patient. If thrombocytopenia is detected, the heparin should be stopped and alternative prophylaxis employed.

DVT prophylaxis: conclusion

The importance of DVT prophylaxis cannot be underestimated, so patient-specific reminders, surgical audit and guidelines should all be used routinely to optimize prevention of a potentially life-threatening complication.

VASCULITIS

'Vasculitis' and 'vasculitides' are terms used to describe a group of conditions characterized by inflammation of the blood vessel wall and subsequent damage to vessel integrity. The vasculitic process may involve only one or many blood vessels and therefore one or many organ systems. In general, the clinical features result in ischaemia of the tissue supplied by the damaged vessel. This is often

Table 3.9 *Clinical pointers to vasculitis in PAOD patients*

- Never smoked
- Young male (< 45 years)
- Premenopausal female
- Ischaemia with fully palpable peripheral pulses (except Takayasu's and Buerger's diseases)
- Associated constitutional features, e.g. fever, weight loss
- Abnormal laboratory markers for inflammation, e.g. plasma viscosity, ESR, C-reactive protein
- Features of vasculitic disorder, e.g. Raynaud's phenomenon, rheumatoid arthritis, photosensitive skin rash

accompanied by constitutional symptoms such as anorexia, weight loss and fever due to widespread inflammation. The vasculitides range from mild obliterative disorders to necrotizing vasculitis, but the classification is confusing because of considerable overlap between the different syndromes and lack of clear aetiology. Diagnosis still requires histological confirmation in the majority of cases, so a classification based on the size of the predominant vessel involved (Table 3.8) and the type of inflammatory change is most frequently used. Vasculitis is an uncommon disorder, detected only infrequently in patients presenting for vascular surgery, and it is to be hoped that the majority will have had the diagnosis made prior to the decision to proceed with surgery. A number of factors should increase the suspicion of vasculitis in patients with vascular disease (Table 3.9), some being similar to the clinical features of thrombophilia. In general, it is the larger vessel vasculitides that are most likely to present to the vascular surgeon, along with connective-tissue diseases which include Raynaud's phenomenon as a major component of the symptomatology.

Takayasu's arteritis

This is an inflammatory and obliterative arteritis which mainly affects the large elastic arteries, but can also involve all levels of the aorta and the pulmonary arteries. It affects women five to nine times more frequently than men (Cupps and Fauci, 1981) and usually presents between the ages of 10 and 30 years, although it can occur in older patients. Symptomatology is divided into two phases, the pre-pulseless (acute systemic) and the pulseless (chronic obliterative) phases. The acute symptoms are often non-specific and include anorexia, weight loss and fever. Flitting joint pains and myalgia are common. The symptoms of the chronic phase are the result of the obliterative arterial lesion and therefore vary with the vessels involved in the obliterative process. Possible findings include diminished or absent arterial pulses, vascular bruits and inequality of blood pressure between arms and legs. Upper limb claudication with ischaemia can occur in association with reduced or absent upper limb pulses.

Laboratory studies in Takayasu's arteritis reflect the inflammatory nature of the disorder. The plasma viscosity, erythrocyte-sedimentation rate (ESR) and C-reactive protein are elevated in the majority of patients during the active phase. Arteriography plays an important role in diagnosis and shows vessel occlusion, stenosis and aneurysm formation, with collateral development around occlusion sites. Biopsy in the acute inflammatory phase shows granulomatous inflammation with patchy involvement of the vessel wall. In the chronic phase, biopsy reveals intimal proliferation and band fibrosis of the adventitia and media. Treatment is by immunosuppression.

Thromboangiitis obliterans (Buerger's disease)

Thromboangiitis obliterans describes a clinical syndrome characterized by segmental thrombotic occlusions of the small or medium-sized arteries usually of the distal lower limb, but occasionally also the upper limb (Buerger, 1908). It usually occurs in young smokers and is frequently associated with both Raynaud's phenomenon and superficial migratory thrombophlebitis. It was previously described only in young men, but the increased prevalence of smoking in women has increased reports of the disorder in the female population (Lie, 1992). The symptoms are usually related to lower limb ischaemia, and include rest pain and tissue loss. Claudication occurs only rarely and, when present, is usually confined to the foot. Femoral or popliteal pulses are usually present, but the pedal pulses are absent (Mills and Porter, 1990). The diagnosis depends to a great extent on the exclusion of other conditions, particularly early-onset atherosclerosis and other vasculitides. Lower limb angiography reveals normal vessels proximal to the popliteal. The tibial and peroneal vessels are frequently normal to a point of sudden occlusion. Thereafter, tortuous corkscrew collaterals may reconstitute patent segments of the distal, tibial or pedal vessels. The management relies on encouraging the patient towards total tobacco abstinence. In patients who do manage to stop smoking, the appearance of new lesions or the development of gangrene requiring amputation is unusual, but persistent smoking leads to progression of the disease. A large number of medical treatments have been proposed and the variety testifies to the fact that none is completely satisfactory. Nearly all have been poorly studied. Corticosteroids, antiplatelet therapy and iloprost infusions (Fiessinger and Schafer, 1990) are just a few of the treatments that have been used.

Giant cell arteritis

This is a systemic granulomatous vasculitis that predominantly affects large and medium-sized blood vessels, usually the cranial branches of the aorta. It is most frequently detected in patients over the age of 50 years and it is an important preventable cause of blindness. However, it is recognized that this disorder, sometimes called 'temporal arteritis', has many different clinical manifestations and extracranial presentations are not uncommon. There is an increased risk in smokers and patients with already established atherosclerotic disease (Machado *et al.*, 1989).

It may present insidiously or acutely. While sudden blindness and headache are the classical symptoms, the constitutional features such as anorexia, fever and fatigue may occur early. Headache is the usual complaint and may be localized to the area over the superficial temporal arteries, or generalized and resembling tension headache. Scalp tenderness, secondary to involvement of the superficial temporal and occipital arteries, can occur and produce difficulty with brushing or combing hair and sleeping on a pillow at night. Jaw claudication occurs in approximately 50 per cent of sufferers secondary to facial and maxillary artery involvement. Tongue claudication and dysphagia have also been reported, and occasionally glossitis and tongue necrosis are seen (Sonnenblick *et al.*, 1989). Sudden blindness is a consequence of disease in the posterior ciliary or ophthalmic arteries and is irreversible once established, but amaurosis fugax, a warning sign of impending blindness, is steroid responsive and should not be confused with carotid territory TIA. Pulmonary, renal and neurological symptomatology have also been reported, as has synovitis, but cutaneous and large-vessel manifestations are rare. Unless they present with amaurosis fugax, patients with this disease are unlikely to come to the attention of the vascular clinician. Diagnosis is by finding an elevated acute phase response, such as plasma viscosity or ESR, although this is not necessarily always the case. Temporal artery biopsy may show granulomatous inflammation, but can be negative in 50 per cent of cases because of intermittent or 'skip' lesions. Therapy is by immunosuppression with corticosteroids.

Polyarteritis nodosa

Polyarteritis nodosa (PAN) is characterized by a systemic necrotizing vasculitis which involves the small and medium-sized muscular arteries. There is a higher incidence of this disease in hepatitis B hyperendemic populations (McMahon *et al.*, 1989) and its prevalence ranges between 5 and 77 per million. PAN is more frequently seen in men, with a ratio of 2 : 1. The average age of diagnosis is between 40 and 60 years, although the disorder can be seen in both childhood and old age. The symptoms depend on the vessel affected, but they are often the constitutional ones which characterize the vasculitides (fever, anorexia and weight loss). Renal disease with proteinuria and progressive failure occurs in about 70 per cent of patients (Conn, 1990). Acute events such as bowel infarction, perforation and haemor-

rhage are rare, but produce the high mortality associated with this condition. Skin manifestations include infarcts (particularly in the nailfold area), purpura and livido reticularis. Mononeuritis multiplex is common and other important sites of involvement include the retina and testis. Damage to the blood vessel wall can result in aneurysm formation. Laboratory findings can be non-specific and make diagnosis difficult, but include an acute phase response and a positive test for antineutrophil cytoplasmic antibody (ANCA). Angiography may be diagnostic, showing characteristic saccular or fusiform aneurysms and arterial narrowing. Corticosteroids are used for treatment, with further immunosuppression (e.g. cyclophosphamide) if control is difficult.

Wegener's granulomatosis

This is also a form of vasculitis which involves mainly the medium and small arteries and veins of the respiratory tract and kidneys. Although it is a systemic necrotizing granulomatous disease, it is classically associated with the triad of upper respiratory tract, kidney and lung involvement. The manifestations and severity of the disease are variable, but the cutaneous vascular features tend to be seen infrequently (Langford and McCallum, 1995). These consist of cutaneous ulcers, subcutaneous nodules and purpura. Laboratory findings reveal an inflammatory response. Sinus X-rays or computed tomography scanning may show evidence of mucosal thickening, sinus opacification or fluid levels. Chest X-ray may also be abnormal. Diagnosis is made by biopsy, but elevated blood c-ANCA levels are strongly associated with Wegener's granulomatosis. Treatment is with immunosuppressant therapy. This disorder is unlikely to present to the vascular clinician except in rare cases of cutaneous ulceration.

Connective-tissue disorders

The connective-tissue disorders are a group of conditions in which an underlying vasculitis often plays a part in the production of symptoms. They are important to the vascular clinician predominantly as a cause of digital ischaemia (Table 3.10) secondary to severe Raynaud's phenomenon (Belch, 1995).

Table 3.10 *Connective tissue disease showing percentage of patients who also suffer from Raynaud's phenomenon.*

Systemic sclerosis (96%)
Mixed connective-tissue disease (85%)
Polymyositis/dermatomyositis (40%)
Systemic lupus erythematosus (30–40%)
Sjögren's syndrome (35%)
Rheumatoid arthritis (10%)

Raynaud's phenomenon severe enough to merit referral to hospital is most likely to be associated with a connective-tissue disorder, especially if associated with digital ulceration (Belch, 1993). The disorder is common amongst young women and most of these probably have primary Raynaud's disease. When Raynaud's develops in an older subject, the likelihood of an underlying connective-tissue disease is increased (Kallenberg, 1990). In patients over 60 years, the larger numbers of secondary cases reflects the higher proportion with atherosclerosis (Friedman, *et al.*, 1988) rather than connective-tissue disease. Features which should alert the clinician to secondary Raynaud's are digital ulceration, severe attacks persisting throughout the summer, abnormal nailfold vessels on capillary microscopy and abnormalities in immunopathological testing.

Systemic sclerosis

Systemic sclerosis is characterized by the appearance of scleroderma (literally 'hard skin') and can be classified as either limited (lSSc) or diffuse (dSSc). Older terminologies such as CREST (calcinosis, Raynaud's, (o)esophageal involvement, sclerodactyly, telangiectasia) for lSSc, are obsolete because they define the patient population poorly. Gastrointestinal manifestations are common, usually being related to oesophageal hypomotility and reflux, but motility defects can occur in all sections of the gastrointestinal tract and produce diarrhoea, constipation and malabsorption. Renal glomerulosclerosis and lung fibrosis account for the early mortality of patients with dSSc, and myocardial fibrosis may also occur (Follansbee *et al.*, 1990). The finding of an anticentromere antibody in the blood is suggestive of lSSc, whilst scleroderma 70 antibody (antitopoisomerase) is diagnostic of dSSC. Treatment of the underlying SSc is difficult, but the Raynaud's phenomenon can be effectively controlled with vasodilator therapy in the majority of patients (Belch, 1996).

Mixed connective-tissue disease

Mixed connective-tissue disease (MCTD) is a discrete entity, but, as its name suggests, symptoms from all the connective-tissue disorders can be present. These subjects have antibodies to RNP in addition to positive antinuclear antibody tests. Raynaud's phenomenon is the most common clinical finding and may precede the main manifestation by months and years (Lundberg and Hedfors, 1991). Ischaemic necrosis or ulceration of the fingertips (common in systemic sclerosis) is rare in MCTD which therefore presents infrequently to the vascular clinician.

Polymyositis and dermatomyositis

Polymyositis and dermatomyositis are chronic inflammatory disorders which primarily affect skeletal muscle, producing proximal weakness. When the characteristic skin rash is present the term 'dermatomyositis' is used. The classical complaint is of insidious progressive pain and proximal muscle weakness over a three- to six-month period. In the older age group these disorders are associated with occult malignancy. It is rare for this condition to present to the vascular clinician because the vascular manifestations are relatively mild. Raynaud's phenomenon can occur, but digital ulceration and gangrene are very rare.

Systemic lupus erythematosus

Systemic lupus erythematosus (SLE) is a chronic autoimmune disease which produces symptoms varying from mild to life threatening. Raynaud's phenomenon may be one of the manifestations, but the clinical features of SLE are multiple and it can produce pathology in any organ. Key components include systemic or constitutional symptoms, a nondestructive and non-deforming arthritis and skin involvement. When the skin is involved, this can be a photosensitive rash (classically a butterfly pattern) occurring in about 60 per cent of patients. Seventy per cent of patients experience alopecia, and oral ulcers reveal mucous membrane involvement. Raynaud's phenomenon can bring the patient to the vascular clinician and the associated skin rashes should raise the index of suspicion. About half the patients with SLE develop renal abnormalities and cerebral lupus is a major problem for those affected by it because it may mimic cerebrovascular disease (Bresnihan *et al.*, 1979). Diagnosis is by identifying antinuclear and anti-DNA antibodies in the blood. Treatment includes symptomatic management and immunosuppression with drugs such as cortico-steroids.

Sjögren's syndrome

Sjögren's syndrome comprises a group of diseases characterized by inflammation and destruction of the exocrine glands. The lacrimal and salivary glands are those principally involved, giving rise to the classical symptoms of dry eyes and mouth. Other glands, including the pancreas, sweat glands and mucous-secreting glands of the bowel, may also be affected. Systemic vasculitis when it occurs in Sjögren's syndrome affects predominantly the small and medium-sized vessels thus most commonly producing symptoms in the skin, although the peripheral nervous system can also be affected. Blood testing for anti-Ro and anti-La antibodies can aid the diagnosis of Sjögren's syndrome. The aetiology is as yet unknown and treatment is directed towards symptomatic relief with artificial tears and saliva.

The vasculitides: conclusion

The vasculitic conditions can present to the vascular clinician because of ischaemic symptoms developing from vessel inflammation. Nevertheless, patients with vasculitis are unlikely to present peri-operatively because it is hoped that the diagnosis would have been established earlier. Furthermore, the predominantly small vessels affected are not usually amenable to operative intervention. However, debridement of digital gangrene secondary to severe Raynaud's phenomenon may mean that the patients present to the vascular surgical team. There must be a high index of suspicion for the connective-tissue disease in those seeing patients for vasospastic symptoms and an understanding of the conditions in all those treating them.

OPPORTUNITIES IN THE PERI-OPERATIVE PERIOD

From this review it can be seen that the peri-operative period provides an ideal opportunity for medical intervention in the vascular surgical patient. In particular, vascular risk modification should be considered and antiplatelet therapy introduced if it can be tolerated. Deep-vein thrombosis prophylaxis is essential for high-risk patients and consideration can be given to a vasculitic element if acute phase markers are elevated or the clinical picture unusual. The golden opportunity provided by surgical admission must be used to manage patients medically as well as operatively.

REFERENCES

Abelin, T. *et al*. 1989. Controlled trial of transdermal nicotine patch in tobacco withdrawal. *Lancet* **1**, 7–10.

Ahn, S.S., Kalunian, K., Rosove, M. *et al*. 1988. Postoperative thrombotic complications in patients with the lupus anticoagulant; increased risk after vascular procedures. *Journal of Vascular Surgery* **7**, 749–756.

Angquist, K.A., Johnson, O., Ericsson, M. and Tollin, C. 1982. Serum lipoproteins and apoliproproteins A1 and A11 in male patients with peripheral arterial insufficiency. *Acta Chirurgica Scandinavica* **148**, 675–678.

Antiplatelet Trialists Collaboration. 1994a. The aspirin papers. Aspirin benefits patients with vascular disease and those undergoing revascularisation. *British Medical Journal* **308**, 71–72.

Antiplatelet Trialists Collaboration. 1994b. Collaborative overview of randomised trials of antiplatelet therapy – I: Prevention of death, myocardial infarction, and stroke by prolonged antiplatelet therapy in various categories of patients. *British Medical Journal* **308**, 81–106.

Antiplatelet Trialists Collaboration. 1994c. Collaborative overview of randomised trials of antiplatelet therapy – II: Maintenance of vascular graft or arterial patency by antiplatelet therapy. *British Medical Journal* **308**, 159–168.

Arcelus, J.I. and Caprini, J.A. 1993. Prevention after hospital discharge. In Goldhaber, S.Z. (ed.),

Prevention of venous thromboembolism. New York: Marcel Dekker, 497–518.

ASPIRE Steering Group. 1996. A British Cardiac Society survey of the potential for the secondary prevention of coronary disease: ASPIRE (Action on Secondary Prevention through Intervention to Reduce Events). *Heart* **75**, 334–342.

Barradas, M.A., Gill, D.S., Fonseca, V.A. *et al.* 1988. Intra-platelet serotonin with diabetes mellitus and peripheral vascular disease. *Eur J Clin Invest* **18**, 399–404.

Beks, P.J., MacKaay, A.J., de Neeling, J.N. *et al.* 1995. Peripheral arterial disease in relation to glycaemic level in an elderly Caucasian population: the Hoorn study. *Diabetologia* **38**(1), 86–96.

Belch, J.J.F. and Ho, M. 1996. Pharmacotherapy of Raynaud's phenomenon. *Drugs* **52**(5), 682–695.

Belch, J.J.F., Lowe, G.D.O., Pollock, J.G. *et al.* 1980. Low dose heparin in the prevention of deep-vein thrombosis after aortic bifurcation graft surgery. *Thrombosis and Haemostasis* **42**, 1429–1433.

Belch, J.J.F., Lowe, G.D.O., Ward, A.G. *et al.* 1981. Prevention of deep vein thrombosis in medical patients by low dose heparin. *Scottish Medical Journal* **26**, 115–117.

Belch, J.J.F., McKay, A., McArdle, B. *et al.* 1983. A double blind study of the effect of prostacyclin infusion in severe peripheral vascular disease. *Lancet* **320**, 315–317.

Belch, J.J.F., Greer, I.A., McLaren, M. *et al.* 1984a. The effects of intravenous infusion of ZK36374, a synthetic prostacyclin derivative, on normal volunteers. *Prostaglandins* **28**(i), 67–77.

Belch, J.J.F., McArdle, B., Burns, P. *et al.* 1984b. The effects of acute smoking on platelet behaviour, fibrinolysis and haemorrheology in habitual smokers. *Thrombosis Haemostasis* **51**, 6–8.

Belch, J.J.F., Mackay, I.R., Hill, A. *et al.* 1995. Oxidative stress is present in atherosclerotic peripheral arterial disease and further increased by diabetes mellitus. *International Angiology* **14**(4), 385–388.

Belch, J.J.F. and Maple, C. 1995. Raynaud's phenomenon. In Belch, J.J.F. and Zurier, R. (eds), *Connective tissue disease*. London: Chapman & Hall, 131–150.

Belch, J.J.F., Mackay, I.R., Hill, A. *et al.* 1996a. Oxidative stress is present in atherosclerotic peripheral arterial disease and further increased by diabetes mellitus. *International Angiology* **14**(4), 385–388.

Belch, J.J.F., Greene, S.A., Litttleford, R. *et al.* 1996b. Impaired skin blood flow response to heat in children with insulin dependent diabetes. *International Journal of Angiology* **5**, 189–191.

Belch, J.J.F., Shaw, J.W., Kirk, G. *et al.* 1997. The white blood cell adhesion molecule E-selectin predicts restenosis in patients with intermittent claudication undergoing percutaneous transluminal angioplasty. *Circulation* **95**, 2027–2031.

Benowitz, N.L. 1988. Pharmacologic aspects of cigarette smoking and nicotine addiction. *New England Journal of Medicine* **319**, 1318–1330.

Bergqvist, D., Almgren, B. and Dickinson, J.P. 1995. Reduction of requirement for leg vascular surgery during long-term treatment of claudicant patients in ticlodipine: results from the Swedish Ticlodipine Multicentre Study (STIMS). *European Journal of Vascular and Endovascular Surgery* **10**, 69–76.

Buerger, L. 1908. Thrombo-angiitis obliterans: a study of the vascular lesions leading to presenile spontaneous gangrene. *American Journal of Medicine* **136**, 567–580.

Bick, R.L. and Baker, W.F. 1992. Anticardiolipin antibodies and thrombosis. *Hematology and Oncology Clinics of North America* **6**, 1287–1299.

Blanchard, J., Carreras, L.O., Kindermans, M. and the EMATAP Group. 1993. Results of EMATAP: a double-blind placebo-controlled multicentre trial of ticlodipine in patients with peripheral arterial disease. *Nouvelle Revue Française d' Hematologie* **35**, 523–528.

Blankenhorn, D.H., Brooks, S.H., Selzer, R.H. *et al.* 1978. The rate of atherosclerosis change during treatment of hyperlipoproteinuria. *Circulation* **57**, 355–361.

Boissel, J.P., Peyrieux, J.C. and Destors, J.M. 1989. Is it possible to reduce the risk of cardiovascular events in subjects suffering from intermittent claudication of the lower limbs? *Thrombosis and Haemostasis* **62**, 681–685.

Brandman, O. and Redisch, W. 1953. Incidence of peripheral vascular changes in diabetes mellitus. *Diabetes* **2**, 194–198.

Bresnihan, B., Hohmeister, R., Cutting, J. *et al.* 1979. The neurophsyciatric disorder in systemic lupus erythematosus: evidence for both vascular and immune mechanisms. *Annals of Rheumatic Diseases* **38**, 301–306.

Bridges, A.B., Fisher, T.C., Scott, N. *et al.* 1992. Circadian rhythm of white blood cell aggregation and free radical status in healthy volunteers. *Free Radical Research Communications* **16**(2), 89–97.

British Society of Haematology. 1990. Guidelines on

oral coagulation: second edition. *Journal of Clinical Pathology* **43**, 177–183.

Brodie, B.C. 1841. Lectures on mortification delivered at the medical theatre of St George's Hospital. Lecture V. In Gazette, S. (ed.), *New Series of London Medicine* **52**, 714.

Brogden, R.N. and Sorkin, E.M. 1990. Ketanserin: a review of its pharmacodynamic and pharmacokinetic properties , and therapeutic potential in hypertension and peripheral vascular disease. *Drugs* **40**, 903–949.

Cameron, H.A., Waller, P.C. and Ramsay, L.E. 1988. Drug treatment of intermittent claudication: a critical analysis of the methods and findings of published clinical trials, 1965–1985. *British Journal of Clinical Pharmacology* **26,** 569–576.

CAPRIE Steering Committee. 1996. A randomised, blinded, trial clopidogrel versus aspirin in patients at risk of ischaemic events (CAPRIE). *Lancet* **348**, 1329–1338.

Cardia, G., Grisorio, D., Impedovo, G. *et al.* 1990. Plasma lipids as a risk factor in peripheral vascular disease. *Angiology* **41**, 19–22.

Clagett, G.P. and Reisch, J.S. 1988. Prevention of venous thromboembolism in general surgical patients. Results of meta-analysis. *Annals of Surgery* **208**, 227–240.

Clagett, G.P., Anderson, F.A., Jr, Levine, M.N. *et al.* 1992. Prevention of venous thromboembolism. *Chest* **102**, Suppl. 391S-407S.

Clyne, C.A.C., Archer, T.J., Atuhaire, L.K. *et al.* 1987. Random control trial of a short course of aspirin and dipyridamole (Persantin) for femorodistal grafts. *British Journal of Surgery* **74**, 246–248.

Colditz, G.A., Tuden, R.L. and Oster, G. 1986. Rates of venous thrombosis after general surgery: combined results of randomized clinical trials. *Lancet* **19**, 143–146.

Coller, B.S., Owen, J., Jesty, J. *et al.* 1987. Deficiency of plasma protein S, protein C, or antithrombin III and arterial thrombosis. *Arteriosclerosis* **7**, 456–462.

Conard, J. and Samama, M.M. 1986. Inhibitors of coagulation, atherosclerosis, and arterial thrombosis. *Seminars in Thrombosis and Hemostasis* **12**, 87–90.

Conn, D.L. 1990. Polyarteritis. *Rheumatoid Diseases Clinics of North America* **16**, 341–362.

Connor, H. 1987. The economic impact of diabetic foot disease. In Connor, H., Boulton, A.J.M. and Ward, J.D. (eds), *The foot in diabetes*. Chichester: John Wiley, 145–149.

Cooke, J.P. and Creager, M.A. 1991. Management of the patient with intermittent claudication. *Vascular Medicine Review* **2**, 19–31.

Cupps, T.R. and Fauci, A.S. 1981. *The vasculitides*. Philadelphia: W.B. Saunders.

Dahlback, B. and Hildebrand, B. 1994. Inherited resistance to activated protein C is corrected by anticoagulant cofactor activity found to be a property of factor V. *Proceedings of the National Academy of Sciences (USA)* **91**, 1396–1400.

Da Silva, A. and Widmer, L.K. 1980. *Occlusive peripheral arterial disease. Early diagnosis, incidence, course, significance*. Bern: Hans Huber.

Da Silva, A., Widmer, L.K., Ziegler, H.W. *et al.* 1979. The Basle longitudinal study: report on the relation of initial glucose level to baseline ECG abnormalities, peripheral arterial disease and subsequent mortality. *Journal of Chronic Disease* **32**, 797–803.

Deckert, T., Poulson, J.E. and Larsen, M. 1978. Prognosis of diabetic with diabetes onset before the age of thirty-one. Survival causes of death and complications. *Diabetologia* **14**, 363–370.

De Frang, R.D., Edwards, J.M., Moneta, G.L. *et al.* 1994. Repeat leg bypass after multiple prior bypass failures. *Journal of Vascular Surgery* **19**, 268–277.

De Stafano, V., Leone, G., Micalizzi, P. *et al.* 1991. Arterial thrombosis as a clinical manifestation of congenital protein C deficiency. *Annals of Hematology* **62**, 180–183.

Donaldson, M.C., Weinberg, D.S., Belkin, M. *et al.* 1990. Screening for hypercoagulable states in vascular surgical practice: a preliminary study. *Journal of Vascular Surgery* **11**, 825–831.

Dormandy, J.A. and Murray, G.D. 1991. The fate of the claudicant – a prospective study of 1969 claudicants. *European Journal of Vascular Surgery* **5,** 131–133.

Eldrup-Jorgensen, J., Brace, L., Flanigan, D.P. *et al.* 1989. Lupus-like anticoagulants and lower extremity arterial occlusive disease. *Circulation* **80** (Suppl III), III54–III58.

Eldrup-Jorgensen, J., Flanigan, D.P., Brace, L. *et al.* 1989. Hypercoaguable states and lower limb ischaemia in young adults. *Journal of Vascular Surgery* **9**, 334–341.

ETDRS Investigators. 1992. Aspirin effects on mortality and morbidity in patients with diabetes mellitus. *Journal of the American Medical Association* **268**, 1292–1300.

European Consensus Statement. 1992. Prevention of venous thromboembolism. *International Angiology* **11**, 151–159.

Fabris, F., Zanocchi, M., Bo, M. et al. 1994. Risk factors for atherosclerosis and ageing. International Angiology 13(1), 52–58.

Fiessinger, J.N. and Schäfer, M. 1990. Trial of iloprost versus aspirin treatment for critical limb ischaemia of thromboangiitis obliterans. Lancet 335, 555–557.

Fiore, M.C. et al. 1990. Methods used to quit smoking in the United States. Journal of the American Medical Association 263, 2760–2765.

Fitzgerald, G.A. 1987. Dipyridamole. New England Journal of Medicine; 316, 1247–57.

FitzGerald, G.A., Smith, B., Pederson, A.K. and Brash, A.R. 1984. Increased prostacyclin biosynthesis in patients with severe atherosclerosis and platelet activation. New England Journal of Medicine 310, 1065–1068.

Follansbee, W.P., Miller, T.R., Curtiss, E.I. et al. 1990. A controlled clinico-pathologic study of myocardial fibrosis in systemic sclerosis (scleroderma). Journal of Rheumatology 17(5), 656–662.

Fowkes, F.G.R., Housley, E., Riemersma, R.A. et al. 1992. Smoking, lipids, glucose intolerence and blood pressure as risk factors for peripheral atherosclerosis compared with ischaemic heart disease in the Edinburgh Artery Study. American Journal of Epidemiology 135, 331–40.

Fowkes, F.G., Allan, P.L., Tsampoulas, C. et al. 1992. Validity of duplex scanning in the detection of peripheral arterial disease in the general population. European Journal of Vascular Surgery 6(1), 31–35.

Fowkes, F.G., Dunbar, J.T. and Lee, A.J. 1995. Risk factor profile of non-smokers with peripheral arterial disease. Angiology 46(8): 657–662.

Friedman, E.I., Taylor, L.M. and Porter, J.M. 1988. Late-onset Raynaud's syndrome: diagnostic and therapeutic considerations. Geriatrics 43, 59–63.

Gerstein, H.C. and Yusuf, S. 1996. Dysglycaemia and risk of cardiovascular disease. Lancet 347, 949–950.

Ginsburg, K.S., Liang, M.H. and Newcomer, L. et al. 1992. Anticardiolipin antibodies and the risk for ischemic stroke and venous thrombosis. Annals of Internal Medicine 117, 997–1102.

Goldhaber, S.Z., Manson, J.E., Stampfer, M.J. et al. 1992. Low-dose aspirin and subsequent peripheral arterial surgery in the Physicians' Health Study. Lancet 340, 143–145.

Goldman, M., Hall, C., Dykes, J. et al. 1983. Does indium-platelet deposition predict patency in prosthetic arterial grafts? British Journal of Surgery 70, 635–638.

Green, R.M., Roedersheimer, L.R. and De Weese, J.A. 1982. Effects of aspirin and dipyridamole on expanded polytetrafluoroethylene graft patency. Surgery 92, 1016–26.

Hauch, O., Jorgensen, L.N., Khattar, S.C. et al. 1990. Fatal pulmonary embolism associated with surgery: an autopsy study. Acta Chirurgica Scandinavica 156, 747–9.

Henningfield, J.E., Radzius, A., Cooper, T.M. and Clayton, R.R. 1990. Drinking coffee and carbonated beverages blocks absorption of nicotine from nicotine polacrilex gum. Journal of the American Medical Association 264, 1560–1564.

Herbert, J.M., Frechel, D., Vallee, E., et al. 1993a. Clopidogrel, a novel antiplatelet and antithrombotic agent. Cardiovascular Drug Review 11, 180–188.

Herbert, J.M., Tissinier, A., Defreyn, G. and Maffrand, J.P. 1993b. Inhibitory effect of clopidogrel on platelet adhesion and intimal proliferation following arterial injury in ravvits. Arteriosclerosis and Thrombosis 13, 1171–1179.

Hess, H., Mietaschk, A. and Deichsel, G. 1985. Drug-induced inhibition of platelet function delays progression of peripheral occlusive arterial disease: a prospective double-blind arteriographically controlled trial. Lancet, i, 415–419.

Hickman, P., McCollum, P.T. and Belch, J.J.F. 1994. Neutrophils may contribute to the morbidity and mortality of claudicants. British Journal of Surgery 81(6), 790–798.

Hirsh, J., Piovella, F. and Pini, M. 1989. Congenital antithrombin III deficiency. American Journal of Medicine 87, 34S-38S.

Hughes, J.R., Hatsukami, D.K. and Skoog, K.P. 1986. Physical dependence on nicotine in gum. Journal of the American Medical Association 255, 3277–3279.

Hughson, W.G., Mann, J.I., Tibbs, D.J. et al. 1978. Intermittent claudication: factors determining outcome. British Medical Journal 1, 377–379.

International Multicentre Trial. 1975. Prevention of fatal postoperative pulmonary embolism by low doses of heparin. Lancet ii, 45–51.

Jacobson, U.K., Dige-Pedersen, H., Gyntelberg, F. and Svendsen, U.G. 1984. 'Risk factors' and manifestations of arteriosclerosis in patients with intermittent claudication compared to normal persons. Danish Medical Bulletin 31, 145–148.

Janzon, L., Bergquist, D., Boberg, J. et al. 1990. Prevention of myocardial infarction and stroke in patients with intermittent claudication: effects of ticlopidine. Results from STIMS, the Swedish

Ticlopidine Multicenter Study. *Journal of Internal Medicine* **227**, 301–308.

Jarvis, M.J. and Russell, M.A.H. 1989. Treatment for the cigarette smoker. *International Review of Psychiatry* **1**, 139–147.

Jennings, P.E., McLaren, M., Scott, N. *et al.* 1991. The relationship of oxidative stress to thrombotic tendency in type 1 diabetic patients with retinopathy. *Diabetic Medicine* **8**, 860–865.

Jonason, T. and Ringqvist, I. 1985. Factors of prognostic importance for subsequent rest pain in patients with intermittent claudication. *Acta Medica Scandinavica* **218**(1), 27–33.

Jones, S.L., Close, C.F., Mattock, M.B. *et al.* 1989. Plasma lipid and coagulation factor concentrations in insulin dependent diabetics with microalbuminuria. *British Medical Journal* **298**, 487–490.

Kallenberg, C.G.M. 1990. Early detection of connective tissue disease in patients with Raynaud's phenomenon. *Rheumatic Diseases Clinics of North America* **16**, 11–30.

Kannel, W.B. and McGee, D.L. 1985. Update on some epidemiological features of intermittent claudication: the Framingham Study. *Journal of the American Geriatric Society* **33**, 13–18.

Karpen, C.W., Cataland, S., Odoriso, T.M. and Panganawala, R.V. 1985. Production of 12–hydroxyeicosatraenoic acid and vitamin E status in platelets from type 1 human diabetic subjects. *Diabetes* **34**, 526–531.

Khan, F. and Belch, J.J.F. 1995. Cholesterol-lowering and endothelial cell function in forearm skin of patients with hypercholesterolaemia and peripheral vascular disease. *International Angiology* **14**(Suppl 1), 356.

Kingsbury, K.J. 1996. The relation between glucose tolerance and atherosclerotic vascular disease. *Lancet* **2**, 1374–1379.

Kohler, T.R., Kaufman, J.L., Kacoyanis, G. *et al.* 1984. Effect of aspirin and dipyridamole on the patency of lower extremity bypass grafts. *Surgery* **96**, 462–466.

Krupski, W.C. 1991. The peripheral vascular consequences of smoking. *Annals of Vascular Surgery* **5**, 291–304.

Laakso, M., Ronnemaa, T., Pyorala, K. *et al.* 1988. Atherosclerotic vascular disease and its risk factors in non-insulin dependent diabetics and non-diabetic subjects in Finland. *Diabetes Care* **11**, 449–463.

Lagarde, M., Burtin, M., Berciaud, P. *et al.* 1980. Increase of platelet thromboxane A_2 formation and

of its plasma half-life in diabetes mellitus. *Thrombosis Research* **19**, 823–830.

Lam, W., Sze, P.C., Sacks, H.S. and Chalmers, T.C. 1987. Meta-analysis of randomised controlled trials of nicotine chewing-gum. *Lancet* **ii**, 27–30.

Langford, C.A. and McCallum, R.M. 1995. Idiopathic vasculitis. In Belch, J.J.F. and Zurier, R.B. (eds), *Connective tissue diseases*. London: Chapman & Hall Medical, 179–217.

Lau, C.S., Scott, N., Brown, J.E. *et al.* 1991a. Increased activity of oxygen free radicals during reperfusion in patients undergoing percutaneous peripheral artery balloon angioplasty. *International Angiology* **10**(4): 244–246.

Lau, C.S., Khan, F., McLaren, M. *et al.* 1991b. The effects of thromboxane receptor blockade on platelet aggregation and digital skin blood flow in patients with secondary Raynaud's syndrome. *Rheumatology International* **11**, 163–168.

Leizorovicz, A., Haugh, M.C., Chapius, F.R. *et al.* 1992. Low molecular weight heparin in the prevention of peroperative thrombosis. *British Medical Journal* **305**, 913–920.

Leng, G.C. and Fowkes, F.G.R. 1993. The epidemiology of peripheral arterial disease. *Vascular Medicine Review* **4**, 5–18.

Levy, L.A. 1989. Smoking and peripheral vascular disease. Epidemiology and podiatric perpective. *Journal of the American Podiatric Medical Association* **79**, 398–402.

Lie, J.T. 1992. Vasculitis 1815–1991: classification and diagnostic specificity. *Journal of Rheumatology* **19**, 83–89.

Loosemore, T.M., Chalmers, T.C. and Dormandy, J.A. 1994. Meta-analysis of randomised placebo control trials in Fontaine stages III and IV peripheral occlusive arterial disease. *International Angiology* **13**(2), 133–142.

Lowe, G.D., Ghafour, M., Belch, J.J.F. *et al.* 1986. Increased blood viscosity in diabetic proliferative retinopathy. *Diabetes Research* **3**(2), 67–70.

Lowe, G.D.O., Donnan, P.T., McColl, P. *et al.* 1991. Blood viscosity, fibrinogen and activation of coagulation and leucocytes in peripheral arterial disease: the Edinburgh Artery Study. *British Journal of Haematology* **7**(Suppl. 1), in press.

Lualdi, J., Goldhaber, S.Z. and Manson, J.E. 1995. The role of antiplatelet agents in patients with peripheral vascular disease. *Vascular Medicine Review* **6**, 109–119.

Lundberg, I. and Hedfors, E. 1991. Clinical course of

patients with anti-RNP antibodies. A prospective study of 32 patients. *Journal of Rheumatology* **18**(10), 1511–1519.

Machado, E.B.V., Gabriel, S.E., Beard, J. *et al*. 1989. A population-based case–control study of temporal arteritis: evidence for an association between temporal arteritis and degenerative vascular disease? *International Journal of Epidemiology* **18**(4), 836–841.

Mangano, D.T., Layug, E.L., Wallace, A. and Tateo, I. 1996. Effect of atenolol on mortality and cardiovascular morbidity after noncardiac surgery. *New England Journal of Medicine* **335**(23), 1713–1720.

McCollom, C., Alexander, C., Kenchington, G. *et al*. 1991. Antiplatelet drugs in femoropopliteal vein bypasses: a multicenter trial. *Journal of Vascular Surgery* **13**, 150–162.

McGill, H.C. 1988. The cardiovascular pathology of smoking. *American Heart Journal* **115**, 250–257.

McKenna, M., Wolfson, S. and Kuller, L. 1991. The ratio of ankle and arm arterial pressure as an independent predictor of mortality. *Atherosclerosis* **87**, 119–128.

McLaren, M., Jennings, P.E., Forbes, C.D. and Belch, J.J.F. 1990. Fibrinolytic response to venous occlusion in diabetic with and without micro-angiopathy compared to normal age and sex matched controls. *Fibrinolysis* **4**(2), 116–117.

McMahon, B.J., Heyward, W.L., Templin, D.W. *et al*. 1989. Hepatitis B-associated polyarteritis nodosa in Alaskan Eskimos: clinical and epidemiologic features and long-term follow-up. *Hepatology* **9**, 97–101.

McTavish, D., Faulds, D. and Goa, K.L. 1990. Ticlopidine: an updated review of its pharmacology and therapeutic use in platelet-dependent disorders. *Drugs* **40**, 238–59.

Mills, J.L. and Porter, J.M. 1990. Thromboangiitis Obliterans (Buerger's Disease). In Churg, A. and Churg J (eds), *Systemic vasculitides*. New York: Igaku-Shoin, 229–239.

Mühlhauser, I. 1990. Smoking and diabetes. *Diabetic Medicine* **7**, 10–15.

Muir, A., Stonebridge, P. and Belch, J.J.F. The diagnosis of 'occult' diabetes in the patient with peripheral arterial disease. Submitted.

Muller, J.E., Stone, P.H., Turi, Z.G. *et al*. 1985. Circadian variation in the onset of acute myocardial infarction. *New England Journal of Medicine* **313**, 1315–1322.

Myers, K.A., King, R.B., Scott, D.F. *et al*. 1978. The effect of smoking of the late patency of arterial reconstruction in the legs. *British Journal of Surgery* **65**, 267–271.

Newman, A.B., Sutton-Tyrrell, K., Vogt, M.T. and Kuller, L.H. 1993. Morbidity and mortality in hypertensive adults with a low ankle/arm blood pressure index. *Journal of the American Medical Association* **270**, 487–489.

Nurmohamed, M.T., Rosendaal, F.T., Buller, H.R. *et al*. 1992. Low molecular weight heparin versus standard heparin in general and orthopaedic surgery: a meta-analysis. *Lancet* **340**, 152–156.

Oswald, G.A., Smith, C.C.T., Delamothe, A.P. *et al*. 1988. Raised concentrations of glucose and adrenaline and increased *in vivo* platelet activation after myocardial infarction. *British Heart Journal* **59**, 663–671.

Patrono, C. 1994. Aspirin as an antiplatelet drug. *New England Journal of Medicine* **330**, 1287–1294.

Pineo, G.F., Hull, R.D. and Raskob, G. 1995. Prevention of venous thrombosis in general surgery and orthopaedics. *Vascular Medicine Review* **6**, 185–192.

Prevention of Atherosclerotic Complications with Ketanserin Trial Group. 1989. Prevention of atherosclerotic complications: controlled trial of ketanserin. *British Medical Journal* **298**, 424–430.

Rees, M.M. and Rodgers, G.M. 1993. Homocysteinemia: association of a metabolic disorder with vascular disease and thrombosis. *Thrombosis Research* **71**, 337–359.

Reid, D.D., Holland, W.W., Hummerfelt, S. and Rose, G. 1966. A cardiovascular survey of British postal workers. *Lancet* **i**, 614–618.

Reidy, M.A., Jackson, C. and Lindner, V. 1992. Neointimal proliferation: control of vascular smooth muscle cell growth. *Vascular Medicine Review* **3**, 156–167.

Rodgers, G.M. and Conn, M.T. 1990. Homocysteine, an atherogenic stimulus reduces protein C activation by arterial and venous endothelial cells. *Blood* **75**, 895–901.

Rosove, M.H. and Brewer, P.M.C. 1992. Antiphospholipid thrombosis: clinical course after the first thrombotic event in 70 patients. *Annals of Internal Medicine* **117**, 303–308.

Rubenstein, I., Murray, D. and Hoffstein, V. 1988. Fatal pulmonary emboli in hospitalised patients: an autopsy study. *Archives of Internal Medicine* **148**, 1425–1426.

Russel, M.A.H. 1990. The nicotine trap: a 40 year sentence for four cigarettes. *British Journal of Addiction* **85**, 293–300.

Sacks, F.M., Pfeffer, M.A., Moye, L.A. *et al*. 1996. The effect of pravastatin on coronary events after myocardial infarction in patients with average cholesterol levels. *New England Journal of Medicine* **335**, 1001–1009.

Salonen, J.T. 1989. Antioxidants and platelets. *Annals of Medicine* **21**, 59–62.

Scandinavian Simvastatin Survival Study Group. 1994. Randomised trial of cholesterol lowering in 4444 patients with coronary heart disease: the Scandinavian Simvastatin Study (4S). *Lancet* **344**, 1383–1389.

Schafer, A.I. and Kroll, M.H. 1993. Nonatheromatous arterial thrombosis. *Annual Review of Medicine* **44**, 155–170.

Schroll, M. and Munck, O. 1981. Estimation of peripheral arteriosclerotic disease by ankle brachial pressure measurements in a population study of 60 year-old men and women. *Journal of Chronic Disease* **34**, 261–269.

Scottish Intercollegiate Guidelines Network (SIGN). *Prophylaxis of venous thromboembolism. A national clinical guideline recommended for use in Scotland.* Pilot Edition, September 1995.

Shepherd, J., Cobbe, S.M., Ford, I. *et al*. 1995. Prevention of coronary heart disease with pravastatin in men with hypercholesterolaemia. *New England Journal of Medicine* **333**, 1301–1307.

Shimada, K., Kawamoto, I., Matsubayashi, K. *et al*. 1992. Diurnal blood pressure variations and silent cerebrovascular damage in elderly patients with hypertension. *Journal of Hypertension* **10**, 875–878.

Silagy, C., Mant, D., Fowler, G. and Lodge, M. 1994. Meta-analysis on efficacy of nicotine replacement therapies in smoking cessation. *Lancet* **343**, 139–142.

Sivenius, J., Laakso, M., Riekkinen, Snr P. *et al*. 1992. European Stroke Prevention Study: Effectiveness of antiplatelet therapy in diabetic patients in secondary prevention of stroke. *Stroke* **23**(6), 851–854.

Smith, F.B., Lowe, G.D., Fowkes, F.G. *et al*. 1993. Smoking, haemostatic factors and lipid peroxides in a population case control study of peripheral arterial disease. *Atherosclerosis* **102**(2), 155–162.

Sonnenblick, M., Nesher, G. and Rosin, A. 1989. Nonclassical organ involvement in temporal arteritis. *Seminars in Arthritis and Rheumatism* **19**(3), 183–190.

Stephens, N.G., Parsons, A., Schofield, P.M. *et al*. 1996. Randomised controlled trial of vitamin E in patients with coronary disease: Cambridge Heart Antioxidant Study (CHAOS). *Lancet* **347**, 781–786.

Stiegler, H., Standl, E., Schulz, K. *et al*. 1992. Morbidity, mortality and albuminuria in type 2 diabetic patients: a three-year prospective study of a random cohort in general practice. *Diabetic Medicine* **9**, 646–653.

Strano, A., Novo, S., Avellone, G. *et al*. 1993. Hypertension and other risk factors in peripheral arterial disease. *Clinical and Experimental Hypertension* **15**(1), 71–89.

Taylor, L.M. Jr. and Porter, J.M. 1993. Elevated plasma homocysteine as a risk factor for atherosclerosis. *Seminars in Vascular Surgery* **6**, 36–45.

Taylor, P., Wolfe, J., Tyrell, M. *et al*. 1990. Graft stenosis: justification for 1–year surveillance. *British Journal of Surgery* **77**, 1125–1128.

Thromboembolic Risk Factors (THRIFT) Consensus Group. 1992. Risk of and prophylaxis for venous thromboembolism in hospital patients. *British Medical Journal* **305**, 567–574.

Turnbull, A., Tundall, V.R., Beard, R.W. *et al*. 1989. Confidential enquiry into maternal deaths in England and Wales 1982–1984. London: HMSO, 28–36.

US Department of Health and Human Services. 1988. *The health consequences of smoking. Nicotine addiction. A report of the Surgeon General.* DHHS publication No. (CDC) 88–8406.

Van Gaal, L., Rillaerts, E., Creten, W. and De Leeuw, I. 1988. Relationship of body fat distribution pattern to atherogenic risk factors in non-insulin dependent diabetes. Preliminary results. *Diabetes Care* **11**, 103–106.

Vianna, J.L., Khamashta, M.A., Ordi-Ris, J. *et al*. 1994. Comparison of the primary and secondary antiphospholipid syndrome: a European multicenter study of 114 patients. *American Journal of Medicine* **96**, 3–9.

Vogt, M.T., McKenna, M., Anderson, S.J. *et al*. 1993. The relationship between ankle arm index and mortality in older men and women. *Journal of the American Geriatric Society* **41**, 523–530.

White, W.B., Schulman, P., McCabe, E.J. *et al*. 1989. Average daily blood pressure, not office blood pressure, determines cardiovascular function in patients with hypertension. *Journal of the American Medical Association* **261**, 873–877.

Wildsmith, J.A.W. and McClure, J.H. 1991. Anticoagulant drugs and central nerve blockade. *Anaesthesia* **46**, 613–614.

Wilson, S., Jennings, P.A. and Belch, J.J.F. 1992. Detection of microvascular impairment in type 1 diabetes by laser Doppler flowmetry. *Clinical Physiology* **12**, 195–208.

Zahavi, J. and Zahavi, M. 1985. Enhanced platelet release reaction, shortened platelet survival time and increased platelet aggregation and plasma thromboxane B2 in chronic obstructive arterial disease. *Thrombosis and Haemostasis* **53**, 105–109.

Zelis, R., Manson, D.T., Braunwald, E. *et al.* 1970. Effects of hyperlipoproteinemias and their treatment on the peripheral circulation. *Journal of Clinical Investigation* **49**, 1007–1013.

4

Normal cardiovascular physiology

MALCOLM O WRIGHT AND GERARD M A KEENAN

INTRODUCTION

The circulation consists of the heart and the blood vessels. It is responsible for the uptake of nutrients from the lungs, gastrointestinal tract and liver and subsequent delivery of these vital substances to all tissues. Waste products are removed and distributed to the liver, kidneys and lungs for excretion. Hormones are also delivered to their target organs as are the mediators of the immune and inflammatory responses. Heat is dispersed from the core to skin where convection, conduction and radiation allow bodily heat loss.

The heart comprises the atria, thin distensible chambers which receive blood from the other tissues, and the muscular ventricles which pump blood into the low-resistance pulmonary and the higher-pressure systemic circulations. The systemic circulation is of high resistance because it consists of many parallel circulatory beds. Consequently the left ventricle, which supplies the systemic circulation, is more muscular than the right, which perfuses the lungs. The volume pumped by each ventricle per minute is the same.

Systemic blood returns to the right atrium through the venae cavae at pressures near zero, passes to the right ventricle through the tricuspid valve and is pumped through the pulmonary valve into the pulmonary artery. It then flows to the pulmonary capillaries, where, at the alveolar–capillary interface, oxygen is taken up and carbon dioxide is liberated in gas exchange. Oxygenated blood returns to the left atrium in the pulmonary veins and passes through the mitral or bicuspid valve into the left ventricle which pumps blood through the aortic valve into the aorta. The aorta and arterial tree distribute blood into the parallel circuits of the systemic circulation (Fig. 4.1). At the termination of the arterial system are the narrow, muscular arterioles which are responsible for the bulk of the peripheral resistance. The precapillary sphincters step down the hydrostatic pressure so that the capillaries are not exposed to a level of pressure which might result in excessive loss of fluid into the interstitium, the space through which nutrients and waste products diffuse between cells and capillaries. From the capillaries, blood drains into the venules and progressively larger veins to reach the superior or inferior venae cavae. Veins are distensible, are at low pressure and are termed the 'capacitance vessels' because they contain around 55 per cent of the circulating blood volume.

The circulation is controlled in many ways. The heart is regulated to maintain the cardiac output according to metabolic requirements. The arterioles constrict or relax to determine regional perfusion.

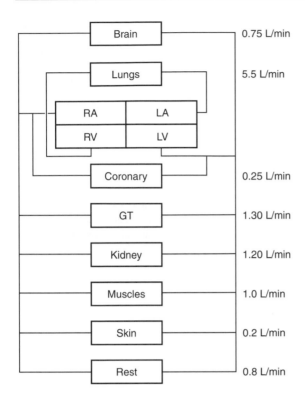

Figure 4.1 *The circulation. RA, right atrium. RV, right ventricle. LA, left atrium; LV, left ventricle. Blood flows are in litres per minute.*

The precapillary sphincters control capillary flow and venoconstriction or venodilation reduce or increase pooling of blood in veins respectively.

OXYGEN TRANSPORT

A major function of the circulation is to deliver sufficient oxygen to the tissues and meet the oxygen demands of cellular metabolism. The metabolic rate is affected by body temperature, exercise and hormones such as catecholamines and thyroxine. At rest, the body requires approximately 250 mL of oxygen per minute.

Oxygen is carried in two ways by the blood. A small amount, proportional to the partial pressure of oxygen in the arterial blood (PaO_2), is dissolved in plasma. However, most oxygen is carried bound to haemoglobin. It is taken up from the alveoli into the pulmonary capillaries where it enters the red blood cells and binds to haemoglobin, the molecule of which has four com-

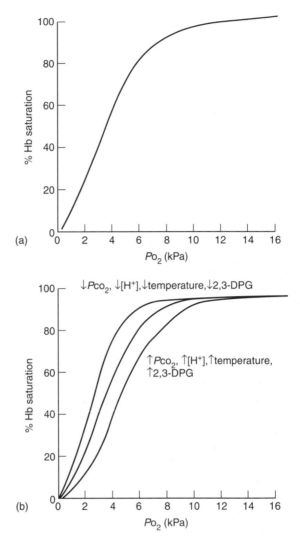

Figure 4.2 *(a) The oxyhaemoglobin dissociation curve. (b) Factors influencing shifts in the curve. 2,3-DPG, 2,3-diphosphoglycerate.*

ponent parts each containing a haem portion attached to a protein chain. The haem group contains a central atom of ferrous iron and the protein chains are classified as α, β, γ or δ according to the amino acid composition. The commonest form of adult haemoglobin is HbA_1 in which there are two α and two β chains each attached to a haem group. There are four binding sites for oxygen on the haemoglobin molecule, each of the four iron atoms being able to bind reversibly with one oxygen molecule.

When the first oxygen molecule binds, there is a conformational change and the two β chains move closer together and facilitate binding of the second molecule. Each oxygen addition is thus progressively faster until saturation occurs. This relationship can be represented graphically as the oxyhaemoglobin dissociation curve, a plot with the Po_2 on the X-axis and haemoglobin saturation percentage on the Y-axis. It is sigmoid in shape and this is physiologically important. At a Po_2 of 13.3 kPa haemoglobin is almost 98 per cent saturated, yet at 9.3 kPa, it is still 94 per cent saturated with oxygen (Fig. 4.2). The horizontal portion acts as a buffer to maintain near normal levels of tissue oxygenation despite lower levels of Pao_2, but below 8 kPa, haemoglobin oxygen saturation decreases significantly.

Blood contains approximately 15 g haemoglobin per 100 mL, each gram combining with 1.34 mL oxygen when fully saturated. At a Pao_2 of 12.7 kPa, haemoglobin is approximately 98 per cent saturated so that there are 19.7 mL oxygen per 100 mL blood in combination, plus 0.29 mL oxygen per 100 mL in solution (0.0225 mL O_2/100 mL blood/kPa). The position of the oxyhaemoglobin dissociation curve is important for tissue oxygen delivery. A rightward shift in the curve results in a reduced affinity for oxygen, so more oxygen is released to the tissues. This can occur when hydrogen ion concentration, $Paco_2$, temperature or 2,3-diphosphoglycerate are increased in the erythrocyte. The opposite conditions result in an increased affinity. Under basal conditions, the arteriovenous oxygen difference is 5 mL/100 mL blood, with venous blood being at a Po_2 of 5.3 kPa, and its haemoglobin 75 per cent saturated.

$$\text{Coefficient of oxygen utilization} = \frac{\text{Tissue oxygen delivery}}{\text{Oxygen content of arterial blood}}$$

For the whole body under basal conditions, this is 25 per cent, but varies in different organs. The coefficient for skin is 5–10 per cent, but for myocardium it is 80–90 per cent.

Available oxygen

Available oxygen is related to cardiac output and arterial oxygen:

Available oxygen =
cardiac output × arterial oxygen content

and is the amount of oxygen available to the tissues per minute (Freeman and Nunn, 1963; Leigh, 1974). At a cardiac output of 5 L/min and a normal arterial oxygen content of 200 ml/L blood, it is (5 × 200) = 1000 mL/min. Around 250 mL/min (25 per cent) is extracted: the oxygen consumption. The unextracted oxygen acts as a reserve for times of need such as exercise. Available oxygen is affected by the cardiac output, the haemoglobin concentration and its percentage saturation. Tissue oxygen delivery may decrease when cardiac output is reduced, anaemia reduces the amount of oxygen carried or problems with pulmonary gas exchange reduce the oxygen saturation of haemoglobin. These abnormalities may all result in tissue hypoxia.

CARDIAC FUNCTION

The heart can initiate its own action and functions with automaticity, impulses passing through its conduction system resulting in synchronized contraction of the atria and ventricles. The volume pumped by each ventricle at rest is 5 L/min, but this can rise to 25–30 L/min in severe exercise.

Cardiac muscle fibres are cross-striated. They branch and interdigitate with each other to form a functional syncytium. The intercalated disc is where the end of one fibre abuts upon another and there are gap junctions which allow the passage of ions, and the spread of excitation, from one cell to the next.

Spontaneous electrical events occur at the sino-atrial node (100–110 per minute), the atrioventricular node (40–60 per minute) and the His–Purkinje system (20–40 per minute). The sino-atrial node, having the highest intrinsic rate, is the normal pacemaker, but the vagus nerve usually maintains a slower rate than that noted above which is for the isolated heart.

Cardiac electrophysiology

In a non-pacemaker cardiac muscle fibre, the resting membrane potential is around –80 mV, the inside of the cell being negative relative to the outside. This potential develops because the membrane has differing ion permeabilities, that for potassium being around 100 times that for sodium. Thus positively charged potassium ions can diffuse down their concentration gradient and out of the cell, but electroneutrality is not maintained because less sodium diffuses inwards. Anions such as proteins and phosphates cannot diffuse out with potassium because of their large size so there is a slight excess of anions intracellularly and of cations extracellularly.

CARDIAC EXCITATION

During excitation of non-pacemaker atrial and ventricular cells, a cardiac action potential passes along the muscle fibre membrane, a process divided into four phases (Fig. 4.3). Phase 4 occurs at rest and is a stable diastolic potential. Phase 0 follows with a partial membrane depolarization to below −60 mV, the threshold for an increase in sodium permeability which allows rapid entry into the cell down its concentration gradient and results in full depolarization to +20 mV (Ross, 1985). Sodium permeability then begins to decrease because some sodium channels close, and so the membrane starts to repolarize. However, a plateau quickly follows during which an increase in calcium permeability, and the residual sodium permeability, maintain the membrane potential at 0 mV for 200–300 ms, calcium also diffusing down its concentration gradient. In phase 3, potassium permeability increases, allowing greater diffusion down its concentration gradient and resulting in repolarization. Muscular contraction commences 10 ms after the action potential upstroke and lasts 1.5 times as long. The fibre is refractory to further stimulation during the action potential and the contractile response is almost 70 per cent complete before another response can commence, so cardiac muscle cannot be tetanized.

In pacemaker cells, the membrane potential during diastole is unstable, slowly depolarizing from −60 mV to the critical firing level of −40 mV, at which point a propagated action potential results. The diastolic membrane potential instability is known as the 'pacemaker potential' and confers intrinsic rhythm upon such cells. It occurs because sino-atrial (SA) node cells have an increased permeability to calcium compared to other myocardial cells. After potassium channel closure at the end of the previous action potential, calcium ions enter the cell and, as a result generate the next impulse (Vassalle, 1977), a cycle that is ongoing and regular. The atrioventricular (AV) node and Purkinje fibres also show pacemaker activity, but the upslope of

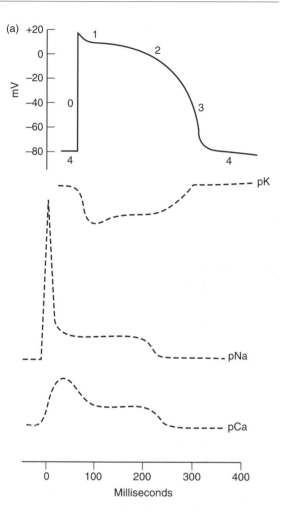

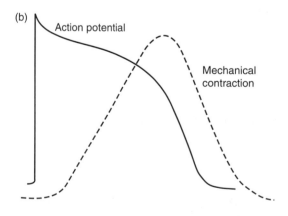

Figure 4.3   *(a) The cardiac action potential and permeabilities to potassium (pK), sodium (pNa) and calcium (pCa). (b) The relationship of action potential to mechanical contraction.*

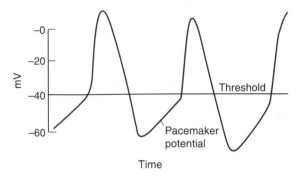

Figure 4.4 *SA node potential showing pacemaker potential.*

depolarization is less, resulting in slower firing and subsequent dominance of pacemaker activity by the SA node (Fig. 4.4).

CARDIAC IMPULSE PROPAGATION

After generation of an action potential at the SA node, the impulse is propagated from cell to cell in an orderly manner via the syncytial, interdigitating network. During excitation at a given moment, when the inside of the cell is positive and the outside negative, the positive charges on the membrane ahead of the cell are drawn into the area of negativity of the action potential which results in depolarization of the next cell to firing level and a new action potential. Circular current flow thus occurs and the action potential spreads throughout the heart by electrotonic depolarization (Fig. 4.5). From the SA node, the cardiac impulse passes to the AV node via the atrial fibres and the three atrionodal tracts. Atrial excitation leads to contraction. About 0.1 s is required for conduction of the impulse through the AV node and this allows sufficient time for 30 per cent of the atrial stroke volume to enter the ventricles before their systole. It also prevents an excess of atrial impulses being transmitted, and so reduces the risk of one reaching the ventricle when it is vulnerable to re-entry type arrhythmias.

From the AV node, the impulse passes to the bundle of His, which has left and right branches. These pass down either side of the interventricular septum and make contact with the Purkinje fibres which form a mesh on the endocardial surface. The ventricles are thus activated from endocardium to epicardium. Impulses in the His–Purkinje system conduct at 1.5–4 m/s, and in the myocardium at

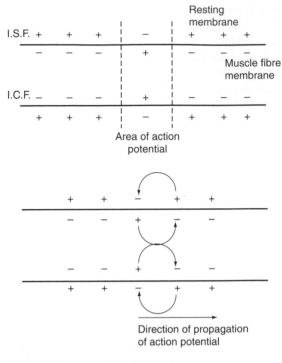

Figure 4.5 *Propagation of the action potential.*

0.5 m/s. This rapid conduction results in a synchronized contraction, and, because the whole ventricle is activated within 0.08 s, the impulse arrives back at its origin during the refractory period and so dissipates. Slower conduction through the ventricle might result in the cells activated first being ready to receive a new impulse as the original impulse returns. Re-entrant arrhythmias might thus occur.

Excitation–contraction coupling

Each myocardial cell contains a nucleus, myofibrils which run the length of the cell, mitochondria, a Golgi apparatus, ribosomes and myoglobin (Somner and Johnson, 1979). On microscopy, the myofibrils are striated with repeating light and dark bands (Fig. 4.6a). On either side of the broad, dark A-band are light I-bands, which are divided by a dark Z-line. The distance between two Z-lines is one sarcomere, the basic unit of striated muscle. In the centre of the A-band is the light H-zone. The myofibrils are made up of adjoined sarcomeres, which consist of interdigitating myofilaments. The thin filaments are attached to the Z-lines and consist of actin, tropomyosin and troponin. They pass longitudinally towards the centre of the sarcomere, where they interdigitate with the myosin molecules in the thick filaments (Hansen and Lang, 1965). The I-bands contain only thin filaments, the A-bands overlapping thick and thin filaments, and the H-zone is an area where actin and myosin do not overlap.

The myosin molecule has a globular head with a filamentous section consisting of two intertwined peptide chains. In the head there is ATPase activity and an actin-binding site. The thick filament contains a number of myosin molecules with their filaments wound together making a rigid structure from which the globular heads protrude (Fig. 4.6b). Actin is a globular protein which is polymerized to form the elongated F-actin. Two chains of this wind helically round each other to form the backbone of the thin filament. In each of the two grooves running longitudinally between the actin is a molecule of tropomyosin. At intervals of around 40 nm along the thin filament is another protein, troponin. It has three components, I, T and C. Troponin I inhibits the actin–myosin interaction, T binds to tropomyosin and C binds to calcium (Fig. 4.6c).

Each myocardial cell has a membrane, the sarcolemma. At Z-lines, invaginations of the sarcolemma form the transverse, or t-tubules. These may be up to half the diameter of the fibre and are continuous with the extracellular space. The intraluminal fluid they contain communicates with the interstitial fluid, allowing the action potential to access the interior of the fibre and activate intracellular structures rapidly.

The sarcoplasmic reticulum is a complex system of anastomosing channels which surround the myofibrils and run longitudinally. Where a portion of this reticulum approaches the t-tubules, it enlarges to form flattened sacs called terminal cisternae. These contain calcium, which is released on muscle fibre activation. During muscular contraction, actin slides over the myosin filaments resulting in contraction of the sarcomere and, consequently, the whole muscle. The muscle action potential results in membrane depolarization including that of the t-tubules. Sodium and calcium concentrations rise in the cell, but this is insufficient to activate contraction until more calcium is released from the terminal cisternae (Fabiato and Fabiato, 1979). This calcium binds to troponin C, which causes the tropomyosin to shift, uncovering actin binding sites which can then bind myosin heads. The myosin

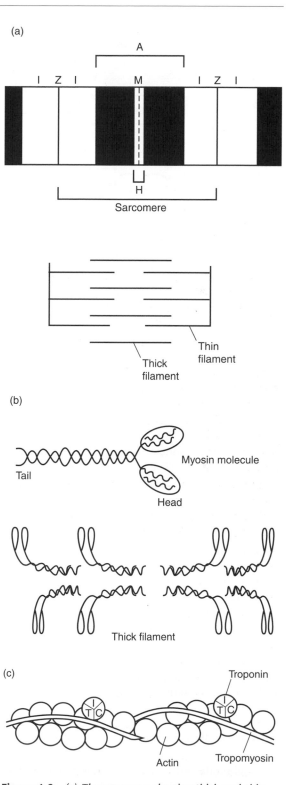

Figure 4.6 (a) The sarcomere showing thick and thin filaments. (b) Myosin and its arrangement in a thick filament. (c) Thin filament with actin, troponin and tropomyosin.

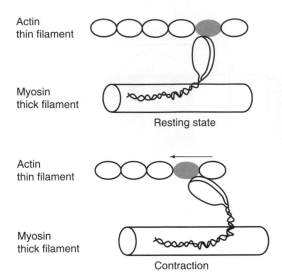

Figure 4.7 *Relationship between actin and myosin during rest and contraction.*

head has bound ATP. After actin binding, myosin ATPase from the head hydrolyses the ATP, releasing energy which causes myosin to swivel causing the thin filament to move towards the sarcomere centre (Fig. 4.7). After a complete swivel, the myosin ejects the hydrolysis products (ADP and phosphate) and binds another ATP. The process continues with further myosin–actin binding, resulting in further shortening (Harrington, 1979). At the end of the action potential, the inward flow of ions ceases and the longitudinal portion of the sarcoplasmic reticulum actively takes up the calcium by means of an ATP pump. This calcium is then stored in the terminal cisternae. Calcium is removed from the cell by a calcium ATPase pump and also a sodium–calcium exchange mechanism. After a decrease in intracellular concentration, calcium detaches from troponin C and tropomyosin returns to its resting position, covering the actin binding sites, inhibiting further binding and allowing relaxation to occur. Both contraction and relaxation require ATP.

The cardiac cycle

The right side of the heart operates at lower pressures, but the events are similar on both sides (Wiggers, 1952).

During ventricular diastole, the atrioventricular valves are open, and blood flows from atria to ven-

tricles. Seventy per cent of ventricular filling is passive, but after excitation, atrial systole occurs and the final 30 per cent passes from atrium to ventricle. Ventricular excitation follows and the atrioventricular valves close. Initial ventricular contraction is isometric because the outlet valves are closed, but the pressure rises rapidly and this isometric phase terminates when the ventricular pressures exceed aortic and pulmonary arterial pressures. The aortic and pulmonary valves open and blood flows through them. This rapid phase of ventricular contraction ejects 70 per cent of the stroke volume into the corresponding vessel, and the left and right intraventricular pressures rise maximally to around 120 mmHg and 25 mmHg, respectively, in normal subjects. After this, the force of contraction diminishes and both intraventricular pressure and blood flow decrease. However, the blood's momentum continues the process to complete the final 30 per cent of ventricular ejection. During the ensuing protodiastole, the pressure in the ventricles decreases rapidly so that the aortic and pulmonary valves snap shut and a period of isometric relaxation occurs until ventricular pressure is below that of the atria again and the AV valves open to start the rapid phase of ventricular filling.

Blood returns to the atria continuously except during atrial systole when there is some regurgitation into the great veins. After excitation, their contraction results in a pressure elevation from 0 to 4 mmHg in the right atrium and 4 to 6 mmHg in the left atrium, giving rise to the A-wave of the atrial pressure curve. During isometric ventricular contraction, the AV valves bulge into the atria, resulting in the C-wave. Ventricular ejection then results in downward movement of the AV septum causing a decrease in atrial pressure, the X descent. Next, continuing venous return fills the atria while the AV valves are closed, and the pressure rises, the V-wave. At the end of isometric ventricular relaxation, atrial pressure exceeds ventricular pressure and the AV valves open allowing rapid ejection of blood so that atrial pressure decreases, the Y descent (Fig. 4.8).

The end-diastolic ventricular volume is around 140 mL, and the stroke volume 70–90 mL. During severe exercise, the maximal end diastolic volume is 200–400 mL and stroke volume 130–170 mL. There are small variations in stroke volume between the two ventricles, usually due to respiratory mechanical effects, but over longer periods, the ventricles must have equal outputs. The ejection fraction (stroke

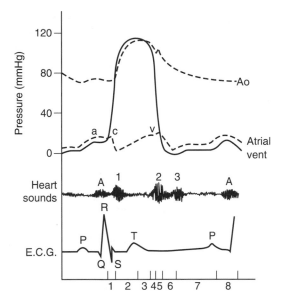

Figure 4.8   *Ventricular (vent), atrial and aortic (Ao) pressure curves. 1, Isometric ventricular contraction. 2, Maximum ejection phase. 3, Reduced ejection phase. 4, Protodiastole. 5, Isometric ventricular relaxation. 6, Rapid ventricular filling. 7, Reduced ventricular filling. 8, Atrial systole.*

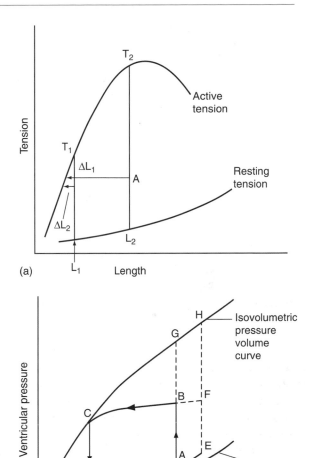

Figure 4.9   *Starling's law. (a) Length–tension diagram. (b) Ventricular pressure–volume loop.*

volume/end diastolic volume) varies between 50 and 70 per cent, increasing during exercise and in the presence of positive inotropic factors.

REGULATION OF CARDIAC OUTPUT

Cardiac output is related to heart rate and stroke volume:

Cardiac output = Heart rate × Stroke volume

and is controlled by a variety of factors. The heart responds to the demands placed upon it by both venous return (which may vary widely) and other factors. Factors affecting heart rate or stroke volume will alter cardiac output.

Stroke volume
Stroke volume is influenced by three factors: preload, afterload and myocardial contractility. The preload is the load placed upon the ventricles prior to contraction by the venous return and atrial systole provides the ventricles with 30 per cent of the stroke volume. In addition, the distensibility of the heart in response to its venous return will affect the preload.

Variations in preload affect the initial length of the muscle fibres in ventricular diastole, which in turn dictates the force of the subsequent contraction by the Frank–Starling mechanism. Starling's law states that, within limits, the force of contraction is a function of the initial length of the muscle fibres (Starling, 1918). The length–tension diagram has two elements (Fig. 4.9a). The resting tension–fibre length curve shows passive resistance to stretch. Resting tension rises slowly initially, then more rapidly during stretching, collagen and elastic tissues providing resistance. The active tension curve results from making the muscle fibres contract isometrically at different lengths. As fibre length increases, so also does the tension generated up to a maximum, after which any increase in length results in a fall in tension. At maximal contractility, actin and myosin are probably at the point at which maximal interdigitation is possible. As fibre length increases, the number of active sites generating force increases and there appears to be an increased sensitivity to calcium (Kirchenberger and Schwartz, 1985). During overstretch, the interdigitation is lost, the actin being pulled out of the myosin. The heart works on the ascending portion of the curve. At resting lengths L_1 and L_2, the tensions produced are T_1 and T_2. If the length exceeds L_2, tension will fall, the situation in ventricular failure.

The ventricular pressure–volume diagram (Sagawa, 1978) (Fig. 4.9b) demonstrates the Frank–Starling mechanism. During diastole, the ventricle fills (point D to A, the end-diastolic volume). Isometric ventricular contraction follows (point A to B). Ventricular pressure then exceeds arterial pressure (afterload) and the aortic and pulmonary valves open so the stroke volume is ejected (B to C, which lies on the isovolumetric pressure–volume curve). Point C corresponds to end-systolic volume and pressure. Isovolumetric relaxation then occurs (C to D). If venous return increases, the ventricle fills from D to E, resulting in increased muscle fibre stretch. If the ventricle were to contract isovolumetrically from E, the pressure would reach H on the isovolumetric pressure curve compared to G if contracting from A. This, the Starling mechanism, shows increased force of contraction upon increased muscle fibre stretching. If the contractility and afterload remain the same as for loop ABCD, the ventricle contracts isovolumetrically from E to F, when the aortic and pulmonary valves open and the muscle fibres thus shorten. The stroke volume is ejected from F to C. An increased preload results in an increase in stroke volume. This mechanism also results in the ability to equalize left and right ventricular outputs. An increase in right ventricular input promotes a greater stroke volume which in turn is received by the left ventricle and, over a few beats, a similar increase in left ventricular stroke volume occurs (Hamilton, 1955).

Myocardial contractility

This may be defined as the change in contractile force for a given fibre length at a given afterload (Fig. 4.10). At normal myocardial contractility, the tension developed on isometric contraction from the resting length L is given by point T_1 on the active length–tension curve. On isotonic contraction at a

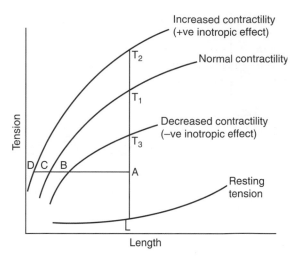

Figure 4.10 Length–tension diagram.

given afterload, the shortening is from A to C. Positive inotropic stimuli shift the length–tension curve upwards and to the left. At the same resting length L, the tension produced is greater on isometric contraction (T_2). At the same afterload, shortening increases (A to D) on isotonic contraction. Conversely, a negative inotropic stimulus will move the curve down and rightwards. This means that tension (T_3) will develop on isometric contraction and shortening occurs from A to B, again at the same afterload. A similar principle applies to the ventricular pressure–volume relationship. During a positive inotropic stimulus, the ventricle will generate a greater pressure during isovolumetric contraction at the same preload, and a lesser pressure at the same preload during a negative inotropic state.

Positive inotropic factors include β-adrenergic stimuli, an increase in heart rate, glucagon, digoxin and inotropic drugs such as catecholamines and phosphodiesterase inhibitors. An increase in intracellular calcium increases the amount available to bind with troponin. The rise in tension is proportional to the amount of calcium made available in the intracellular fluid (Langer, 1968). Sympathetic stimulation increases heart rate and contractility. The increase in heart rate shortens diastole. This reduces the extrusion time for calcium from the intracellular space to the extracellular space. Consequently, intracellular calcium rises along with contractility. During a negative inotropic stimulus, the amount of muscle shortening is reduced and end-systolic volume is increased, so decreasing ejection fraction. Factors causing this state include acidosis, hypoxia, hypercapnia, hyperkalaemia (which can occur during reperfusion of an ischaemic region of the body as in, for example, aortic surgery), cardiac failure and drugs such as anaesthetic agents and antiarrhythmics, including β_1-antagonists.

Afterload
The afterload is that tension against which the ventricular muscle must contract in order to exceed the pressures within the aortic and pulmonary arteries so that the stroke volume may be ejected. This, in the presence of competent aortic and pulmonary valves, is a function of the vascular resistance of the systemic or pulmonary vessels, their visco-elastic properties and their diameters. For a given level of contractility, the amount of muscle fibre shortening and stroke volume varies directly with preload and inversely with afterload.

Heart rate
The heart rate adjusts to pump the venous return so that atrial pressure does not increase, and much of the cardiac reserve is due to the capacity to increase rate. The SA node is under neural, humoral and mechanical influences. It is innervated by the parasympathetic (vagal) and sympathetic nervous systems. The vagus nerve releases acetylcholine at post-ganglionic nerve endings to act on muscarinic receptors on the nodal cells. This slows heart rate by increasing potassium permeability, so facilitating its efflux and reducing the slope of the pacemaker potential (Ross, 1985). More calcium ions have to enter the cells to depolarize them to threshold. Atrial contractility and AV nodal conduction rate are also reduced.

The sympathetic nerves to the SA and AV nodes arise from the first five segments of the thoracic spinal cord and release noradrenaline at the SA node. Catecholamines from the adrenal medulla also have an effect. β_1-receptor stimulation increases the slope of the pacemaker potential by increasing calcium permeability (Ross, 1985). Atrial and ventricular contractility are also increased, as is the speed of transmission through the AV node. At rest, the vagus predominates and the resting heart rate is 70–80 beats per minute.

Heart rate is affected by changes in vagal or sympathetic activity at the SA node. Anger and fear initiate sympathetic activity, but pain may precipitate either tachycardia or bradycardia depending on the type of stimulus. Hypoxia or hypercapnia produce

tachycardia through the chemoreceptors. The baroreceptors in the carotid and aortic sinuses produce reflex bradycardia during an increase in blood pressure, and tachycardia during a decrease. These effects contribute to the integrated response of the cardiovascular system in maintaining homeostasis (Folkow and Neil, 1971). Distension of the atria from an increase in venous return results in stretch of the SA nodal cells with an increase in the prepotential slope. The Bainbridge reflex (Bainbridge, 1915) occurs when the atria are stretched. This produces an increase in vagal afferent transmission to the vasomotor centre with a reduction in parasympathetic, and an increase in sympathetic, activity. An increased heart rate results, so that cardiac output increases to avoid an increase in filling pressure.

Pyrexia increases heart rate by 7 beats/min/°C. This may be due to a direct nodal effect or to reflexes mediated through the hypothalamus (Jose *et al.*, 1970). Thyroid hormones also increase heart rate.

Changes in heart rate are very important in exercise. Cardiac output is influenced by heart rate in a curvilinear manner, in that output increases with rate up to a maximum beyond which further increases result in a decrease (Sagimoto *et al.*, 1966). At rates of up to 150 beats per minute, only the slow phase of ventricular filling is affected during the shorter diastole and so output increases overall because the effect of heart rate on contractility, as well as increased rate, override the small decrease in stroke volume. At heart rates above 150, cardiac output declines because the rapid phase of ventricular filling is affected as diastole shortens and the stroke volume decreases. In addition, coronary flow occurs mostly during diastole so, if it shortens, ventricular perfusion time is reduced and the thick left ventricular wall may become ischaemic, especially in the presence of coronary artery disease or ventricular hypertrophy. Cardiac output may also decrease at heart rates of less than 45 beats per minute because the ventricle may be maximally filled and unable to increase stroke volume with respect to preload, so output will be rate-dependent. Finally, at large end-diastolic volumes coronary perfusion pressure will lessen because of increased ventricular wall tension.

Myocardial oxygen requirement

The resting adult myocardium requires about 25 mL oxygen per minute. As oxygen extraction from coronary blood is almost maximal, any increase in oxygen demand must be met by an increase in flow. Factors influencing cardiac oxygen requirement (Gibbs and Chapman, 1979) include:

- Heart rate: the increase in oxygen requirement is almost linear with heart rate.
- Intramyocardial tension: an increase in peak systolic pressure results in an increase in work.
- Outflow impedance changes: an increase in arterial blood pressure causes an increased end-diastolic volume, and myocardial tension rises due to the increased force of contraction by Starling's law.
- Contractility changes: an increased force of contraction for a given fibre length requires more oxygen.

Twenty per cent of the total oxygen requirement is for non-contractile functions such as molecular synthesis and 0.05 per cent for production of the action potential.

THE PERIPHERAL CIRCULATION

During ventricular contraction, blood is ejected into the aorta. The aorta, and the other large vessels, contain a large proportion of elastic tissue, so during systole they distend and create a source of potential energy. Then, as aortic pressure decreases after ventricular systole, the elastic tissues recoil and convert potential energy into kinetic energy which maintains forward flow during diastole and thus throughout the cardiac cycle. As the arteries branch and become smaller, the elastic tissue content decreases and the smooth muscle content increases. The arterioles contain a substantial proportion of smooth muscle and contraction of this will affect vessel calibre. Because the arterioles as a group have a large surface area, the effect of constriction on afterload is substantial, and they are termed the 'resistance vessels'. They regulate blood flow to the various organs.

The pressure pulse wave is transmitted through the circulation in a sequential manner. During systole, blood is ejected into the elastic aorta. This distends because the inertia of the column of blood within it prevents that blood from moving immediately. The inertia is then overcome and some blood moves into a more distal segment. The same course

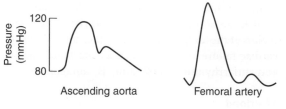

Figure 4.11 *Ascending aorta and femoral artery pressure waveforms.*

of events follows and the pressure wave passes along the arterial tree. The pressure wave is conducted rapidly, but blood flow lags behind because of the inertia of the system. The shape of the arterial pressure waveform (Fig. 4.11) changes with the cardiac cycle (McDonald, 1960). In the ascending aorta, pressure rises rapidly from 80 to 120 mmHg as 70 per cent of the stroke volume is expelled during the rapid ejection phase. Pressure then decreases during the period of reduced contraction, when only 30 per cent is expelled, and continues to decrease during protodiastole, when the left ventricle begins to relax. Once ventricular pressure is below that of the proximal aorta slight backward flow closes the aortic valve. The blood flowing retrogradely now 'collides' with the valve and produces the dicrotic notch. Pressure then decreases further during diastole as blood is conducted distally.

The difference between systolic and diastolic pressure is the pulse pressure. Mean arterial pressure is not the average of systolic and diastolic pressures because the duration of diastole exceeds that of systole, and the pressure decline in diastole is not linear. Thus mean pressure is calculated from the diastolic pressure plus one third of the pulse pressure, giving a mean of 93 mmHg at a blood pressure of 120/80 mmHg.

The femoral arterial pressure curve is different. It has a steeper upstroke and downstroke, with slightly higher systolic and lower diastolic pressures. Thus pulse pressure is higher and mean pressure slightly lower. The systolic portion of the curve is narrower and there is no discrete incisura, but a rise in pressure occurs in diastole. Reasons for these differences include:

- Vessel compliance affects the transmission velocity of the pressure pulse, compliance being reduced in smaller arteries and as blood pressure increases. This leads to an increased velocity of pulse propagation, producing a narrower and taller waveform.

- Reflected waves from vessel branches and arterioles, especially when they are constricted, are superimposed upon the basic.

Factors influencing blood pressure

Ohm's law states that:

Voltage = Current × Resistance

Applied to the vasculature, this gives an analogous equation of:

Blood pressure = Cardiac output ×
Peripheral resistance

The pressure within the arterial system depends upon the rate at which blood enters it and the rate of outflow through the arterioles. The larger the stroke volume, the greater the vessel distension and the higher the pressure. Also, the compliance of the vessel affects pressure. The more compliant, the less the pressure. Ageing vessels are less compliant so a greater rise in pressure occurs per given stroke volume. Compliance represents the volume change per unit pressure change or:

$C = \Delta V/\Delta P$

Diastolic pressure is affected by:

- The elastic recoil of the vessels which are distended during systole.
- Peripheral resistance. Arteriolar constriction reduces outflow from the circulation and diastolic pressure increases. Vasodilatation results in the reverse. Poiseuille's law states that:

$Q = \pi \Delta P r^4/8\rho l$,

where Q is flow, ΔP the pressure difference along the vessel, r the radius, l the length and ρ the viscosity. Substituting in the formula:

Pressure = Flow × Resistance,

we find that:

resistance = $8l\rho/\pi r^4$.

This formula, although strictly relating to laminar flow of a perfect fluid in a rigid tube, can be used with limitations, and it can be seen that a small change in arteriolar radius will have a large

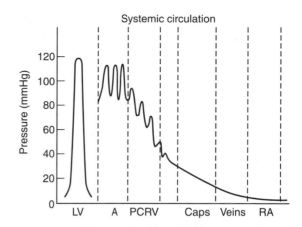

Figure 4.12 *Blood pressures throughout the circulation. LV, left ventricle. A, arteries. PCRV, precapillary resistance vessels. Caps, capillaries. RA, right atrium.*

effect on peripheral resistance. The viscosity of blood is affected by the haematocrit, an increase in which also increases viscosity and resistance.

- Diastolic pressure increases with heart rate because of the shorter time for arteriolar run-off.

The microcirculation

The arterioles divide into the small, but muscular metarterioles, then into pre-capillary sphincter vessels, 10–15 μm in diameter, which possess some smooth muscle. In some vascular beds, the metarteriole has a direct connection to the venule. The arterioles step down the hydrostatic pressure to 30–35 mmHg (Fig. 4.12) and serve to control the total peripheral resistance, the degree of which depends upon the proportion of arterioles in the dilated or constricted state. In this way, the blood flow distribution may be varied from one vascular bed to another. Also, the formation and turnover of interstitial fluid is affected by the amount of flow permitted through the arterioles.

SMOOTH MUSCLE

Smooth muscle is found in the media of arteries, in spiral array in larger vessels and circumferentially in arterioles. The cells contain few mitochondria and their sarcoplasmic reticulum, which contains calcium, is poorly developed. Where one cell connects to another, there are gap junctions, specialized areas that allow greater ionic conductance. Thus the electrochemical processes spread rapidly and smooth muscle may behave as a syncytium.

The innervation is mainly sympathetic, the postganglionic nerves forming plexuses with branches that have intermittent swellings, or varicosities, containing vesicles of transmitter. The distance between the varicosities and the smooth muscle cells is 80–120 μm, with the area of muscle adjacent to the varicosity having receptors, not only for the transmitter, but also for hormones and factors mediating local chemical control.

CONTROL OF PRECAPILLARY RESISTANCE VESSELS

The relative importance of neural and humoral mechanisms in the control of precapillary resistance vessels varies according to the organ involved. For example, the skin and splanchnic circulations are mainly under neural control, whereas the cerebral and coronary circulations are influenced more by other mechanisms.

Vasoconstriction

Post-ganglionic sympathetic fibres innervate all blood vessels except capillaries, precapillary sphincters and perhaps metarterioles, with the arterioles being the most densely innervated. The sphincters and metarterioles can, however, respond to circulating vasoactive substances. Within the adventitia of the vessel, the post-ganglionic fibres form a ground plexus which sends fibres to the outer aspect of the media. Noradrenaline released from the vesicles must diffuse from the outer to the inner part of the media where the receptors lie. As one muscle cell is activated, so are the adjacent cells through the gap junctions (Johansson and Somlyo, 1980), and the degree of vasoconstriction is proportional to the rate of sympathetic discharge. A steady rate of discharge in the nerves to the arterioles maintains a background degree of vasoconstriction, and thus resistance, known as the 'vascular tone'. This is under the control of the vasomotor centre in the medulla and is part of the baroreceptor reflex maintaining blood pressure (see below).

Circulating substances also affect the resistance vessels, with noradrenaline activating α_1-receptors in the cutaneous, splanchnic and muscular circulations, and adrenaline (at physiological concentrations) causing vasoconstriction in the skin. In response to reduced renal blood flow, renin is secret-

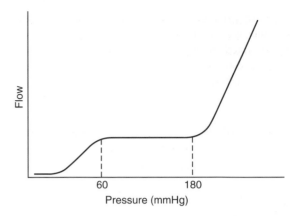

Figure 4.13 *Pressure–flow curve showing autoregulation.*

ed from the juxtaglomerular apparatus and catalyses production of angiotensin II, a potent vasoconstrictor acting at specific receptors. Vasopressin acts at V_1 receptors, especially after blood loss when concentrations of circulating vasoconstrictors are elevated. Endothelin (ET) is now considered to be the most potent endogenous vasoconstrictor and is released from endothelium in response to local hypoxia. There are three main types: ET-1, -2 and -3, and even small increases in ET-1 result in vasoconstriction (Schini and Vanhoutte, 1991). It also has an inotropic effect (Moracev *et al.*, 1989).

Local effects on vascular tone produce autoregulation, the ability of some tissues to regulate their own blood flow (Haddy and Scott, 1977). For a given level of metabolic activity, blood flow will remain relatively constant despite changes in perfusion pressure (Fig. 4.13). Tissues vary, but the range of mean arterial pressures over which autoregulation is maintained is of the order of 60–180 mmHg. Outside these limits, flow varies with perfusion pressure and autoregulation fails. Between the limits, flow increases transiently when pressure increases, but then reflex smooth muscle contraction increases local arteriolar resistance to flow and reduces flow. Conversely, flow decreases initially when perfusion pressure falls, but this results in accumulation of vasodilator metabolites. These concepts are known as the 'myogenic' and 'metabolic' theories respectively, and, in the coronary vasculature, the delay in response is around 10 s. A 'tissue pressure' theory of local blood flow control has been proposed. An increase in capillary hydrostatic pressure increases fluid flux into the interstitium. This increases tissue tension and the resistance to flow through the capillary (Johnsson, 1980). Autoregulation occurs in metabolically active tissue at a higher pressure and the curve is shifted upwards (Stainsby, 1962).

Local factors

Any increase in local oxygen tension, or decrease in either carbon dioxide tension or hydrogen ion concentration, leads to arteriolar and precapillary sphincter constriction. When skin is cooled, the arterioles in it become more sensitive to adrenaline and noradrenaline. When vessels are damaged, platelets adhere to the site and degranulate to release serotonin and thromboxane A_2 which cause local vasoconstriction and reduce blood flow to the injured area.

CRITICAL CLOSING PRESSURE

In rigid tubes flow and the pressure gradient are directly related, but in blood vessels flow ceases before the pressure gradient reaches zero because of vessel closure at what is known as the 'critical closing pressure' (Nichol et al., 1951) This phenomenon occurs because the elasticity of the vessel wall tending to close the vessel overcomes the distending tension of the intravascular pressure. Sympathetic stimulation increases the critical closing pressure which may range from 15 to 60 mmHg.

VASODILATATION

A decline in sympathetic activity results in vasodilatation in most tissues. However, skeletal muscle arterioles have dual innervation, receiving both sympathetic vasoconstrictor and sympathetic vasodilator fibres. The latter follow an anatomically sympathetic route, but secrete acetylcholine from their endings to increase blood flow. This system is activated at the beginning of exercise and by strong emotional stimuli. A few other arterioles also receive a cholinergic innervation, e.g. the coronary, pulmonary and renal circulations. In the salivary glands and the erectile tissue of the penis, parasympathetic nerve endings release vasoactive intestinal polypeptide which dilates their arterioles. Skin irritation causes impulses to pass along pain fibres to the spinal cord to activate pathways signalling pain, but these impulses also pass antidromically along branches of the same axon to nerve endings which release substance P. This causes arteriolar dilatation in the area of irritation (the axon reflex).

CIRCULATING VASODILATOR SUBSTANCES

At physiological concentrations, adrenaline causes vasodilatation in liver and skeletal muscle by an action at β_2-receptors. The kinins (bradykinin, and lysyl bradykinin formed from kininogen by the action of kallikrein) are potent vasodilators that also increase capillary permeability. They are produced by the salivary glands, sweat glands and the pancreas during secretion, and also by inflamed tissue. Histamine, from mast cells, also causes arteriolar dilatation, as does the natriuretic peptide released by the atria when they are distended. de Bold et al. (1981) demonstrated that this peptide produces natriuresis, hypotension, an increase in haematocrit and that it has a brief half-life. Brain natriuretic peptide (BNP) is produced primarily in the cardiac ventricles in response to stretch. C-type natriuretic peptide causes vasodilation and seems to be produced by brain tissue and endothelium. It also appears to inhibit the vascular proliferative response to injury. The plasma concentrations of natriuretic peptides may indicate the severity of cardiac insufficiency (Nicholls, 1994).

LOCAL EFFECTS

Autoregulation results in vasodilatation when perfusion pressure decreases as long as pressure remains within the range described earlier. Hypoxia, hypercapnia and acidosis cause vasodilatation, which results in 'washout' of metabolites and an increase in tissue oxygen delivery. Centrally, hypoxia and hypercapnia stimulate the vasomotor centre and result in peripheral vasoconstriction, but the local factors are more important in the cerebral and coronary circulations, and hypercapnia is dominant in the cutaneous circulation. Thus vasodilatation still occurs in these tissues.

Pyrexia causes vasodilatation, as does an increased local potassium concentration, with metabolic acidosis predisposing to cellular potassium release. In the coronary circulation, adenosine is an important local vasodilator and may be the agent responsible for dilatation during myocardial hypoxia. Prostacyclin produced by endothelial cells, and other prostaglandins such as PGE_2 and PGD_2 released in inflammatory conditions, also cause dilatation.

Palmer et al. (1988) have shown that nitric oxide is synthesized in endothelial cells from L-arginine by the enzyme nitric oxide synthase. It seems that there is a nitric oxide-dependent physiological vasodilator tone, and that nitric oxide is responsible for the effects previously ascribed to endothelium-derived relaxing factor. It is thus vital in the control of blood pressure and flow. Stimuli for its release may be pulsatile flow and shear stress upon endothelial cells (Moncada, 1992). Nitric oxide binds to the ferrous iron in the haem prosthetic group of the soluble guanylate cyclase in vascular smooth muscle cells and increases the concentration of cyclic GMP leading to vascular relaxation (Waldman and Murad, 1988). Haemoglobin is an important inactivator of nitric oxide, binding it in a similar way. Potent vasodilators such as sodium nitroprusside and glyceryl trinitrate release nitric oxide (Feelisch, 1991), which is also known to inhibit platelet aggregation and adhesion. Platelets also generate nitric oxide and this may inhibit further their own activation (Radomski and Moncada, 1991).

THE CAPILLARIES

The capillaries are the exchange vessels, transporting nutrients to the interstitium and receiving waste products to be delivered to the venous system. There are around 4×10^{10} systemic capillaries with around a thousand times the cross-sectional area of the aorta. They are lined by a single layer of endothelium, which is usually unfenestrated. However, endocrine and exocrine glands, the renal glomeruli and the choroid plexus have fenestrated endothelium, with pores in the peripheral cytoplasm through which proteins and electrolytes may pass. In bone marrow, liver and spleen, there are large gaps between the endothelial cells through which proteins and erythrocytes pass. In the resting state, around 25 per cent of these small vessels are patent, and between them they usually contain about 5 per cent of the circulating blood volume. Blood flows through them slowly (0.3 mm/s) and the transit time is 2–3 s, the tone of the arterioles and precapillary sphincters determining flow. When metabolite concentrations increase in active tissues, the precapillary sphincters relax and capillary pressure exceeds critical closing pressure to increase the size of the capillary bed.

CAPILLARY/INTERSTITIUM TRANSPORT

Diffusion
Oxygen, glucose and other nutrients diffuse from the blood into the interstitium, with carbon dioxide

and lactic acid moving in the opposite direction. All of these substances diffuse passively along their concentration gradients.

Micropinocytosis
This active process transports large molecules across endothelial cells. The substance attaches to a receptor and is drawn into a vesicle within the cell (endocytosis). It is then transported across the cell within the vesicle before being released by exocytosis into the interstitium.

Filtration/absorption
Fluid is filtered from plasma to intersitium at the arterial end of the capillary and is reabsorbed at the venous end, the quantities filtered or reabsorbed being influenced by hydrostatic and osmotic (Starling) forces. The hydrostatic pressure of the capillaries favours filtration, and averages 32 and 12 mmHg at the arterial and venous ends respectively, with the decrease representing 25 per cent of total peripheral resistance. Capillaries in the renal glomeruli are at a higher pressure, but it is lower in the pulmonary capillaries and hepatic sinusoids. Although very low, the interstitial fluid hydrostatic pressure (varying between –6 and +2 mmHg; mean 0 mmHg) opposes that of the capillary. The overall pressure producing filtration is the difference between the hydrostatic pressures of the capillary and the interstitium.

Plasma has a higher osmotic pressure (25 mmHg) than the interstitium (5 mmHg) because of the difference in protein concentrations. The difference (an inward-directed osmotic gradient) opposes the effect of filtration, the osmotic pressure of the interstitium remaining low because any proteins reaching it are removed by the lymphatics. The formula for net filtration is:

$$A \times P[(\mathrm{HP_C} - \mathrm{HP_{ISF}}) - (\mathrm{OP_C} - \mathrm{OP_{ISF}})]$$

where A is surface area for capillary exchange, P is capillary permeability, $\mathrm{HP_C}$ is capillary hydrostatic pressure, $\mathrm{HP_{ISF}}$ is interstitial fluid hydrostatic pressure, $\mathrm{OP_C}$ and $\mathrm{OP_{ISF}}$ are the oncotic pressures in the capillary and interstitial fluid respectively. Assuming that A and P remain constant, the net pressure at the arterial end of the capillary will be

$$[(32 - 0) - (25 - 5)] = +12 \text{ mmHg},$$

so there will be net filtration from capillary to interstitium. At the venous end of the capillary, the net pressure will be

$$[(12-0)-(25-5)] = -8 \text{ mmHg,}$$

so the osmotic forces predominate, and fluid is drawn back into the capillary. Vasoconstriction decreases capillary hydrostatic pressure and fluid moves from the interstitium to the capillary. Conversely, vasodilatation increases capillary hydrostatic pressure, and thus fluid filtration from capillary to interstitium.

THE VENOUS SYSTEM

Blood from the capillaries drains into the venules, small vessels with an endothelial lining and a media containing a small amount of smooth muscle. They feed into progressively larger veins, and then into the superior or inferior venae cavae which return blood to the right atrium. Increasing the amount of blood in the lumen of an artery will produce a linear increase in pressure, but a larger volume of blood is required to produce a similar change in pressure in a vein. The veins are thin walled, and thus more distensible, allowing them to act as capacitance vessels. The venous system has three times the capacity of the arterial circulation and normally contains 55–60 per cent of the circulating blood volume. The veins are innervated by sympathetic vasoconstrictor fibres.

Factors influencing venous return

Venous return is a major factor controlling cardiac output. In the horizontal position, the pressure in the venules is around 12 mmHg, compared to 0–4 mmHg in the right atrium, this depending on the phases of respiration and the cardiac cycle. Blood returns to the heart down this pressure gradient with right atrial pressure being affected by blood volume, right ventricular function and venous tone.

The mean systemic pressure is that pressure at which equilibrium would be reached if the heart stopped beating. It is normally 7 mmHg and is an indication of vascular filling (Guyton et al., 1976). Venomotor tone is due to continuous sympathetic discharge and allows adjustment of the venous capacity. This α-adrenoceptor stimulation prevents venous pooling and maintains venous return. On assuming the erect position, blood pools in the dependent veins

and this causes decreases in venous pressure, venous return and cardiac output. Venous pressure also decreases after haemorrhage. In both situations, hypotension leads to a decrease in discharge from the baroreceptors and, through the vasomotor centre, an increase in sympathetic outflow. Venoconstriction shifts blood to the arterial side of the circulation to maintain pressure and perfusion.

Venous drainage from the leg is both superficial (the saphenous veins) and deep (a network of sinuses within soleus and gastrocnemius muscles), the two systems being connected by the perforating veins. All of these vessels have valves which normally permit only unidirectional flow. When the calf muscles contract, blood is squeezed into the popliteal and femoral veins. During muscle relaxation, blood is drawn from the superficial to the empty deep veins to be pumped onwards with the next muscle contraction. This is the calf muscle pump. Ninety per cent of lower limb blood flow returns in the deep system, and the rest in the superficial.

During normal inspiration, intrathoracic pressure changes from –2 to –6 mmHg and causes an increase in venous return. As noted above, gravity also affects venous return, with blood diverting from the central veins to those in the legs on standing. Gravity affects pressures as well with venous and arterial figures increasing by 0.77 mmHg/cm below heart level in the lower limbs, and decreasing by the same amount above heart level (Fig. 4.14). The pressure in the foot veins may approach 95 mmHg in the erect position and increase fluid transfer from the capillaries to the interstitium.

Any factors increasing venous return, such as an increase in blood volume or arteriolar dilatation will increase cardiac output. When arterioles dilate, more blood flows through the capillaries so that venous pressure and venous return increase. This is known as *vis a tergo*, and is seen in exercise, thyrotoxicosis, the presence of an arteriovenous fistula and anaemia, where tissue hypoxia leads to vasodilatation. The increase in venous return produces a hyperdynamic circulation because the heart must pump the venous return in full. The increased right atrial and ventricular end diastolic pressures cause the muscle fibres to lengthen and stroke volume to increase by the Frank–Starling mechanism. The Bainbridge reflex also increases heart rate to maintain right atrial pressure within normal limits. If the heart is unable to pump the blood it receives there is a resultant rise in right atrial and venous pressures.

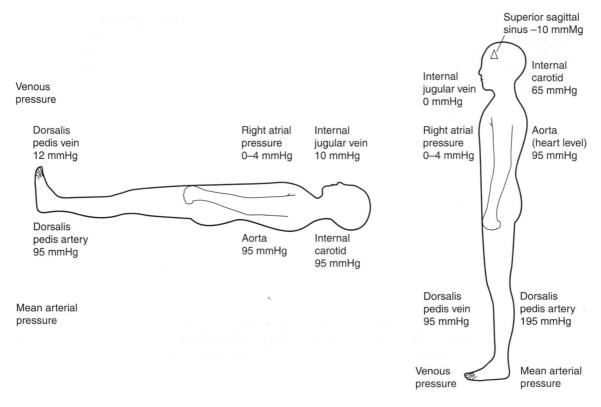

Figure 4.14 *The circulation and posture.*

Finally, the heart must be able to distend when venous return increases preload, and the pericardial sac, normally containing 20 mL fluid, must be loose. Any increase in pericardial fluid volume, from either ventricular leakage or effusion, will restrict ventricular filling, as will constrictive pericardial fibrosis.

CONTROL OF BLOOD PRESSURE

Blood pressure is the force exerted per unit area of vessel wall. In arteries it is pulsatile and varies between 100 and 130 mmHg systolic and 70 and 90 mmHg diastolic, although many factors may cause these figures to vary. Homeostasis is maintained to permit normal flow through vascular beds, and in the supine position, arterial pressure is approximately the same in all regional circuits. As noted earlier, blood pressure is the product of cardiac output and peripheral resistance and any change in these will affect it.

Short-term control

Blood pressure may be influenced by changes in posture as well as by the Valsalva manoeuvre or straining. Arterial pressure is monitored by the baroreceptors present in the carotid and aortic sinuses (Folkow and Neil, 1971). These stretch receptors respond to pressure increase, but are also sensitive to both the average pressure and its rate of change (Covell, 1985). The afferent fibres start to transmit at a threshold of 50 mmHg, but do so minimally up to 70 mmHg, above which there is a linear relationship between pressure and the resultant decrease in heart rate. At 170 mmHg, the response is maximal.

The afferent fibres run in the glossopharyngeal and vagus nerves to the medulla where they synapse in the nucleus of the tractus solitarius and the nucleus ambiguus (Fig. 4.15). The latter has a cardioinhibitory role and supplies parasympathetic vagal efferents to the heart. The nucleus of the tractus solitarius has hypothalamic projections as well as

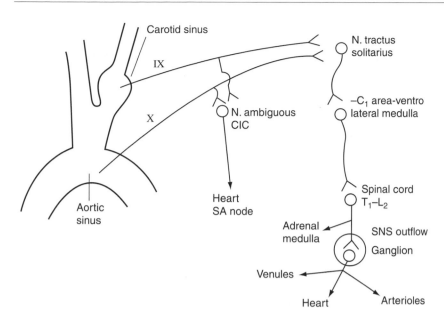

Figure 4.15 *The baroreceptor system. CIC, cardio-inhibitory centre; SNS, sympathetic nervous system.*

synapses with inhibitory interneurones which descend to the ventrolateral medulla at C_1 (the vasomotor centre). From there, fibres descend to the intermediolateral grey matter of the spinal cord from T_1 to L_2, with relays passing to the heart, adrenals, arterioles and venules. The system constantly sends out low-frequency impulses to the arterioles and venules to maintain peripheral resistance and prevent venous pooling, respectively.

An increase in arterial pressure produces activity in the glossopharyngeal and vagus nerves and stimulation of the nucleus ambiguus and the nucleus of the tractus solitarius. Activation of the former leads to bradycardia, and of the latter to a reduction in sympathetic activity by way of the inhibitory interneurone connections to C_1. Cardiac rate, contractility and output decrease, as does peripheral resistance. There is peripheral venous pooling and a decrease in venous return, so that blood pressure returns to normal within 10–20 s of the increase. The reverse set of events occurs when blood pressure decreases, as for example on assuming the erect posture. Vasomotor centre activity is also influenced by the hypothalamus in response to stimuli such as the emotions, pain and temperature changes. The chemoreceptors in the carotid and aortic bodies are stimulated by hypercapnia, hypoxia and acidosis mainly to affect respiration but also to produce vasoconstriction and tachycardia. Carbon dioxide depresses the isolated myocardium and dilates isolated arterioles, but these effects are overridden by the neural reflexes of the intact human subject. Thus hypercapnia, by producing vasomotor centre activation, increases sympathetic outflow so that heart rate and cardiac output increase as cutaneous, cerebral and coronary vessels dilate.

Long-term control

Longer-term influences are mediated through control of sodium, chloride and water balance by renin, angiotensin, aldosterone and antidiuretic hormone (ADH; vasopressin) (Miller, 1981). The total extracellular fluid (ECF) osmolarity is around 280 mosmol/L, with 96 per cent of this being due to sodium and its salts. Osmolarity is homeostatically regulated so that an increase produces water retention, and increased vascular volume, venous return, cardiac output and blood pressure.

The juxtaglomerular apparatus of the kidney consists of a portion of the afferent arteriole with some glomerular cells and the macula densa, a segment of the nephron at the junction of the ascending limb of the loop of Henle with the distal convoluted tubule. Renin is secreted from the myoepithelial cells of the afferent arteriole in response to afferent arteriolar hypotension, reduced sodium concentration at the macula densa, sympathetic stimulation and reduced stimulation of the atrial volume receptors (Davis and Freeman, 1976). Renin cleaves the hepatically produced globulin angiotensinogen to yield the decapeptide angiotensin I, which is converted to the octapeptide angiotensin II by angiotensin converting enzyme mainly in the lung.

Angiotensin II is a potent constrictor of skin, splanchnic and skeletal muscle arterioles, and acts at angiotensin receptors. It is also a venoconstrictor.

Additionally, angiotensin stimulates thirst and the release of catecholamines from the adrenal medulla, ADH from the posterior pituitary and aldosterone from the adrenal cortex. Aldosterone increases sodium, chloride and bicarbonate reabsorption from the distal convoluted tubule and the collecting duct of the kidney in exchange for potassium and hydrogen ions, which are secreted. The retention of sodium, chloride and bicarbonate promotes hypothalamic osmoreceptors to stimulate the release of ADH from the posterior pituitary in addition to the direct effect of angiotensin II. ADH increases water reabsorption from the collecting ducts and osmolarity returns to normal. So ECF and plasma volumes, venous pressure, cardiac output and blood pressure increase. It takes about 20 minutes from renin release for aldosterone to become functional at the distal nephron.

Vascular volume is sensed by the type B atrial stretch receptors stimulated by increased venous pressure during atrial filling. Vagal afferent impulses travel via the medullary cardiovascular centres to the hypothalamus so that thirst and ADH secretion are reduced. In addition, sympathetic efferent activity decreases to produce vasodilatation. Renal blood flow and glomerular filtration rate increase, renin secretion declines and reduced aldosterone levels decrease sodium, chloride and water reabsorption by the kidney. Loss of sodium and water from the kidney is enhanced by the natriuretic peptide released from the myocytes on atrial distension (Lange *et al.*, 1985). It causes vasodilatation, renal sodium, chloride and water loss, and inhibits the renin–angiotensin–aldosterone system. ECF and plasma volumes decrease. Arteriolar dilatation raises capillary hydrostatic pressure and fluid transfers to the interstitium.

The reverse of these changes occurs when blood volume decreases (Gauer and Henry, 1976).

ORGAN BLOOD FLOW

In a specific organ,

$$\text{Flow} = \frac{(\text{Arterial pressure} - \text{Venous pressure})}{\text{Vascular resistance}}$$

with local vascular resistance having extravascular as well as intravascular components. For example, intracranial pressure compresses cerebral vessels, and contraction does the same in skeletal and cardiac muscle.

Coronary circulation

The heart is unique in that it supplies itself with blood and its perfusion declines in systole. Myocardial metabolism is mainly aerobic and coronary blood oxygen extraction is almost maximal at rest. Glycolysis is hardly used as an energy source. In cardiac muscle, myoglobin acts as a small reservoir for oxygen supply to mitochondria under hypoxic conditions. The dissociation curve of myoglobin lies to the left of that of haemoglobin, so it has a greater affinity for oxygen. It takes up oxygen from the capillaries and transfers it to the mitochondria where the P_{O_2} is much lower.

The coronary arteries are the first branches of the aorta and run around the outside of the heart. The vessels derived from them pass from epicardial to endocardial surface and give rise to arterioles and capillaries. Venous drainage is via the coronary sinus, coronary veins or venae cordae minimi directly into a ventricle. The coronary blood flow is 250 mL/min at rest, and can increase to 1.5 L/min during exercise, but it is not constant. Flow varies through the cardiac cycle, with the subendocardial parts of the left ventricle being particularly susceptible to the effects of extraneous compression.

During isometric ventricular contraction, coronary blood flow declines rapidly, increases somewhat during systolic ejection because aortic pressure increases, but decreases again late in systole. The flow increases again during isometric ventricular relaxation, and peaks during early diastole. Systolic coronary flow is 15–60 per cent that of diastolic. An adequate diastolic pressure is thus important for left ventricular perfusion, but any increase in left ventricular end diastolic pressure will increase intramural tension and may reduce flow. Right ventricular flow peaks during both systole and diastole, because vessel compression is less on the lower pressure side of the heart.

The coronary arterioles possess both α- and β-receptors, but sympathetic stimulation generally produces vasodilatation, perhaps because increased cardiac activity leads to accumulation of vasodilator metabolites. Coronary flow is autoregulated between 60 and 150 mmHg, decreases below 60 mmHg, and is linearly related to perfusion pressure above 150 mmHg (Mosher *et al.*, 1964). Because oxygen extraction is maximal at rest, any increase in oxygen supply must be met by an increase in coronary flow which is usually linearly related to oxygen consumption. If the myocardium is hypoxic, ADP accumulates and is converted to adenosine by 5'-nucleotidase on the sarcolemma of muscle cells. Adenosine then dilates the coronary vessels to increase blood flow and thus oxygen delivery (Berne and Rubio, 1979). Local acidosis, hypercarbia and potassium also dilate these vessels.

Cerebral circulation

The cerebral circulation is supplied by the internal carotid and vertebral arteries. The two vertebral arteries unite to form the basilar artery which links to the two internal carotids at the circle of Willis, from which specific vessels supply the brain. Venous drainage is by superficial and deep veins into dural sinuses and then into the internal jugular veins. Flow is relatively constant at around 750 mL/min (54 ml/100 g/min), regardless of posture or exercise, and ischaemic symptoms develop if the flow is less than 40 per cent of normal, the brain requiring 45 mL of oxygen per minute.

Cerebral perfusion pressure (CPP) = MAP − ICP,

where MAP is mean arterial pressure and ICP is intracranial pressure. Although α-adrenoceptors which mediate vasoconstriction are present in the cerebral vessels, their effect is weak and autoregulation is all important, flow varying little at CPP between 50 and 130 mmHg. Normally, blood flow decreases only when CPP is less than 50 mmHg, but in hypertension the autoregulation curve is shifted to the right, so that ischaemia is more likely at a higher pressure if hypotension occurs, as for example during haemorrhage.

CPP is normally about 85 mmHg in the horizontal position. On standing, both the arterial and venous pressures decreases (as does the intracranial pressure) so that perfusion pressure is relatively unchanged. In addition, arterial hypotension activates baroreceptor reflexes to increase heart rate and blood pressure, thus helping to maintain cerebral blood flow in the face of postural changes. The internal jugular pressure may decrease from 10 mmHg to zero, and the vessels col-

lapse, but the dural sinuses have rigid walls which cannot collapse, so the pressure within them can become subatmospheric. Pressure in the superior sagittal sinus is approximately −10 mmHg in the upright position and this acts as a syphon, drawing blood into the venous circulation. A mean arterial pressure below 50 mmHg leads to a decrease in cerebral blood flow and causes ischaemia. Hypoxia and hypercapnia activate the sympathetic nervous system to restore blood pressure to normal. Ischaemia for 3–5 minutes produces neuronal death.

Cerebral vascular resistance is controlled by intra- and extravascular factors. Because this circulation lies within the rigid skull, the volume of the brain, blood and CSF must remain constant (Monro-Kellie doctrine). If the volume of any one of the constituents increases, there must be a corresponding reduction in the other two. Intracranial pressure (ICP) is about 10 mmHg in the supine position, but decreases on standing as CSF transfers to the spinal theca. This ICP change is another factor maintaining perfusion if hypotension occurs on standing up. An intracranial mass will, initially, compress adjacent cerebral structures and displace venous blood and CSF extracranially. However, once these initial compensatory mechanisms have reached their limit, ICP increases. At a critical ICP of about 33 mmHg, cerebral blood flow decreases and the brain becomes hypoxic and hypercapnic. This stimulates the vasomotor centre and causes widespread vasoconstriction, the coronary and cerebral circulations excepted. Systemic hypertension follows, stimulates the baroreceptors and results in bradycardia. This reaction to ICP increase is known as the Cushing response (Ganong, 1997).

Pulmonary circulation

The pulmonary circulation is a low-pressure system, with the pulmonary vascular resistance being one-tenth of the systemic vascular resistance. Normal pulmonary arterial pressure is 25/10 mmHg (mean 15 mmHg) and lung perfusion pressure is mean pulmonary artery pressure minus pulmonary venous pressure (15 − 6 mmHg = 9 mmHg). Extravascular resistance is provided by the alveoli which compress the pulmonary capillaries lining the alveoli and affect flow through them (West, 1974).

In the upright position, blood flow increases from apex to base because of gravity. The pulmonary artery enters the lung at its middle position and the pressure decreases by 0.77 mmHg/cm vertical height above this level, and similarly increases below it. Alveolar pressure varies between -1 mmHg on inspiration and $+1$ mmHg on expiration. Thus in the erect position the apex of the lung receives blood only at peak systolic pressure and during inspiration. This is because the alveolar pressure, which is relatively high in the apex, resists flow by extraneous compression of the capillaries. Blood flow to this area further decreases during pharmacological hypotension or haemorrhage. In the mid-zone, alveolar pressure is the same, but arterial pressure is higher and exceeds alveolar pressure. The flow is thus influenced by the arterio-alveolar pressure difference. In the base, venous pressure is above alveolar pressure and flow is due to the arteriovenous pressure difference. In the supine position, flow is greatest posteriorly, again because of gravity.

As pulmonary blood flow increases, so pulmonary vascular resistance decreases because of passive vasodilatation and recruitment of additional vessels, internal pressure exceeding critical closing pressure. Inspiration also decreases vascular resistance because the vessels are pulled open by radial traction from the surrounding elastic fibres. However, at very high lung volumes, resistance increases. The microcirculation is compressible and the capillaries become stretched and narrowed. Sympathetic stimulation has a weak effect on the pulmonary circulation, although receptors in the pulmonary arterioles can mediate vasoconstriction. However, an alveolar PO_2 of less than 9.3 kPa has a direct vasoconstrictor effect on pulmonary arterioles (the hypoxic pressor response) which is potentiated by acidosis. This diverts blood away from unventilated alveoli to reduce shunt (West, 1985).

Renal circulation

The renal arteries divide progressively into smaller vessels which eventually give rise to the interlobular arteries of the cortex. From these, the afferent arterioles branch and then split into a cluster of parallel capillaries called a 'glomerulus'. Each glomerulus invaginates the Bowman's capsule of a nephron, the blood draining from the glomerulus into an efferent arteriole which leads to a second, peritubular set of capillaries, surrounding the proximal and distal convoluted tubules of the nephron. These capillaries

drain into tributaries of the renal vein. The efferent arterioles of those nephrons which are juxtamedullary in position give rise to the vasa recta which descend into the medulla to surround the loops of Henle prior to draining into the interlobular veins.

Renal blood flow is around 1–1.2 L/min, being controlled by factors affecting the arteriovenous pressure difference and the renal vascular resistance. Blood flow is autoregulated and varies less than 10 per cent between systolic pressures of 80 and 180 mmHg. This keeps glomerular hydrostatic pressure near 45 mmHg so that a constant salt and water load is delivered to the nephrons (Shipley and Stady, 1951). An increase in blood pressure produces afferent arteriolar constriction through the myogenic response to stretch, and the reverse occurs when blood pressure decreases, but neural and humoral effects may override this autoregulation. Sympathetic vasoconstrictor fibres supply both afferent and efferent arterioles of cortical nephrons, and the efferent arterioles of the juxtamedullary nephrons. Mild sympathetic stimulation, as occurs in posture-induced changes in activity, causes efferent arteriolar constriction at both cortical and juxtamedullary nephrons to maintain glomerular capillary pressure and glomerular flow rate in the presence of reduced renal blood flow. Greater degrees of hypotension result in the recruitment of the afferent vessels as part of the whole-body response to maintain peripheral resistance. Reduced atrial volume receptor stimulation also produces this effect. The blood is diverted more to the juxtamedullary nephrons because their afferent arterioles are less sensitive to sympathetic stimuli.

Skin circulation

The primary determinant of skin blood flow is not its own metabolic requirement, but the body's need to lose or preserve heat. Pyrexia causes the hypothalamus to decrease sympathetic outflow, the skin vessels dilate and heat is lost by conduction, convection and radiation. Increased blood flow is also needed for sweat production. The reverse occurs when body temperature decreases.

Liver and gastrointestinal circulation

The liver receives its blood supply from the hepatic artery and the portal vein (300 and 1000 mL/min, respectively), the latter draining blood from the intestinal tract between lower oesophagus and rectum, as well as from the pancreas and spleen. Portal blood mixes with that from the hepatic artery in the hepatic sinusoids, which drain into the central veins, the hepatic veins and the inferior vena cava. The liver receives 25–30 per cent of cardiac output and uses 20 per cent of the body's oxygen consumption at rest, 60 per cent of this coming from the portal vein and 40 per cent from the hepatic artery. However, the hepatic artery provides more during digestion because portal venous oxygen saturation decreases when the bowel is active. The bowel receives blood from the coeliac, superior and inferior mesenteric arteries.

The portal vein and its radicals (as well as the hepatic arterioles) have smooth muscle in their walls which are supplied by sympathetic fibres acting through α-adrenoceptors. During stimulation, vasoconstriction occurs and portal pressure rises (Jacobson and Lanciault, 1979). Up to 350 mL blood may be 'transfused' into the general circulation.

REFERENCES

Bainbridge, F.A. 1915. The influence of venous filling upon the rate of the heart. *Journal of Physiology* **50**, 65–84.

Berne, R.M. and Rubio R. 1979. Coronary circulation. In Berne, R.M. (ed.), *Handbook of physiology, Section 2*, Vol.1, Chapter 1, Washington DC: American Physiological Society, 873–952.

Covell, J.W. 1985. Cardiovascular control and integrated responses. In West, J.B. (ed.), *Best and Taylor's physiological basis of medical practice*, 11th edn, Chapter 16, Baltimore: Williams and Wilkins, 263-283.

Davis, J.O. and Freeman R.H. 1976. Mechanisms regulating renin release. *Physiological Review* **56**, 1–56.

de Bold, A.J., Borenstein, H.B., Veress, A.T. and Sonnenberg, H. 1981. A rapid and potent natriuretic response to intravenous injection of atrial myocardial extract in rats. *Life Sciences* **28**, 89–94.

Fabiato, A. and Fabiato, F. 1979. Calcium and cardiac excitation–contraction coupling. *Annual Review of Physiology* **41**, 473–484.

Feelisch, M. 1991. The biochemical pathways of nitric oxide formation from nitrovasodilators: appropriate choice of NO donors and aspects of preparation and handling of aqueous NO solutions. *Journal of Cardiovascular Pharmacology* **17** (Suppl. 3), S25–S33.

Folkow, B. and Neil, E. 1971. *Circulation*. New York: Oxford University Press.

Freeman, J. and Nunn, J.F. 1963. Ventilation–perfusion relationships after haemorrhage. *Clinical Science* **24**, 135–147.

Ganong, W.F. 1997. Circulation through special regions. *Review of medical physiology*, 18th. edn, Chapter 32. Norwalk, CT: Appleton & Lange, 567–585.

Gauer, O.H. and Henry, J.P. 1976. Neurohormonal control of plasma volume. In Guyton, A.C. and Cowley, A.P (eds), *International review of physiology: cardiovascular physiology II*, Vol. 9. Chapter 4. Baltimore, MD: University Park Press, 145–190.

Gibbs, C.L. and Chapman, J.B. 1979. Cardiac energetics. In Berne, R.M. (ed.), *Handbook of physiology, Section 2*, Vol. 1, Chapter 22. Washington DC: American Physiological Society, 775–804.

Guyton, A.C., Cowley, A.W., Young, D.B. *et al.* 1976. Integration and control of circulatory function. In Guyton, A.C. and Cowley, A.W. (eds), *International review of physiology: cardiovascular physiology II*, Vol. 9, Chapter 9. Baltimore, MD: University Park Press, 341–385.

Haddy, F.J. and Scott, J.B. 1977. Active hyperaemia, reactive hyperaemia and autoregulation of blood flow. In Kaley, G. and Altura, B.M. (eds), *Microcirculation*, Vol. 2. Baltimore, MD: University Park Press.

Hamilton, W.F. 1955. The role of the Starling concept in regulation of the normal circulation. *Physiological Review* **35**, 161–168.

Hansen, J. and Lang, J. 1965. Molecular basis of contractility in muscle. *British Medical Bulletin* **21**, 264–271.

Harrington, W.F. 1979. Contractile proteins of muscle. In Neurath, H. and Hill, R.L. (eds), *The proteins*, 3rd edn, Vol. IV, Chapter 3. New York: Academic Press, 245–409.

Jacobson, E.O. and Lanciault, G. 1979. The gastrointestinal vasculature. In Duthie, H.L. and Wormslie, K.G. (eds), *Scientific basis of gastroenterology*, Chapter 2. Edinburgh: Churchill Livingstone, 26–48.

Johansson, B. and Somlyo, A.P. 1980. Electrophysiology and excitation–contraction coupling. In Bohr, D.F., Somlyo, A.P. and Sparks, H.V. (eds), *Handbook of physiology, Section 2*, Vol. II, Chapter 12. Bethesda, MD: American Physiological Society, 301–323.

Johnsson, P.C. 1980. The role of intravascular pressure in regulation of the microcirculation. In Novacs, A.G.B., Hamar, J. and Szabo, L. (eds), *Advances in physiological science*, Vol. 7. Budapest: Pergamon Press, 17–34.

Jose, A.D., Stitt, F. and Collison, D. 1970. The effects of exercise and changes in body temperature on the intrinsic heart rate in man. *American Heart Journal* **79**, 488–498.

Kirchenberger, M.A. and Schwartz, I.L. 1985. Excitation and contraction of skeletal muscle. In West, J.B. (ed.), *Best and Taylor's physiological basis of medical practice*, Chapter 4. Baltimore, MD: Williams and Wilkins, 58–106.

Lange, R.E., Tholken, H., Ganten, D. *et al.* 1985. Atrial natriuretic factor: a circulating hormone stimulated by volume loading. *Nature* **314**, 264–266.

Langer, G.A. 1968. Ion fluxes in cardiac excitation and contraction and their relation to myocardial contractility. *Physiological Review* **48**, 708–757.

Leigh, J.M. 1974. Oxygen therapy at ambient pressure. In Scurr, C. and Feldman, S. (eds), *Scientific foundations of anaesthesia*, Chapter 5. London: Heinemann, 253–262.

McDonald, D.A. 1960. *Blood flow in arteries*. London: Edward Arnold.

Miller, E.D. 1981. The role of the renin angiotensin aldosterone system in circulatory control and in hypertension. *British Journal of Anaesthesia* **53**, 711–718.

Moncada, S. 1992. The L-arginine:nitric oxide pathway. *Acta Physiologica Scandinavica* **145**, 201–227.

Moracev, C.S., Reynolds, E.E., Stewart, R.W. and Bond, M. 1989. Endothelin is a positive inotropic agent in human and rat heart *in vitro*. *Biochemical and Biophysical Research Communications* **159**, 14–18.

Mosher, P., Ross, J., McFate, P.A. and Shaw, R.F. 1964. Control of coronary blood flow by an autoregulatory mechanism. *Circulation Research* **14**, 250–259.

Nichol, J., Girling, F., Jerard, W. *et al.* 1951. Fundamental instability of the small blood vessels and critical closing pressures in vascular beds. *American Journal of Physiology* **164**, 330–344.

Nicholls, M.G. 1994. The natriuretic peptide hormones. *Journal of Internal Medicine* **235**, 507–514.

Nunn, J.F. 1977. Oxygen. In *Applied respiratory physiology*, 2nd edn, Chapter 12. London: Butterworths, 375–444.

Palmer, R.M.J., Ashton, D.S. and Moncada, S. 1988. Vascular endothelial cells synthesise nitric oxide from L-arginine. *Nature* **333**, 664–666.

Radomski, M.W. and Moncada, S. 1991. Biological role of nitric oxide in platelet function. In Moncada, S., Higgs, E.A. and Berrazueta, J.R. (eds), *Clinical relevance of nitric oxide in the cardiovascular system*. Madrid: Edicomplet, 45–46.

Ross, J. 1985. Electrical impulse formation and conduction in the heart. In West, J.B. (ed.), *Best and Taylor's physiological basis of medical practice*, 11th edn, Chapter 8. Baltimore, MD: Williams and Wilkins, 148–162.

Sagawa, K. 1978. The ventricular pressure–volume diagram revisited. *Circulation Research* **43**, 677–687.

Sagimoto, T., Sagawa, K. and Guyton, A.C. 1966. Effect of tachycardia on cardiac output during normal and increased venous return. *American Journal of Physiology* **211**, 288–292.

Schini, V.B. and Vanhoutte, P.M. 1991. ET-1: a potent vasoactive peptide. *Pharmacology and Toxicology* **69**, 303–309.

Shipley, R.E. and Stady, R.S. 1951. Changes in renal blood flow, extraction of inulin, GFR, tissue pressure and urine flow with acute alterations of renal artery pressure. *American Journal of Physiology* **167**, 676–688.

Somner, J.R. and Johnson, E.A. 1979. Ultrastructure of cardiac muscle. In Berne, R.M. (ed.), *Handbook of physiology*, Section 2, Vol. 1, Chapter 5. Washington, DC: American Physiological Society, 113–186.

Stainsby, W.N. 1962. Autoregulation of blood flow in skeletal muscle during increased metabolic activity. *American Journal of Physiology* **202**, 273–276.

Starling, E.H. 1918. The Linacre Lecture on the Law of the Heart. Given at Cambridge, 1915. London: Longman's Green.

Vassalle, M. 1977. Cardiac automaticity and its control. *American Journal of Physiology* **233**, H625–H634.

Waldman, S.A. and Murad, F. 1988. Biochemical mechanisms underlying vascular smooth muscle relaxation: the guanylate cyclase-cyclic GMP system. *Journal of Cardiovascular Pharmacology* **12**, Suppl. 5, S115–S118.

West, J.B. 1974. Blood flow. In *Respiratory physiology: the essentials*, Chapter 4. Baltimore: Williams and Wilkins, 33–50.

West, J.B. 1985. Uptake and delivery of respiratory gases. In West, J.B. (ed.), *Best and Taylor's physiological basis of medical practice*, 11th edn, Chapter 36. Baltimore: Williams and Wilkins, 546–571.

Wiggers, C.J. 1952. *Circulatory dynamics*. New York: Grune & Stratton.

5

Cardiovascular dysfunction

PIERRE FOËX AND S J HOWELL

INTRODUCTION

The major aspects of cardiovascular dysfunction considered in this chapter include myocardial ischaemia, arterial hypertension and the effects of drug therapy. In addition, the implications of left ventricular failure will be considered.

MYOCARDIAL ISCHAEMIA

For many years, it was thought that myocardial ischaemia resulted almost exclusively from an imbalance between myocardial oxygen demand and myocardial oxygen supply. Because myocardial oxygen extraction is almost maximal at all times, any increase in oxygen demand has to be matched by a commensurate increase in oxygen supply, but while the coronary arteries are normal, even very large changes in oxygen requirement can be met by increases in blood flow. The main determinants of flow in normal coronary arteries are the aortic diastolic pressure, left ventricular end-diastolic pressure, duration of diastole and the ability of the coronary arteries to dilate. Because coronary vasodilatory capacity is large, flow reserve is of the order of six-fold and blood supply can be maintained at a level that matches the oxygen requirements over a very wide range of haemodynamic situations (Opie, 1991). Thus, even the combination of hypertension (increased demand) and tachycardia (reduced duration of diastolic perfusion) is tolerated during maximum exercise.

However, when the coronary arteries are narrowed, the flow reserve is reduced and haemodynamic aberrations may cause acute myocardial ischaemia. Tachycardia is poorly tolerated because of the reduction in the duration of diastole which impairs diastolic coronary flow. Hypertension is also poorly tolerated. The increase in diastolic pressure leads to an increase in coronary flow and oxygen delivery, but this is exceeded by the greater oxygen demand because of increased systolic wall stress. When hypertension is associated with tachycardia, the imbalance between oxygen demand and oxygen supply is worse than with hypertension alone. Also, in effort angina coronary blood flow may increase, but as its velocity increases across the stenosis, the pressure drop is accentuated (Brown et al., 1984) and subendocardial perfusion worsens. Hypotension compromises the oxygen supply more than it reduces oxygen demand because a low diastolic pressure causes an excessive reduction of the coronary perfusion pressure. Again, the combination of hypotension and tachycardia is worse than hypotension alone. Acute increases in left ventricular diastolic

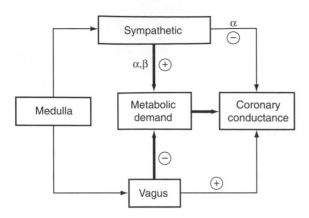

Figure 5.1 *Schematic representation of the effects of autonomic activity on coronary conductance. Direct effects (thin arrows) are usually overshadowed by the effects on metabolic demand. α and β denote α and β adrenoceptor-mediated effects.*

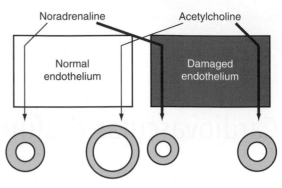

Figure 5.2 *Diagrammatic representation of the effects of noradrenaline and acetylcholine on the calibre of arterioles when the endothelium is intact (thin arrows) and when it is damaged (thick arrows). Endothelial damage increases the vasoconstriction caused by noradrenaline, while it replaces by vasoconstriction the vasodilatation normally caused by acetylcholine.*

pressure decrease coronary blood flow at a time when diastolic wall stress and myocardial oxygen demand are augmented. Many episodes of myocardial ischaemia result from haemodynamic aberrations such as these, but it is now recognized that ischaemia may occur in their absence (Slogoff and Keats, 1985). This suggests that myocardial oxygen supply may be decreased by non-haemodynamic factors.

It is now recognized that changes in coronary vascular tone do not occur exclusively as a consequence of local metabolism (local regulation) and that they also occur in response to changes in autonomic nervous system activity (Fig. 5.1) (Baumgart *et al.*, 1995). Under most circumstances changes in sympathetic or parasympathetic activity cause their major coronary effect through changes in oxygen demand. Coronary blood flow is then adjusted by local regulation. Sympathetic activation has inotropic, chronotropic and vasomotor effects which increase oxygen demand and, therefore, coronary blood flow. Where metabolic demand is controlled, α-adrenoceptor-mediated coronary vasoconstriction is uncovered (Young *et al.*, 1990). Similarly, parasympathetic activation slows the heart, decreases blood pressure, reduces oxygen demand and, therefore, coronary blood flow (Reid *et al.*, 1985). Again, it is only where metabolic demand is controlled, that acetylcholine-mediated vasodilatation becomes apparent.

The endothelium plays a very important role in the regulation of coronary blood flow because it synthesizes and releases a number of mediators which alter vascular tone (van Hinsberg, 1992; Bassenge *et al.*, 1995). When the endothelium is damaged, the effects of autonomic nervous system activity are modified. The vasoconstriction caused by noradrenaline is more pronounced when the endothelium is damaged than when it is intact because noradrenaline stimulates the production of nitric oxide, a coronary vasodilator. For acetylcholine, the role of endothelial integrity is even more important because the vasodilator effect of acetylcholine is apparent only when the endothelium is capable of synthesizing nitric oxide. Where the endothelium is damaged, acetylcholine causes vasoconstriction. The presence of endothelial damage, a feature of coronary atheromatosis, may therefore exaggerate the effects of sympathetic activity (vasoconstriction) and reverse the effects of parasympathetic activity (vasoconstriction instead of vasodilatation) (Fig. 5.2). This may create a situation where modest changes in autonomic nervous system activity cause marked changes in coronary blood flow even though global haemodynamics are little altered.

In the presence of endothelial damage, the release of local mediators such as nitric oxide or prostacyclin may also be altered so that less vasodilatation occurs than in normal conditions. Similarly, endothelial dysfunction may result in excess release of thromboxane A_2 or of endothelins resulting in inappropriate vasoconstriction. Such local imbalances between vasodilator and vasoconstrictor agencies may explain why ischaemia can occur in the absence of gross haemodynamic aberrations. This is made more likely as vascular stenoses may not be fixed but dynamic. This means that part of the vessel wall is still anatomically intact and remains responsive to agencies which alter vascular smooth muscle tone. In a dynamic stenosis small changes in vascular tone may cause large changes in flow.

Pathophysiology of coronary disease

Ischaemic heart disease results from coronary atherosclerosis, a focal intimal disease which starts with fatty streaks and evolves into a raised fibrolipid plaque. Many plaques are situated eccentrically and a regional area of normal vessel persists opposite the plaque resulting in a dynamic stenosis. Although arteries may remodel themselves, the lumen is usually compromised and the plaque causes a limitation of blood flow. Clinical symptoms may result from flow reduction (see above) and also from local thrombosis.

Of special interest to anaesthetists are the possible implications of a distribution of coronary artery lesions termed 'steal-prone' anatomy (Buffington *et al.*, 1988). This is defined by the presence of the occlusion of one coronary artery, the stenosis of another and collaterals between these vessels. Such features have been found in approximately 25 per cent of patients with angiographically documented coronary artery disease. Where 'steal-prone' anatomy is present, there is the risk of myocardial ischaemia when a dilator of the coronary resistance vessels is administered. This may be relevant to agents such as isoflurane (Buffington *et al.*, 1987; Priebe and Foëx, 1987; Cutfield *et al.*, 1988), desflurane (Hartman *et al.*, 1992), and sevoflurane (Harkin *et al.*, 1994). However, the importance of the 'steal-prone' anatomy has been questioned (Leung *et al.*, 1992).

Thrombosis may occur because of either endothelial damage over the plaque or the presence of microfissures. In response to thrombus formation, there is local smooth muscle proliferation and replacement by collagen tissue. Plaques that undergo thrombosis are unstable, and there is an increased risk of further thrombosis and/or occlusion.

Effect of ischaemia

The objective effects of ischaemia include four categories: electrical; mechanical; biochemical/hormonal; and ultrastructural.

ELECTROPHYSIOLOGICAL EFFECTS

Ischaemia causes potassium and chloride ions to leak across the myocyte causing an imbalance of electrical potentials at the boundaries between ischaemic and non-ischaemic tissue. This causes a current to flow from injured to non-injured tissue during repolarization, and from non-injured to injured tissue during depolarization, such currents being seen as ST-segment changes on the electrocardiogram (ECG). Another important effect is the establishment of re-entry circuits leading to ventricular arrhythmias and possibly ventricular fibrillation. Re-entry occurs because a conduction delay in the ischaemic area makes it possible for currents to reach recently repolarized myocardial fibres.

MECHANICAL EFFECTS

Regional myocardial ischaemia reduces the amount of shortening and thickening of the affected segments (hypokinesia, akinesia) and can cause paradoxical lengthening and thinning (dyskinesia). While a reduction of coronary flow by 10–20 per cent is sufficient to reduce systolic shortening, abolition of wall motion requires an 80 per cent, and paradoxical wall motion a 95 per cent, reduction of flow (Vatner *et al.*, 1980). Post-systolic shortening is a type of dyskinesia which has been well described (Lowenstein *et al.*, 1981) and is a marker of potential recovery after reperfusion (Takayama *et al.*, 1988).

BIOCHEMICAL AND HORMONAL EFFECTS

Leakage of potassium ions is the first recordable metabolic abnormality of myocardial ischaemia and represents impairment of an energy-requiring ion pump. In the later stages of ischaemia, plasma catecholamine levels are elevated and this causes potassium to enter the cells and produce hypokalaemia. The latter is associated with ventricular arrhythmias. In the absence of oxygen, pyruvate is produced and reduced to lactate, because production of high-energy phosphates then depends upon anaerobic glycolysis. The accumulation of lactate lowers intracellular pH and excess lactate spills over into the coronary sinus blood. Macromolecules, including myocardial enzymes, myosin and troponins, are released by severely injured cells and used clinically as markers of cell injury.

ULTRASTRUCTURAL DAMAGE

This predominates at the subendocardium and is usually patchy because of the variable and patchy nature of collateral blood flow.

Recovery from ischaemia

The success of thrombolytic therapy has brought reperfusion to the forefront. Thrombolysis reduces mortality and improves left ventricular function in survivors. However, reperfusion does not mean immediate recovery of function. Usually a state of temporary depression of function termed 'stunning' is observed (Braunwald and Kloner, 1982). This is generally attributed to injury caused by oxygen free radicals. Recovery may be delayed for several weeks.

Myocardial hibernation

In this state, the hypoperfused myocardium stops contracting so that its energy requirements are greatly reduced, but it remains viable so that function returns when the myocardium is reperfused (Rahimtoola, 1989).

High-risk coronary disease

Patients with previous myocardial infarction are five to ten times more likely to suffer post-operative re-infarction than patients without this history. For many years, the major risk factor was thought to be the delay between previous infarction and surgery. From studies published in the early seventies, it was estimated that surgery within three months of a previous infarction carried an almost 40 per cent risk of re-infarction (Tarhan et al., 1972; Steen et al., 1978). However, in more recent years it has been thought that invasive monitoring and aggressive management of haemodynamic aberration during the peri-operative period will reduce this risk very substantially (Rao et al., 1983, Shah et al., 1990) (Table 5.1). This improvement in post-operative morbidity has many causes, one of which is the better anaesthetic management of patients with ischaemic heart disease, with this including maintenance of drug therapy throughout the peri-operative period. Another is the management of myocardial infarction itself.

Table 5.1 *Risk of post-operative re-infarction*

Elapsed time	Tarhan et al. (1972)	Steen et al. (1978)	Rao et al. (1983)	Shah et al. (1990)
< 3 months	37%	27%	6%	4%
4–6 months	16%	11%	2%	0%
> 6 months	7%	4%	1.5%	6%

When the early studies were published, there was no treatment for myocardial infarction other than rest, a far cry from the current situation with thrombolysis, early coronary angiography, angioplasty and coronary bypass surgery all available.

However, the consequences of a previous infarction must also be taken into consideration. Transient left ventricular failure, impaired left ventricular function, presence of a ventricular aneurysm, and dysrhythmias all indicate a higher risk of cardiovascular complications of anaesthesia and surgery. The risk of complications remains high when such sequelae have been observed, irrespective of the delay that has elapsed since the previous infarction. Mortality of emergency surgery has been shown to relate to the presence, at any time, of left ventricular failure, rather than to the time since previous myocardial infarction (Dirksen and Kjøller, 1988). It has also been clearly demonstrated that a patient with a low ejection fraction is much more at risk of peri-operative infarction than one with normal left ventricular function (Pasternack et al., 1984).

While body surface surgery carries a relatively low risk of re-infarction, intrathoracic, intra-abdominal, and vascular surgery all carry a much greater risk, especially if surgery is prolonged. When considering patients with previous infarction, it is important to take into consideration all three factors: time that has elapsed since infarction, the type of surgery to be undertaken, and the consequences of the previous infarction.

Patients suffering from well-controlled, stable angina have a relatively low risk of post-operative infarction, while patients with disabling angina are at a high risk (Johnston and Scobie, 1988). In patients with unstable angina or disabling angina, detailed pre-operative assessment is essential and it is almost imperative to obtain a coronary angiogram with a view to coronary angioplasty and possible coronary stenting or bypass surgery. The experience of the last decade is that after successful coronary artery bypass surgery, the risk of peri-operative cardiac complications is significantly lower than in patients who have not benefited from revascularization procedures (Foster *et al.*, 1986; Gersh *et al.*, 1991; Eagle *et al.*, 1997). If the coronary lesions are not amenable to reperfusion measures, medical treatment should be optimized in the hope of minimizing the risk of adverse cardiac outcome.

The role of silent myocardial ischaemia during the peri-operative period has been emphasized in a number of American studies. Silent myocardial ischaemia (SMI) was recognized about forty years ago (Holter, 1961). It is similar to symptomatic myocardial ischaemia in all respects except that it does not cause pain. It may occur in totally asymptomatic patients (type 1 SMI), in patients with previous myocardial infarction (type 2 SMI) and in patients with angina (type 3 SMI). In the latter group, 75–90 per cent of all episodes of ischaemia may be silent (Deanfield *et al.*, 1983; Egstrup, 1988). Several studies in surgical patients have shown an association between silent ischaemia and major peri-operative adverse outcomes including cardiac death, myocardial infarction, new angina, unstable angina and left ventricular failure (Raby *et al.*, 1989; Ouyang *et al.*, 1989; Mangano *et al.*, 1990; McCann and Clements, 1991; Raby *et al.*, 1992). Post-operative silent ischaemia often precedes cardiac complications by several hours. A number of factors contribute to the development of post-operative silent ischaemia: tachycardia, increased coagulability and hypoxaemia. Indeed, several studies have shown an association between peri-operative (mostly) nocturnal hypoxaemia and silent ischaemia (Rosenberg *et al.*, 1990; Reeder *et al.*, 1991; Gill *et al.*, 1992).

As a result of studies demonstrating the relationship between peri-operative ischaemia and adverse outcome, several multicentre trials of the efficacy of peri-operative administration of drugs which can decrease ischaemia have been undertaken (Hollenberg *et al.*, 1994). Intensive analgesia (Mangano *et al.*, 1992), administration of the adenosine modulator acadesine (Leung *et al.*, 1994), or the α_2-adrenoceptor agonist dexmedetomidine (Talke *et al.*, 1995) appear to reduce the risk of silent ischaemia and adverse outcome. Stühmeier and colleagues have demonstrated a reduction in the incidence of intra-operative myocardial ischaemia with clonidine, but they did not find a statistically significant difference in the incidence of adverse events (Stühmeier *et al.*, 1996).

HYPERTENSIVE HEART DISEASE

All patients with arterial hypertension have either an increased contractile state or increased mass of vascular smooth muscle in arterioles and venules (Frohlich *et al.*, 1992). Systemic vascular resistance is increased while venous compliance is reduced. The causes of increased vascular tone include enhanced catecholamine output, increased release of angiotensin II, vasoactive intestinal peptide, endothelins and ions (calcium). The final common pathway for all these factors is an increased intracytoplasmic calcium concentration. In addition, growth factors contribute to increased smooth muscle mass (Dzau and Gibbons, 1991). The increased systemic vascular resistance causes left ventricular hypertrophy and dysfunction (Frohlich, 1991). Usually the intravascular volume is decreased and the interstitial fluid volume increased (Tarazi *et al.*, 1970).

Altered autonomic nervous function is a characteristic of hypertension. Baroreceptor sensitivity is reduced and there is both increased release of, and sensitivity to, noradrenaline. Responsiveness to catecholamines and to stressful stimuli is increased. The renin–angiotensin–aldosterone system is involved in renovascular hypertension and is suppressed in hyperaldosteronism. Patients with high plasma renin activity may be more likely to develop myocardial infarction (Alderman *et al.*, 1991).

Complications of hypertension

The most prominent cardiac alteration is left ventricular hypertrophy (LVH), which is necessary to overcome the excessive systemic vascular resistance (Frohlich *et al.*, 1992). Left ventricular hypertrophy impairs diastolic function, hence the atrial gallop rhythm (fourth heart sound). In the elderly, left ventricular failure may occur solely because of diastolic dysfunction, with systolic function being maintained. Left ventricular hypertrophy is an independent risk factor for sudden death and may also lead to end-stage renal failure. Renal damage must be suspected, especially if patients are anaemic. Myocardial ischaemia and myocardial infarction are also major complications of hypertension. Myocardial ischaemia is caused by the combination of excessive wall stress and co-existent atherosclerosis, because hypertension is a recognized accelerator of the latter (MacMahon *et al.*, 1990). Malignant hypertension has become less common thanks to better drug management, but the mortality remains extremely high if it is present. Stroke is also a major complication of hypertension, but the advent of antihypertensive therapy has substantially reduced the risk.

Treatment of hypertension

Blood pressure is the product of cardiac output and systemic vascular resistance, so all antihypertensive drugs must either reduce one or the other. The first stage of treatment includes moderate sodium restriction, plus weight reduction in the obese. When drug therapy is necessary, a diuretic is generally advocated first, although many practitioners use a β-adrenoceptor blocking agent (Raison *et al.*, 1986) or, more recently, an angiotensin-converting enzyme (ACE) inhibitor (Psaty *et al.*, 1993). In patients with overt coronary artery disease, there is a strong case for using a β-adrenoceptor-blocking agent as first-line treatment.

Recently, two problems have come to light. The first is the increased risk of sudden death in hypertensive patients taking non-potassium-sparing, as opposed to potassium-sparing, diuretics (Hoes *et al.*, 1995), an effect that appears to be dose-related (Siscovick *et al.*, 1994). The second is the increase in the risks of myocardial infarction in hypertensive patients treated with moderate or high doses of calcium channel-blocking agents (Psaty *et al.*, 1995). This effect is dose-related. Conversely, the risk of infarction is reduced by β-adrenoceptor blocking agents. With ACE inhibitors alone, the risk of infarction is the same as with diuretics alone, but their combination reduces it. Because the adverse effects of non-potassium-sparing diuretics and calcium channel-blocking agents are dose-related it makes sense to use only low doses and to combine them with other drugs if they prove ineffective as single medications. Two features of ACE inhibitors deserve special mention. The effect of the first dose can be quite dramatic in patients with high renin levels, and there is a risk of hyperkalaemia so they should not be given with potassium-sparing diuretics. Recently, angiotensin II receptor-blocking agents have been introduced. The rationale is that angiotensin II causes vasoconstriction which is implicated in essential hypertension, renal hypertension and the rare renin-secreting tumours. Losartan, a specific competitive inhibitor at the angiotensin-1 receptor (AT_1) is an effective hypotensive agent (Weber *et al.*, 1995), especially where combined with a diuretic (Brunner, 1995). Like ACE inhibitors, losartan may cause hyperkalaemia and, therefore, should not be used with a potassium-sparing diuretic (Dahløf *et al.*, 1995).

Alpha-2 adrenoceptor agonists have become of renewed relevance to anaesthesia. Clonidine and dexmedetomidine are effective in decreasing sympathetic outflow and, thereby, arterial pressure. What has also become clear is that clonidine minimizes the release of catecholamines during surgery, and makes the circulation more stable (Quintin *et al.*, 1991). Clonidine potentiates the effects of opioids (Engleman *et al.*, 1989) and inhalational anaesthetics (Gabriel *et al.*, 1995) and improves the quality of regional anaesthesia (Liu *et al.*, 1995). However, there is a risk of increased need for vasopressor and inotropic support after coronary artery surgery (Abi-Jaoude *et al.*, 1993). Dexmedetomidine has similar properties, but again there is a price to pay for haemodynamic stability: the need for more intra-operative pharmacological intervention.

The aims of antihypertensive therapy are to promote the regression of left ventricular hypertrophy, and to prevent the early morning increase in blood pressure which is associated with a risk of acute myocardial infarction and stroke. Finally, another aim is to control or prevent acute severe hypertensive crises. In this respect, sublingual nifedipine is often regarded as standard medication. In the long term, treatment of hypertension reduces overall cardiovascular morbidity, mostly by reducing stroke mortality (Collins *et al.*, 1980), the risk of coronary artery disease not being convincingly reduced by treatment of hypertension.

Treatment of hypertension in the elderly is a particular concern. Several trials have shown that protection against stroke and left ventricular failure is better in the elderly than in the middle-aged patient (Joint National Committee, 1993), and there is clear evidence that the isolated systolic hypertension frequently found in the elderly should be treated actively (STOP study, 1991). However, the diastolic blood pressure must be watched carefully in patients over the age of 75 years because excessive reductions may increase mortality.

Hypertensive disease in surgical patients

Arterial hypertension is generally regarded as a risk factor for cardiovascular complications of anaesthe-

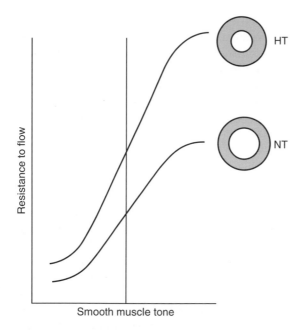

Figure 5.3 *Alterations in the structure of arterioles in hypertension (HT) exaggerates the changes in resistance to flow in response to changes in vascular smooth muscle tone, by comparison with the responses observed in normotensive subjects (NT) (inspired by Folkow, 1987).*

sia and surgery. There is concern that the long-term consequences of arterial hypertension, i.e. coronary artery disease, cerebrovascular disease, left ventricular hypertrophy and impaired renal function, render the patient less fit for anaesthesia and surgery. Indeed, hypertension was found to increase the odds ratio for post-operative death to 3.8 in a multivariate analysis of risk factors (Browner and Mangano, 1992). Haemodynamic instability (presenting as exaggerated hypotension on induction of anaesthesia, excessive pressor responses to laryngoscopy, endotracheal intubation and extubation, or hypertensive crises during the peri-operative period) can be blamed for the increased cardiovascular morbidity and mortality in hypertensive patients. Clearly, this results almost directly from an exaggerated vascular responsiveness to changes in autonomic activity (Fig. 5.3) (Folkow, 1987).

It was established in the early seventies that treated hypertensive patients exhibit smaller responses to anaesthesia and awakening than untreated hypertensive patients (Prys-Roberts *et al.*, 1971a,b), especially if they are treated with beta-blocking agents (Prys-Roberts *et al.*, 1973). These almost abolish the

risk of myocardial ischaemia and dysrhythmias, even when a single dose is given with the premedication (Stone *et al.*, 1988). The better stability of the treated hypertensives suggests that all hypertensive patients should be properly controlled before elective surgery. Of course, such a policy results in a large number of operations being cancelled because, even now, a large proportion of hypertensive patients are untreated or are not properly controlled (Fahey and Peters, 1996).

Several epidemiological studies, including those of Goldman and colleagues (1977) and Detsky and colleagues (1986), have failed to identify hypertension as a significant predictor of adverse outcome, so an empirical approach has evolved. Patients with severe hypertension (diastolic arterial pressure greater than 115 mmHg) are referred for treatment, those with moderate hypertension (diastolic arterial pressure between 100 and 115 mmHg) are considered for treatment if they have signs of coronary artery disease, cerebrovascular disease, or impaired renal functions; and those with mild hypertension are not usually cancelled. This approach reduces the number of operations cancelled, but does not necessarily prevent complications because some patients with untreated mild or moderate hypertension can be extremely unstable. Careful, individual assessment may be necessary, but a major problem in establishing guidelines for the peri-operative management of hypertensive patients is that no study has, as yet, shown conclusively that treatment brings about a significant improvement in outcome. Indeed, Goldman and Caldera (1979) found no difference in outcome whether patients with mild-to-moderate hypertension were treated or not.

Two recent studies may shed some light on the issue. A case–control study showed that hypertension was present in 43 per cent of patients who died within three months of surgery, and in only 19 per cent of matched patients who survived the operation (Howell *et al.*, 1996); hypertension remained a significant predictor of death even after other factors such as myocardial infarction had been taken into consideration (Howell *et al.*, 1998). However, the level of blood pressure at admission was the same in both cases and in controls. This suggests that the hypertensive disease itself is the major risk factor rather than the level of blood pressure at the time of surgery, although pressure becomes a significant determinant of complication when a soft measure of outcome such as silent myocardial ischaemia is taken into consideration (Allman *et al.*, 1994; Howell *et al.*, 1997). This suggests that the quality of blood pressure control matters, and not just the presence of the hypertensive disease.

Although the need to treat all hypertensive patients before elective surgery is still unsettled, it seems clear that treatment, when given, should be maintained throughout the peri-operative period, because its benefit is thought to derive in part from the prevention of intra-operative cardiovascular instability. Early studies showed that β-adrenoceptor blockade makes the patients more stable and minimizes the risk of peri-operative myocardial ischaemia (Prys-Roberts *et al.*, 1973; Stone *et al.*, 1988; Dodds *et al.*, 1994; Wallace *et al.*, 1994). With the newer drugs such as calcium-channel blockers, ACE inhibitors, α-adrenoceptor antagonists and $α_2$-adrenoceptor agonists, it is generally agreed that interactions with anaesthesia are predictable from their pharmacology. In a study of patients suffering from mild hypertension, a comparison of the haemodynamic responses to induction of anaesthesia, laryngoscopy and intubation in patients on single-drug therapy (diuretics, beta-blocking agents, calcium channel-blocking agents or ACE inhibitors) revealed no difference except for slower heart rates in patients on beta-blocking agents. Neither calcium channel-blocking agents nor ACE inhibitors were associated with exaggerated hypotension (Sear *et al.*, 1994). However, exaggerated hypotension or an increased need for vasopressor therapy has been reported in patients who had received an ACE inhibitor up until the morning of surgery (Myles *et al.*, 1993; Coriat *et al.*, 1994). This may suggest that ACE inhibitors should be withheld on the morning of surgery, but this may not be necessary when relatively low doses are used.

Peri-operative risks and their management

In hypertensive patients, induction of anaesthesia is often associated with marked hypotension. This is of particular concern in patients about to undergo vascular surgery because of the widespread nature of the atheromatous disease. The major risks are myocardial or cerebral ischaemia with the possibility of myocardial infarction or stroke. Induction of anaesthesia should be carefully controlled with the smallest effective doses of drugs. Fluid loading and/or small doses of vasopressors (e.g. ephedrine or methoxamine) may be required in order to maintain an acceptable blood pressure. The hypertensive response to laryngoscopy and intubation has been well described. It is minimized by β-adrenoceptor blockade, but it is not abolished even in patients on long-term therapy and many measures may be employed to ablate this undesirable response. In the context of surgery of large abdominal aortic aneurysms, prevention of blood-pressure overshoot after induction is important because a hypertensive crisis might cause the aneurysm to rupture.

Post-operative rebound hypertension may result in bleeding from arteriotomy suture lines, cerebral haemorrhage and myocardial infarction, with the mortality of such accidents being as high as 50 per cent (Leslie, 1993). In the extreme situation a potent and rapidly acting vasodilator such as sodium nitroprusside may be indicated, administered at an initial infusion rate of 0.3–0.5 mg/kg/min and then titrated to effect (Friederich and Butterworth, 1995). If the situation is less acute, esmolol may be used as well as vasodilators such as phentolamine, glyceryl trinitrate and nifedipine. The last is very effective when administered sublingually. However, excessive hypotension may occur and accidents have been reported (Grossman *et al.*, 1996).

CARDIAC FAILURE

Cardiac failure is the inability of either or both ventricles to maintain cardiac output in the face of an increase in the resistance (or impedance) to ejection (ejection failure), or impaired filling (filling failure). Many pathological processes result in cardiac failure, including coronary heart disease (ischaemia), hypertensive heart disease, the cardiomyopathies, myocarditis, ageing and valvular disease. Myocardial ischaemia is the commonest process which diminishes myocardial function because it decreases systolic function and increases myocardial stiffness to cause both systolic and diastolic failure. Dysrhythmias and/or conduction disorders further impair systolic function. Ageing causes cardiac damage essentially because of stiffening of arterial walls. This increases systolic pressure and increases wave reflection in the large arteries (i.e. the aorta and its branches) and results in a dynamic afterload on the left ventricle. Failure may result from the excessive workload of the heart. In addition, atheroma in the coronary arteries causes myocardial ischaemia (Lakatta and Fleg, 1986).

Cardiomyopathy

There are three distinct types of cardiomyopathy: hypertrophic, dilated and constrictive (Goodwin, 1982).

- Hypertrophic (obstructive) cardiomyopathy is characterized by massive ventricular hypertrophy. The ventricles relax irregularly and slowly, so impeding filling. By contrast, systolic function is powerful and blood is ejected rapidly from the ventricles. In the face of positive inotropic stimulation, a pressure gradient can develop within the cavity of the left ventricle. Obstruction can be alleviated by drugs which decrease left ventricular performance (i.e. beta-blocking agents and verapamil).
- Dilated cardiomyopathy is characterized by a marked dilatation of both ventricles resulting in impaired contractile performance. Excessive alcohol intake and previous viral myocarditis are the main causes. The ejection fraction is extremely low (10–30 per cent). Pulmonary venous engorgement, pulmonary hypertension and subsequent right ventricular failure result from the failure of the right ventricle to eject.
- Constrictive cardiomyopathy results from the deposition of organic material in the endomyocardium. This results in an inflow obstruction to the ventricles. Filling in early diastole is still rapid, but it almost ceases in the later part of diastole because of the excessive stiffness of the endomyocardium.

Valvular heart disease

Stenosis or incompetence of a cardiac valve is likely to result in failure of the ventricle adjacent to that valve.

AORTIC STENOSIS

The aortic valve is not supported by a fibrous ring, but by the base of the left ventricle and the aorta, the normal orifice being 2.1–3.6 cm^2 during systole. The most common causes of isolated aortic stenosis are calcification of congenital valve abnormalities,

degenerative calcification of normal valves, and isolated rheumatic disease of the valve (6 per cent of cases) (Normand et al., 1988). There is usually a very long asymptomatic period and the mean age of presentation is over 60 years, but after the onset of angina or syncope life expectancy is reduced to three years. The most common causes of death include sudden death, congestive heart failure, and bacterial endocarditis. Generally, a valve area of less than 0.7 cm^2 and a peak systolic gradient of more than 50 mmHg are regarded as indications for valve replacement, but the benefits of valve replacement or valvuloplasty in asymptomatic patients have been questioned (Pellika et al., 1990).

Delayed upstroke of the carotid pulse, narrowed pulse pressure, diamond-shaped systolic murmur, electrocardiographic signs of left ventricular hypertrophy and conduction delays are characteristic features. Doppler echocardiography and colour-flow mapping allow an accurate assessment of the severity of the stenosis. Obstruction to left ventricular ejection causes both pressure overload and a pressure gradient between ventricle and aorta. Concentric ventricular hypertrophy allows stroke volume to be maintained unless the reduction of diastolic compliance impedes filling (Danielsen et al., 1991). Because the systolic intraventricular pressure greatly exceeds the aortic pressure, there is a basic imbalance between high oxygen demand and relatively reduced oxygen supply because of the low diastolic aortic pressure (Fig. 5.4). Coronary flow

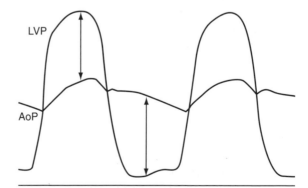

Figure 5.4 *In aortic stenosis, the systolic pressure gradient between left ventricular and aortic pressures indicates the severity of the stenosis. The gradient between aortic and ventricular pressures during diastole is reduced and an imbalance between oxygen demand (high) and supply (compromised) facilitates the development of acute myocardial ischaemia.*

reserve is decreased and angina may occur in the absence of coronary artery disease because of increased oxygen demand from increased muscle mass.

The central venous pressure often underestimates the left ventricular end-diastolic pressure because of the left ventricular diastolic dysfunction. Maintenance of sinus rhythm is important because the contribution of atrial contraction to filling may be as high as 40 per cent. Tachycardia is potentially harmful because it increases the risk of ischaemia (reduced duration of diastole). Bradycardia is poorly tolerated because the obstruction limits the stroke volume: cardiac output may be rate-dependent. As ventricular compliance is reduced the range of effective preload is decreased. Reductions of peripheral vascular resistance may be poorly tolerated because the reduction of the diastolic arterial pressure reduces coronary blood flow. Finally, venodilators can cause an excessive reduction of left ventricular preload.

AORTIC REGURGITATION

Aortic root dilatation, damage to valve leaflets, or loss of commissural support may cause aortic insufficiency, but aortic dissection is the most common cause, followed by infective endocarditis. Chronic aortic insufficiency may have a very prolonged latent period: up to thirty years may elapse between haemodynamically significant alterations and the appearance of symptoms (Yousof et al., 1988). The most common presentation in chronic aortic insufficiency is dyspnoea on exertion. Myocardial ischaemia is not as common as in aortic stenosis because volume work requires less energy than pressure work. The widened pulse pressure, low diastolic pressure and diastolic murmur are characteristic features, while the ECG remains normal except in advanced cases when left ventricular hypertrophy may be noted. The volume overloading results in elongation of sarcomere with replication in series (eccentric hypertrophy). This contrasts with pressure overloading of aortic stenosis that causes the sarcomeres to thicken with replication in parallel (concentric hypertrophy).

The main feature of aortic incompetence is that forward flow during systole is followed by regurgitant flow during diastole. This leads to a marked flow–volume overload of the left ventricle, with dilatation more marked than hypertrophy. Forward flow is facilitated by a low resistance to ejection while it is impeded by increases in vascular resistance. Tachycardia decreases the regurgitant flow and favours forward output. This explains why exercise may be relatively well tolerated, while increases in vascular resistance can reduce cardiac output dramatically.

Acute aortic regurgitation results in an acute volume overload with an acute increase in left ventricular end-diastolic pressure with little change in volume so that forward flow decreases. Modest reductions in afterload increase forward output, but there is the risk of excessive reduction of the coronary pressure gradient. Adequacy of preload is very important because it must be utilized to maintain forward flow. Increases in heart rate may benefit forward flow but, in the absence of increase in contractility, the effect of tachycardia on cardiac output is minimal.

MITRAL STENOSIS

The majority of cases of mitral stenosis are caused by rheumatic fever. The latency period may extend to twenty-five years and progression of the symptoms is very slow (Selzer and Cohn, 1972). Typically, patients experience dyspnoea (especially on exertion because tachycardia reduces the diastolic filling time of the left ventricle), but atrial fibrillation and haemoptysis may occur before dyspnoea. Development of atrial fibrillation decreases the survival rate, and a major complication of mitral stenosis is systemic arterial embolization. Most of the emboli involve the cerebral vasculature. Important features include P mitrale on the ECG, and signs of left atrial enlargement or pulmonary hypertension on the chest X-ray. Interstitial pulmonary oedema may be demonstrated by Kerley B lines.

When the mitral valve area is less than 2 cm^2, a pressure gradient develops across the stenosis. When the valve area is 1.2 cm^2 or less, dyspnoea worsens, with orthopnoea and/or paroxysmal nocturnal dyspnoea occurring. A valve area of less than 1 cm^2 is associated with pulmonary oedema. The development of pulmonary hypertension tends to reduce cardiac output and is an indication for surgery (Brandenburg et al., 1991).

Filling of the left ventricle requires increases in both driving pressure and time so strict control of heart rate is essential. Control of preload is also very important and may be best achieved by monitoring the pulmonary artery occlusion pressure (PAOP). The latter overestimates the left ventricular end-diastolic pressure, but is a useful monitor of trends. It is also essential to avoid conditions that may exacerbate pulmonary hypertension, especially hypoxia and hypercarbia.

Mitral stenosis causes flow though the narrowed mitral valve to depend upon the left atrial pressure and the duration of diastole. The picture is of outflow obstruction for the left atrium and inflow obstruction for the left ventricle. Tachycardia impairs ventricular filling because of the reduced diastolic time. Atrial fibrillation compromises late diastolic filling and may, when it appears for the first time, cause pulmonary oedema. The operational range for left atrial pressure is decreased. Mean left atrial pressure is usually above 15 mmHg. Any factor that promotes overfilling of the atria can cause pulmonary oedema, especially in the early stages of the disease. In the later stages pulmonary hypertension develops and is associated with right ventricular failure. Note that hypovolaemia is poorly tolerated because a low atrial pressure reduces left ventricular inflow and, therefore, stroke volume.

MITRAL REGURGITATION

The pathogenesis of mitral regurgitation is complex and includes defects in the annulus, leaflets or commissures, chordae or papillary muscles. Rheumatic heart disease, mitral valve prolapse, myocardial ischaemia or infective endocarditis may cause mitral insufficiency. The development of regurgitation is usually very slow unless it is caused by rupture of a chordae tendineae or papillary muscle. Early symptoms of chronic mitral regurgitation include fatigue due to low cardiac output. Pulmonary congestion is rare because left atrial dilatation protects the pulmonary circulation from the regurgitant flow. The chest X-ray shows signs of left atrial and left ventricular enlargement. Regurgitant flow is noted during left ventricular isovolumic contraction and during ejection, with total cardiac output being normal or elevated, but with forward flow decreased. Bradycardia increases the magnitude of the regurgitant flow. Preload should be carefully controlled and measurement of the PAOP may be useful.

Mitral regurgitation results in dilatation of both left ventricle and atrium, with the regurgitant flow causing marked pressure and volume overload of the left atrium during systole. Any increase in systemic vascular resistance will limit forward left ventricular flow and encourage retrograde flow into the left atrium, while a low systemic vascular resistance will encourage forward flow.

TRICUSPID STENOSIS

Most commonly, tricuspid stenosis results from rheumatic heart disease (Wooley, 1981) and it is generally associated with mitral and aortic valve disease. Dyspnoea, fatigue and systemic venous hypertension are major features, with a valve orifice of less than 2 cm^2 indicating significant stenosis. Inotropes, vasodilators and diuretics may be required. Atrial fibrillation can cause a dramatic reduction in cardiac output.

TRICUSPID REGURGITATION

The most common aetiology is again rheumatic fever (Waller, 1987), and other valves are usually involved. The reversal of flow from the right ventricle is well tolerated as long as pulmonary arterial pressure is normal. If pulmonary hypertension develops regurgitation is exacerbated and forward output is reduced. Interventions that increase pulmonary artery pressure should be avoided (hypoxia, hypercarbia) and preload should be carefully controlled.

Haemodynamics of ventricular failure

Understanding of ventricular failure is facilitated by consideration of the dynamic relationships between pressure and volume (Fig. 5.5). For a normal heart, the end-systolic pressure–volume relationship (termed 'maximum elastance', E_{max}) is relatively steep, while for the failing heart it is flatter. The end-diastolic pressure–volume relationship is also altered. It is steeper for the ischaemic or hypertrophic heart than for the normal heart. Thus, the failing heart responds to changes in vascular resistance by smaller increases in systolic pressure and greater decreases in stroke volume than the normal heart (Laskey et al., 1985). In addition, larger increases in end-diastolic pressure are observed (Fig. 5.5). Drugs which impair left ventricular contractility further flatten the end-systolic pressure–volume relationship and cause stroke volume to decrease. In the presence of valvular heart disease, the dynamic

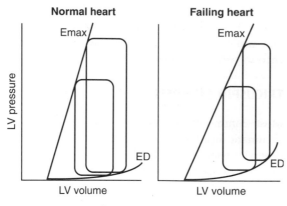

Figure 5.5 *The dynamic relationship between pressure and volume in the left ventricle is altered in the failing heart. Two important modifications are represented. The flatter end-systolic pressure–volume relationship (E_{max}) indicates the loss of contractility. The steeper end-diastolic pressure–volume relationship (ED) indicates that ventricular compliance is reduced. As a result, the loops are narrower for the failing heart, indicating reduced stroke volume (and stroke work). In addition, increases in pressure cause a marked reduction in the width of the loop for the compromised heart, demonstrating that increased resistance reduces stroke volume.*

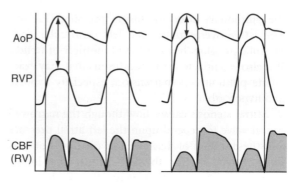

Figure 5.6 *Diagrammatic representation of the effect of right ventricular hypertension on the pressure gradient between aortic and right ventricular pressure and on systolic and diastolic right ventricular coronary blood flow (CBF(RV)). The left-hand panel represents normal conditions, while the right-hand panel represents the effect of acute right ventricular hypertension. Note the decreased systolic coronary flow. AoP, aortic pressure; RVP, right ventricular pressure.*

pressure–volume relationships of the left ventricle are profoundly altered, but the same principles apply. The anaesthetic management of patients with a failing heart must minimize any negative inotropic intervention, prevent increases in vascular resistance and maintain adequate filling. Monitoring of these variables can be improved by the use of a balloon-tipped pulmonary artery catheter because measurement of PAOP is an indirect estimate of left ventricular end-diastolic pressure provided there is no mitral valve stenosis.

RIGHT VENTRICULAR FAILURE

Right ventricular failure may be caused by extensive right ventricular infarction, pulmonary valvular stenosis or most frequently, by pulmonary hypertension secondary to chronic obstructive airway disease. Other causes include repeated pulmonary thromboembolism, mitral valve disease and chronic left ventricular failure. Hypoxia may precipitate acute pulmonary hypertension (acute pulmonary arteriolar constriction) so short episodes of hypoxia associated with difficult intubation or inadequate ventilation

during recovery from anaesthesia can precipitate right ventricular failure in patients with pre-existing pulmonary hypertension. A possible mechanism for acute right ventricular failure is acute right ventricular myocardial ischaemia caused by decrease in the pressure gradient between aorta and right ventricle associated with acute right ventricular hypertension (Fig. 5.6). Though coronary flow may increase during diastole because of local control, the reduction in systolic coronary flow prevents the matching of oxygen demand and oxygen supply. Another factor of risk is systemic hypotension, because this decreases coronary perfusion pressure and may, in turn, compromise function of the hypertrophic right ventricular wall.

REFERENCES

Abi-Jaoude, F., Brusset, A., Ceddaha, A. *et al*. 1993. Clonidine premedication for coronary artery bypass grafting under high-dose alfentanil anesthesia: intraoperative and post-operative hemodynamic study. *Journal of Cardiothoracic and Vascular Anesthesia* **7**, 35–40.

Alderman, M.H., Madhavan, S. and Ooi, W.L. 1991. Association of the renin sodium profile with the risk of myocardial infarction in patients with hypertension. *New England Journal of Medicine* **324**, 1098–1104.

Allman, K.G., Muir, A., Howell, S.J. *et al*. 1994. Resistant hypertension and preoperative silent myocardial ischaemia in surgical patients. *British Journal of Anaesthesia* **73**, 574–578.

Bassenge, E. 1995. Control of coronary blood flow by autacoids. *Basic Research in Cardiology* **90**, 125–141.

Baumgart, D. and Heusch, G. 1995. Neuronal control of coronary blood flow. *Basic Research in Cardiology* **90**, 142–159.

Brandenburg, R., Giuliani, E., Nishimura, R. and McGoon, D. 1991. Acquired valvular heart disease: mitral stenosis. In Giuliani, E., Fuster, V., Gersh, B., McGoon, M. and McGoon, D. (eds), *Cardiology: fundamentals and practice*. St Louis: Mosby Year Book, 1543–1561.

Braunwald, E. and Kloner, R.A. 1982. The stunned myocardium: prolonged, postischemic ventricular dysfunction. *Circulation* **66**, 1146–1149.

Brown, B.G., Bolson, E.L. and Dodge, H.T. 1984. Dynamic mechanisms in human coronary stenosis. *Circulation* **70**, 917–922.

Browner, W.S. and Mangano, D.T. 1992. In-hospital and long-term mortality in male veterans following noncardiac surgery. The Study of peri-operative Ischemia Research Group. *Journal of the American Medical Association* **268**, 228–232.

Brunner, H.R. 1995. Anti-hypertensive therapy by losartan. How effective is AT1 receptor blockade? *Journal of Human Hypertension* **9**, 859–860.

Buffington, C., Davis, K., Gillispie, S. and Pettinger, M. 1988. The prevalence of steal-prone coronary anatomy in patients with coronary artery disease: an analysis of the coronary artery surgery study registry. *Anesthesiology* **69**, 721–727.

Buffington, C.W., Romson, J.L., Levine, A. *et al*. 1987. Isoflurane induces coronary steal in a canine model of chronic coronary occlusion. *Anesthesiology* **66**, 280–292.

Collins, R., Peto, R., MacMahon, S. *et al*. 1990. Blood pressure, stroke, and coronary heart disease. Part 2, Short-term reductions in blood pressure: overview of randomised drug trials in their epidemiological context. *Lancet* **335**, 827–838.

Coriat, P., Richer, C., Douraki, T. *et al*. 1994. Influence of chronic angiotensin-converting enzyme inhibition on anesthetic induction. *Anesthesiology* **81**, 299–307.

Cutfield, G.R., Francis, C.M., Foëx, P. *et al*. 1988. Isoflurane and large coronary artery haemodynamics: an experimental study. *British Journal of Anaesthesia* **60**, 784–790.

Dahlöf, B., Keller, S.E., Makris, L. *et al*. 1995. Efficacy and tolerability of losartan potassium and atenolol in patients with mild to moderate essential hypertension. *American Journal of Hypertension* **8**, 578–583.

Danielsen, R., Nordrehaug, J. and Vik-Mo, H. 1991. Clinical and haemodynamic features in relation to severity of aortic stenosis in adults. *European Heart Journal* **12**, 791–795.

Deanfield, J.E., Selwyn, A.P., Chierchia, S. *et al*. 1983. Myocardial ischaemia during daily life in patients with stable angina: its relation to symptoms and heart rate changes. *Lancet* **ii**, 753–758.

Detsky, A.S., Abrams, H.B., Forbath, N. *et al*. 1986. Cardiac assessment for patients undergoing non-cardiac surgery: a multifactorial clinical risk index. *Archives of Internal Medicine* **146**, 2131–2134.

Dirksen, A. and Kjoller, E. 1988. Cardiac predictors of death after non-cardiac surgery evaluated by intention to treat. *British Medical Journal* **297**, 1011–1013.

Dodds, T.M., Stone, J.G., Coromilas, J. *et al*. 1993. Prophylactic nitroglycerin infusion during noncardiac surgery does not reduce peri-operative ischaemia. *Anesthesia and Analgesia* **76**, 705–713.

Dzau, V.J. and Gibbons, G.H. 1991. Endothelium and growth factors in vascular remodelling of hypertension. *Hypertension* **18**(3), 115–121.

Eagle, K.A., Rihal, C.S., Mickel, M.C. *et al*. 1997. Cardiac risk of noncardiac surgery: influence of coronary disease and type of surgery in 3368 operations. CASS Investigators and University of Michigan Heart Care Program. Coronary Artery Surgery Study. *Circulation* **96**, 1882–1887.

Egstrup, K. 1988. Randomized double-blind comparison of metoprolol, nifedipine, and their combination in chronic stable angina: effects on total ischemic activity and heart rate at onset of ischemia. *American Heart Journal* **116**, 971–978.

Engelman, E., Lipszyc, M., Gilbart, E. *et al*. 1989. Effects of clonidine on anesthetic drug requirements and hemodynamic response during aortic surgery. *Anesthesiology* **71**, 178–187.

Fahey, T.P. and Peters, T.J. 1996. What constitutes controlled hypertension? Patient based comparison of hypertension guidelines. *British Medical Journal* **313**, 93–96.

Folkow, B. 1987. Structure and function of the arteries in hypertension. *American Heart Journal* **114**, 938–948.

Foster, E.D., Davis, K.B., Carpenter, J.A. *et al*. 1986. Risk of noncardiac operation in patients with defined coronary disease: The Coronary Artery Surgery Study (CASS) Registry experience. *Annals of Thoracic Surgery* **41**, 42–50.

Friederich, J.A. and Butterworth, J.F. 1995. Sodium nitroprusside: twenty years and counting. *Anesthesia and Analgesia* **81**, 152–162.

Frohlich, E.D. 1991. The heart in hypertension: a 1991 overview. *Hypertension* **18**(3), 62–68.

Frohlich, E.D., Apstein, C., Chobanian, A.V. *et al*. 1992. The heart in hypertension. *New England Journal of Medicine* **327**, 998–1008.

Gabriel, A.H., Faryniak, B., Sojka, G. *et al*. 1995. Clonidine: an adjunct in isoflurane N_2O/O_2 relaxant anaesthesia. Effects on EEG power spectra, somatosensory and auditory evoked potentials. *Anaesthesia* **50**, 290–296.

Gersh, B.J., Rihal, C.S., Rooke, T.W. and Ballard, D.J. 1991. Evaluation and management of patients with both peripheral vascular and coronary artery disease. *Journal of the American College of Cardiology* **18**, 203–214.

Gill, N.P., Wright, B. and Reilly, C.S. 1992. Relationship between hypoxaemic and cardiac events in the perioperative period. *British Journal of Anaesthesia* **68**, 471–473.

Goldman, L. and Caldera, D.L. 1979. Risks of general anesthesia and elective operation in the hypertensive patient. *Anesthesiology* **50**, 285–292.

Goldman, L., Caldera, D.L., Nussbaum, S.R. *et al*. 1977. Multifactorial index of cardiac risk in noncardiac surgical procedures. *New England Journal of Medicine* **297**, 845–850.

Goodwin, J.F. 1982. The frontiers of cardiomyopathy. *British Heart Journal,* **48**, 1–18.

Grossman, E., Messerli, F.H., Grodzicki, T. and Kowey, P. 1996. Should a moratorium be placed on sublingual nifedipine capsules given for hypertensive emergencies and pseudoemergencies? *Journal of the American Medical Association* **276**, 1328–1331.

Harkin, C.P., Pagel, P.S., Kersten, J.R. *et al*. 1994. Direct negative inotropic and lusitropic effects of sevoflurane. *Anesthesiology* **81**, 156–167.

Hartman, J.C., Pagel, P.S., Proctor, L.T. *et al*. 1992. Influence of desflurane, isoflurane and halothane on regional tissue perfusion in dogs. *Canadian Journal of Anaesthesia* **39**, 877–887.

Hoes, A.W., Grobbee, D.E., Lubsen, J. *et al*. 1995. Diuretics, beta-blockers, and the risk for sudden cardiac death in hypertensive patients. *Annals of Internal Medicine* **123**, 481–487.

Hollenberg, M. and Mangano, D.T. 1994. Therapeutic approaches to post-operative ischemia. The Study of peri-operative Ischemia Research Group. *American Journal of Cardiology* **73**, 30B-33B.

Holter, N.J. 1961. New method for heart studies. *Science* **134**, 1214–1220.

Howell, S.J., Hemming, A.E., Allman, K.G. *et al*. 1997. Predictors of post-operative myocardial ischaemia: the role of intercurrent arterial hypertension and other cardiovascular risk factors. *Anaesthesia* **52**, 107–111.

Howell, S.J., Sear, Y.M., Yeates, D. *et al*. 1996. Hypertension, admission blood pressure and perioperative cardiovascular risk. *Anaesthesia* **51**, 1000–1004.

Howell, S.J., Sear, Y.M., Yeates, D. *et al*. 1998. Risk factors for cardiovascular death after elective surgery under general anaesthesia. *British Journal of Anaesthesia* **80**, 14–19.

Joint National Committee. 1993. The fifth report of the Joint National Committee on detection, evaluation, and treatment of high blood pressure (JNC V). *Archives of Internal Medicine* **153**, 154–183.

Johnston, K.W. and Scobie, T.K. 1988. Multicenter prospective study of nonruptured abdominal aortic aneurysms. I. Population and operative management. *Journal of Vascular Surgery* **7**, 69–81.

Lakatta, E.G. and Fleg, J.L. 1986. Aging of the adult cardiovascular system. In Stephen, C.R. and Assaf, R.A.E. (ed.), *Geriatic anesthesia principles and practice*. Boston: Butterworths, 1–26.

Laskey, W.K., Kussmaul, W.G., Martin, J.L. *et al*. 1985. Characteristics of vascular hydraulic load in patients with heart failure. *Circulation* **72**, 61–71.

Leslie, J.B. 1993. Incidence and aetiology of perioperative hypertension. *Acta Anaesthesiologica Scandinavica* **Suppl 99**, 5–9.

Leung, J.M., Hollenberg, M., O'Kelly, B.F. *et al*. 1992. Effects of steal-prone anatomy on intraoperative myocardial ischemia. The SPI Research Group. *Journal of the American College of Cardiology* **20**, 1205–1212.

Leung, J.M., Stanley, T., Mathew, J. *et al*. 1994. An initial multicenter, randomized controlled trial on the safety and efficacy of acadesine in patients undergoing coronary artery bypass graft surgery. SPI Research Group. *Anesthesia and Analgesia* **78**, 420–434.

Liu, S., Chiu, A.A., Neal, J.M. *et al*. 1995. Oral clonidine prolongs lidocaine spinal anesthesia in human volunteers. *Anesthesiology* **82**, 1353–1359.

Lowenstein, E., Foëx, P., Francis, C.M. *et al*. 1981. Regional ischemic ventricular dysfunction in myocardium supplied by a narrowed coronary artery with increasing halothane concentration in the dog. *Anesthesiology* **55**, 349–359.

MacMahon, S., Cutler, J.A. and Stamler, J. 1989. Antihypertensive drug treatment. Potential, expected, and observed effects on stroke and on coronary heart disease. *Hypertension* **13 (Suppl I)**, 45–50.

Mangano, D.T., Browner, W., Hollenberg, M. *et al.* 1990. Association of peri-operative myocardial ischaemia with cardiac morbidity and mortality in men undergoing noncardiac surgery. *New England Journal of Medicine* **323**, 1781–1788.

Mangano, D.T., Siliciano, D., Hollenberg, M. *et al.* 1992. post-operative myocardial ischemia. Therapeutic trials using intensive analgesia following surgery. The Study of peri-operative Ischemia (SPI) Research Group. *Anesthesiology* **76**, 342–353.

Mangano, D.T., Layug, E.L., Wallace, A. and Tateo, I. 1996. Effect of atenolol on mortality and cardiovascular morbidity after noncardiac surgery. Multicenter Study of Perioperative Ischemia Research Group. *New England Journal of Medicine* **335**, 1713–1720.

McCann, R.L. and Clements, F.M. 1991. Silent myocardial ischemia in patients undergoing peripheral vascular surgery: incidence and association with peri-operative morbidity and mortality. *Journal of Vascular Surgery* **9**, 583–587.

Myles, P.S., Olenikov, I., Bujor, M.A. and Davis, B.B. 1993. ACE-inhibitors, calcium antagonists and low systemic vascular resistance following cardiopulmonary bypass. A case-control study. *Medical Journal of Australia* **158**, 675–677.

Normand, J., Loire, R. and Zambartas, C. 1988. The anatomical aspects of aortic stenosis. *European Heart Journal* **9** (Suppl E), 31–36.

Opie, L.H. 1991. Oxygen supply: coronary flow. In Opie, L.H (ed.), *The heart, physiology and metabolism*, 2nd edn. New York: Raven Press, 277–300.

Ouyang, P., Gerstenblith, G., Furman, W.R. *et al.* 1989. Coronary artery disease: frequency and significance of early post-operative silent myocardial ischemia in patients having peripheral vascular surgery. *American Journal of Cardiology* **64**, 1113–1116.

Pasternack, P.F., Imparato, A.M. and Bear, G. 1984. The value of radionuclide angiography as a predictor of peri-operative myocardial infarction in patients undergoing abdominal aortic aneurysm resection. *Journal of Vascular Surgery* **1**, 320–325.

Pellikka, P., Nishimura, R., Bailey, K.R. and Tajik, A.J. 1990. The natural history of adults with asymptomatic, hemodynamically significant aortic stenosis. *Journal of the American College of Cardiology* **15**, 1012–1017.

Priebe, H-J. and Foëx, P. 1987. Isoflurane causes regional myocardial dysfunction in dogs with critical coronary artery stenoses. *Anesthesiology* **66**, 293–300.

Prys-Roberts, C., Greene, L., Meloche, R. and Foëx, P. 1971a. Studies of anaesthesia in relation to hypertension. II. Haemodynamic consequences of induction and endotracheal intubation. *British Journal of Anaesthesia* **43**, 531–547.

Prys-Roberts, C., Meloche, R. and Foëx, P. 1971b. Studies of anaesthesia in relation to hypertension. I. Cardiovascular responses of treated and untreated patients. *British Journal of Anaesthesia* **43**, 122–137.

Prys-Roberts, C., Foëx, P., Biro, G.P. and Roberts, J.G. 1973. Studies of anaesthesia in relation to hypertension. V: Adrenergic beta-receptor blockade. *British Journal of Anaesthesia* **45**, 671–680.

Psaty, B.M., Heckbert, S.R., Koepsell, T.D. *et al.* 1995. The risk of myocardial infarction associated with antihypertensive drug therapies. *Journal of the American Medical Association* **274**, 620–625.

Psaty, B.M., Savage, P.J., Tell, G.S. *et al.* 1993. Temporal patterns of antihypertensive medication use among elderly patients. *Journal of the American Medical Association* **270**, 1837–1841.

Quintin, L., Roudot, F., Roux, C. *et al.* 1991. Effect of clonidine on the circulation and vasoactive hormones after aortic surgery. *British Journal of Anaesthesia* **66**, 108–115.

Raby, K.E., Barry, J., Creager, M.A. *et al.* 1992. Detection and significance of intraoperative and post-operative myocardial ischemia in peripheral vascular surgery. *Journal of the American Medical Association* **268**, 222–227.

Raby, K.E., Goldman, L., Creager, M.A. *et al.* 1989. Correlation between preoperative ischemia and major cardiac events after peripheral vascular surgery. *New England Journal of Medicine* **321**, 1296–1300.

Rahimtoola, S.H. 1989. The hibernating myocardium. *American Heart Journal* **117**, 211–221.

Raison, J., Achimastos, A., Asmar, R. *et al.* 1986. Extracellular and interstitial fluid volume in obesity with and without associated systemic hypertension. *American Journal of Cardiology* **57**, 223–226.

Rao, T.L., Jacobs, K.H. and El-Etr, A.A. 1983. Re-infarction following anesthesia in patients with myocardial infarction. *Anesthesiology* **59**, 499–505.

Reeder, M.K., Muir, A.D., Foëx, P. *et al*. 1991. Post-operative myocardial ischaemia: temporal association with nocturnal hypoxaemia. *British Journal of Anaesthesia* **67**, 626–631.

Reid, J.V., Ito, B.R., Huang, A.H, Buffington, C.W. and Feigl, E.O. 1985. Parasympathetic control of transmural coronary blood flow in dogs. *American Journal of Physiology* **249**, H337–H343.

Rosenberg, J., Rasmussen, V., van Jensen, F. *et al*. 1990. Late post-operative episodic and constant hypoxaemia and associated ECG abnormalities. *British Journal of Anaesthesia* **65**, 684–691.

Sear, J.W., Jewkes, C., Tellez, J-C. and Foëx, P. 1994. Does the choice of antihypertensive therapy influence haemodynamic responses to induction, laryngoscopy and intubation. *British Journal of Anaesthesia* **73**, 303–308.

Selzer, A. and Cohn, K. 1972. Natural history of mitral stenosis: a review. *Circulation* **45**, 878–890.

Shah, K.B., Kleinman, B.S., Sami, H. *et al*. 1990. Reevaluation of peri-operative myocardial infarction in patients with prior myocardial infarction undergoing noncardiac operations. *Anesthesia and Analgesia* **71**, 231–235.

Siskovick, D.S., Raghunathan, T.E., Psaty, B.M. *et al*. 1994. Diuretic therapy for hypertension and the risk of primary cardiac arrest. *New England Journal of Medicine* **330**, 1852–1857.

Slogoff, S. and Keats, A.S. 1985. Does peri-operative myocardial ischemia lead to post-operative myocardial infarction? *Anesthesiology* **62**, 107–114.

Steen, P.A., Tinker, J.H. and Tarhan, S. 1978. Myocardial infarction after anesthesia and surgery. *Journal of the American Medical Association* **239**, 2566–2570.

Stone, J.G., Foëx, P., Sear, J.W. *et al*. 1988. Myocardial ischemia in untreated hypertensive patients: effects of a single small oral dose of beta-adrenergic blocking agent. *Anesthesiology* **68**, 495–500.

STOP Study. Ekbom, T., Dahlof, B., Hansson, .L *et al*. 1991. Morbidity and mortality in the Swedish Trial in Old Patients with Hypertension (STOP-Hypertension). *Lancet* **338**, 1281–1285.

Stühmeier, K-D., Mainzer, B., Cierpka, J. *et al*. 1996. Small, oral dose of clonidine reduces the incidence of intraoperative myocardial ischemia in patients having vascular surgery. *Anesthesiology* **85**, 706–712.

Takayama, M., Norris, R.M., Brown, M.A. *et al*. 1988. Post-systolic shortening of acutely ischemic canine myocardium predicts early and late recovery of function after coronary artery reperfusion. *Circulation* **78**, 994–1007.

Talke, P., Li, J., Jain, U. *et al*. 1995. Effects of peri-operative dexmedetomidine infusion in patients undergoing vascular surgery. The Study of peri-operative Ischemia Research Group. *Anesthesiology* **82**, 620–633.

Tarazi, R.C., Dustan, H.P., Frohlich, E.D. *et al*. 1970. Plasma volume and chronic hypertension. Relationship to arterial pressure level in different hypertensive diseases. *Archives of Internal Medicine* **125**, 835–842.

Tarhan, S., Moffitt, E.A., Taylor, W.F. and Giuliani, E.R. 1972. Myocardial infarction after general anesthesia. *Journal of the American Medical Association* **220**, 1451–1454.

van Hinsbergh, V.W. 1992. Regulatory functions of the coronary endothelium. *Molecular and Cellular Biochemistry* **116**, 163–169.

Vatner, S.F. 1980. Correlation between acute reductions in myocardial blood flow and function in conscious dog. *Circulation Research* **47**, 201–207.

Waller, B. 1987. Etiology of pure tricuspid regurgitation. *Cardiovascular Clinics* **17**, 53–95.

Weber, M.A., Byyny, R.L., Pratt, H. *et al*. 1995. Blood pressure effects of the angiotensin II receptor blocker, losartan. *Archives of Internal Medicine* **155**, 405–411.

Wooley, C. 1981. Rediscovery of the tricuspid valve. *Current Problems in Cardiology* **6**, 1–41.

Young, M.A., Vatner, D.E. and Vatner, S.F. 1990. Alpha- and beta-adrenergic control of large coronary arteries in conscious calves. *Basic Research in Cardiology* **85** (Suppl 1), 97–109.

Yousof, A.M., Mohammed, M.M., Shuhaiber, H. and Cherian, G. 1988. Chronic severe aortic regurgitation: a prospective followup of 60 asymptomatic patients. *American Heart Journal* **116**, 1262–1267.

6

Pre-operative assessment of patients at risk of peri-operative cardiovascular complications

R BUTLER, ANDREW D MORRIS AND A D STRUTHERS

INTRODUCTION

Pre-operative assessment of patients at high risk of peri-operative cardiac complications is a major dilemma. Accurate prediction and optimal management in individual patients who may develop peri-operative cardiac complications remains unsatisfactory. Various risk-reduction strategies, including intensive peri-operative anti-ischaemic therapy, monitoring and prophylactic revascularization have been proposed, although the efficacy of these techniques has not been adequately investigated and their benefits remain unproven. The aim here is to consider current views on two distinct and separate aspects. First, the need to assess the functional state of the cardiovascular system prior to the stress of major surgery; and second, consideration of the drugs taken by the patient and the scope for optimizing this therapy pre-operatively.

FUNCTIONAL STATE OF THE CARDIOVASCULAR SYSTEM BEFORE SURGERY

Recognition of cardiovascular disease

A thorough history and examination are of the utmost importance. Prior to major surgery, a pre-operative 12-lead electrocardiograph (ECG) and a standard postero-anterior chest radiograph (CXR) are useful to provide baseline information in case of post-operative changes. They may also help define the patient's pre-operative status and should be performed in all vascular surgical patients over the age of 40 years. However, much more could be done, but requires critical analysis.

CARDIOVASCULAR INVESTIGATION

This is a complex matter, and there has been much

debate, not only about which are the best investiga-tions, but even about the aims of performing them. Which is more important pre-operatively: to detect occlusive coronary artery disease and areas of ischaemia, or to estimate left ventricular function? The answer may depend on the precise nature of the intercurrent problem, and each of the different con-ditions which may co-exist with peripheral vascular disease needs to be discussed.

Ischaemic heart disease

Coronary artery disease is commonly associated with occlusive peripheral vascular disease. Underlying the overt disease, patients may have a constellation of risk factors including smoking, hyperlipidaemia, hypertension, diabetes mellitus and genetic predisposition, but three separate clini-cal entities are of relevance here: angina pectoris, myocardial ischaemia and myocardial infarction.

Angina pectoris   Stable angina pectoris usually denotes significant (>70 per cent) occlusive coronary disease in 90 per cent of men and women over the ages of 40 and 60 years, respectively (Diamond *et al.*, 1979). However, its role as predictor of adverse coro-nary events after non-coronary surgery remains in dispute. A number of workers (Driscoll *et al.*, 1961; Tarhan *et al.*, 1972; Larsen *et al.*, 1987; Von Knorring, 1981) all consider angina as a predictor of adverse cardiac events in the peri-operative period. However, neither Goldman and colleagues (1977) nor Foster and colleagues (1986) found a relationship, although the latter group did find that the pre-operative use of nitrates was associated with increased risks of peri-operative cardiovascular events.

Thus there is controversy about whether stable angina pectoris even affects peri-operative morbidi-ty. One probable explanation is that many episodes of ischaemia, perhaps as many as 75 per cent (Cohn *et al.*, 1986), are painless and therefore angina itself may be a poor indicator of the presence or absence of ischaemia. This is even more important in the patient with diabetes mellitus whose potential for silent myocardial ischaemia is even higher. This may suggest that documenting evidence of myocardial ischaemia may be a more specific prognostic investi-gation than the presence or otherwise of sympto-matic angina.

Myocardial ischaemia   The pre-operative demon-stration of myocardial ischaemia by treadmill exer-cise testing or dipyridamole–thallium scanning, or the detection of occlusive coronary disease by angiography, have not been shown to be associated with poor clinical outcomes. For example, dipyri-damole–thallium scanning has been used to stratify patients undergoing major non-cardiac surgery. Redistribution defects, which indicate areas of myocardium with inadequate blood supply, could be used to sensitively predict adverse cardiac events, but were not specific. Many subjects with an ischaemic myocardium did not suffer adverse car-diovascular events (Boucher *et al.*, 1985; Leppo *et al.*, 1987; Hendel *et al.*, 1990; Mangano *et al.*, 1991).

Myocardial infarction   A previous myocardial infarction is undoubtedly a strong and consistent predictor of adverse post-operative outcome. The re-infarction rate after surgery is generally 0.1–0.7 per cent (Knapp *et al.*, 1962; Topkins and Artusio, 1964; Tarhan *et al.*, 1972, Steen *et al.*, 1978), but rises to 5–8 per cent (Plumlee and Brettner, 1972; Tarhan *et al.*, 1972; Rao *et al.*, 1983) in those with a myocar-dial infarction within the last six months. If the infarction occurred within three months of opera-tion, the re-infarction rate increases to 30 per cent; at three to six months it is 15 per cent and at greater than six months it is 6 per cent (Knapp *et al.*, 1962; Topkins and Artusiol, 1964; Tarhan *et al.*, 1972; Steen *et al.*, 1978; Goldman, 1983).

However, the Coronary Artery Surgery Study (CASS) (Foster *et al.*, 1986) refutes this. Foster found no adverse risk associated with a previous myocardial infarction, but rather found that poor left ventricular function, pre-operative nitrate use (presumably a surrogate for degree of angina), male sex, diabetes, age, dyspnoea on exertion and electro-cardiographic left ventricular hypertrophy were fac-tors which predicted an adverse outcome. An inter-esting observation from the CASS registry was that beta-blocking agents were beneficial when contin-ued through the operative period. Prior to this time these agents had been routinely stopped weeks in advance.

Interestingly, data from the CASS showed no dif-ference between the operative complications of those patients without significant angiographically determined coronary artery disease and those who had undergone coronary artery bypass grafting (CABG). The CABG group had less post-procedural chest pain than those with coronary artery disease but without prior CABG, but no greater incidence of cardiovascular complications. However, in the Cleveland Clinic, Hertzer and colleagues (1984) showed that myocardial infarction occurred in approximately 3.8 per cent of patients undergoing peripheral vascular surgery, and was a leading cause of death. Further study showed that in those patients who were assessed by coronary angiography and then revascularized prior to their vascular operation, survival figures were improved.

Heart failure

Heart failure produces an enormous cost to the healthcare system. It is common, occurring in approximately 0.5–1 per cent of the population (McKee *et al.*, 1971; Sutton, 1990), accounts for approximately 5 per cent of all hospital admissions (Sutton, 1990) and has a 50 per cent five-year mortality rate when the ejection fraction is less than 30 per cent (McKee *et al.*, 1971). It has been universally accepted as a strong predictor of a poor cardiovascular outcome in terms of post-operative myocardial infarction, re-infarction and worsening left ventricular dysfunction (Goldman *et al.*, 1977; Foster *et al.*, 1986; Larsen *et al.*, 1987).

The only conflict has been in which *clinical* sign of heart failure most strongly predicts an adverse outcome (Mangano, 1990). Goldman and colleagues (1977) suggested the presence of a third heart sound and a raised jugular venous pulse have predictive value, whereas cardiomegaly does not. Foster and colleagues (1986) suggested that the presence of a third heart sound, paroxysmal nocturnal dyspnoea, exertional dyspnoea and orthopnoea were univariate predictors, but only an abnormal left ventricular score indicating ventricular wall motion abnormalities or poor function overall was a strong multivariate predictor of poor operative outcome. The left ventricular score (indicating left ventricular dysfunction) was the strongest predictor of an adverse outcome in the data in the CASS registry.

Hypertension

Whether mild-to-moderate hypertension is a predictor of adverse outcome after non-cardiac surgery is still contentious. Some (Goldman *et al.*, 1977; Rao *et al.*, 1983) suggest that it is not; others (Foster *et al.*, 1986) that it is a univariate predictor, or that it predicts post-operative myocardial infarction (Prys-Roberts *et al.*, 1971) and other adverse cardiovascular events in the peri-operative period such as blood pressure lability, arrhythmias, transient myocardial

and cerebral ischaemia (Driscoll *et al.*, 1961; Tarhan *et al.*, 1972; Steen *et al.*, 1978).

Arrhythmias

The significance of dysrhythmias in patients with coronary artery disease or left ventricular dysfunction is undoubted. After myocardial infarction the presence of multifocal premature ventricular complexes, ventricular tachycardia and conduction disturbances are predictors of a poor outcome.

However, there is little evidence available to indicate the role of such dysrhythmias in the peri-operative period. Atrial fibrillation and premature atrial or ventricular complexes would appear to have little effect unless the atrial fibrillation rate is uncontrolled or the ventricular complexes are multifocal or very frequent. Foster and colleagues (1986) found no link between arrhythmias and an adverse outcome after anaesthesia, although the numbers in the study were small. Even complex conduction problems such as left axis deviation, right bundle branch block and complete trifascicular block appear to have no adverse risk, unless associated with an acute myocardial infarction (Mangano, 1990).

Valvular heart disease

There are few data on the impact of valvular heart disease on post-operative complications. An exception is aortic stenosis, moderate or severe degrees of which are associated with an increased post-operative mortality (Goldman *et al.*, 1977; O'Keefe, 1989). Goldman and colleagues found little evidence to suggest that aortic regurgitation, mitral or tricuspid valve disease conferred any significant increased risk of death, although mitral valve disease was associated with an increased risk of post-operative congestive heart failure. However, significant valvular disease seldom exists alone and concomitant ventricular dysfunction, arrhythmia or pulmonary hypertension make it difficult to know whether the original valve disease *per se* increases risk.

AN OVERVIEW

In summary, the only definite risk factors for increased morbidity and mortality in the peri-operative period would appear to be recent myocardial infarction (under six months), heart failure or severe aortic stenosis. Data on most other factors (angina pectoris, hypertension and arrhythmia) are conflicting.

Table 6.1 *The ASA Classification of Physical Status*

1. A normal healthy patient
2. A patient with a mild systemic disease
3. A patient with a severe systemic disease that limits activity, but is not incapacitating
4. A patient with an incapacitating systemic disease that is a constant threat to life
5. A moribund patient not expected to survive 24 hours with or without operation

In the event of emergency operation, precede the number with an E.

(Adapted from ASA, 1963)

Many attempts have been made to devise scoring systems for operative risk based on a composite of clinical examination and easily performed investigations, but such risk stratification is complex. Patients may have classical histories of stable angina pectoris with exertional central chest pain radiating to the arms and jaw, and this may occur with or without breathlessness on exertion, but many individuals have no such warning features. The patient may appear clinically well and have a normal ECG, but

still have a significant stenosis of the left main stem or proximal left anterior descending artery. They may even complain of atypical symptoms which draw attention away from the critical underlying problem.

In spite of the problems, a number of scoring systems have been developed to assist pre-operative risk stratification. Perhaps the earliest attempt was the American Society of Anesthesiologists (ASA, 1963) system (Table 6.1), and it is now over twenty years since Goldman and colleagues (1977) developed their clinical risk scoring system (Table 6.2). This is more specific than the original ASA system, identifying nine factors, five cardiovascular, which were shown to be independently associated with post-operative cardiac complications. This system was subsequently modified by Detsky and colleagues (1986) to take the current classification of angina into account, and to simplify the scoring process (Table 6.3). However, such systems (apart from the ASA one) are rarely used outwith the research setting, yet myocardial infarction remains a leading cause of death after surgery (Aitkenhead, 1987) and non-fatal myocardial infarction accounts for considerable morbidity (Gajraj and Jamieson, 1994).

Table 6.2 *The Goldman Multifactorial Risk Index*

Criteria	Multivariate discriminant-function coefficient	Points
1. History		
Age >70 years	0.191	5
MI in previous 6 months	0.384	10
2. Physical examination		
S_3 gallop or JVD	0.451	1
Important VAS	0.119	3
3. Electrocardiogram		
Rhythm other than sinus or PAC on last pre-operative ECG	0.283	7
>5 PVC/min documented at any time before operation	0.278	7
4. General status		
Po_2 <60 or Pco_2 >50 mmHg, K^+ <3.0 or HCO_3^- <20 mEq/L, BUN >50 or Cr >3.0 mg/dL, abnormal SGOT, signs of chronic liver disease, or patient bedridden from non-cardiac disease	0.132	3
5. Operation		
Intraperitoneal, intrathoracic or aortic operation	0.123	3
Emergency operation	0.167	4
Total		53

Abbreviations: MI, myocardial infarction; JVD, jugular vein distension; VAS, valvular aortic stenosis; PAC, premature atrial contractions; ECG, electrocardiogram; PVC, premature ventricular contractions; Po_2, partial pressure of oxygen; Pco_2, partial pressure of carbon dioxide; K^+, potassium; HCO_3^-, bicarbonate; BUN, blood urea nitrogen; Cr, creatinine; SGOT, serum glutamic–oxaloacetic transaminase.
(Adapted from Goldman *et al.*, 1977)

Table 6.3   *The Modified Multifactorial Cardiac Risk Index*

Variables	Points
CAD	
MI within 6 months	10
MI more than 6 months	5
Canadian Cardiovascular Society angina	
Class 3	10
Class 4	20
Alveolar pulmonary oedema	
Within 1 week	10
Ever	5
Valvular disease	
Suspected critical aortic stenosis	
Arrhythmias	
Sinus plus atrial premature beats or	
rhythm other than sinus on last	
pre-operative ECG	5
>5 ventricular premature beats at	
any time before surgery	5
Poor general medical status*	5
Age >70 years	5
Emergency operation	10

*Oxygen pressure <60 mmHg; carbon dioxide pressure >50 mmHg; serum K^+ <3.0 mmol/L; serum HCO_3^- <20 mmol/L; serum urea >18 mmol/L; serum creatinine >260 mmol/L; aspartate aminotransferase, abnormal; signs of chronic liver disease; and/or bedridden because of non-cardiac disease.

(Adapted from Detsky *et al.*, 1986)

An extensive review of peri-operative cardiac morbidity by Mangano (1990) suggested that the highest risk patient is one who has current congestive cardiac failure or has suffered a recent myocardial infarction. Age and a history of stable angina were poorer predictors of an adverse outcome in the peri-operative period and suggested that more invasive monitoring was likely to minimize the incidence of peri-operative infarction.

Cardiovascular investigation

Identifying the high-risk patient, either with a scoring system or by the presence of the three most serious prognostic factors (recent myocardial infarction, heart failure and severe aortic stenosis), is but the first step. The next stage is the question of what is the best and most cost-effective objective method of identifying and quantifying these risk factors, and

then whether is it safe to ignore all others. It could be argued that history, examination, ECG and transthoracic echocardiography should be sufficient to delineate the three main risk factors. However, symptoms that arise from ischaemic heart disease, left ventricular dysfunction and valvular heart disease commonly overlap, and are difficult to ascribe to one pathological entity in many cases. The major symptoms are dyspnoea, chest pain, palpitations, dizziness and syncope, but there are less common ones such as fatigue, nocturia, polyuria, cyanosis and cardiac cachexia.

Besides the more obvious symptoms and signs, there are some interesting anomalies in the clinical signs of heart failure. Tachycardia is a non-specific sign and may be absent, even in severe heart failure (Stevenson and Perloff, 1989), and a third heart sound is not specific to heart failure (Folland *et al.*, 1992). The cardiac apex beat is often difficult to palpate, and this makes it a poor index of cardiomegaly (O'Neil *et al.*, 1989). Among non-specialists there is often disagreement about whether the jugular venous pressure (JVP) is elevated or not (Butman *et al.*, 1993). Furthermore, the JVP is not always elevated, even in severe heart failure (Stevenson and Perloff, 1989). Heart failure itself may be quite advanced before oedema is evident, especially in men (Stevenson and Perloff, 1989), and oedema is typically of right or biventricular origin. In essence, the severity of the symptoms and signs of severe heart failure do not correlate well with the severity of left ventricular dysfunction (Marantz *et al.*, 1988).

Because the only confirmed predictors of adverse risk are a myocardial infarction within the last six months, heart failure or aortic stenosis of moderate to severe severity, it seems unnecessary currently to perform cardiac investigations to detect asymptomatic coronary disease *per se*. The presence of a recent myocardial infarction (i.e. within the last six months) should be discerned from the history and/or the case records. The ECG may show a typical Q-wave infarct, but the absence of such should not preclude the diagnosis. Investigation with exercise testing is controversial. It may be inappropriate because the majority of patients with peripheral vascular disease are unable to reach 85 per cent of the maximum heart rate (McPhail *et al.*, 1988) or the information garnered has no impact on outcome (Carliner *et al.*, 1985). However, others have found that exercise testing has predicted perioperative myocardial infarction (Cutler *et al.*, 1981). Perhaps, as suggested by Mangano and Goldman (1995), it is the response to exercise and ability to reach the age-specific target heart rate if possible, that is important, not the ischaemic changes themselves. Ambulatory ECG monitoring has been shown to be an independent indicator of adverse outcomes, but is not sensitive enough to identify low risk groups (Mangano *et al.*, 1990).

Defining the area of impaired blood flow with thallium scanning (Baron *et al.*, 1994) or coronary angiography (Foster *et al.*, 1986), followed by the appropriate revascularization procedure, has not altered the risk of adverse peri-operative outcome. Thus the diagnosis of reversible ischaemia does not appear to matter. The main investigation should be therefore the diagnosis of pre-operative heart failure. The assessment of cardiac function is primarily by transthoracic echocardiography, though nuclear cardiac scanning is probably more sensitive. Newer, specialist investigations are transoesophogeal echocardiography, myocardial Doppler echocardiography, dobutamine stress echocardiography, positron emission tomography (PET) scans and blood tests such as measurement of brain or B-type natriuretic peptide (BNP).

ASSESSING CARDIAC FALIURE

Previously, the only method available to the physician or anaesthetist to assess heart size was the chest radiograph. Attempts to improve the predictive accuracy of chest radiographs included the use of the Ungerleider table, which combined the cardiothoracic ratio and the patient's height and weight. However, there is little correlation between radiographic findings and measured left ventricular dimensions and echocardiography is required to differentiate reliably between cardiac chamber dilatation, hypertrophy or pericardial disease (Madsen *et al.*, 1984; Alam *et al.*, 1989).

Echocardiography
The advent of echocardiography has greatly assisted the ability to diagnose heart failure. It is a technique which is widely available, cheap, simple and safe. Three main modes are in common current use: M-mode, two-dimensional and Doppler echocardiography.

- M-mode echocardiography was the first modality to be used, but has now been largely superseded by two-dimensional studies. It is still the mode of choice for delineating the timing of early mitral valve closure in aortic regurgitation and for the systolic anterior motion of the anterior mitral leaflet in hypertrophic obstructive cardiomyopathy. It also has a major role in determining wall thickness and chamber sizes.
- Two-dimensional (2-D) echocardiography allows assessment of all the features that M-mode can display. Additionally, it can be used to assess cardiac valves, calculate ventricular volumes, assess systolic and diastolic function, left ventricular mass and ventricular wall motion. It also has the advantage that pericardial abnormalities can be demonstrated.
- Doppler imaging allows blood flow velocities across stenotic valves to be documented, giving a measure of maximum pressure drop and regurgitant flow. An indirect measure of pulmonary artery pressure can be calculated if a degree of tricuspid regurgitation is present. The combination of 2-D and Doppler echocardiography gives an excellent combination for assessing ventricular function and valvular disease in the same study.

Systolic LV dysfunction is a common finding on echocardiography, and this may be subdivided into global and regional wall motion abnormalities. An area may be described as hypokinetic, akinetic or dyskinetic depending on the severity of myocardial disease in that area. In large epidemiological studies of patients with heart failure or who have suffered myocardial infarction, the risk of death from pump failure or sudden arrhythmic death rises dramatically as ejection fraction decreases. In the first Veterans Administration Co-operative Heart Failure Trial (V-HeFT I) of mild and moderate left ventricular dysfunction, the one-year mortality rate was 19.5 per cent (Cohn, 1986), whereas in studies of severe heart failure (Massie and Conway, 1987; CONSENSUS-I Trial Study Group, 1987), the one-year mortality rate was 40–60 per cent.

In older patients, the typical symptoms of heart failure can occur in the presence of normal left ventricular systolic function and the heart failure may be attributed to diastolic dysfunction. Diastolic dysfunction occurs as the ventricular wall becomes stiff and non-compliant and this is accentuated by advancing age and systemic hypertension. The symptoms occur because poor left ventricular filling leads to a reduced cardiac output. The normal pat-

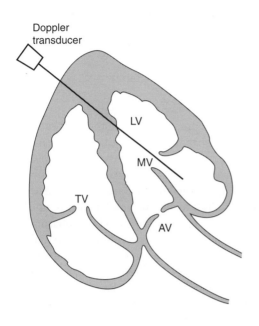

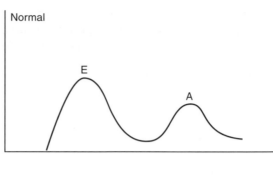

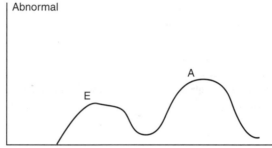

Figure 6.1   *E:A reversal on Doppler echocardiographic assessment of the mitral valve.*

tern of blood flow through the mitral valve is altered and the E : A ratio is reversed, that is the early phase (E) of ventricular filling is diminished but the late phase (A) caused by atrial contraction is maintained or exaggerated (Fig. 6.1).

Echocardiographic assessment of any valve relies upon getting a good-quality picture that can be lined up with the Doppler probe. If the angle between blood flow and the Doppler beam is greater than 20 per cent then the degree of stenosis will be greatly underestimated. The valve can often be seen to be thickened or heavily calcified both on the M-mode and 2-D picture. Results are often quoted as a maximum pressure change across the valve which usually gives a figure approximately 20 mmHg greater than the peak-to-peak gradient obtained at cardiac catheterization. This is because it measures an instantaneous gradient between the left ventricle and the aorta. With significant stenosis there is a lag between the rise in ventricular pressure and its transmission through the stenotic valve to the aortic root. Figure 6.2 represents the pressure–time relationship schematically. Measurement of left ventricular and aortic pressures will give an aortic gradient A–B, whereas from echocardiographic assessment it will be A–C. This is because it measures an instantaneous pressure difference between LV and aorta.

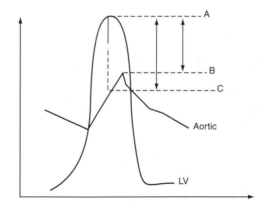

Figure 6.2   *Composite of catheter- and echocardiographic-derived pressure traces.*

Transoesophageal echocardiography is a rapidly developing field. Most of the views available via the transthoracic approach can be reproduced, but many others can be added. It has the advantage that it is not fixed to particular windows where the heart is visible between bone and lung tissue and is therefore particularly useful for patients with a high body mass index. It has a higher frequency transducer which allows better resolution of cardiac structures and is especially useful for assessing the left atrium, left atrial appendage, aortic valve and root, left ventricle and pulmonary artery. It is invaluable at looking for clot in the left atrial appendage and for vegetations on valves in cases of suspected endocarditis.

Despite left ventricular dysfunction and valvular heart disease being independent predictors of adverse cardiac events (Mangano, 1990), the evidence seems to suggest that neither pre-operative transthoracic or transoesophageal echocardiography routinely add appreciably to information on cardiovascular risk (Mangano and Goldman, 1995). The exceptions seem to be those patients who would justify echocardiographic assessment on the grounds of the severity of their cardiovascular disease alone, rather than because they were being assessed for a major operation.

There is a growing trend for intra-operative transoesophageal echocardiography as a method for assessing segmental wall motion abnormalities as an early indicator of myocardial ischaemia. It has been shown to be more sensitive than ECG monitoring for picking up regional myocardial ischaemia (Wohlgelernter et al., 1985; Smith et al., 1985) and has demonstrated that segments progress from hypokinesia to akinesia to dyskinesia rapidly if the ischaemic insult is not relieved. Interestingly, there is evidence that ischaemia demonstrated by this technique may adversely affect peri-operative morbidity. A small study found that four patients who suffered a myocardial infarction after surgery had wall motion abnormalities whereas only one had ECG evidence of ischaemia (Smith et al., 1985).

Stress echocardiography is another technique which relies on inducing an increase in myocardial oxygen demand either with exercise or by infusion of dobutamine. The normal patient will respond with an increase in ventricular wall motion eventually to hyperkinesis. The patient with no wall motion abnormalities at rest may develop abnormalities under stress. It is similar to the exercise ECG in sensitivity and specificity (Marcovitz and Armstrong, 1992), and a study of 302 patients suggested that stress echocardiography identifies the high-risk population awaiting surgery (Poldermans et al., 1995). However, there is as yet little consensus on whether it is better than the exercise ECG in predicting adverse outcomes during non-cardiac vascular operations.

Nuclear cardiology

Myocardial imaging can be divided into three broad areas:

- Imaging the areas of the heart that are perfused during both rest and exercise.
- Locating the site of an infarct using radiolabelled pyrophosphate.
- Radionuclide ventriculography.

Evidence already presented suggests that perfusion imaging has little predictive role in the assessment of patients with ischaemic heart disease prior to major vascular surgery, although is useful for deciding whether a coronary artery lesion is producing myocardial ischaemia or to confirm a borderline treadmill test. The technique consists of a period of myocardial stress (induced by exercise or pharmacologically) followed by an injection of the radioisotope thallium-201. Imaging begins within 10–15 minutes and, if a perfusion defect is seen, repeated at 3–24 hours to see if the defect has filled in. If the defect is reversible, it suggests that the area is ischaemic rather than an area of infarction. Younis and colleagues (1990) suggested that both a previous history of angina and reversible perfusion defects were predictors of non-fatal myocardial infarction and death, although Baron and colleagues (1994) have refuted this.

Radionuclide angiography has certain advantages over echocardiography, the inter- and intra-observer variabilities both being low: 2 per cent and 5 per cent respectively (Wackers et al., 1979). However, Himelman and colleagues (1982) found that the ejection fraction varied by 15 per cent when assessed by different operators, and that studies were less than ideal in 30 per cent, being very difficult in approximately 10 per cent of patients.

Most nuclear ventriculography studies are equilibrium, rather than first pass, studies which rely on gathering information on a bolus of tracer as it passes through the heart. First-pass studies need gamma cameras with high count rates or multicrystal units. Both of these are scarce in the majority of units. Equilibrium studies are synchronized on the R-wave of the ECG and then sixteen frames are sampled per cardiac cycle for normal systolic function studies, and thirty-two frames per cycle for diastolic function studies. The average length of study is 200–800 cardiac cycles.

Early studies suggested that this method of assessing ventricular function was promising in its ability to identify patients at risk (Pasternack et al., 1984) of adverse cardiovascular outcomes. However, this has not been borne out by later work which identified older age and definite clinical evidence of coronary artery disease as the most important predictors (Baron *et al.*, 1994).

Positron emission tomography (PET)

Positron emitters can be used to label naturally occurring elements such a hydrogen, nitrogen and oxygen. The emitted positron travels a short distance before colliding with an electron and this reaction causes the release of two gamma photons, which can be detected by an array of gamma detectors. It remains a research tool, available only to those fortunate to work near a cyclotron which is necessary to generate the tracers. It is expensive and the tracers are short lived. Its advantages include the labelling of naturally occurring chemicals, low radiation dose and the sensitivity of the test. Its main contribution has been to add weight to the hypothesis of hibernating myocardium, which suggests that if the supply of oxygen is diminished, then myocardial cells will cease to contract and will switch from their preferred energy source, fatty acids, to anaerobic glycolysis. On a nuclear perfusion scan they may appear as fixed defects during both stress and reperfusion phases and as akinetic or dyskinetic wall motion abnormalities on echocardiographic studies, but on PET scanning with the glucose analogue, ^{18}F-fluorodeoxyglucose, there is still evidence of cellular activity, which means that revascularization could improve ventricular function (Dicarli *et al.*, 1993).

Neuroendocrine evaluation

There is epidemiological evidence that renin, angiotensin II, aldosterone and norepinephrine concentrations are related to the severity and prognosis of heart failure (Swedberg *et al.*, 1990). However, their usefulness in individual patients is unclear. Therapy with diuretics causes activation of the renin–angiotensin–aldosterone axis, but recent studies have shown that there may be a role for measuring natriuretic peptides in the identification of patients who are asymptomatic, but have reduced left ventricular function (Motwani *et al.*, 1993). Whether natriuretic peptides have a role in assessing the peri-operative has yet to be determined.

Summary

In summary, it would appear prudent for the patient with left ventricular dysfunction to be assessed initially by history and examination, and then investigated with echocardiography, which should delineate ventricular function and valve pathology. If there are significant technical difficulties with echocardiography then a radionuclide ventriculogram should be obtained. The only time coronary angiography should be considered is when the patient has severe or unstable coronary disease, or is being assessed for valve surgery and direct measurement of pressure gradients is needed.

PERI-OPERATIVE CARDIOVASCULAR DRUG THERAPY

The short time before surgery during which a routine anaesthetic assessment is made is not the ideal time to alter medication. However, cardiovascular medications are often prescribed over a prolonged period of time and the number of drugs accumulates, often with a large number of tablets being prescribed with little discernible benefit. Therefore, with a major operation and its appreciable risks in prospect, critical appraisal of the patient's medication is expected.

The major aim in prescribing for cardiovascular disease of all degrees is to combine three outcomes: first to alleviate symptoms; second to improve the prognosis; and third to aid compliance. Many cardiovascular drugs, with the exception of digoxin and warfarin (where therapeutic levels can be achieved and maintained safely and effectively), are difficult to monitor.

Ischaemic heart disease

ASPIRIN

Aspirin improves outcome when prescribed for unstable angina or in the early stages of myocardial infarction, when the mortality reduction equals that of intravenous streptokinase (ISIS-2, 1988). However, its effects when given in the recovery period (between one and six months) after myocardial infarction, or as prophylaxis in stable angina pectoris, are less impressive. PARIS-II (Klimt, 1986) was the only large study to show benefits of reduced cardiovascular deaths (24 per cent) and non-fatal infarction (placebo 11.8 vs. drug 9.0 per cent). There was no difference in all cause mortality. It relied upon a meta-analysis of 31 randomized trials, covering 29 000 patients, which showed a 15 per cent reduction in cardiovascular mortality and a 30 per cent reduction in the incidence of stroke and myocardial infarction (Antiplatelet Trialists Collaboration, 1988). There was no evidence that one dose of aspirin was better than any other or that the addition or substitution of other antiplatelet agents (dipyridamole) was of any advantage. However, 300 mg of aspirin has demonstrable effects in hours, whereas 75 mg may take days to exert an initial effect. Primary prevention studies with aspirin (Peto *et al.*, 1986; Physicians Health Study, 1989) have revealed no effect on overall mortality, with a trend towards increased haemorrhagic stroke and a small trend towards a lower incidence of myocardial infarction. At this time, there is no convincing evidence that stable angina pectoris should be prophylactically treated with antithrombotic agents unless the patient is at high risk because of other co-existing factors.

BETA-BLOCKADE

The main cardiovascular effects of beta-blockade are decreases in heart rate and myocardial contractility. These reduce myocardial oxygen demand, and improve its delivery by increasing the diastolic time period. First-generation beta-blocking agents inhibited both β_1- and β_2-receptors, second-generation drugs were more specific for β_1-receptors, and the third-generation agents also have vasodilator properties, chiefly produced by intrinsic sympathomimetic activity (ISA) at β_2-receptors in peripheral arterioles. At this stage, there is no convincing evidence that these additional effects produce any definite benefits, except for the suggestion that, during the acute stages of myocardial infarction, non-selective beta-blockers should theoretically be better anti-arrhythmic agents. The different side-effect profiles may be important for individual patients. For example, those with early morning angina may well benefit from long-acting agents, and those with peripheral vascular disease may be able to tolerate beta-blockade if there is concomitant vasodilatation.

In trying to tailor therapy, it is usual to try and achieve a resting heart rate of 55–60 beats per minute, although rates of 50 beats per minute may be well tolerated. Another guide is to decrease the exercise heart rate to 100–110 beats per minute. A

caveat to this is that newer agents with ISA (pindolol, celiprolol) will not reduce heart rate to the same degree as the older ones because of the peripheral vasodilatation. Indeed, total peripheral vascular resistance would be markedly reduced in some cases, causing hypotension before the heart rate decreased to the same degree.

There is no evidence that beta-blockade has any prognostic effect in patients with stable angina pectoris. However, the benefits of beta-blockade after myocardial infarction are well documented by several large studies (BHAT, 1982, 1983; ISIS-1, 1986). The drugs produced significant reductions in all cause and cardiovascular mortality, and there was also a sustained reduction in the risk of sudden cardiac death and non-fatal reinfarction in the 25 months follow-up period in BHAT.

More recently, Mangano and colleagues (1996) have shown that beta-blocking agents should not only be continued peri-operatively in patients with coronary artery disease, but that therapy should be initiated in those patients with known coronary disease. This conferred a significant survival advantage which was still present at two years. This confirms findings from the CASS study, which showed that these agents should be continued throughout the surgical period (Foster *et al.*, 1986).

NITRATES

Nitrates are a mainstay of treatment of acute exertional angina pectoris, being widely used in sublingual, buccal and oral preparations. They act as donators of nitric oxide, causing vasodilatation of epicardial arteries and acting on both stenotic arteries and collaterals. This prevents the coronary steal effects which are seen with some other vasodilators. The circulatory effects include reduced preload through dilation of venous capacitance vessels. To a lesser degree they also dilate arteriolar resistance vessels and reduce afterload. Therefore the resulting effect is decreased oxygen consumption because of decreased myocardial work and increased myocardial oxygen delivery because of epicardial arterial vasodilatation. However, some of these beneficial effects are offset by the reflex increase in heart rate seen with the reduction in afterload.

Tolerance to nitrate therapy has led to the development of long-acting preparations, taken once daily, which ensure that there is an eight-hour 'nitrate free' interval. If patients wish to persist with older preparations then the need for an eccentric dosing pattern to prevent tolerance must be emphasized. Nitrates appear to have no prognostic effects on chronic stable angina or acute myocardial infarction. Again, there is no survival benefit in unstable angina, where therapy with intravenous nitrates is necessary and tolerance does develop over a period of days. However, they were shown to improve mortality when combined with hydralazine in heart failure (Cohn, 1986).

CALCIUM-CHANNEL BLOCKADE

All calcium-channel blockers act by inhibiting the voltage-dependent L-channels which allow calcium entry from the sarcoplasmic reticulum. There are two major groups of drugs: verapamil and diltiazem; and the dihydropyridines (nifedipine, amlodipine, felodipine).

Verapamil
Verapamil was the first calcium-channel blocker, its major effects including arteriolar vasodilatation and reduced afterload, epicardial artery dilatation and increased oxygen supply, depression of sino-atrial and atrioventricular nodes with decreased heart rate, and increased atrioventricular conduction. It is particularly negatively inotropic. The net effect is vasodilatation without a reflex tachycardia, but a varying degree of bradycardia. Certainly, in patients with chronic stable angina pectoris, the heart rate is usually unchanged when compared to placebo. There appears to be no prognostic advantage with intravenous verapamil during acute myocardial infarction, but in the DAVIT-II study (1990) there was a small, but significant improvement in survival when verapamil was started 4–6 weeks after myocardial infarction.

Diltiazem
Diltiazem has similar actions to verapamil, but its effect upon the atrioventricular node is less, and on the sino-atrial node greater so it has a larger potential for causing sinus bradycardia. It still causes peripheral vasodilatation with afterload reduction, and epicardial vasodilatation with improved myocardial oxygen supply. Diltiazem has less of a negative inotropic effect than verapamil. Again, the net negative chronotropic effect is small in monotherapy in a patient with a normal conduction system because vasodilatation acts reflexly to increase heart rate.

Dihydropyridines
The first generation dihydropyridine, nifedipine, has its greatest effects on vascular smooth muscle and has no effect upon nodal tissue. In monotherapy, it is a powerful arteriolar vasodilator and its main indication is hypertension. Its role in chronic angina pectoris is limited by the initial reflex tachycardia, which could in theory increase myocardial oxygen consumption and worsen angina. However, once the patient is established on these agents, the baroreflex becomes blunted and heart rate is unchanged. For this reason, patients with unstable angina pectoris may proceed to myocardial infarction if given an unopposed short-acting dihydropyridine (HINT, 1986). Nifedipine has a negative inotropic effect similar to the other calcium channel-blocking agents. The use of sublingual nifedipine for severe hypertension is popular because it often brings blood pressure under control quickly, and it is easier and cheaper than nitroprusside infusion (Franklin et al., 1986). However, it has the disadvantage that the hypotensive effect may be too great in some patients and it is not easy to reverse.

The second-generation dihydropyridines act on the same dihydropyridine receptor as nifedipine, although they are more cardio-specific. Short-acting agents such as nicardipine have similar indications and side effects, but longer-acting agents such as amlodipine and felodipine may produce less side effects because of their slower onset. Certainly the reflex tachycardia is less.

COMBINATION THERAPY FOR ANGINA PECTORIS

There is an ascending pyramid of treatment for chronic exertional angina pectoris with normal ventricular function. Patients with a minor degree of angina pectoris are treated with sublingual glyceryl trinitrate as required. Therafter, most physicians would add a beta-blocking agent and titrate it against heart rate at rest and on exercise. If this therapy alone does not afford symptomatic relief, a second regular agent should be added. Whether this is a calcium channel-blocking drug or an oral nitrate preparation is a matter for personal preference. The most haemodynamically sound combination is a beta-blocking agent with a dihydropyridine, such as nifedipine. This combines the heart rate-limiting effect of the beta-blocking agent (minimizing oxygen consumption and preventing reflex tachycardia) with the afterload reduction produced by the calcium channel-blocking agent. More recently, there has been a move to add diltiazem to a beta-blocking agent, and this combination is both effective and suprisingly well tolerated. Adding a third agent does not always increase control of symptoms and can merely add to the side-effect profile.

Angina pectoris with left ventricular dysfunction is more difficult to treat effectively. The patient would still benefit from beta-blockade, but this might provoke a worsening of heart failure symptoms. Here there is a rationale for the newer agents with vasodilatatory action, perhaps in combination with a nitrate rather than a calcium channel-blocking agent.

Heart failure

There are two separate issues in the treatment of heart failure: relief of symptoms; the improvement of prognosis.

DIURETICS

Initial therapy almost always involves diuretics. Loop diuretics are usually more powerful than the thiazides and still work in renal impairment. They will reduce preload even before producing a diuretic effect.

Loop diuretics work on the ascending loop of Henle, inhibiting the sodium/potassium/chloride ($Na^+/K^+/Cl^-$) co-transporter system, diminishing the passage of Cl^- across the tubular lining cells. There is little to choose between frusemide and bumetanide, both acting intraluminally after being excreted by the proximal tubule. Consequently, larger doses may be necessary in chronic renal failure and severe heart failure to overcome impairment of both renal blood flow and proximal tubular secretion. The diuretic action starts within 10 minutes of an intravenous dose, although venous dilatation occurs even sooner.

The dose used is completely dependent on the response of the patient, some may need as little as 20 mg of frusemide, while others require 2 g daily. Diuretic requirement also changes and it is important that regular checks are made of both the clinical state of the patient and the biochemical profile. A common cause of lethargy and breathlessness is dehydration associated with overzealous diuretic

therapy leading to hypovolaemia with decreases in filling pressures and cardiac output. Identifying the correct dose of diuretic therapy can be difficult, but may be helped by establishing a target weight and allowing the patient to alter the dose according to a simple algorithm. Alternatively, there may be a role for the use of natriuretic peptide assays in helping to optimize diuretic therapy.

Thiazide diuretics are the traditional first-line agents for mild hypertension in which they may take up to three months to exert a maximal effect. They can be effective as monotherapy in mild heart failure, and in combination with a loop diuretic if failure is severe. They exert their action at the distal tubule, inhibiting the resorption of Na^+ and K^+.

The crucial difference between the two types of agent is in the degree of diuresis, the thiazides producing approximately one-third of the loop diuretics. Low thiazide doses would seem to produce a maximum diuretic effect quite quickly, and higher doses are only marginally more effective while increasing side effects disproportionately. Thiazides, perhaps with the exception of metolazone, are much less effective when the glomerular filtration rate is below 20 mL/min.

Potassium-sparing agents are weak diuretics in their own right and include amiloride, triamterene and spironolactone. Amiloride and triamterene act by inhibition of Na^+ resorption in the distal tubule and the collecting duct so that there is no direct loss of K^+. Spironolactone antagonizes the aldosterone-governed Na^+/K^+ exchange in the distal tubule, and has a role where there is activation of the renin–angiotensin–aldosterone axis as in heart failure and chronic liver disease. It is a more potent diuretic than amiloride and triamterene. Problems can occur when compound drugs which contain potassium or potassium-sparing diuretics are co-prescribed with other drugs such as angiotensin-converting enzyme (ACE) inhibitors and nephrotoxic agents.

DIGOXIN

Digoxin has three main actions: first, it is traditionally thought of as a positive inotrope, although this is now controversial; second, it is negatively chronotropic; and third, it has a recently described sympatholytic action. The inotropic effect may not always be beneficial because oxygen consumption might increase with myocardial contraction and this can cause problems if cardiac oxygen delivery is already maximal. However, the bradycardic effect is beneficial because it should decrease myocardial oxygen consumption while increasing delivery during the longer diastolic time period.

Digoxin inhibits the Na^+/K^+ exchange system to increase intracellular Na^+ which, in turn, is exchanged for Ca^{2+}. A higher intracellular Ca^{2+} concentration increases force of myocardial contraction. There are also direct autonomic effects. Vagal tone is increased so that activity decreases at both sino-atrial and atrioventricular nodes, and sympathetic activity is decreased.

There is no doubt about the efficacy of digoxin in the control of atrial fibrillation with a rapid ventricular response. In the presence of atrial fibrillation and heart failure, digoxin has a significant role to play. However, the position in sinus rhythm is less clear. The results of the recent DIG (1996) trial suggest that there is no prognostic advantage for digoxin in sinus rhythm, but patients' symptoms are better controlled on digoxin. It does not, in itself, cause reversion of recent onset atrial fibrillation, and it is relatively ineffective in controlling ventricular rate in atrial flutter or atrial fibrillation due to sympathetic stimulation as in sepsis.

Digoxin toxicity can be a major problem, especially with elderly patients, low serum K^+ and concurrent drug administration. The elderly patient is at risk mainly because serum digoxin increases before creatinine when the glomerular filtration rate starts to decrease. Lower skeletal and lean body masses are also associated with higher concentrations, and a low serum K^+ renders the heart more susceptible to digoxin toxicity.

Drug interactions are commonplace and concomitant administration of quinidine, quinine, verapamil and amiodarone all increase serum concentrations. Diuretic therapy may cause hypokalaemia and increase the likelihood of digoxin toxicity. An important feature of toxicity associated with hypokalaemia is that the digoxin effect may manifest as atrioventricular block and therefore prophylactic pacing may be necessary.

ACE INHIBITORS

While diuretics are the mainstay of symptomatic relief, angiotensin-converting enzyme (ACE) inhibitors have the major role in preventing deterioration in left ventricular function. They act by inhibiting the conversion of angiotensin-I to angiotensin-II, and consequently prevent the multiple effects of angiotensin-II, as well as inhibiting the breakdown of the vasodilator, bradykinin. Angiotensin-II increases release of aldosterone from the adrenal medulla, and has direct effects on arteriolar wall tone through activation of specific receptors. It also has indirect effects, increasing the release of noradrenaline and preventing its re-uptake. Therefore, interrupting this cycle will firstly decrease afterload (loss of angiotensin-II and noradrenaline action) and subsequently decrease preload through less aldosterone-mediated Na^+ and water retention, and increased vasodilatation because of higher concentrations of bradykinin.

All trials have shown that ACE inhibition is effective in both preventing deterioration of heart failure and improving symptom control (CONSENSUS-I, 1987; SOLVD-treatment, 1991; Cohn et al., 1991; SOLVD-prevention, 1992). There seems to be little to choose between different agents, although there is, in renal impairment, a slight preference for short-acting drugs which allow the renal vasculature time to recover.

Other vasodilators have only a moderate role in the management of heart failure, although Cohn and colleagues (1986) did show that the combination of the arterial vasodilator, hydralazine, with the predominantly venodilator, isosorbide dinitrate, reduces mortality. Nitrates are commonly used to reduce preload and consequently the degree of dyspnoea that patients feel. Hydralazine is now rarely used in the UK, especially with the advent of ACE inhibitors.

Side effects include first-dose hypotension (which should not affect peri-operative management) and interactions with other drugs, especially potassium-sparing diuretics and, to a lesser degree, with other agents that reduce afterload such as the calcium channel-blocking agents.

The treatment of angina associated with heart failure is very difficult, but the combination of diuretic, ACE inhibitor, nitrate and, if possible, a beta-blocking agent is reversible.

Hypertension

Currently, the treatment of hypertension is complex. Previously, a stepped-care process was accepted practice, but has become increasingly criticized. This typically involved the prescription of a diuretic agent or beta-blocking agent, followed by their combination, and then by a vasodilator. This has now been changed and now almost any drug can be used as a first-line agent. However, current data on prognosis suggest that only diuretics and beta-blocking agents decrease the risk of myocardial infarction, stroke or premature death from hypertension (Collins *et al.*, 1990), although data from the Captopril Primary Prevention Project group (1990) should be available soon.

Drug choice is governed by patients' individual needs. Those with hypertension and coronary artery disease ought to have their angina pectoris treated first by the combination of a beta-blocking agent and a vasodilator. The latter should be a calcium channel-blocking drug rather than a nitrate.

Studies have shown that treating hypertension in the elderly (SHEP, 1991; MRC-elderly hypertensives, 1992), and treating isolated systolic hypertension (Dahlöf *et al.*, 1991) does reduce mortality. Interestingly, diuretics appeared better than beta-blocking agents in the MRC trial of elderly hypertensives. Black hypertensive patients seem to respond better to diuretics and vasodilators than to beta-blockade.

CONCLUSION

Extensive investigation has culminated in the American College of Cardiology and the American Heart Association producing guidelines for practitioners in this area (Task force of the ACC/AHA, 1996), and the broad themes of these have been covered in this chapter.

The routine use of expensive pre-operative evaluation in patients undergoing non-cardiac surgery can no longer be justified. Patients with no history of symptomatic heart disease do not need further evaluation and their risk of death from cardiac causes is less than 1 per cent. Even patients with stable angina pectoris who are in class I or II functional status, do not need further investigation (risk of death 2 per cent).

Further cardiac investigation should be carried out (irrespective of the proposed surgery) in patients who have disease that is not controlled as well as it can be. The major factors governing increased risk of adverse cardiovascular events in the peri-operative period in a non-cardiac operation are heart failure, myocardial infarction within six months or significant aortic stenosis. These entities should be sought by history and examination in all patients and simple transthoracic echocardiography in suspect patients. In those in whom a transthoracic echocardiograph is unsatisfactory then alternative procedures should be undertaken such as transoesophageal echocardiography for valve pathology and/or left ventricular function, a radionuclide ventriculogram for left ventricular function or a left heart cardiac catheter for valve pathology and/or left ventricular function.

However, the key is that treatment regimes should be optimized before surgery is contemplated. Even though the CASS registry data show no difference in survival in patients treated with CABG, the patient should be listed for bypass grafting if the severity of their coronary disease merits it, and this should take precedence over the non-cardiac surgery.

Optimization of drug therapy should be performed with a full background knowledge of the patient's history, and of the haemodynamic and side effects of each drug. Changes to medication should not be undertaken by junior staff without discussing the case with senior physicians. In addition, adequate assessment of patients with significant co-existing cardiovascular disease should be undertaken well in advance of major surgery, and not simply in the few days before it.

REFERENCES

Aitkenhead, A.R. 1987. Post-operative ischaemia, cardiac morbidity after non-cardiac surgery. *Lancet* **341**, 731–732.

Alam, M., Rosenhamer, G. and Hoglund, C. 1989. Comparability of echocardiography and chest X-ray following myocardial infarction. *Journal of Internal Medicine* **226**, 171–175.

Antiplatelet Trialists Collaboration. 1988. Secondary prevention of vascular disease by prolonged antiplatelet treatment. *British Heart Journal* **296**, 320.

ASA. 1963. New classification of physical status. *Anesthesiology* **24**, 111.

Baron, J-F., Mundler, O. and Bertrand, M. 1994. Dipyridimole–thallium scintigraphy and gated radionuclide angiography to assess cardiac risk before abdominal aortic surgery. *New England Journal of Medicine* **330**, 663–669.

Boucher, C.A. *et al.* 1985. Determination of cardiovascular risk by dipyridamole–thallium imaging before peripheral vascular surgery. *New England Journal of Medicine* **312**, 389–394.

BHAT 1 (The β-Blocker Heart Attack Trial Research Group) 1982. A randomised trial of propranolol in patients with acute myocardial infarction. I. Mortality results. *Journal of the American Medical Association* **247**, 1707–1714.

BHAT 2 (The β-Blocker Heart Attack Trial Research Group) 1983. A randomised trial of propranolol in patients with acute myocardial infarction. I. Morbidity results. *Journal of the American Medical Association* **250**, 2814–2819.

Butman, S.M., Ewy, G.A., Standen, J.R. *et al.* 1993. Bedside cardiovascular examination in patients with severe chronic heart failure: importance of rest or inducible jugular venous distension. *Journal of the American College of Cardiology* **22**, 968–974.

Captopril Primary Prevention Project group (CAPPP) 1990. The Captopril Primary Prevention Project: a prospective intervention trial of angiotensin converting enzyme inhibition in the treatment of hypertension. *Journal of Hypertension* **8**, 985–990.

Carliner, N.H., Fisher, M.L., Plotnick, G.D. *et al.* 1985. Routine pre-operative exercise testing in patients undergoing major non-cardiac surgery. *American Journal of Cardiology* **56**, 51–58.

Cohn, P.F. 1986. Silent myocardial ischaemia. Dimensions of the problem in patients with and without angina. *American Journal of Medicine* **80** (Suppl. 4C), 3–8.

Cohn, J.N., Archibald, D.G., Ziesche, S. *et al.* 1986. Effects of vasodilator therapy om mortality in chronic congestive heart failure. *New England Journal of Medicine* **314**, 1547–1552.

Cohn, J.N., Johnson, G., Ziesche, S. *et al.* 1991. A comparison of enalapril with hydralazine–isosorbide dinitrate in the treatment in the treatment of congestive heart failure. *New England Journal of Medicine* **325**, 303–310.

Collins, R., Peto, R., Macmahon, S. *et al.* 1990. Blood pressure, stroke and coronary heart disease. Part 2. Short term reductions in blood pressure: Overview of randomised drug trial in their epidemiological context. *Lancet* **335**, 827–838.

CONSENSUS-I Trial Study Group 1987. Effects of enalapril on mortality in severe congestive heart failure. *New England Journal of Medicine* **316**, 1429–1435.

Cutler, B.S., Wheeler, H.B., Paraskos, J.A. and Cardullo, P.A. 1981. Applicability and interpretation of electrocardiographic stress testing in patients with peripheral vascular disease. *American Journal of Surgery* **141**, 501–506

Dahlöf, B., Lindholm, L.H., Hansson, L. *et al.* 1991. Morbidity and mortality in the Swedish Trial in Old People with Hypertension (STOP-Hypertension). *Lancet* **338**, 1281–1285.

DAVIT-II, The Danish Study Group on Verapamil in Myocardial Infarction 1990. Effect of verapamil on mortality and major events after acute myocardial infarction. *American Journal of Cardiology* **66**, 779–785.

Detsky, A.S., Abrams, H.B., Forbath, N. *et al.* 1986. Cardiac assessment for patients undergoing non-cardiac surgery. *Archives of Internal Medicine* **146**, 2131–2134.

Diamond, G.A. and Forrester, J.S. 1979. Analysis of probability as an aid in the clinical diagnosis of coronary heart disease. *New England Journal of Medicine* **300**, 1350–1358.

Dicarli, M., Khanna, S. and Davidson, M. 1993. The value of PET for predicting the improvement in heart failure symptoms in patients with coronary disease and severe left ventricular dysfunction. *Journal of the American College of Cardiology* **21**, 129A.

DIG (Digitalis Investigation Group) trial 1997. The effect of digoxin on mortality and morbidity in patients with heart failure. *New England Journal of Medicine* **336**, 525.

Driscoll, A.C., Hobika, J.H., Etsten, B.E. and Proger, S. 1961. Clinically unrecognised myocardial infarction following surgery. *New England Journal of Medicine* **264**, 633–639.

Folland, E.D., Kriegel, B.J., Henderson, W.G. and participants of the Veterans Affairs Cooperative Study on Valvular Heart Disease 1992. Implications of third heart sounds in patients with valvular heart disease. *New England Journal of Medicine* **327**, 458–462.

Foster, E.D., Davis, K.B., Carpenter, J.A. *et al.* 1986. Risk of noncardiac operations in patients with defined coronary disease: The Coronary Artery Surgery Study (CASS) Registry experience. *Annals of Thoracic Surgery* **41**, 42–50.

Franklin, C., Nightingale, S. and Mamdani, B. 1986. A randomised comparison of nifedipine and sodium nitroprusside in severe hypertension. *Chest* **90**, 500–503.

Gajraj, H. and Jamieson, C.W. 1994. Coronary artery disease in patients with peripheral vascular disease. *British Journal of Surgery* **81**, 333–342.

Goldman, L. 1983. Cardiac risks and complications of non-cardiac surgery. *Annals of Internal Medicine* **98**, 504–513.

Goldman, L., Caldera, D.L., Nussbaum, S.R. *et al*. 1977. Multifactorial index of cardiac risk in noncardiac surgical procedures. *New England Journal of Medicine* **297**, 845–850.

Hendel, R.C. *et al*. 1990. Prognostic value of dipyridamole–thallium scintigraphy for evaluation of ischaemic heart disease. *Journal of the American College of Cardiologists* **15**, 109–116.

Herzer, N.R. *et al*. 1984. Coronary artery disease in peripheral vascular disease patients: a classification of 1000 coronary angiograms and results of surgical management. *Annals of Surgery* **199**, 223.

Himelman, R.B., Cassidy, M.M., Landzberg, J.S. and Schiller, N.B. 1988. Reproducibility of quantitative two-dimensional echocardiography. *American Heart Journal* **115**, 425–431.

HINT research group (Holland Interuniversity Nifedipine/Metoprolol Trial) 1986. Early treatment of unstable angina in the coronary care unit: a randomised, placebo controlled comparison of recurrent ischaemia in patients treated with nifedipine or metoprolol or both. *British Heart Journal* **56**, 400–413.

ISIS-1 1986. First International Study of Infarct Survival Collaborative Group. Randomised trial of intravenous atenolol among 16027 cases of suspected acute myocardial infarction. *Lancet* **ii**, 57–66.

ISIS-2 1988. Second International Study of Infarct Survival Collaborative Group. Randomised trial of intravenous streptokinase, oral aspirin, both or neither among 17187 cases of suspected acute myocardial infarction. *Lancet* **ii**, 349–360.

Klimt, C.R. *et al*. 1986. Persantin–Aspirin Reinfarction Study. Part II. Secondary coronary prevention with Persantin and aspirin. *Journal of the American College of Cardiology* **7**, 251.

Knapp, R.B., Topkins, M.J. and Artusio, J.F. 1962. The cerebrovascular accident and coronary occlusion in anaesthesa. *Journal of the American Medical Association* **182**, 332–334.

Von Knorring, J. 1981. Post-operative myocardial infarction: a prospective study in a risk group of surgical patients. *Surgery* **90**, 55–60.

Larsen, S.F., Olesen, K.H., Jacobsen, E. *et al*. 1987. Prediction of cardiac risk in non-cardiac surgery. *European Heart Journal* **8**, 179–185.

Leppo, J. *et al*. 1987. Noninvasive evaluation of cardiac risk before elective vascular surgery. *Journal of the American College of Cardiology* **9**, 269.

Madsen, E.B., Gilpin, E., Slutsky, R.A. *et al*. 1984. Usefulness of the chest X-ray for predicting abnormal left ventricular function after acute myocardial infarction. *American Heart Journal* **108**, 1431–1436.

Mangano, D.T. 1990. Perioperative cardiac morbidity. *Anesthesiology* **72**, 153–184.

Mangano, D.T. and Goldman, L. 1995. Preoperative assessment of patients with known or suspected coronary disease. *New England Journal of Medicine* **333**, 1750–1766.

Mangano, D.T. *et al*. 1991. Dipyridamole–thallium-201 scintigraphy as a preoperative screening test: a reexamination of its predictive potential. *Circulation* **84**, 493–502.

Mangano, D.T., Browner, W.S., Holenberg, M. *et al*. 1990. Association of perioperative myocardial ischaemia with cardiac morbidity and mortality in men undergoing noncardiac surgery. *New England Journal of Medicine* **323**, 1781–1788.

Mangano, D.T., Layug, E.L., Wallace, A. and Tateo, I. for the Multicenter Study of Perioperative Ischaemia Research Group 1996. Effect of atenolol on mortality and cardiovascular morbidity after noncardiac surgery. *New England Journal of Medicine* **335**, 1713–1720.

Marantz, P.R., Tobin, J.N. and Wassertheil-Smoller, J.R. 1988. The relationship between left ventricular systolic function and congestive heart failure diagnosed by clinical criteria. *Circulation* **77**, 607–612.

Markovitz, P.A. and Armstrong, W.F. 1992. Accuracy of dobutamine stress echocardiography in detecting coronary artery disease. *American Journal of Cardiology* **69**, 1269.

Massie, B.M. and Conway, M. 1987. Survival of patients with congestive heart failure: past, present and future prospects. *Circulation* **75** (Suppl. IV), 11–19.

McKee, P.A., Castelli, W.P., McNamara, P.M. and Kannel, W.B. 1971. The natural history of congestive heart failure. *New England Journal of Medicine* **285**, 1441–1446.

McPhail, N., Calvin, J.E., Shariatmadar, J.A. *et al*. 1988. The use of preoperative exercise testing to predict cardiac complications after arterial reconstruction. *Journal of Vascular Surgery* **7**, 60–68.

Motwani, J., McAlpine, H., Kennedy, N. and Struthers, A.D. 1993. Plasma BNP as an indicator for ACE inhibition after myocardial infarction. *Lancet* **341**, 1109–1113.

MRC Working Party 1992. Medical Research Council trial of treatment of hypertension in older adults: principal results. *British Medical Journal* **304**, 405–412.

O'Keefe, J.H. 1989. Risk of non-cardiac surgical procedures in patients with aortic stenosis. *Mayo Clinical Proceedings* **64**, 400–403.

O'Neil, T.W., Barry, M., Smith, M. and Graham, I.M. 1989. Diagnostic value of the cardiac apex beat. *Lancet* **1**, 410–411.

Pasternack, P.E., Imparato, A.M., Bear, G. *et al*. 1984. The value of radionuclide angiography as a predictor of perioperative myocardial infarction in patients undergoing abdominal aortic aneurysm resection. *Journal of Vascular Surgery* **1**, 320–325.

Peto, R., Gray, R. and Collins, R. 1988. Randomised trial of prophylactic aspirin in British male doctors. *British Medical Journal* **296**, 313–316.

Physician Health Study (Steering Committee) 1989. Final Report on the aspirin component of the ongoing Physician Health Study. *New England Journal of Medicine* **321**, 129–135.

Plumlee, J.E. and Boettner, R.B. 1972. Myocardial infarction during and following anaesthesia and operation. *South African Medical Journal* **65**, 886–889.

Poldermanns, D., Arnese, M., Fiorettie, P. *et al*. 1995. Improved cardiac risk stratification in major vascular surgery with dobutamine–atropine stress echocardiography. *Journal of the American College of Cardiology* **26**, 648–653.

Prys-Roberts, C., Meloche, R. and Foëx, P. 1971. Studies of anaesthesia in relation to hypertension. I. Cardiovascular responses to treated and untreated patients. *British Journal of Anaesthetics* **43**, 122–137.

Rao, T.K., Jakobs, K.H. and EL-Etr, A.A. 1983. Reinfarction following anaesthesia in patients with myocardial infarction. *Anesthesiology* **59**, 499–505.

SHEP Cooperative Research Group 1991. Prevention of stroke by antihypertensive drug treatment in older persons with isolated systolic hypertension. Final results of the Systolic Hypertension in the Elderly Program (SHEP). *Journal of the American Medical Association* **265**, 3255–3264.

Smith, J.S., Cahalan, M.K., Benefiel, D.J. *et al*. 1985. Intraoperative detection of myocardial ischaemia in high risk patients: electrocardiographic versus two-dimensional transoesophogeal echocardiography. *Circulation* **72**, 1015–1021.

SOLVD-treatment 1991. The SOLVD Investigators. Effect of enalapril on survival in patients with reduced left ventricular ejection fractions and congestive heart failure. *New England Journal of Medicine* **325**, 293–302.

SOLVD-prevention 1992. The SOLVD Investigators. Effect of enalapril on mortality and on the development of heart failure in asymptomatic patients with reduced left ventricular ejection fractions. *New England Journal of Medicine* **327**, 685–691.

Steen, P.A., Tinker, J.H. and Tarhan, S. 1978. Myocardial reinfarction after anaesthesia and surgery. *Journal of the American Medical Association* **239**, 2566–2570.

Stevenson, L.W. and Perloff, J.K. 1989. The limited reliability of physical signs for estimating hemodynamics in chronic heart failure. *Journal of the American Medical Association* **261**, 884–888.

Sutton, G.C. 1990. Epidemiological aspects of heart failure. *American Heart Journal* **120** (6 part 2), 1538–1540.

Swedberg, K., Eneroth, P., Kjekshus, J. and Wilhelmson, L. for the CONSENSUS Trial Study Group 1990. Hormones regulating cardiovascular function in patients with severe congestive heart failure and their relative mortality. *Circulation* **82**, 1730–1736.

Tarhan, S., Moffitt, E., Taylor, W.F. and Guiliani, E.R. 1972. Myocardial infarction after general anaesthesia. *Journal of the American Medical Association* **220**, 1451–1454.

Task force of the ACC/AHA 1996. Guidelines for perioperative cardiovascular evaluation for noncardiac surgery. *Circulation* **93**, 1278–1317.

Topkins, M.J. and Artusio, J.F. 1964. Myocardial infarction and surgery: a five year study. *Anesthesia Analgesia* **43**, 716–720.

Wackers, F.J., Berger, H.J. and Johnstone, D.E. 1979. Multiple gated cardiac blood pool imaging for left ventricular ejection fraction: validation of the technique and assessment of variability. *American Journal of Cardiology* **43**, 1159–1165.

Wohlgelernter, D., Cleman, M., Highman, H.A. *et al*. 1985: Regional myocardial dysfunction during coronary angioplasty: evaluation by two-dimensional echocardiography and 12 lead electrocardiography. *Journal of the American College of Cardiology* **7**, 1245–1254.

Younis, I.T., Aguirre, F., Byers, S. and Dowell, S. 1990. Perioperative and long term prognostic value of intravenous dipyridamole thallium scintigraphy in patients with peripheral vascular disease. *American Heart Journal* **119**, 1287–1292.

7

Pre-operative assessment and preparation

CHARLES S REILLY

INTRODUCTION

The pre-operative assessment of a patient presenting for vascular surgery is a critical part of management, embracing medical, surgical and anaesthetic care. From the medical point of view, it allows co-existing disease to be identified and the treatment optimized. From the surgical point of view, it allows the decision to be made on the nature of the surgery to be undertaken with a broader view of the patient's general status. From the anaesthetic point of view it allows decisions on peri-operative monitoring and the choice of anaesthetic technique to be made with full knowledge of the patient's general health. Indeed, all three disciplines should be involved in the decision regarding the risk–benefit of the proposed operation for the individual patient. That is, will a patient with severe co-existing disease benefit from a major vascular operation with its attendant risks?

Patients with peripheral vascular disease are quite rightly regarded as being at higher risk than those in a general population. In a review of peri-operative myocardial ischaemia Haagensen and Steen (1988) quoted ten studies looking at the incidence of peri-operative myocardial infarction in patients undergoing vascular surgery. These studies included a total of over 3500 patients and revealed post-operative myocardial infarction rates of 2.3–25 per cent, the mortality after infarction being 20–79 per cent. This can be compared with four studies (cited in the same review) which included approximately 58 000 operations in patients with no previous history of myocardial infarction where the post-operative myocardial infarction rate was between 0.13 and 0.66 per cent, and mortality 27–69 per cent. Indeed, the incidence of post-operative myocardial infarction in the vascular surgery group was of the same magnitude as that found in studies involving patients who had previously had a myocardial infarction where the post-operative myocardial infarction rate was between 2 and 16 per cent.

The aims of this chapter are to describe the methods for assessing the cardiac risk for an individual undergoing vascular surgery, and the relationship of this assessment to the risk–benefit analysis. It will, in addition, deal with the management of co-existent disease and the influence of all these factors on the choice of anaesthetic technique and peri-operative management.

Cardiac risk

It would be useful to have a method of assessing a patient pre-operatively which came up with an cal population is not yet clear, with studies supporting and refuting the link.

SMOKING

Cigarette smoking is a causal factor in both ischaemic heart disease and peripheral vascular disease (Wood, 1988). Smokers have approximately three times the risk of non-smokers of developing ischaemic heart disease, but in studies of operative cardiac risk, cigarette smoking has not been shown to be an independent factor.

HYPERCHOLESTEROLAEMIA

Markedly raised blood cholesterol levels are associated with up to a threefold increase in the risk of developing ischaemic heart disease. Patients with this are likely to develop ischaemic heart disease at a younger age.

Application of cardiac risk to vascular surgery patients

Because patients undergoing peripheral vascular surgery are obviously a high-risk group for adverse cardiac events, it is important to look at the application of the risk factors noted above. It is likely that in such a selected group the relationship of the risk factors described above will differ from those in a general population.

ISCHAEMIC HEART DISEASE

The incidence of ischaemic heart disease in this group of patients is high. In a study of 566 patients undergoing major vascular operations, Cooperman and colleagues (1978) found that 21 per cent had had a previous myocardial infarction, 7 per cent a history of congestive heart failure, 3.7 per cent an arrhythmia and 60 per cent an abnormal pre-operative ECG. Bunt (1992), in a study of 630 patients undergoing elective vascular surgery, found that 68 per cent had clinical evidence of ischaemic heart disease as demonstrated by a positive history or ECG findings. This incidence is in keeping with the well-known study by Hertzer and colleagues (1983) who undertook coronary angiograms on 1000 consecutive patients presenting for vascular surgery. The angiograms were classified into five groups: (1) normal coronary arteries; (2) mild to moderate disease

Table 7.2 *Classification by coronary angiography of 1000 patients presenting for vascular surgery. For classification, see text. (Based on Hertzer et al., 1984)*

Presenting feature (%)				Clinical suspicion of CAD (%)	
CAD	AAA	LLI	CVD	No	Yes
1	6	10	9	14	4
2	29	33	32	49	18
3	29	29	27	22	34
4	31	21	26	14	34
5	5	7	6	1	10

AAA, abdominal aortic aneurysm; CVD, cerebrovascular disease; LLI, lower limb ischaemia; CAD, degree of coronary artery disease (see text).

(< 70 per cent stenosis); (3) advanced, but compensated disease (> 70 per cent stenosis, but not requiring intervention); (4) severe, but correctable disease; and (5) severe, but inoperable disease (multiple stenosis or ventricular impairment). As can be seen (Table 7.2) only 8 per cent of these patients had normal coronary arteries and 60 per cent had grade 3, 4 or 5 disease. The incidence of each class was consistent across the different surgical groups: aortic aneurysm, lower limb or cerebral vascular disease. Another important finding in this study was that 37 per cent of the 446 patients who were classified before angiography as having no clinical indicators of coronary artery disease had category 3 to 5 disease on angiography, and only 14 per cent had normal coronary arteries. However, only 4 per cent of the 554 patients who were classified as having clinical suspicion of coronary artery disease had normal coronary arteries, and 78 per cent had category 3 to 5 disease. This emphasizes the importance of clinical findings.

Angina is a relatively common finding in vascular surgery patients, occurring in up to 45 per cent of patients (Tomatis et al., 1972; Cunningham, 1989). There is some controversy about the significance of stable angina as a risk factor for post-operative cardiac events in a general population, but there is evidence that it is associated with an increased risk in vascular surgical patients. Cooperman and colleagues (1978) found angina to be the significant factor in multivariant analysis of risk in their study population. Similarly congestive cardiac failure, which has been shown to be present in up to 15 per cent of peripheral vascular surgery patients, adds a significant risk (Cooperman et al., 1978; Cunningham, 1989).

HYPERTENSION

Population studies of patients with peripheral vascular disease suggest that up to 60 per cent may have co-existent hypertension (Bunt, 1992). Because arterial hypertension is a causal factor in both ischaemic heart disease and peripheral vascular disease, this is perhaps not surprising, but hypertension does not appear to be an independent risk factor for the development of post-operative cardiac complications, perhaps because of its prevalence in this group.

ARRHYTHMIAS

As in the general population, the presence of arrhythmias in vascular surgery patients indicates an increased risk of cardiac events. For example, Cooperman and colleagues (1978) found that around 4 per cent of patients had pre-operative arrhythmias and that one-third of these had cardiac complications in the peri-operative period.

AGE

It is generally accepted that increasing age confers an increasing risk of peri-operative ischaemia. Goldman's (1977) original study found a significant increase in risk over the age of 70 years, and subsequent studies have demonstrated that age over 70 or 65 years is an independent risk factor (Eagle *et al.*, 1989; Baron *et al.*, 1994). This is an important aspect to consider in vascular disease patients because a number of current reviewers have commented on the steady increase in the upper age limit of patients who would be considered for major vascular surgery over the past three decades. If we consider the 1000 patients enrolled sequentially in the study by Hertzer and colleagues (1983), 71 were under the age of 50 years, 252 aged 50–59 years, 399 aged 60–69 years, 245 aged 70–79 years and 33 were over the age of 80 years.

SMOKING

Previous population studies have shown that up to 95 per cent of patients with occlusive arterial disease are smokers (Coffman, 1983). This is a higher percentage than is found in population studies of ischaemic heart disease with which there is also a causal relationship.

HYPERCHOLESTEROLAEMIA

As mentioned above, there have been no studies which have looked at hypercholesterolaemia as an independent factor in the development of peri-operative ischaemia. However, the incidence will be higher within this group because it is an aetiological factor in both ischaemic heart disease and peripheral vascular disease. Indeed, in the study by Tomatis and colleagues (1972), 13 per cent of patients had a cholesterol > 7.6 mmol/L and 23 per cent had a level between 6.6 and 7.6 mmol/L. To put this in perspective, the current recommendation in the UK is to treat hypercholesterolaemia to achieve a level below 5.5 mmol/L.

DIABETES MELLITUS

As indicated above diabetes appears to confer a higher risk of peri-operative events. The prevalence of diabetes is higher in a vascular surgery population than in a general surgical population with some studies showing an incidence as high as 40 per cent. There are also a number of other important consequences of diabetes which further influence the risk. These are dealt with later.

GENERAL MEDICAL CONDITION

The peripheral vascular disease population may show a higher incidence of concurrent medical problems at pre-operative assessment. In view of the association between cigarette smoking and the development of peripheral vascular disease it would be expected that there would be a high incidence of associated respiratory disease. Indeed some studies have shown the incidence of chronic obstructive airways disease to be as high as 50 per cent in a peripheral vascular surgery population (Cunningham, 1989). As would be expected with the relatively high incidence of diabetes, there is a corresponding increase in the number of patients with evidence of renal impairment pre-operatively.

INVESTIGATIONS

Assessment of myocardial function

A wide range of tests can be used to assess patients' myocardial function (Table 7.3) (Edwards and

Table 7.3   *Methods used for the pre-operative investigation of cardiac disease*

12-lead ECG
Ambulatory ECG
Exercise ECG
Echocardiography
Functional
Stress
Ventriculography
Dipyridamole–thallium scan
Coronary angiography

Reilly, 1994). It can be seen that there is considerable variation in the prognostic value of the information obtained, the invasiveness of the test and the cost. In this section the potential value of each will be reviewed and the rationales that have been applied to their discriminating use will be discussed.

12-LEAD ECG

Over the past forty years a considerable number of studies have demonstrated a relationship between abnormalities detected on the pre-operative ECG and an adverse post-operative cardiac outcome. One of the difficulties of applying this information is in defining what is 'abnormal'. While the changes of a previous myocardial infarction or ST elevation (> 2 mm) or depression (> 1 mm) are strongly suggestive of ischaemic heart disease, other abnormalities such as conduction defects, arrhythmias and T-wave abnormalities only hold an association with ischaemic heart disease and may have other causes. Using all of these criteria a survey of 354 consecutive general surgery patients in Sheffield showed that 16 per cent of patients had abnormalities on the pre-operative ECG (Callaghan *et al.*, 1994). The incidence of abnormalities increased with age.

The relationship between pre-operative ECG abnormality and the incidence of coronary artery disease on angiography was explored by Tomatis and colleagues (1972). They found that 63 per cent of vascular surgery patients had abnormal pre-operative ECGs and 37 per cent had apparently normal traces. Of those with abnormal ECGs, 22 per cent did not have significant coronary artery disease, but 30 per cent of those with apparently normal ECGs had severe coronary artery disease.

AMBULATORY ECG

In the past ten years, there have been considerable advances in the technology of ambulatory ECG monitoring with the development of small portable monitors which are capable of real-time analysis. By examining a digitized ECG signal on an inbuilt microcomputer, these systems avoid the distortions introduced by the older tape recording and play back methods. Use of such systems has become established in cardiological practice and their application reported in a good number of studies of peri-operative myocardial ischaemia. These studies have established that there is a high incidence of silent ischaemic episodes in patients with coronary artery disease, and that patients experiencing silent ischaemic episodes in the peri-operative period have an increased risk of post-operative cardiac events.

The use of this technique as part of pre-operative assessment has been examined in a number of studies of elective vascular surgery patients. Raby and colleagues (1989) identified 32 patients (18 per cent) who had pre-operative ischaemia, 12 of whom had post-operative cardiac events. Of the 144 patients who did not have pre-operative ischaemia only 1 patient had a post-operative cardiac event. Similarly, 78 (39 per cent) of 200 patients had pre-operative ischaemia, and 9 of these had a post-operative myocardial infarction (Pasternack *et al.*, 1989). None of the patients who did not have pre-operative ischaemia had a post-operative myocardial infarction. However, other studies have been less supportive of this method. Fleisher and colleagues (1991) found that 9 out of 24 patients who had pre-operative ischaemia developed post-operative cardiac events, as did 8 of 122 patients without pre-operative ischaemia. Kirwin and colleagues (1993) concluded that silent myocardial ischaemia was not predictive of post-operative cardiac problems in this group of patients. An interesting sequel to the use of this technique is a subsequent study by Raby and colleagues (1990) who followed up their original group of patients for three years. Over 90 per cent of patients who had no ischaemia on ambulatory monitoring in the peri-operative period had a cardiac event-free survival over the subsequent three years which compared with an event-free survival of just over 60 per cent in the group who did have ischaemia.

There are some limitations to the use of ambulatory ECG monitoring which relate to the presence of other variables which may effect the ST segment such as conduction abnormalities, pacing, ventricular hypertrophy, electrolyte imbalance and digoxin therapy.

EXERCISE ECG

The aim of exercise ECG testing is to have the patient perform a graded increase in exercise on a treadmill to achieve a maximum heart rate or until ischaemic changes develop. Exercising to produce an increase in oxygen demand, heart rate and arterial pressure may not seem a good model for the cardiovascular changes which take place during anaesthesia and in the post-operative period, but a number of studies have shown that exercise-induced ECG change is a good predictor of post-operative cardiac problems. Cutler and colleagues (1979) looked at 100 patients undergoing peripheral vascular surgery and found that 14 of the 73 patients with a normal resting ECG developed ischaemia on exercise; 48 of the patients proceeded to surgery and all 6 patients who developed post-operative myocardial infarction had an abnormal exercise ECG. In a study of 808 patients presenting for peripheral vascular surgery, 17 per cent had a positive pre-operative exercise test (Arous et al., 1984); 56 of the patients with positive exercise tests subsequently underwent surgery and 18 suffered a post-operative myocardial infarction. It is interesting that 5 patients of those who developed post-operative myocardial infarction had both no history of coronary artery disease and a normal resting ECG pre-operatively.

However, studies in a general population did not find the method to be a predictor of post-operative outcome (Carliner et al., 1985). It must be remembered that exercise may be limited in vascular surgery patients by the development of claudication before ECG changes, but it is possible to use an arm ergomometer to continue the exercise. Two studies of vascular surgery patients (Cutler et al., 1981; McPhail et al., 1988) have noted an increase in adverse outcome in the patients who were unable to achieve either 75 or 85 per cent of predicted maximal heart rate response during an exercise test. The overall incidence of post-operative cardiac events was 2 and 7 per cent, whereas in the groups who were unable to raise heart rate satisfactorily the complication rates were 11 and 24 per cent respectively. The combination of inability to achieve 75 or 85 per cent of maximal heart rate response with the devel-

opment of ischaemic ECG changes resulted in an even higher incidence of post-operative cardiac events.

VENTRICULOGRAPHY

The technique of using a radionuclide for gated blood-pool scanning can measure ventricular ejection fraction as an indicator of compromised cardiac function. Two studies by Pasternack and colleagues (1984, 1985) demonstrated that an ejection fraction < 35 per cent carried a 75 per cent risk of post-operative complications, compared to patients who had an ejection fraction greater than 56 per cent and no post-operative cardiac complications. Those with an ejection fraction between 35 and 56 per cent had an intermediate risk (19 per cent overall). These studies established ejection fraction as a pre-operative predictor and the threshold of 35 per cent is the most commonly used (Wong and Detsky, 1992). However, a number of subsequent studies, while supporting the value of detecting a low ejection fraction, have demonstrated that the sensitivity of this test is not as high as might be expected from the original studies (Franco et al., 1989; McPhail et al., 1990).

ECHOCARDIOGRAPHY

Echocardiographic examination of the heart can be used to assess ventricular filling and ejection, ventricular wall thickness and hence contractility. These measures are perhaps the most frequent additional investigation undertaken for vascular surgery patients in many centres. Other than identifying patients with low ejection fraction, simple transthoracic echocardiography contributes little to the overall assessment, the figures giving an assessment of the myocardium in its resting state only. The presence of an ischaemic area is associated with abnormalities in the motion of the wall of the ventricle. It follows that if the myocardium becomes ischaemic during a period of stress, such as would occur during exercise, wall motion abnormalities should occur. It is possible, but technically difficult, to undertake echocardiography during physical exercise, but a useful alternative to physical exercise is pharmacological stress as produced by either vasodilatation with dipyridamole, or by an inotrope such as dobutamine.

In the last few years there has been considerable interest in the use of stress echocardiography in the pre-operative assessment of patients with vascular disease. Tischler and colleagues (1991) used dipyridamole in 109 patients and found that 7 of the 9 patients who had positive tests (that is, developed wall motion abnormalities) had post-operative cardiac events compared with 1 of the 100 patients who had a normal scan. Similarly, three studies using dobutamine as the stressing agent have demonstrated a good predictive value for this test (Eichelberger et al., 1991; Lalka et al., 1992; Poldermans et al., 1993). Dobutamine is infused to produce a graded increase in heart rate to a predetermined level. In one of these studies, 11 of 38 patients with an abnormal scan suffered a post-operative cardiac complication compared with only 1 of the 22 patients with a normal scan (Lalka et al., 1992). It is interesting to note an inability to achieve the target heart rate also indicated an increased risk. This finding is in agreement with the response noted in the exercise testing studies described above.

DIPYRIDAMOLE–THALLIUM SCINTIGRAPHY (DTS)

This method involves the uptake of the radioisotope thallium into the myocardium following intravenous injection in the presence of dipyridamole which produces coronary arterial vasodilatation. The resulting scan can show areas without uptake (a perfusion defect). A repeat scan is performed up to 4 hours later to see whether any perfusion defects are still present. The defects can then be classed as irreversible (indicating an area of infarction) or reversible (indicating an area of ischaemia). There has been considerable interest in the use of DTS as a pre-operative predictor of post-operative cardiac problems, the majority of studies being favourable to such use (Wong and Detsky, 1992). However, it is an expensive test and is associated with a number of complications including (rarely) myocardial infarction and bronchospasm. It is obvious that this test is not appropriate or specific enough to be applied to all potential patients.

The problem of specificity was addressed in an important study by Eagle and colleagues (1989). They used the presence of any one of five clinical markers (previous myocardial infarction, congestive cardiac failure, angina, diabetes or Q-waves on the ECG) to assess the use of DTS in pre-operative assessment. Of the 32 patients who had one or more risk factors, 15 patients demonstrated reversible defects on DTS and 7 patients had post-operative ischaemic events. None of the patients with no demonstrable defect had a post-operative event. In their patients without risk factors, only 3 of the 28 developed reversible defects on DTS and one of these had an ischaemic event post-operatively. Again none of those with no defects had an ischaemic event. This is an important study both in its findings and in the contribution it makes to the discriminative use of pre-operative tests.

Application of pre-operative tests

Given that we are dealing with an at-risk population and that a range of investigations is available to apply to our assessment, there are a number of important questions which have to be addressed.

- First, which patients should any or all of these tests be applied to?
- Second, which test or tests produce the most useful information?
- Third, what benefits derive from undertaking these tests? It must be shown that they produce useful information which contributes to the risk–benefit decision process regarding the operation.
- Further, the cost effectiveness of any such investigation must be considered.

It would be appropriate for each institution or team to work through these questions in devising protocols for the assessment of their own patients, based on knowledge of the local surgical population and the techniques available.

WHO TO TEST?

In reviewing the literature regarding the pre-operative testing of peripheral vascular surgery patients there is a spectrum of practice which ranges from a minimalist approach on one hand to a universal invasive investigation policy on the other (Wong and Detsky, 1992; Fleisher and Barash, 1992; Krupski and Bensard, 1995). In looking further at these policies they can be banded into three groupings which could be broadly categorized as: (1) symptom-driven policy; (2) those guided by pre-set criteria; and (3) investigation driven policy. Each of these three approaches has its own algorithm.

Table 7.4   *Clinical predictors for use in pre-operative assessment of cardiac risk stratification (Eagle et al., 1989; ACC/AHA Task Force, 1996)*

Major predictors	Intermediate predictors	Minor predictors
Unstable angina	Mild angina	Age
Decompensated cardiac failure	Previous myocardial infarction	Abnormal ECG
Significant arrythmias	Compensated cardiac failure	Rhythm other than sinus
Severe vascular disease	Diabetes mellitus	Poor exercise tolerance
		Previous stroke
		Poorly controlled arterial hypertension

Symptom-driven policy

A good example of the symptom-based approach was described by Taylor and colleagues (1992) who studied approximately 500 patients undergoing elective or emergency vascular surgery. The screening process for detection of coronary artery disease was history, physical examination and a 12-lead ECG. Only patients with severe symptomatic coronary artery disease (e.g. unstable angina, severe arrhythmias or severe congestive failure) had further investigations. The authors found that over 60 per cent of their patients had evidence of coronary artery disease, but less than 6 per cent of the total required further investigation with either DTS or coronary angiography. Thus only 24 out of 69 patients with a history or symptoms of angina, and 3 out of 70 with congestive failure, had further investigations. The overall incidence of peri-operative myocardial infarction was 2.8 per cent, which is comparable with that of many other studies in similar groups of patients, many of whom have had more intensive investigation. The authors recommended that invasive screening should be restricted to selected patients.

Predetermined criteria approach

The second approach is to use a set of predetermined criteria to categorize the risk for an individual patient, using the 'Goldman' or 'Detsky' scores as a basis. Both of these scoring systems were derived for a general population, but have been applied to vascular surgery patients. It has been suggested that patients with a Goldman score >12 or a Detsky score >15 carry a high risk of post-operative complications (Wong and Detsky, 1992), but a low score does not necessarily imply a low risk. A further adaptation of this approach was proposed by Eagle and colleagues (1989) after the studies referred to above. This group used five criteria (age

>70 years; diabetes; angina; Q-waves on the ECG; ventricular arrhythmias) to classify the patients into three risk groups. Those with none of the criteria could be classed as low risk, those with one or two as intermediate risk, and those with three or more as high risk. Those at intermediate risk underwent DTS which, if positive, would grade them as high risk or, if negative, as low risk. Those at low risk could safely proceed to surgery while those at high risk should be considered for coronary angiography as the next step.

Investigation-orientated approach

The third approach, the more investigation-orientated approach, was demonstrated in a study by Bunt (1992). All patients had history, ECG and radionuclide studies as baseline. If no abnormalities were detected in any of these three areas, the patient was regarded as class I and proceeded to surgery. If one or more were present they were regarded as class II and investigated with DTS. If this was negative they proceeded to surgery, but if the test was positive they were regarded as class III and put forward for cardiac catheterization. Using this algorithm in 630 patients presenting for elective vascular procedures, 32 per cent were class I and required no further investigation, but 68 per cent underwent DTS which was normal in 93 per cent. Therefore only 44 of the total of 428 patients who had DTS went on to coronary angiography. This policy resulted in an impressively low incidence of post-operative myocardial infarction (< 1 per cent). However, there are considerable cost implications in this approach, particularly as over 90 per cent of the DTS studies were negative.

A unified approach to this problem may be based on the guidelines produced jointly by the American College of Cardiology and the American Heart

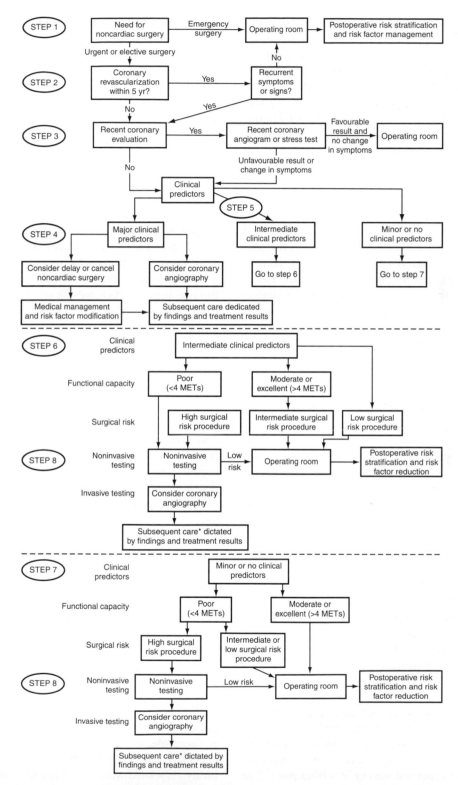

Figure 7.1 *Stepwise approach to pre-operative cardiac assessment. *Subsequent care may include cancellation or delay of surgery, coronary revascularization followed by non-cardiac surgery, or intensified care. MET, metabolic equivalent; 4 METs = walking up one flight of stairs.*

Association for peri-operative cardiovascular evaluation in patients presenting for non-cardiac surgery (1996). This proposal stratifies clinical predictors as major, intermediate and minor (Table 7.4) and uses them to enter patients into one of three separate algorithms. These algorithms follow a sequence of steps based on the functional capacity (that is exercise tolerance), the surgical risk (that is the severity of the procedure – high, medium or low) and the results of non-invasive and, if necessary, invasive testing (Fig. 7.1).

WHICH TEST?

One of the most commonly used tests in the pre-operative evaluation of vascular surgery patients in the UK is the transthoracic echocardiogram. This is surprising because there is little evidence to suggest that it is of any benefit as a predictor of outcome. Of the tests described above, a number of them seem to have been used more frequently in the assessment of patients for vascular surgery. These are ambulatory ECG, radionuclide ventriculography, DTS and stress echocardiography. Mantha and colleagues (1994) have undertaken a meta-analysis of studies involving these techniques for pre-operative assessment. They looked at over fifty studies which had used one or more of these techniques and identified twenty which allowed comparative assessment. As a measure of the efficacy of these tests as predictors, they described a relative risk which was the probability of an adverse cardiac outcome when the test was positive rather than negative. A relative risk of 1 would mean that there was no difference in overall risk if a test was positive or negative, whereas a relative risk of 10 would mean that a positive result carried a ten times greater risk than a negative result. Using this methodology, they found that ambulatory ECG had a relative risk index of 2.7 (95 per cent confidence interval, 1.4–5.1), radionuclide ventriculography an index of 3.7 (1.6–8.3), DTS an index of 4.6 (2.1–10.4) and stress echocardiography an index of 6.2 (1.7–22.8). Their conclusion was that all of the tests are effective, but they were unable to determine an optimal test method because of the overlap in confidence intervals. However, they were supportive of stress echocardiography as a method worthy of further study. The majority of algorithms that have been described in the above section tend to use DTS as the preferred method of investigation.

BENEFITS DERIVED FROM TESTS

When establishing a protocol for the pre-operative evaluation of vascular surgery patients, it is important that the team has a clear understanding of the implications of the test results, and that the protocol includes strategies for the management of patients with abnormal findings. To justify undertaking an invasive and/or expensive test on a patient, it must be clear that the result of this test will be important in the treatment plan for the patient. That is, if a test produces a result showing significant impairment of function, the patient's surgery will be deferred while therapeutic measures are taken to improve cardiovascular (or respiratory) function or the proposed surgery is modified to a less invasive procedure. If the response to abnormal findings is to be, 'Well, we will give it a try anyway!', there is little point in undertaking the investigation in the first place.

An important consequence of pre-operative testing is the decision on the management of a patient who has been shown to have significant myocardial ischaemia. This patient could be referred for coronary angiography and, if appropriate, coronary artery grafting. Alternatively, the patient could undergo the scheduled procedure with intensive per- and post-operative monitoring or undergo a modified procedure. There is reasonably good evidence to support the hypothesis that patients who have had successful coronary artery grafting have a lower risk during subsequent non-cardiac surgery (Hertzer et al., 1984). This must be balanced against the risks associated with coronary angiography and cardiac surgery (Krupski and Bensard, 1995). The urgency of the surgery and the natural progression of vascular disease must, of course, be factors in this decision (Hertzer, 1991) and the management of a patient with a small stable aneurysm of the aorta will be different from that of a patient with a large or expanding one.

The benefit of essentially normal results of pre-operative tests is in identifying the patients at low risk of peri-operative problems. The point here is the cost–benefit of undertaking these tests. To give an example, the study by Bunt (1992) used an expensive test (DTS) which has a measurable morbidity associated with it, and found it to be normal in 90 per cent of the patients. Does the reassurance of identifying low-risk patients justify the costs involved?

CONCURRENT MEDICAL PROBLEMS

In addition to considering the influence of cardiac disease on the outcome of surgery, it is important to address the problem of other medical conditions which may be present before surgery. Chapter 6 has dealt with the optimization of current cardiovascular therapy within this population, but it must be remembered that they also have a high incidence of other conditions, particularly pulmonary disease and diabetes mellitus which must be considered as part of the pre-operative preparation.

Pulmonary disease

As mentioned earlier, over 90 per cent of the vascular surgical population are smokers and it is estimated that some 50–60 per cent will have evidence of chronic pulmonary disease (Cunningham, 1989). The changes in respiratory physiology which occur after abdominal surgery are well recognized, there being marked decreases in functional residual capacity, peak expired flow (FEV_1) and forced vital capacity (FVC). These changes are maximum during the first 48 hours after surgery, but may take up to five days to recover and are potentially detrimental in two ways.

First, the combination of an abdominal wound, decreased respiratory reserve, opioid administration and the supine posture results in a high possibility of hypoxaemia during the first two to three days. Indeed, a study of around 30 patients after abdominal vascular surgery found that 38 and 52 per cent had overall mean oxygen saturations < 90 per cent on the second and third post-operative nights, respectively (Reeder et al., 1992). A significant number of patients had periods with a saturation below 85 per cent, particularly on the second and third post-operative nights when oxygen had not, at that time, been routinely prescribed. As has been shown previously, there is a relationship between hypoxaemic episodes and the development of myocardial ischaemia (Gill et al., 1992). It is interesting to note that there is a temporal relationship between the maximum hypoxaemic effect of changed respiratory function and the highest incidence of post-operative myocardial infarction, with both peaking on the second and third post-operative days.

The second influence of decreased respiratory function is that it will increase the likelihood of post-operative respiratory infection. The many smokers in this group will also have decreased ciliary function and many have clinical evidence pre-operatively of chronic obstructive airways disease.

PRE-OPERATIVE TESTS OF PULMONARY FUNCTION

Clinical
There is reasonable evidence in the literature that the information obtained by careful clinical history-taking and examination is the most useful predictor of likely post-operative pulmonary complications (Derrington and Smith, 1987). In particular, this should be guided toward detecting any evidence of acute or chronic airways disease, evidence of bronchospasm or of current upper respiratory tract infection.

Chest X-ray
A chest X-ray should be taken in all patients presenting for vascular surgery in view of the high incidence of complications. While a chest X-ray in itself may not contribute much to the pre-operative evaluation, it will serve as a baseline which will make further subsequent interpretation of post-operative chest X-rays easier. It can be of use in detecting active lung disease including bronchial carcinomas and may also contribute to the cardiac evaluation if there is radiological evidence of cardiac failure.

PULMONARY FUNCTION TESTS

In patients with known pulmonary disease the use of simple pulmonary function tests which measure FVC, FEV_1 and peak flow measurements can make a significant contribution to pre-operative evaluation. For example, in a patient requiring a major abdominal vascular operation the presence of severe chronic obstructive airways disease would have a significant negative influence on the risk–benefit analysis pre-operatively. It is important that, in the presence of any asthmatic symptoms, pulmonary function tests should be undertaken before and after the administration of bronchodilators. Any improvement in these tests after bronchodilators suggests that the current therapy is not adequate and should be optimized before proceeding to surgery. There are a number of other increasingly sophisticated tests of pulmonary function which probably would contribute relatively little to the overall decision process and management of a vascular surgery patient.

It is interesting to note that a number of studies have shown that there is little relationship between pre-operative pulmonary function tests and the likelihood of developing post-operative pulmonary complications (Tisi, 1979). In fact, a number of studies have shown that there is a relationship between the incidence of post-operative cardiac complications and the likelihood of developing pulmonary complications (Williams-Russo *et al.*, 1992).

Diabetes mellitus

As has been noted, a significant percentage of patients presenting for vascular surgery have diabetes. To the anaesthetist, the most immediate is the peri-operative management of the blood sugar. However, it must be appreciated that these patients have a high incidence of coronary artery disease, hypertension, renal disease and autonomic neuropathy. Coronary artery disease is the most common cause of death in diabetics, and hypertension is also common. The incidence of coronary artery disease and arterial hypertension has been shown to parallel the development of nephropathy in both type I and type II diabetes (UK Prospective Diabetes Study, 1985). This can be illustrated with the findings of a Danish study of type II (non-insulin-dependent) diabetics (Gall *et al.*, 1991) where the incidence of coronary artery disease increased from 22 per cent in those who had normal renal function, to 26 per cent in those with microalbuminuria, and 46 per cent in those with macroalbuminuria. The incidence of arterial hypertension was 48, 68 and 85 per cent in these three groups, respectively. This study also refuted the popular misconception that type II diabetes is a milder disease, with fewer complications. In the Danish study, and a similar one in type I diabetics (Norgaard *et al.*, 1990), the mean time from diagnosis of diabetes in the patients with macroalbuminuria was 25 years for type I, and 10 years for type II. It is known that hyperinsulinaemia and hyperlipidaemia may be present for some considerable time before diagnosis of type II diabetes and that significant macrovascular disease may already be present at that time.

Autonomic neuropathy is estimated to occur in up to 40 per cent of patients with long-standing diabetes, and it is more likely to be present if there is evidence of neuropathy, retinopathy and peripheral sensory neuropathy (Ewing *et al.*, 1980). Autonomic neuropathy has been shown to increase both the peri-operative cardiac and respiratory morbidity, its effect being to alter both parasympathetic and sympathetic input to the heart. This leads to increased haemodynamic instability during anaesthesia and it has been associated with sudden death during anaesthesia (Burgos *et al.*, 1989; Latson *et al.*, 1994). This event (which has been called 'sudden death syndrome') is characterized by sudden, profound bradycardia and hypotension, and is refractory to pharmacological intervention. It has occurred during both anaesthesia and the immediate post-operative period in patients who have had otherwise uneventful and well-monitored procedures (Page and Watkins, 1978). It has also been shown that autonomic neuropathy will affect the ventilatory responses to hypoxaemia, and this may be a factor in the significantly increased risk that diabetics have of post-operative respiratory problems (Rose *et al.*, 1994). It is likely that these effects are of a mild nature in the awake patient, but become apparent in the presence of anaesthetic agents and respiratory depressant drugs such as opioids.

TESTING FOR AUTONOMIC DYSFUNCTION

In the light of this evidence, there is an argument for screening all diabetics pre-operatively for autonomic dysfunction as well as for the presence of coronary artery disease, hypertension and renal dysfunction. There are a number of factors in the patient's history which may be suggestive of a degree of autonomic dysfunction, including postural hypotension (which is often treated with fludrocortisone), gastric stasis, diarrhoea, excessive sweating, urinary retention and impotence (Ewing and Clarke, 1982).

Clinical tests which measure the integrity of the autonomic nervous system are based primarily on cardiovascular reflexes. It is thought that abnormalities detected in the cardiovascular reflexes will reflect damage to other autonomic reflexes. Cardiac autonomic dysfunction can be detected by either simple clinical tests or analysis of the ECG. The two most useful tests are the heart rate response to the Valsalva manoeuvre (which tests parasympathetic integrity), and the blood-pressure response to the change from lying to standing (which tests sympathetic function) (Ewing and Clarke, 1982). During a Valsalva manoeuvre, the blood pressure decreases and heart rate increases. On release, the blood pressure overshoots its resting value and the heart rate slows. In patients with autonomic damage, the blood pressure changes occur slowly and do not overshoot, and there is no change in heart rate. If the ECG is recorded during the manoeuvre the result can be expressed as a ratio of the longest R–R interval after the manoeuvre to the shortest one during. In the normal individual, this ratio will be >1, but in the abnormal it will be < 1.1.

The change in blood pressure normally associated with moving from the lying to the standing position is normally < 10 mmHg, whereas in a patient with autonomic neuropathy the decrease would be > 30 mmHg. The heart-rate response to this change in posture is a tachycardia maximal at about the 15th beat after standing, followed by a brief bradycardia maximal around the 30th beat. This response is mediated by the vagus nerve, and the ratio of the ECG R–R intervals at the 15th and 30th beats is normally > 1.04. A clearly abnormal ratio is < 1.

More recently, a system which can undertake power spectral analysis of heart-rate variability has been used to detect abnormalities in cardiac autonomic function (Latson et al., 1994). It has been shown that high- and low-frequency oscillations on the ECG wave form correspond to the integrity and activity of parasympathetic and sympathetic reflexes respectively. These measurements have been shown to correlate well with abnormalities detected during clinical testing.

THE ROLE OF PRE-OPERATIVE ASSESSMENT IN DECISION-MAKING

To be of value, pre-operative assessment has to contribute to the decision-making process in the patient's management. It can do this in a number of ways. First, accurate assessment of pre-operative clinical status can allow the team to make informed decisions on when to operate (i.e. can the status be improved?), on what is the appropriate operation for the patient, or indeed whether to operate. The second contribution of assessment is to anaesthetic management decisions such as the choice of technique, peri-operative monitoring, and the level of post-operative care. The potential contribution of pre-operative assessment to the decision-making process has largely been dealt with in the above sections. It is important that the findings of pre-operative investigations are used in the decision process.

Whether the approach is minimalist or extensive, tests are of no value if they have no influence on the decision-making. It would seem appropriate that (as well as devising a protocol for the chain of investigations to be undertaken pre-operatively), each team or institution should have a protocol for the subsequent management and that this has an input from the results of pre-operative assessment.

Anaesthetic technique

The anaesthetic techniques for various vascular surgical procedures are dealt with elsewhere in this book. However, the findings of pre-operative assessment may influence the choice of technique. The main area of controversy within this is the choice between regional and general anaesthetic techniques, but the issue remains unresolved and is considered later. Multifactorial analysis of cardiac risk or cardiac ischaemia factors suggests there is no overall difference between anaesthetic techniques (Mangano, 1990). A recent study of 423 patients having spinal, epidural or general anaesthesia for lower limb vascular operations demonstrated no difference in the incidence of peri-operative cardiac events (Bode et al., 1996). The main concern in using a regional technique is that there may be sudden hypotension and that the methods used to treat this present potential problems. Fluid loading may precipitate cardiac failure, or treatment with vasoconstrictors induce a tachycardia. However, there is evidence that high-risk patients who have an epidural as part of their peri-operative management have a better surgical outcome with fewer graft failures (Yeager et al., 1987; Tuman et al., 1991).

Monitoring

In general, the greater the peri-operative risk, the greater the level of monitoring that is undertaken. This is appropriate only if the information provided by the monitoring is used to maintain haemodynamic stability throughout the procedure. The benefit of such interventional treatment has been demonstrated in patients undergoing surgery after recent myocardial infarction (Rao et al., 1983). The ECG should be monitored continuously in an ST trend mode. The accuracy of modern systems is reasonable and, even if the figures for ST-segment depression are not exact, changes will give a reliable indication that intervention is needed. A study by London and colleagues suggested that the most accurate leads for identifying ST-segment changes are V5, V4 and II. Indeed, as an alternative, the concurrent use of all three leads should identify over 95 per cent of ST-segment changes. Transoesophageal echocardiography is potentially a useful monitor for the management of these patients. Detection of wall motion abnormalities predates the development of ST-segment changes and therefore allows earlier treatment of ischaemic changes. It is, however, a much more expensive technique and requires training in its use and interpretation.

Post-operative care

Pre-operative assessment can also contribute to decisions on post-operative management. Patients regarded as high risk must be monitored during the post-operative period, most appropriately in a high-dependency unit where continuous ECG and invasive arterial pressure monitoring are available. It is important to remember that the peak incidence of myocardial infarction and ischaemia, and possibly hypoxaemic episodes, is on the second and third post-operative days. It is obvious that high-risk patients should be monitored through this period, and the need for early intervention recognized (Shoemaker et al., 1983).

SUMMARY

Patients presenting for vascular surgery are at significantly greaterer risk than the general surgical population. They have a higher incidence of concomitant disease, including coronary artery disease, arterial hypertension, chronic obstructive airways disease and diabetes mellitus. A number of methods can be used in the pre-operative assessment of myocardial function, ranging from straightforward clinical methods to invasive techniques. Each of these has its own merits and disadvantages. However, each of these investigative techniques is only useful if the information provided is used in the decision-making process for the individual patient. It is appropriate that each team or institution establishes a protocol for the pre-operative assessment and decision-making processes for its vascular surgery patients. The findings should allow the surgical, anaesthetic and post-operative care to be tailored to the individual patient's needs.

REFERENCES

ACC/AHA Task Force Report 1996. Guidelines for perioperative evaluation for noncardiac surgery. *Journal of the American College of Cardiology* **27**, 910–948.

Arous, E.S., Baum, P.L. and Culter, B.S. 1984. The ischaemic exercise test in patients with peripheral vascular disease. *Archives of Surgery* **119**, 780–783.

Baron, J.F., Mundler, O. and Bertrand, M. 1994. Dipyridamole–thallium scintigraphy and gated radionuclide angiography to assess cardiac risk before abdominal aortic surgery. *New England Journal of Medicine* **330**, 663–669.

Bode, R.H., Lewis, K.P., Zarich, S.W. et al. 1996. Cardiac outcome after peripheral vascular surgery. Comparison of general and regional anaesthesia. *Anesthesiology* **84**, 3–13.

Bunt, T.J. 1992. The role of a defined protocol for cardiac risk assessment in decreasing peri-operative myocardial infarction in vascular surgery. *Journal of Vascular Surgery* **15**, 626–634.

Burgos, L.G., Ebert, T.J., Asiddao, C. et al. 1989. Increased intraoperative cardiovascular morbidity in diabetics with autonomic neuropathy. *Anesthesiology* **70**, 591–597.

Callaghan, L.C., Edwards, N.D. and Reilly, C.S. 1994. Utilisation of the pre-operative ECG. *Anaesthesia* **50**, 488–490.

Carliner, N.H., Fisher, M.L., Plotnick, G.D. et al. 1985. Routine pre-operative exercise testing in patients undergoing major noncardiac surgery. *American Journal of Cardiology* **56**, 51–58.

Coffman, J.D. 1983. Principles of conservative treatment of occlusive arterial disease. *Cardiovascular Clinics* **13**, 1–13.

Cooperman, M., Pflug, B., Martin, E.W. jr. and Evans, W.E. 1978. Cardiovascular risk factors in patients with peripheral vascular disease. *Surgery* **84**, 505–509.

Cunningham, A.J. 1989. Anaesthesia for abdominal aortic surgery – a review. *Canadian Journal of Anaesthesia* **36**, 568–577.

Cutler, B.S., Wheeler, H.B., Paraskos, J.A. and Cardullo, P.A. 1979. Assessment of operative risk with electrocardiographic exercise testing in patients with peripheral vascular disease. *American Journal of Surgery* **137**, 484–490.

Cutler, B.S., Wheeler, H.B.,Paraskos, J.A. and Cardullo, P.A. 1981. Applicability and interpretation of electrocardiographic stress testing in patients with peripheral vascular disease. *American Journal of Surgery* **141**, 501–506.

Derrington, M.C. and Smith, G. 1987. A review of studies of anaesthetic risk, morbidity and mortality. *British Journal of Anaesthesia* **59**, 815–833.

Detsky, A.S., Abrams, H.B., Forbath, N. *et al*. 1986. Cardiac assessment for patients undergoing noncardiac surgery. A multifactorial clinical risk index. *Archives of Internal Medicine* **146**, 2131–2134.

Eagle, K.A., Coley, C.M., Newell, J.B. *et al*. 1989. Combining clinical and thallium data optimizes pre-operative assessment of cardiac risk before major vascular surgery. *Annals of Internal Medicine* **110**, 859–866.

Edwards, N.D. and Reilly, C.S. 1994. Detection of peri-operative myocardial ischaemia. *British Journal of Anaesthesia* **72**, 104–115.

Eichelberger, J.P., Schwarz, K.Q., Black, E.R. *et al*. 1991. Predictive value of dobutamine echocardiography just before noncardiac vascular surgery. *American Journal of Cardiology* **72**, 602–607.

Ewing, D.J., Campbell, I.W. and Clarke, B.F. 1980. The natural history of diabetic autonomic neuropathy. *Quarterly Journal of Medicine* **49**, 95–108.

Ewin,g D.J. and Clarke, B.F. 1982. Diagnosis and management of diabetic autonomic neuropathy. *British Medical Journal* **285**, 916–918.

Fleisher, L.A. and Barash, P.G. 1992. Preoperative cardiac evaluation for noncardiac surgery: a functional approach. *Anesthesia and Analgesia* **74**, 586–598.

Fleisher, L.A., Rosenbaum, S.H., Nelson, A.H. and Barash, P.G. 1991. The predictive value of pre-operative silent ischaemia for post-operative ischaemic events in vascular and nonvascular surgery patients. *American Heart Journal* **122**, 980–986.

Foster, E.D., Davis, K.B., Carpenter, J.A. *et al*. 1986. Risk of noncardiac operation in patients with defined coronary disease: The Coronary Artery Surgery Study (CASS) registry experience. *Annals of Thoracic Surgery* **41**, 42–50.

Franco, C.D., Goldsmith, J., Veith, F.J. *et al*. 1989. Resting gated pool ejection fraction: a poor predictor of peri-operative myocardial infarction in patients undergoing vascular surgery for infrainguinal bypass grafting. *Journal of Vascular Surgery* **10**, 656–661.

Gall, M.A., Rossing, P., Skott, P. *et al*. 1991 Prevalence of micro- and macroalbuminuria, arterial hypertension, retinopathy and large vessel disease in European Type 2 diabetic patients. *Diabetologia* **34**, 655–661.

Gill, N.P., Wright, B. and Reilly, C.S. 1992. Relationship between peri-operative ischaemic and hypoxic events in patients with cardiovascular disease. *British Journal of Anaesthesia* **68**, 471–473.

Goldman, L., Caldera, D.L., Nussbaum, S.R. *et al*. 1977. Multifactorial index of cardiac risk in noncardiac surgical procedures. *New England Journal of Medicine* **297**, 845–850.

Haagensen, R. and Steen, P.A. 1988. Perioperative myocardial infarction. *British Journal of Anaesthesia* **61**, 24–37.

Hertzer, N.R., Beven, E.G., Young, J.R. *et al*. 1983. Coronary artery disease in peripheral vascular patients. a classification of 1000 coronary angiograms and results of surgical management. *Annals of Surgery* **199**, 223–233.

Hertzer, N.R. 1991. The natural history of peripheral vascular disease. *Circulation* **83**, I-12–I-19.

Kirwin, J.D., Ascer, E. and Gennaro, M. 1993. Silent myocardial ischaemia is not predictive of myocardial infarction in peripheral vascular surgery patients. *Annals of Vascular Surgery* **7**, 27–32.

Krupski, W.C. and Bensard, D.D. 1995. Preoperative cardiac risk management. *Surgical Clinics of North America* **75**, 647–663.

Lalka, S..G, Sawada, S.G., Dalsing, M.C. *et al*. 1992. Dobutamine stress echocardiography as a predictor of cardiac events associated with aortic surgery. *Journal of Vascular Surgery* **15**, 831–842.

Latson, T.W., Ashmore, T.H., Reinhart, D.J. *et al*. 1994. Autonomic reflex dysfunction in patients presenting for elective surgery is associated with hypotension after anesthesia induction. *Anesthesiology* **80**, 326–337.

Mangano, D.T. 1990. Perioperative cardiac morbidity. *Anesthesiology* **72**, 153–184.

Mantha, S., Roizen, M.F., Barnard, J. *et al*. 1994. Relative effectiveness of four pre-operative tests for predicting adverse cardiac outcomes after vascular surgery: a meta analysis. *Anesthesia Analgesia* **79**, 422–433.

McPhail, N., Calvin, J.E., Shariatmadar, A. *et al*. 1988. The use of pre-operative exercise testing to predict cardiac complications after arterial reconstruction. *Journal of Vascular Surgery* **7**, 60–68.

McPhail, N.V., Ruddy, T.D., Calvin, J.E. *et al*. 1990. Comparison of left ventricular function and myocardial perfusion for evaluating peri-operative cardiac risk of abdominal aortic surgery. *Canadian Journal of Surgery* **33**, 224–8.

Norgaard, K., Feldt-Rasmussen, B., Borch-Johnsen, K. *et al*. 1990. Prevalence of hypertension in type 1 diabetes mellitus. *Diabetologia* **33**, 407–410.

Page, M.M. and Watkins, P.J. 1978. Cardiorespiratory arrest and diabetic autonomic neuropathy. *Lancet* **I**, 14–16.

Pasternack, P.F., Imparato, A.M., Bear, G. *et al*. 1984. The value of radionuclide angiography as a predictor of peri-operative myocardial infarction in patients undergoing abdominal aortic aneurysm resection. *Journal of Vascular Surgery* **1**, 320–325.

Pasternack, P.F., Imparato, A.M., Riles, T.S. *et al*. 1985. The value of the radionuclide angiogram in the prediction of peri-operative myocardial infarction in patients undergoing lower extremity revascularization procedures. *Circulation* **72**, 13–17.

Pasternack, P.F., Grossi, E.A., Baumann, F.G. *et al*. 1989. The value of silent myocardial ischaemia monitoring in the prediction of peri-operative myocardial infarction in patients undergoing peripheral vascular surgery. *Journal of Vascular Surgery* **10**, 617–625.

Poldermans, D., Fioretti, P.M., Forster, T. *et al*. 1993. Dobutamine stress-echocardiography for assessment of peri-operative cardiac risk in patients undergoing major vascular surgery. *Circulation* **87**, 1506–1512.

Raby, K.E., Goldman, L., Creager, M.A. *et al*. 1989. Correlation between pre-operative ischaemia and major cardiac events after peri-operative vascular surgery. *New England Journal of Medicine* **321**, 1296–1300.

Rao, T.L., Jacobs, K.H. and El-Etr, A.A. 1983. Reinfarction following anaesthesia in patients with myocardial infarction. *Anesthesiology* **59**, 499–505.

Raby, K.E., Goldman, L., Cook, E.F. *et al*. 1990. Long term prognosis of myocardial ischaemia detected by Holter monitoring in peripheral vascular disease. *American Journal of Cardiology* **66**, 1309–1313.

Reeder, M.K., Goldman, M.D., Loh, L. *et al*. 1992. Postoperative hypoxaemia after major abdominal vascular surgery. *British Journal of Anaesthesia* **68**, 23–26.

Rose, D.K., Cohen, M.M., Wigglesworth, D.F. and

DeBoer, D.P. 1994. Critical respiratory events in the post anaesthesia care unit. Patient, surgical and anaesthetic factors. *Anesthesiology* **81**, 410–418.

Shaper, A.G., Pocock, S.J., Walker, M. *et al*. 1985. Risk factors for ischaemic heart disease: the prospective phase of the British Regional Heart Study. *Journal of Epidemiology and Community Health* **39**, 197–209.

Shoemaker, W.C., Appel, P. and Bland, R. 1983. Use of physiologic monitoring to predict outcome and to assist in clinical decisions in critically ill post-operative patients. *American Journal of Surgery* **146**, 43–50.

Taylor, L.M., Yeager, R.A., Moneta, G.L. *et al*. 1992. The incidence of peri-operative myocardial infarction in general vascular surgery. *Journal of Vascular Surgery* **15**, 52–61.

Tischler, M.D., Lee, T.H., Hirsch, A.T. *et al*. 1991. Prediction of major cardiac events after peripheral vascular surgery using dipyridamole echocardiography. *American Journal of Cardiology* **68**, 593–597.

Tisi, G.M. 1979. Preoperative evaluation of pulmonary function. Validity, indications and benefits. *American Review of Respiratory Disease* **119**, 293–310.

Tomatis, L.A., Fierens, E.E. and Verbrugge, G.P. 1972. Evaluation of surgical risk in peripheral vascular disease by coronary arteriography: a series of 100 cases. *Surgery* **71**, 429–435.

Tuman, K.J., McCarthy, R.J., March, R.J. *et al*. 1991. Effects of epidural anaesthesia and analgesia on coagulation and outcome after major vascular surgery. *Anesthesia and Analgesia* **73**, 696–704.

United Kingdom Prospective Diabetes Study 1985 Prevalence of hypertension and hypotensive therapy in patients with newly diagnosed diabetes. *Hypertension* **7**, 8–13.

Williams-Russo, P., Charlson, M.E., MacKenzie, R. *et al*. 1992. Predicting post-operative pulmonary problems. *Archives of Internal Medicine* **152**, 1209–1213.

Wong, T. and Detsky, A.S. 1992. Preoperative cardiac risk assessment for patients having peripheral vascular surgery. *Annals of Internal Medicine* **116**, 743–753.

Wood, D.A. 1988. Aetiology of ischaemic heart disease. *British Journal of Anaesthesia* **61**, 3–10.

Yeager, M.P., Glass, D.D., Neff, R.K. and Brinck-Johnsen, T. 1987. Epidural anaesthesia and analgesia in high risk surgical patients. *Anesthesiology* **66**, 729–736.

8

Peri-operative management of the cardiovascular system

NEAL D EDWARDS

INTRODUCTION

Over recent years there have been enormous advances in the monitoring available to the anaesthetist for assessing cardiovascular parameters during surgery. These range from improvements in the technology of electrocardiography (ECG) and pulmonary artery monitoring, to the development of exciting new monitors such as transoesophageal echocardiography and Doppler ultrasonography. This chapter considers their advantages, disadvantages and potential pitfalls, the interpretation of their findings, and their use in the management of patients undergoing vascular surgery. Although arterial blood pressure monitoring (invasive and non-invasive) is extremely important in the cardiovascular management of all vascular surgical patients, it is well established, and the reader is referred elsewhere for further detail (Sykes *et al.*, 1991).

The importance of cardiovascular monitoring and management in high-risk surgical patients has been highlighted in recent years. Two studies (Shoemaker *et al.*, 1988; Boyd *et al.*, 1993) have emphasized the value of optimizing tissue perfusion peri-operatively, whilst the importance of promptly detecting and treating peri-operative myocardial ischaemia to reduce post-operative cardiac complications has become increasingly apparent (Mangano, 1990). The aim of anaesthetic management during surgery should be to maximize tissue perfusion while maintaining cardiovascular stability and an advantageous myocardial oxygen supply/demand ratio. This involves optimizing the cardiac output and avoiding tachycardia, hypertension and excessive hypotension. These objectives apply to anaesthesia for all types of surgery, but are of particular importance in patients undergoing vascular procedures because:

- they tend to be elderly and have a high incidence of cardiovascular disease;
- there is a high incidence of intra-operative haemodynamic stress related to vascular clamping and release;
- there is the potential for major blood loss; and
- the operations are often of long duration.

The management of patients undergoing these procedures does not end with surgery, but must be continued into the post-operative period.

In monitoring for myocardial ischaemia, it should be appreciated that the earliest manifestations are functional abnormalities of myocardial contraction and relaxation (Labovitz *et al.*, 1987; Wohlgelernter *et al.*, 1987), and that ECG changes appear relatively late. Consequently, once myocardial ischaemia is detected, it should be treated promptly to avoid further cardiac complications.

When monitoring myocardial performance, it is imperative that the anaesthetist understands the relationship between ventricular end diastolic pressure and volume (see Chapters 4–6), and considers both the ventricular function curve and the way that therapeutic manipulations may alter this. Information on heart rate, blood pressure, intravascular volume, ventricular function and vascular resistance can be integrated to assess cardiovascular performance in terms of preload, myocardial function and afterload. These can then be adjusted to achieve the desired effect, while avoiding manipulations likely to impair the myocardial oxygen supply/demand ratio and increase the risk of ischaemia. For example

- Preload is decreased in hypovolaemia and intravascular volume needs to be restored with the appropriate fluid, but blood pressure can be maintained temporarily (if necessary) with a vasoconstrictor to increase afterload and maintain perfusion.
- If, on the other hand preload is too high, then a venodilator, inotrope (bearing in mind the resulting increased myocardial work) or both, may be appropriate, depending upon ventricular function.
- If cardiac output is high but mean arterial pressure is low, this implies a low systemic vascular resistance, in which case arterial vasoconstrictors are appropriate.
- If cardiac output is low but mean arterial pressure normal or high, the careful use of an arterial vasodilator to reduce afterload may help to improve stroke volume and cardiac output without increasing myocardial oxygen requirement or adversely affecting arterial blood pressure.

Intra-operative monitoring of cardiovascular parameters is vital if such control is to be exercised, and invasive monitoring will often detect abnormalities before they become clinically apparent. In fact, continuing such monitoring into the post-operative period may be more important than its use during surgery in influencing patient outcome (Mangano, 1992).

The particular type of monitoring used to assess cardiovascular performance and detect myocardial ischaemia may depend upon:

- the particular operation;
- the pre-operative medical condition of the patient;
- the equipment available within the hospital;
- the preference of the anaesthetist; and
- the facilities available post-operatively.

However, of probably greater importance than the choice of monitoring device is that the anaesthetist is familiar with the equipment and understands its limitations.

ELECTROCARDIOGRAPHY

Intra-operative ECG monitoring is used for two reasons. First, and most importantly, it is used to demonstrate heart rate and rhythm. Second, it can, if used appropriately, detect myocardial ischaemia. In order to get the best from the ECG, the anaesthetist should understand the origins of the signal, the importance of lead selection, and its limitations.

Origins of the ECG signal

Each lead measures the electrical potential between two electrodes, one 'negative' and one 'positive'. Current flowing towards the positive electrode results in an upward deflection, and current flowing away from it a downward deflection. Eindhoven originally described the detection of current between electrodes placed on the two arms and the left leg. These connections produce three bipolar limb leads which form an equilateral triangle around the heart (lead I: right arm negative, left arm positive; lead II: right arm negative, left leg positive; lead III: left arm negative, left leg positive). Unipolar leads were then added which measured the potential between an exploring positive electrode and a common terminal located at the 'centre' of the heart and formed by connecting both the arm and left leg leads. Subsequently it was found that the amplitude of the potential recorded from the limb leads was augmented if the connection to the limb from which the potential was being recorded was omitted from the combined electrode. These leads were termed augmented limb leads (aVR, aVL and aVF). The addition to these first six leads of six unipolar praecordial leads (V_1 to V_6) gave rise to the modern 12-lead ECG.

When ECG monitoring was introduced into the operating theatre, the large number of leads and the requirement for continuous display, made monitoring of each impossible. The first systems available for theatre use had three leads, but were capable of monitoring only one at a time. Then Mason and colleagues (1966) showed (during exercise ECG testing) that placing the right- and left-arm electrodes on the right and left shoulders and the left leg lead on the left hip did not affect the ECG unduly, and these placements became common in the operating theatre. Although, modern systems allow several leads to be monitored at one time, continuous monitoring of all 12 leads remains neither practical nor particularly desirable.

The environment in which the ECG is monitored also presents problems. Within the operating theatre there is much electrical 'noise' which can interfere with the ECG signal at both high (e.g. diathermy) and low (e.g. patient movement with respiration) frequencies. Filters are incorporated to reduce this noise, but unfortunately they also remove some of the high- and low-frequency waveforms which contribute to the ECG signal and may thus change its shape. When using the ECG in theatre, the anaesthetist should consider carefully the capabilities of the system and decide precisely what it is being used to detect. The electrodes are then placed appropriately and the relevant leads monitored.

Monitoring heart rate and rhythm

The ECG was first used in the theatre environment to detect and characterize disturbances in heart rate, rhythm and conduction. The best lead for this is lead II, because its vectoral plane passes through the left atrium, giving a greater P-wave amplitude than other leads so it has become the standard lead used for monitoring rhythm (Tyers *et al.*, 1988).

Monitoring for myocardial ischaemia

Whilst ECG monitoring of heart rate and rhythm is relatively easy, monitoring for myocardial ischaemia is more difficult. Its success depends upon the equipment used, the lead selected and the ability of the observer to detect subtle changes (Edwards and Reilly, 1994). Myocardial ischaemia produces characteristic

changes: subendocardial ischaemia results in ST-segment depression, whilst transmural ischaemia results in ST-segment elevation. It has therefore become increasingly popular to monitor the ST segment to detect myocardial ischaemia peri-operatively. However, other factors may also lead to ST-segment changes. Conduction abnormalities (particularly left bundle branch block), ventricular hypertrophy, electrolyte imbalance and the presence of drugs such as digoxin, may all affect the ST segment. Consequently, ECG ST-segment analysis is of little value in such conditions, yet these patients may be at most risk of developing myocardial ischaemia.

EQUIPMENT

The ECG signal is the sum of a series of sine waves with a wide range of frequencies. The voltages generated by the myocardium are relatively small and the signal must be amplified. In addition, for reasons noted above, the signal has to be filtered. Such amplification and filtering need to be equal across a large range of frequencies to avoid signal distortion. It is therefore recommended that ECG devices have a flat amplitude response across a frequency range of 0.05 to 100 Hz (Pipberger *et al.*, 1975). However, the level of electrical noise in the theatre environment means that a more stable signal is obtained with greater filtering, and a flat amplitude response across a narrower frequency range (0.5 to 40 Hz). Unfortunately, increased low frequency filtering can change the signal and produce apparent ST-segment depression (Berson and Pipberger, 1966). The anaesthetist should therefore know the filter band of the monitor. Some instruments now have two modes: one for monitoring with a low frequency cut-off at 0.5 Hz; and a diagnostic mode with a low frequency cut-off at 0.05 Hz to allow ST-segment analysis.

LEAD SELECTION

The best ECG leads for detecting myocardial ischaemia depend upon the area affected: leads V_4 and V_5 best detect anterior ischaemia; leads II, III and aVf inferior ischaemia; lead V_4R right ventricular ischaemia; and an oesophageal lead posterior ischaemia (Tyers *et al.*, 1988). Because about 90 per cent of myocardial ischaemia during exercise ECG monitoring is detected by V_5, this lead was originally suggested as the most appropriate for detecting intra-operative myocardial ischaemia (Kaplan and

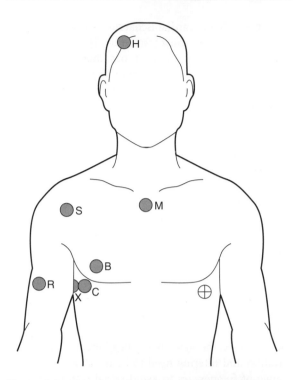

Figure 8.1 *Negative references for commonly used bipolar lead systems. The positive reference is at the V_5 position. First prefix in all leads is C. Letters shown in the diagram stand for second prefix (i.e. CM_5, CS_5, CB_5, CC_5, CH_5, CX_5, CR_5). (From Froelicher et al., 1976.)*

King, 1976). Indeed, London and colleagues (1988) have shown that 75 per cent of myocardial ischaemia occurring intra-operatively will be shown in lead V_5. Combining leads V_4 and V_5 increases the detection rate to 90 per cent, and the further addition of lead II increases detection to 96 per cent.

BIPOLAR LEAD SYSTEMS

Monitoring of a true V_5 requires a five-lead system. Although monitors which use five or more leads and allow observation of more than one lead at a time are now available for theatre, most systems in current use provide only a three-lead system and allow observation of only one lead. With such systems, it is therefore necessary to use bipolar configurations to detect myocardial ischaemia. Several such configurations have been assessed and would appear to be satisfactory alternatives to a true lead V_5 for detecting ischaemia (Fig. 8.1). The ideal combination during and, if necessary, after surgery would seem to be lead

II (arrhythmia detection and inferior myocardial ischaemia) and V_5 (anterior myocardial ischaemia), but many alternative arrangements have been suggested (Griffin and Kaplan, 1987). A five-lead system is obviously preferable, because both can be monitored, but if only a three-lead system is available and only one lead can be observed at a time, there is an alternative (Bazaral and Norfleet, 1981). This is to monitor lead CB_5 (Fig. 8.1, positive electrode V_5 position, negative electrode on back just beneath right scapula) which allows easy P-wave recognition and reliable detection of ischaemia. Alternatively, the right-arm electrode can be placed on the right shoulder, the left-arm electrode at the V_5 position, and the left-leg electrode on the left hip. Selection of lead I enables continuous monitoring of bipolar lead CS_5, whilst giving the capability to switch to lead II periodically or at any suggestion of an arrhythmia.

ST-SEGMENT MONITORS

Monitoring for myocardial ischaemia also depends upon the ability of the observer to detect ST-segment changes. It has been shown that even when myocardial ischaemia is detected using standard ECG monitoring, the rate of observation by anaesthetists is poor (London *et al.*, 1988). This may be due to several factors such as the duration of the ischaemia, the anaesthetist being busy in other ways, or simply not regarding observed changes as important. The development of monitoring devices capable of continuous ST-segment analysis should improve this detection rate. Such systems allow better identification of the beginning and end of each QRS complex, reliable measurements of the ST segments, and also allow the anaesthetist to alter the point at which ST measurements are made (Weinfurt, 1990). Despite these technological advances, ST-segment analysis may still be misleading and as such should always be used in conjunction with other monitoring findings. ST-segment monitors are best regarded as alarms that cause increased vigilance.

CENTRAL VENOUS PRESSURE (CVP) AND PULMONARY CAPILLARY WEDGE PRESSURE (PCWP) MEASUREMENT

These pressures are used as aids for assessing intravascular volume and blood loss, guiding fluid management and optimizing cardiac function. However, both readings are influenced by more than intravascular volume and cardiac function, so it is very important that the underlying principles are understood, and the limitations recognized, if these measures are to be used appropriately for patient management.

- CVP is the blood pressure at the junction of the vena cavae with the right atrium, and the normal trace has been described previously (Chapter 4). This trace indicates the filling pressures of the right atrium and ventricle, and generally gives an accurate reflection of right ventricular preload. CVP monitoring can thus be used to assess right-sided cardiac function.
- PCWP is usually measured using a catheter passed through the right atrium, tricuspid valve, right ventricle and pulmonary valve into the pulmonary artery. When the balloon at the end of a pulmonary artery catheter is inflated, the catheter is carried by the flow of blood and becomes 'wedged' within a pulmonary vessel. Flow through this vessel ceases, and the pressure waveform measured at the tip of the catheter is similar to that of the CVP, with A, C and V waves reflecting left atrial pressure changes. The mean pressure (the PCWP), is therefore assumed to reflect the pressure in the left atrium.

Measurement of cardiac filling/preload

Cardiac performance depends to a large extent upon filling of the right and left ventricles during diastole. The extent of filling, or 'preload', is generally accepted as being best reflected by the volume of the ventricle immediately prior to systole, the end-diastolic volume. At constant aortic pressure, an increase in end-diastolic volume produces an increase in stroke volume until a maximal figure is reached. Beyond this, further increases in end-diastolic volume overstretch the ventricle and stroke volume may start to fall (Starling's law). Monitoring of cardiac filling can therefore be used to optimize preload and hence cardiac function. Unfortunately, left ventricular end-diastolic volume (LVEDV) has, until recently, been extremely difficult to measure in the clinical situation, particularly intra-operatively, and left ventricular end-diastolic pressure (LVEDP) has usually been taken as a reasonable approximation. Left atrial catheters can be used to estimate LVEDP after car-

diac surgery, but in other situations preload is usually assessed by monitoring CVP and PCWP. Their use as monitors of intravascular volume makes two assumptions: first that LVEDP accurately reflects LVEDV; and second that CVP and PCWP accurately reflect LVEDP. Unfortunately, this is not always the case and anyone interpreting CVP and PCWP data needs to be aware of the potential pitfalls.

CVP indicates the pressure at the right atrium and also gives a fairly accurate reflection of right ventricular preload because right atrial and ventricular pressures are almost equal when the tricuspid valve is open at the end of ventricular diastole. CVP measurement can therefore be used to assess right-sided cardiac function, but it is a much less reliable reflection of left ventricular preload. In patients with healthy ventricles the function curves are similar (although not parallel), so that CVP monitoring provides a reasonable reflection of left ventricular filling. However, when either ventricle is compromised, the function curves are neither equal nor parallel. CVP monitoring in such circumstances is unreliable and the CVP reading can be higher *or* lower than LVEDP, making interpretation difficult (Rice *et al.*, 1978; Ansley *et al.*, 1987).

The use of a pulmonary artery catheter to measure PCWP has several advantages. CVP does not always give an accurate reflection of PCWP, whereas PCWP is usually in close agreement with left atrial pressure and LVEDP (Tuman *et al.*, 1989). Thus PCWP gives a better indication of left heart filling pressure, particularly in conditions of increased pulmonary vascular resistance or impaired right heart function. In addition the pulmonary artery catheter allows measurement of mixed venous oxygen saturation, and can also be used to determine cardiac output using the thermodilution technique. Other factors such as systemic and pulmonary vascular resistance can then be calculated, allowing selective manipulation of haemodynamic parameters. This has resulted in the pulmonary artery catheter being used in the diagnosis, treatment and monitoring of a variety of serious medical conditions. However, PCWP is certainly not a panacea despite being superior to the CVP as a measure of left ventricular preload. First, it has important technical limitations, and second, interpretation of PCWP readings depends upon an understanding of the relationships between PCWP and ventricular preload, venous tone and ventricular function.

Table 8.1 *Conditions in which pulmonary capillary wedge pressure (PCWP) may not accurately reflect left ventricular end-diastolic pressure (LVEDP)*

Overestimates	Underestimates
Positive pressure ventilation	Non-compliant left ventricle
Positive end-expiratory pressure	
Increased intrathoracic pressure	Aortic regurgitation
Tachycardia	Pulmonary embolism
Increased PVR	
Chronic obstructive airway disease	
Mitral valve disease	
Pulmonary vein compression	
Left-to-right intracardiac shunt	

Accuracy of PCWP measurement

For the pressure reading from a 'wedged' pulmonary artery catheter to accurately reflect LVEDP, there must be a continuous column of blood from catheter tip to aortic valve. At the end of diastole, there should be a minimal pressure gradient so that PCWP, pulmonary artery diastolic pressure, left atrial pressure and LVEDP should be virtually the same. Unfortunately, there are several factors which can interfere with this (Table 8.1; Tuman *et al.*, 1989).

POSITION OF CATHETER WITHIN THE LUNG

West and colleagues (1964) have defined zones within the lung that relate to the relationships between alveolar, arterial and venous pressures.

- In zone I, alveolar pressure is greater than arterial and venous pressures, so that there is no blood flow. Should the pulmonary artery catheter tip lie in such a zone, it will reflect alveolar rather than vascular pressure.
- Zone II describes that part of the lung in which alveolar pressure is less than arterial pressure, but greater than venous. If the catheter tip lies there, the inflated balloon may obstruct blood flow and produce a zone I relationship.
- In zone III alveolar pressure is less than both arterial and venous pressure so that the capillaries will remain open when the balloon is inflated and the measurement will accurately reflect left atrial pressure.

When the patient is supine, the zone III situation pertains throughout most of the lung and a flotation catheter will tend to enter such an area because most blood flows there. However, the pressure relationship may change to another pattern because of factors such as hypovolaemia, or the use of positive pressure ventilation and positive end-expiratory pressure (PEEP). These can lead to false interpretation of readings so it is essential to confirm that the catheter tip is in a zone III situation. The following criteria are useful in confirming this: the tracing should be phasic with A and V waveforms; blood can be easily aspirated from the catheter; mean PCWP should be less than or equal to pulmonary artery diastolic pressure and less than mean pulmonary arterial pressure.

INTRATHORACIC PRESSURE

Changes in intrathoracic pressure can significantly affect PCWP and, regardless of whether ventilation is spontaneous or controlled, intrathoracic pressure is closest to atmospheric at the end of expiration. Thus pulmonary artery pressure readings should be taken at the end of expiration to minimize the effects of changes in intrathoracic pressure. PEEP is often used to improve patient oxygenation, and is also used intra-operatively by some anaesthetists to reduce post-operative atelectasis. The resulting increase in alveolar pressure can affect PCWP in two ways. First, the pressure is transmitted to the pulmonary capillaries so that PCWP is increased. Second, pulmonary capillary blood flow is reduced so that a zone III relationship is converted to a zone II or I situation. The amount of PEEP transmitted to the PCWP is proportional to pulmonary compliance; in patients with low compliance, the effect is less.

VALVULAR HEART DISEASE

Abnormalities of the left heart valves often affect the PCWP reading. For example, in mitral stenosis, obstruction to the flow of blood into the left ventricle may result in PCWP exceeding LVEDP. In aortic regurgitation, flow of blood back into the left ventricle during diastole causes premature closure of the mitral valve and PCWP will underestimate LVEDP. Mitral regurgitation can affect the PCWP tracing by producing large V waves (see below). In a similar way, abnormalities of right heart valves will affect CVP readings.

TACHYCARDIA

Tachycardia reduces both diastolic filling time and ventricular filling. When heart rate increases sufficiently, the left atrium contracts against a partially closed mitral valve and PCWP exceeds LVEDP.

PULMONARY VASCULAR RESISTANCE

Increases in pulmonary vascular resistance may lead to distortion of the pressure waveform between the right atrium and the tip of the pulmonary artery catheter, and this can result in the PCWP and pulmonary artery diastolic pressure exceeding LVEDP.

CONDITIONS THAT PRODUCE LARGE V WAVES

Blood flow into the atrium towards the end of ventricular systole when the mitral valve is closed, generates the V wave of the PCWP tracing. Some clinical conditions (e.g. mitral regurgitation, mitral stenosis with poor left ventricular compliance, or whenever preload is increased in a patient with poor left atrial compliance) can produce large V waves and lead to problems in data interpretation. The large waves can result in the mistaken view that the catheter has not wedged, but this error can be avoided by observing the relationship of the pressure tracing to the T wave of the ECG. A pulmonary artery trace shows the systolic peak to be synchronous with the T wave, but the peak of the PCWP V wave occurs *after* the T wave.

CVP and PCWP as measures of preload

CVP and PCWP are dependent upon intravascular fluid volume, intrinsic tone of the large veins, and right- and left-sided myocardial function. Interpretation of the readings depends on an understanding of their relationships with these factors. Essentially, PCWP is used as an estimate of LVEDP. However, the degree of ventricular wall stretching correlates better with LVEDV than LVEDP. Whilst LVEDP gives a reasonable reflection of LVEDV in many instances, there are circumstances in which this may not be the case because of the non-linear relationship between LVEDV and LVEDP. At low LVEDV, a large increase in volume results in a small change in LVEDP, but at larger volumes small changes can result in much larger pressure changes. In addition, the relationship between the two can be altered by changes in left ventricular compliance. Reduced compliance usually means that at any given end-diastolic volume, the end-diastolic pressure is greater than in ventricles of normal compliance. In such circumstances, LVEDP may need to be somewhat greater than normal to achieve an adequate preload. Thus the change in LVEDP occurring as a result of a change in volume will depend upon the initial LVEDV and the ventricular compliance. For example, increased PCWP could represent either increased preload in a compliant ventricle, or normal preload in a ventricle with reduced compliance. Similarly, an increase in PCWP may be due to an increase in intravascular volume, or to reduced left ventricular compliance as may occur with myocardial ischaemia or sepsis.

INFLUENCE OF VENOUS TONE

Whilst a low CVP or PCWP is usually indicative of reduced cardiac preload, reflex responses to fluid and blood loss mean that hypovolaemia can exist despite normal, or even high, right- and left-sided filling pressures. This is because the large veins of the body act as an extremely compliant reservoir for the storage of blood and alterations in vessel wall tone in response to changes in blood volume help to maintain filling pressures. Loss of fluid leads to venous constriction so that CVP and PCWP are reasonably maintained even though blood volume is effectively reduced. In addition, arteriolar constriction maintains systemic blood pressure while reducing stroke volume. Cardiac output is effectively maintained by an increase in heart rate. If a bolus of fluid is given in this situation, an initial increase in PCWP is followed by a decrease as the compensatory venoconstriction is reduced. In addition, arterial constriction may decrease, so that stroke volume will increase and heart rate decrease. Thus it is the lack of a significant change in filling pressures and the pattern of haemodynamic change in response to a fluid bolus which indicate that the patient is hypovolaemic, rather than a low initial PCWP or CVP.

Insufficient appreciation of the various factors determining CVP and PCWP can lead to misinterpretation of the clinical situation by inexperienced medical staff, and either inappropriate or inadequate treatment. In particular it is essential to recognize that the change in CVP or PCWP in response to treatment, particularly fluid, is of far greater importance than the absolute value. The situation can often occur in vascular surgery, particularly when there has been a large volume loss and fluid shift, when the blood pressure is low despite a normal or even increased PCWP. In such circumstances, significant blood loss and transfusion requirement, with subsequent acidosis and hypothermia, may lead to alterations in left ventricular compliance. The challenge is therefore to decide whether the most appropriate treatment is further fluid administration to increase ventricular preload, or inotropic support to increase myocardial contractility. By observing the response to a rapid infusion of fluid (3–5 mL/kg), it is possible to estimate the relationship between LVEDV and LVEDP. A small increase in PCWP implies that LVEDV is increasing without a substantial increase in LVEDP, and that fluid treatment is appropriate. However, a large increase in PCWP implies that a small increase in LVEDV results in large increase in LVEDP and that further fluid is unlikely to improve cardiac function.

Monitoring of cardiac output and stroke volume

The management of the situations described above is never easy, and additional information to guide therapy is always welcome. With a pulmonary artery catheter, this can be provided by measuring cardiac output and stroke volume by thermodilution. Monitoring cardiac output and stroke volume gives a better indication of left ventricular function than PCWP, and it is in this use that pulmonary artery catheterization is arguably of greatest value. By using the relationship between PCWP and stroke volume, the ventricular function curve can be determined much more easily. Quite simply, if fluid challenges fail to increase stroke volume and cardiac output then further fluid therapy alone is inappropriate.

The recent introduction of continuous cardiac output monitoring has made such readings easily available 'on line' in theatre and represents a major advance in monitoring, particularly in circumstances of major blood loss. A filament coiled over part of the catheter which lies in the right atrium and ventricle is heated intermittently. A thermistor at the tip of the catheter detects changes in blood temperature which are analysed to produce a thermodilution curve. The heating sequence is repeated every

minute and the displayed value (based upon about six determinations) is updated every minute. The direct observation of changes in stroke volume and cardiac output in response to fluid challenges and other therapeutic interventions provides a far greater facility for optimizing cardiac function than simply relying on PCWP, and this is of immense value when managing difficult cases.

PCWP and myocardial ischaemia

Abnormalities in myocardial function caused by myocardial ischaemia increase PCWP, and produce new A–C or V waves. Kaplan and colleagues (1981) have shown that the appearance of large V waves in the PCWP trace can be associated with the onset of myocardial ischaemia and suggested that detection of these may be an additional function of the pulmonary artery catheter. However, as previously mentioned, large V waves can be caused by a wide variety of factors other than myocardial ischaemia. Indeed, Haggmark and colleagues (1989), in comparing different indicators of intra-operative myocardial ischaemia, showed that such changes are not very specific and that the pulmonary artery catheter (on its own) is of little value for detecting myocardial ischaemia. In addition, PCWP cannot be used continuously because the catheter must be wedged. Thus a pulmonary artery catheter is only of benefit in the detection of myocardial ischaemia when used in conjunction with other monitors.

Indications for pulmonary artery catheterization in vascular anaesthesia?

There is great diversity of opinion on the indications for pulmonary artery catheters. Some excellent anaesthetists never use them, but others, equally able, use them at any indication. The technique certainly has the potential for complications (Shah et al., 1984), and should not be used unless the these risks have been considered and balanced against the potential benefits. A study from the United States (Conners et al., 1996) strongly questioning the value of the pulmonary artery flotation catheter in intensive care has provoked much debate (Dalen and Bone, 1996; Soni, 1996). A major argument against the technique is the lack of any study showing improved outcome, and the potential benefit should always be assessed on an individual basis. Such benefit is more likely to be gained when major haemodynamic insults, blood loss and fluid shifts are likely, particularly in patients with significantly impaired cardiac function. In addition, a major advantage over other methods of assessing cardiovascular status is that this monitoring can easily be extended well into the post-operative period.

Every individual anaesthetizing patients for vascular surgery should consider the arguments and decide his or her own practice. The present author prefers to insert a pulmonary artery catheter in all patients undergoing emergency aortic aneurysm surgery as soon as is practical; in those undergoing thoracic or suprarenal aortic aneurysm repair; in patients with pulmonary artery hypertension, or significantly impaired ventricular function undergoing infrarenal aortic surgery. In contrast, there seems little indication in patients undergoing peripheral procedures where little haemodynamic insult or fluid shift occurs. However, there have been studies (Rao *et al.*, 1983; Berlauk *et al.*, 1991) indicating that pre-operative optimization of cardiovascular function guided by pulmonary artery catheterization improves outcome in peripheral vascular surgery, and in patients undergoing surgery after a recent myocardial infarction. Thus the option might be considered in particularly high-risk patients.

TRANSOESOPHAGEAL ECHOCARDIOGRAPHY

Transoesophageal echocardiography (TOE) is likely to become an increasingly important monitoring and diagnostic tool in anaesthesia. With the development of a transducer which can be positioned in the oesophagus it has become possible to assess cardiac function directly intra-operatively using two-dimensional echocardiography. Echocardiography uses frequencies in the range of 1 to 7 MHz, the higher ones giving high resolution, but having low penetration, whereas lower frequencies penetrate well but at the expense of decreased resolution. Because there is no need to penetrate the chest wall, TOE utilizes frequencies between 3.5 and 7 MHz, affording excellent resolution.

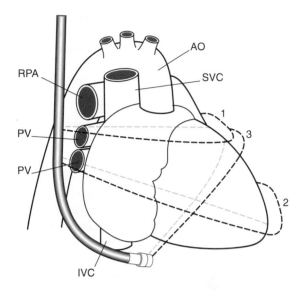

Figure 8.2 *The three basic imaging planes of the heart that can be obtained with transoesophageal echocardiography. AO = aorta, IVC = inferior vena cava, PV = pulmonary vein, RPA = right pulmonary artery, SVC = superior vena cava.*

TOE can be performed in an awake patient under local anaesthesia, but in surgical patients the probe is usually placed after induction of anaesthesia and intubation. The transducer is inserted through the mouth and advanced 35–40 cm initially to obtain basal short axis views of the heart and allow imaging of the aortic and pulmonary valves, left and right atria, the ascending aorta and the pulmonary trunk. Further advancement then allows all four heart chambers, the mitral and tricuspid valves, to be viewed. Finally, by angling the transducer forward, and advancing it a further 2–5 cm, a cross-sectional image of the left ventricle, including a short-axis view at the level of the papillary muscle, is obtained (Cahalan *et al.*, 1987; Werner and Mugge, 1995) (Fig. 8.2). The technique is minimally invasive and appears to be extremely safe, although it is not recommended in patients with a history of oesophageal disease.

TOE provides the anaesthetist with an immense amount of previously unavailable information. By far the greatest value of this new monitoring technique can be seen in cardiothoracic surgery because it allows vastly improved imaging of cardiac structures and can be used to assess valvular function, and detect intracardiac defects and residual ventricular air. However, the ability of TOE to monitor cardiac function and detect myocardial ischaemia indicates considerable potential for its use during non-cardiac vascular surgery (Abel *et al.*, 1987; London *et al.*, 1990).

Monitoring of cardiac function

TOE allows continuous measurement of ventricular preload and assessment of cardiac function. Ventricular preload can be determined more reliably than with other monitoring techniques because it allows direct assessment of LVEDV compared to indirect estimates of ventricular preload using pressure data (Stoddard *et al.*, 1994). Whilst some studies have questioned the accuracy of TOE in assessing left ventricle volume status (Urbanowicz *et al.*, 1990), there is little doubt that it is far more reliable than the pulmonary artery catheter. In addition, measurement of left ventricular end-systolic volume also allows determination of ejection fraction. Cardiac function can be further assessed by measuring shortening fraction or determining end-systolic left ventricular diameter/pressure–volume relationships (Heinrich *et al.*, 1987), and cardiac output measured by Doppler ultrasound of aortic blood flow shows excellent correlation with thermodilution techniques (Terai *et al.*, 1985). This provides the possibility of optimization of intravascular fluid volume and cardiac function to an extent never previously available. Such monitoring offers significant potential benefit, particularly in surgery of the thoracic aorta and in the management of aortic rupture, where large haemodynamic insult and fluid shifts are inevitable. Indeed, in suprarenal aortic surgery, Roizen and colleagues (1984) have shown that TOE can allow identification and treatment of significant myocardial dysfunction undetected by other monitoring techniques.

Monitoring for myocardial ischaemia

TOE also has potential value in the detection of intra-operative myocardial ischaemia which can result in pronounced alterations in ventricular wall motion. A reduction in regional coronary blood flow results in reduced contractile function in that area of the myocardium. Contractile function can be assessed using TOE by observing ventricular wall thickening and movement towards the centre of the ventricle which occur during systole (systolic wall thickening

and endocardial excursion). Changes in ventricular function observed in this way are known as systolic wall motion abnormalities (SWMA), and are particularly sensitive to subendocardial blood flow. SWMA have been shown to occur within seconds of changes in blood flow, as compared with ECG changes which can take several minutes to appear (Battler *et al.*, 1980). In monitoring wall motion with TOE, the ventricle is divided into segments based upon the distribution of the coronary arteries and a scoring system is used to define the severity of SWMA. The short-axis view at the level of the papillary muscle is most commonly used and allows detection of SWMA in the anterior, septal, posterior and lateral walls, permitting assessment of areas supplied by all three major coronary arteries. If the heart is not enlarged, a cross-sectional view of both ventricles can frequently be obtained. However, SWMA in the apical and basal areas may be missed. The introduction of the biplanar TOE probe, capable of scanning the left ventricle in both short axis and longitudinal views without changing transducer position addresses this problem (Shah *et al.*, 1991).

Limitations of TOE

Whilst the detection of SWMA is a very sensitive indicator of myocardial ischaemia, it is poorly specific. Previous myocardial infarction can result in dyskinetic segments, making interpretation difficult and factors other than ischaemia (particularly increases in ventricular afterload and decreases in contractility) can cause or exaggerate such abnormalities (Ross, 1986). These factors may limit the value of TOE in detecting myocardial ischaemia. Indeed, if clinicians are to be encouraged to use the findings of TOE to alter intra-operative management, it is necessary that studies investigate the relationship between the development of intra-operative SWMA and outcome. An initial study (Smith *et al.*, 1985) in patients undergoing cardiac and major vascular surgery was promising, showing a significant correlation between the development of SWMA and poor outcome. However, later studies have been less encouraging, suggesting that intra-operative SWMA are common during vascular surgery and that their presence has a low predictive value for post-operative cardiac complications (Gewertz *et al.*, 1987; London *et al.*, 1990; Watters *et al.*, 1991). Indeed, one study (Eisenberg *et al.*, 1992) showed that the detection of myocardial ischaemia with TOE provided little additional value over two-lead Holter ECG recording in predicting post-operative cardiac risk. There remains considerable debate therefore as to the true value of TOE in detecting myocardial ischaemia. In particular, the criteria describing the significance of SWMA in terms of duration and type (hypokinesis, akinesis or dyskinesis) need validation.

TOE has other important limitations (Vandenberg, 1990):

• monitoring does not usually begin until the probe has been positioned *after* induction of anaesthesia, by which time many ischaemic episodes may have occurred (Edwards *et al.*, 1994);
• probe position and orientation must be very carefully attended to throughout surgery, and high-quality scans of both ventricles are required for accurate detection of wall motion abnormalities and this is not always possible;
• the technique relies heavily upon the skill of the operator;
• it cannot be used post-operatively once the patient is extubated.

Finally, the costs of providing TOE mean that it is unlikely to be available for non-cardiac theatre use in all but the largest centres (Townend and Hutton, 1996). At the present time, an echo Doppler system costs approximately £100 000 and the probe, costing £30 000, has a lifespan of about 500 procedures. When the additional expense of training sufficient skilled operators to provide a comprehensive TOE service is also added, the overall cost becomes prohibitive.

Despite its considerable potential, current research does not support the routine use of TOE in vascular surgery, with the possible exceptions of monitoring volume when extensive blood loss is expected and suprarenal aortic surgery. However, improving technological development and a greater understanding of the relevance of its findings mean that TOE remains the cardiovascular monitor of the future.

TRANSOESOPHAGEAL DOPPLER ULTRASOUND

The advent of transoesophageal Doppler ultrasound has provided another potentially valuable tool for assessing fluid volume status. It is a safe, non-invasive technique which allows continuous measurement and analysis of aortic blood flow allowing estimation of cardiac output (Singer *et al.*, 1989). In addition, analysis of the waveform can be used to assess left ventricular filling, myocardial contractility and afterload (Singer and Bennett, 1991). Compared to TOE, it is cheaper, easier to use, and far less reliant on operator skill. In clinical use, transoesophaegeal Doppler has been shown to give a good indication of changes in cardiac output (Patel and Singer, 1993) and intravascular volume shifts (Evans *et al.*, 1992).

Functional principles

An oesophageal probe is used to direct a continuous beam of ultrasound at the descending aorta. The frequency at which this beam is reflected from the blood cells travelling down the aorta is proportional to their velocity. The reflected waves are translated into a waveform recording the velocity of blood against time. An estimate of cardiac output and stroke volume is then calculated by using an estimated aortic diameter, based upon the patient's height, weight

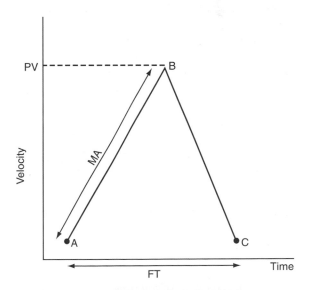

Figure 8.3 *Systolic flow waveform detected by transoesophageal Doppler in the descending thoracic aorta. A = Start of systolic flow; B = Peak of systolic flow; C = End of systolic flow; FT = Systolic flow time (time from A to C); PV = Velocity at peak of systole (B); MA = Mean acceleration (gradient of slope A to B).*

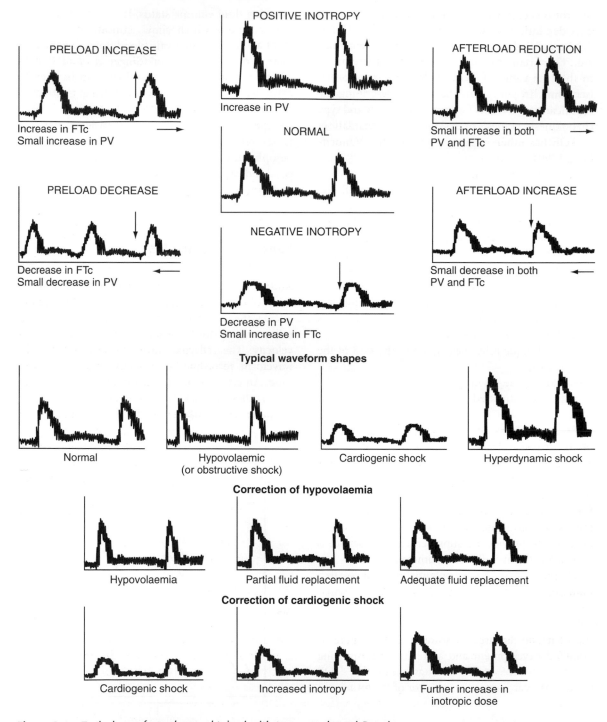

Figure 8.4 *Typical waveform shapes obtained with transoesophageal Doppler.*

and age. The probe is inserted to a distance of 35–40 cm and is then rotated, inserted or withdrawn until the characteristic descending aortic waveform is seen. An audible signal can also be used to help with accurate placement. The probe is then further adjusted until the clearest and sharpest waveform is obtained. This is displayed continuously along with an estimate of cardiac output and stroke volume.

Probably of more value in assessing volume status than the derived cardiac output and stroke volume figures, is the shape of the waveform itself. In recognition of this, oesophageal Doppler devices also display the parameters determined from the waveform which can help in determining the patient's haemodynamic status. These include the velocity at the peak of systole (peak velocity (PV)) and mean acceleration (the gradient of the upslope (MA)) which give an indication of myocardial contractility, and the systolic flow time corrected for heart rate (FTc) which gives an indication of preload (Fig. 8.3).

Figure 8.4 shows some examples of waveforms obtained in different haemodynamic situations. For example, hypovolaemia, or a reduced preload results in a decrease in FTc with a small decrease in PV; myocardial depression (cardiac failure) results in a decrease in PV with a small decrease in FTc; a hyperdynamic circulation, such as may be seen in sepsis, results in an increase in PV with a small increase in FTc.

Uses and limitations

Such a device has some clear advantages for all types of anaesthesia, primarily in monitoring those patients in whom more invasive monitoring is not deemed necessary, but in whom it would be desirable to have some indication of fluid balance or cardiac status. Indeed, Mythen and Webb (1995) have shown the value of optimizing intravascular volume per-operatively on outcome, and suggested that transoesophageal Doppler may be superior to CVP monitoring in this aspect. Unfortunately, transoesophageal Doppler has some limitations similar to those of TOE:

• it can only be used in sedated or anaesthetized patients and it is unsuitable for monitoring the conscious patient;
• the signal is positional, and changes may be due to alterations in the probe position rather than in the patient's condition;
• cardiac output and stroke volume readings are only estimates, although changes are of more importance than the actual figures; and
• because it monitors blood flow through the descending aorta, *it is inaccurate during aortic cross clamping*.

Thus transoesophageal Doppler monitoring would seem most useful in patients undergoing peripheral vascular procedures under general anaesthesia. Its value in aortic surgery is obviously more limited although it may still prove useful in patients undergoing repair of an abdominal aneurysm, and in whom pulmonary artery catheterization is thought unnecessary.

OVERVIEW

Until recently, the emphasis on the care of the anaesthetized patient has been on 'monitoring' the patient and only intervening with treatment when undesirable changes occur. This is certainly the case with myocardial ischaemia which should be looked for and treated promptly should it occur. Although the ECG remains the simplest and most reliable method of detecting myocardial ischaemia, there are several limitations to its use. However, improvements in ECG technology and the development of newer monitoring techniques should improve the ability to detect and treat myocardial ischaemia in the future.

In contrast to the traditional expectant approach to monitoring, recent work suggests that the emphasis should change. The information available may be used to guide therapy in order to achieve predetermined cardiovascular goals. Evidence that optimizing cardiovascular state to maximize tissue perfusion leads to improved outcome is available (Shoemaker et al., 1988; Boyd et al., 1993). In these studies, patients were monitored with pulmonary artery catheters pre-operatively, and inotropes were used specifically to increase cardiac output to supranormal levels. There is no doubt that patients undergoing vascular surgery should be regarded as a high-risk group, but exactly how far these aims should be pursued in each patient is less clear. Caution should always be used when applying the results of one institution to another because of differences in practice between them.

Despite these reservations, there are certain principles which can be applied universally to optimize intra-operative cardiovascular status. Undoubtedly, the first priority should be to optimize preload. Vasodilators, vasoconstrictors and inotropes can then be used as necessary to control arterial blood pressure and cardiac output to maintain tissue perfusion, whilst avoiding myocardial ischaemia. Such therapy necessarily requires close monitoring of the cardiovascular system. Whilst the particular type of monitoring used will depend upon several factors, the application of sound physiological principles together with a thorough knowledge of the monitoring equipment being used, will ensure that the patients are provided with optimal care. Whilst CVP and PCWP are currently the commonest methods for assessing preload, monitors which give an estimate of cardiac output and stroke volume may be better, particularly if therapies aimed at achieving cardiovascular goals are intended. The advent of continuous cardiac output monitoring, transoesophageal Doppler and transoesophageal echocardiography may lead to a radical change in the way intra-operative cardiovascular performance is assessed and managed.

REFERENCES

Abel, M.D., Nishimura, R.A., Callahan, M.J. et al. 1987. Evaluation of intra-operative transesophageal two-dimensional echocardiography. Anesthesiology 66, 64–68.

Ansley, D.M., Ramsay, J.G. and Whalley, D.G. 1987. The relationship between central venous pressure and pulmonary capillary wedge pressure during aortic surgery. Canadian Journal of Anaesthesia 34, 594–600.

Battler, A., Froelicher, V.F., Gallagher, K.P. et al. 1980. Dissociation between regional myocardial dysfunction and ECG changes during ischaemia in the conscious dog. Circulation 62, 735–744.

Bazaral, M.G. and Norfleet, E.A. 1981. Comparison of CB_5 and V_5 leads for intra-operative electrocardiographic monitoring. Anesthesia and Analgesia 60, 849–853.

Berlauk, J.F., Abrams, J.H., Gilmour, I.J. et al. 1991. Preoperative optimisation of cardiovascular hemodynamics improves outcome in peripheral vascular surgery. Annals of Surgery 214, 289–297.

Berson, A.S. and Pipberger, H.V. 1966. The low-frequency response of electrocardiographs, a frequent source of recording errors. American Heart Journal 71, 779–789.

Boyd, O., Grounds, R.M. and Bennett, E.D. 1993. A randomized clinical trial of the effect of deliberate peri-operative increase of oxygen delivery on mortality in high-risk surgical patients. Journal of the American Medical Association 270, 2699–2707.

Cahalan, M.K., Litt, L., Botvinick, E.H. and Schiller, N.B. 1987. Advances in noninvasive cardiovascular imaging: implications for the anesthiologist. Anesthesiology 66, 356–372.

Connors, A.F., Speroff, T., Dawson, N.V. et al. 1996. The effectiveness of right heart catheterisation in the initial care of critically ill patients. Journal of the American Medical Association 276, 889–897.

Dalen, J.E. and Bone, R.C. 1996. Is it time to pull the pulmonary artery catheter? Journal of the American Medical Association 276, 916–918.

Edwards, N.D., Alford, A.M., Dobson, P.M. et al. 1984. Myocardial ischaemia during tracheal intubation and extubation. British Journal of Anaesthesia 73, 537–539.

Edwards, N.D. and Reilly, C.S. 1994. The detection of peri-operative myocardial ischaemia. British Journal of Anaesthesia 72, 104–115.

Eisenberg, M.J., London, M.J., Leung, J.M. et al. 1992. Monitoring for myocardial ischemia during noncardiac surgery. A technological assessment of transesophageal echocardiography and 12–lead electrocardiography. Journal of American Medical Association 268, 210–216.

Evans, J.W.H., Singer, M., Chapple, C.R. et al. 1992. Haemodynamic evidence for cardiac stress during transurethral prostatectomy. British Medical Journal 304, 666–671.

Froelicher, V.F., Wolthius, R., Keiser, N. et al. 1976. A comparison of two bipolar exercise ECG leads to lead V_5. Chest 70, 611–616.

Gewertz, B.L., Kresmer, P.C., Zarins, C.K. et al. 1987. Transesophageal echocardiographic monitoring of myocardial ischemia during vascular surgery. Journal of Vascular Surgery 5, 607–613.

Griffin, R.M. and Kaplan, J.A. 1987. Myocardial ischaemia during non-cardiac surgery. A comparison of different lead systems using computerised ST segment analysis. Anaesthesia 42, 155–159.

Haggmark, S., Hohner, P., Ostman, M. et al. 1989. Comparison of hemodynamic, electrocardiographic, mechanical and metabolic indicators of intra-operative myocardial ischemia in vascular surgical patients with coronary artery disease. Anesthesiology 70, 19–25.

Heinrich, H., Foesel, T.H., Fontaine, L. et al. 1987. Assessment of contractility changes in humans by transoesophageal echocardiography. The peak systolic pressure end-systolic diameter relationship (PSPESDRS). International Journal of Clinical Monitoring and Computing 4, 243–248.

Kaplan, J.A. and King, S.B. 1976. The precordial ECG lead (V₅) in patients who have coronary-artery disease. *Anesthesiology* **45**, 570–574.

Kaplan, J.A. and Wells, P.H. 1981. Early diagnosis of myocardial ischemia using the pulmonary artery catheter. *Anesthesia and Analgesia* **60**, 789–793.

Labovitz, A.J., Lewen, M.K., Kern, M. *et al.* 1987. Evaluation of left ventricular systolic and diastolic dysfunction during transient myocardial ischemia produced by angioplasty. *Journal of the American College of Cardiology* **10**, 748–755.

London, M.J., Hollenberg, M., Wong, M.G. *et al.* and the SPI Research Group. 1988. Intraoperative myocardial ischemia: localisation by continuous 12–lead electrocardiography. *Anesthesiology* **69**, 232–241.

London, M.J., Tubau, J.F., Wong, M.G. *et al.* and the SPI research group 1990. The 'natural history' of segmental wall motion abnormalities in patients undergoing noncardiac surgery. *Anesthesiology* **73**, 644–655.

Mangano, D.T. 1990. Perioperative cardiac morbidity. *Anesthesiology* **72**, 153–184.

Mason, R.E. and Likar, I. 1966. A new system of multiple-lead exercise electrocardiography. *American Heart Journal* **71**, 196–205.

Mythen, M.G. and Webb, A.R. 1995. Perioperative plasma volume expansion reduces the incidence of gut mucosal hypoperfusion during cardiac surgery. *Archives of Surgery* **130**, 423–429.

Patel, M. and Singer, M. 1993. The optimal time for measuring the cardiorespiratory effects of positive end-expiratory pressure. *Chest* **104**, 139–142.

Pipberger, H.V., Arzbaecher, R.C., Berson, A.S. *et al.* 1975. Recommendations for standardisation of leads and of specifications for instruments in electrocardiography and vectorcardiography. Report of the Committee on Electrocardiography, American Heart Association. *Circulation* **52**, 11–31.

Rao, T.L., Jacobs, K.H. and El-Etr, A.A. 1983. Reinfarction following anesthesia in patients with myocardial infarction. *Anesthesiology* **59**, 499–505.

Rice, C.L., Hobelman, C.F. and John, D.A. 1978. Central venous pressure or pulmonary capillary wedge pressure as the determinant of fluid replacement in aortic surgery. *Surgery* **84**, 437–440.

Roizen, M.F., Beaupre, P.N., Alpert, R.A. *et al.* 1984. Monitoring with two-dimensional transesophageal echocardiography. Comparison of myocardial function in patients undergoing supraceliac, suprarenal-infraceliac or infrarenal aortic occlusion. *Journal of Vascular Surgery* **1**, 300–305.

Ross, J. 1986. Assessment of ischemic regional myocardial dysfunction and its reversibility. *Circulation* **74**, 1186–1190.

Shah, K.B., Rao, T.L.K., Laughlin, S. and El-Etr, A.A. 1984. A review of pulmonary artery catheterisation in 6245 patients. *Anesthesiology* **61**, 271–275.

Shah, P.M., Kyo, S., Matsumura. M. and Omoto, R. 1991. Utility of biplane transesophageal echocardiography in left ventrivular wall motion analysis. *Journal of Cardiothoracic and Vascular Anaesthesia* **5**, 316–319.

Shoemaker, W.C., Appel, P.L., Kram, H.B. *et al.* 1988. Prospective trial of supranormal values of survivors as therapeutic goals in high-risk surgical patients. *Chest* **94**, 1176–1186.

Singer, M., Clarke, J. and Bennett, E.D. 1989. Continuous hemodynamic monitoring by oesophageal doppler. *Critical Care Medicine* **17**, 447–452.

Singer, M. and Bennett, E.D. 1991. Noninvasive optimisation of left ventricular filling using esophageal doppler. *Critical Care Medicine* **19**, 1132–1137.

Smith, J.S., Cahalan, M.K., Benefiel, D.J. *et al.* 1985. Intraoperative detection of myocardial ischemia in high-risk patients: electrocardiography versus two-dimensional transesophageal echocardiography. *Circulation* **72**, 1015–1021.

Soni, N. 1996. Swan song for the Swan–Ganz catheter? *British Medical Journal* **313**, 763–764.

Stoddard, M.F., Keedy, D.L. and Longaker, R.A. 1994. Two-dimensional transesophageal echocardiographic characterisation of ventricular filling in real time by acoustic quantification: comparison with pulsed doppler echocardiography. *Journal of the American Society of Echocardiography* **7**, 116–131.

Sykes, M.K., Vickers, M.D. and Hull, C.J. 1991. *Principles of measurement and monitoring in anaesthesia and intensive care*. Oxford: Blackwell Scientific Publications.

Terai, C., Uenishi, M., Sugimoto, H. *et al.* 1985. Transesophageal echocardiographic dimensional analysis of four cardiac chambers during positive end expiratory pressure. *Anesthesiology* **63**, 640–646.

Townend, J.N. and Hutton, P. 1996. Transoesophageal echocardiography in anaesthesia and intensive care. *British Journal of Anaesthesia* **77**, 137–139.

Tuman, K.J., Carroll, G.C. and Ivankivich, A.D. 1989. Pitfalls in interpretation of pulmonary artery catheter data. *Journal of Cardiothoracic Anesthesia* **3**, 625–641.

Tyers, M.R., Russell, W.J. and Runciman, W.B. 1988. Electrocardiographic monitoring in anaesthesia. *Anaesthesia and Intensive Care* **16**, 66–69.

Urbanowicz, J.H., Shaaban, M.J., Cohen, N.H. *et al.* 1990. Comparison of transesophogeal and scintigraphic estimates of left ventricular end-diastolic volume index and ejection fraction in patients following coronary artery bypass grafting. *Anesthesiology* **72**, 607–612.

Vandenberg, B.F. and Kerber, R.E. 1990. Transesophageal echocardiography and intra-operative monitoring of left ventricular function. *Anesthesiology* **73**, 799–801.

Watters, T.A., Botvinick, E.H., Dae, M.W. *et al.* 1991. Comparison of the findings on pre-operative dipyridamole perfusion scintigraphy and intra-operative transesophageal echocardiography: implications regarding the identification of myocardium at ischemic risk. *Journal of American College of Cardiology* **18**, 93–100.

Weinfurt, P.T. 1990. Electrocardiography: an overview. *Journal of Clinical Monitoring* **6**, 132–138.

Werner, G.D. and Mugge, A. 1995. Transesophageal echocardiography. *New England Journal of Medicine* **332**, 1268–1279.

West, J.B., Dollery, C.T. and Naimark, A. 1964. Distribution of blood flow in isolated lung: relation to vascular and alveolar pressures. *Journal of Applied Physiology* **19**, 713–724.

Wohlgelernter, D., Jaffe, C.C., Cabin, H.S. *et al.* 1987. Silent ischemia during coronary occlusion produced by balloon inflation: relation to regional myocardial dysfunction. *Journal of the American College of Cardiology* **10**, 491–498.

9

Regional anaesthesia and vascular surgery

MEGAN GRAY AND MICHAEL J COUSINS

INTRODUCTION

The choice between regional and general anaesthesia, or a combination of the two, for major vascular surgery is a matter of some controversy and debate. The high incidence of intercurrent disease in the patients often gives rise to the view that regional anaesthesia is beneficial, and the physiological effects of the techniques are generally beneficial. However, physiological advantage does not necessarily translate into a positive effect on outcome, and concerns about potential complications (notably cardiovascular effects and the impact of drugs affecting coagulation) have to be addressed. Thus this review will concentrate on the advantages and disadvantages of central nerve block (CNB) compared with general anaesthesia. Detailed aspects of technique will not be dealt with here, but certain block complications have particular relevance in the vascular patient and will be considered. Some aspects of the use of other regional blocks for vascular surgery will also be reviewed.

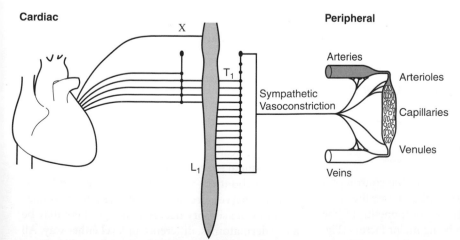

Figure 9.1 *Sympathetic blockade: 'central' (cardiac) and 'peripheral' components. These consist of T1–T4 cardiac sympathetic fibres and T1–L2 'peripheral' sympathetic fibres. Note important innervation of veins and venules. Vagal cardiac fibres are also shown. (Redrawn with permission from M. Cousins and P. Bridenbaugh,* Neural Blockade, *1998: 261.)*

Table 9.1   *Mechanisms for physiological effects of epidural analgesia*

By way of absorption of local anaesthetic (LA) or epinephrine (EPI)	By way of direct neural blocking effects or indirect results of blockade

Receptor
  β-stimulation by EPI
  α-stimulation by EPI or phenylephrine
Smooth muscle
  Blood vessels, LA or EPI
  Heart, LA or EPI
  Other organs, LA or EPI
Cardiac muscle
  By LA or EPI
Neural tissue
  CNS, by LA
  Conducting system of heart, by LA
Miscellaneous
  Neuromuscular junction by LA
	Spinal nerves (roots and trunks) by axonal blockade
	  Sympathetic
	    Efferent blockade
	      Peripheral (T1–L2) vasoconstrictor
	      'Adrenal' (T6–L1)
	      'Central' (T1–T4) cardiac sympathetic
	  Sensory
	    Afferent blockade
	      Reduced peripheral sensation
	      Blockade of visceral pain fibres
	      Reduced efferent neurohumoral response to surgical or other stimulus within the blocked area
	  Motor
	    Efferent blockade
	      Varying degrees of motor paralysis
	      Reflex muscle relaxation without paralysis (de-afferentation)
	
	Spinal cord
	  Axons
	    Superficial, sensory tracts blocked (e.g. bupivacaine, lidocaine and etidocaine)
	    Deep motor paths blocked (e.g. etidocaine)
	      Dorsal horn modulation of pain transmission (? axons, ? cells)
	      Possibility of 'anti-analgesic' effect owing to block of inhibitory paths
	  Cell bodies: 'selective' blockade, by opioids
	  Secondary changes in parasympathetic activity
	    Sympathetic block to T5 + ↓ venous return may → ↑↑ vagus
	    Sympathetic block to T1 → unopposed vagus
	  Secondary changes in vasoactive hormones
	    Sympathetic block to T1 → blockade of ↑ renin but not ↑ vasopressin, that usually helps maintain blood pressure in response to ↓ blood pressure challenge

Modified, with permission, from M. Cousins and P. Bridenbaugh, *Neural blockade*, 1998.

THE PHYSIOLOGY OF CENTRAL NERVE BLOCK (CNB)

The cardiovascular system

The cardiovascular system is under the control of a number of neural and hormonal systems, the sympathetic and parasympathetic components of the autonomic nervous system being major factors (Fig. 9.1). The cardiovascular changes which occur with CNB are mainly due to sympathetic block, but systemic absorption of local anaesthetics, vasoconstrictors or other drugs after epidural injection may also have significant physiological effects that are not seen in spinal anaesthesia. CNB with local anaesthetics takes about 20–30 minutes to develop, and sympathetic nerves are usually blocked to a similar extent as the sensory nerves, although there may be a few dermatomes, difference in level either way. All

Table 9.2 *Cardiovascular effects of epidural blockade*

Mechanism	Effect
Neural effects	
'Peripheral' sympathetic block (T10–L2)	Arteriolar dilatation. Increased venous capacitance and
Blockade of vasoconstrictor fibres to lower limbs	pooling of blood in lower limbs → decreased venous return → ↓ CO
Reflex increase in vasoconstrictor fibre activity in upper limbs via baroreceptors	Increased vasomotor tone in upper limbs → ↑ venous return → ↑ CO
Reflex increase in cardio-accelerator nerve activity	↑ HR ↑ CO
Reduced right atrial pressure, due to ↓ venous return*	? ↓ HR (note ↓↓ RA pressure → ↓↓ HR*
Adrenal medullary sympathetic block (T6–L1) (blockade of splanchnic nerves)	
Vasoconstrictor fibres to abdominal viscera	Pooling of blood in gut → decreased venous return
Adrenal medullary catecholamine secretion	Decreased levels of circulating catecholamines → ↓ HR ↓ CO
'Central' sympathetic block (T1–T4)	
Blockade of:	
Cardiac sympathetic outflow from vasomotor centre	↓ HR ↓ CO
Cardiac sympathetic reflexes at segmental level	
Vasoconstrictor fibres to head, neck, and arms	Vasodilatation in upper limbs. Blockade of compensatory lower-limb vasoconstriction if T5–L1 is also blocked
Vagal predominance	'Inappropriate bradycardia'; 'sudden bradycardia'; vagal arrest
Effects of drug absorption	
Absorbed local anaesthetic	Usually no measurable effects on HR, CO, MAP or TPR even in patients with vascular disease
Moderate blood levels	Lidocaine may → ↑ CO, which is balanced ↓ TPR, so
Anti-arrhythmic	that MAP is unchanged
Maintenance of normal CO	
Minimal reduction in vascular tone	
High blood levels (toxic)	↓ CO ↓ HR
Decreased contractility	↓ MAP
If convulsions occur hypoxia results in further reduction in CO	
Cardiac conducting tissue, ? unidirectional blockade	Bupivacaine (very high levels) → VT, VF, and cardiac arrest
Vascular dilatation	↓ TPR
Absorbed epinephrine	↑ CO ↑ HR ↓ TPR
β-stimulation	MAP may be unchanged or slightly reduced. Antagonism of reflex vasoconstriction above level of blockade because of β-effects on muscle vasculature (→ ↓ TPR)

CO, cardiac output; HR, heart rate; MAP, mean arterial pressure; TPR, total peripheral resistance; VT, ventricular tachycardia; VF, ventricular fibrillation.
*Decreased venous return was associated with increased vagal activity in one study. This may offset any increases in sympathetic activity.
Modified, with permission, from M. Cousins and P. Bridenbaugh, *Neural Blockade*, 1998: 265.

of these factors interact to produce the effects seen in clinical practice (Tables 9.1 and 9.2).

THE RESPONSE TO CNB

Vasodilatation is the major haemodynamic change and will be greatest during the first 30 minutes after the onset of the block. Healthy subjects respond to the resultant decrease in arterial pressure with a reflex increase in sympathetic outflow above the level of the block. This results in vasoconstriction above the level of the block and catecholamine release from the adrenals if the relevant fibres (T6 to Ll) have not been blocked. Other hormonal systems will be activated and dilated precapillary sphincters will contract under autoregulation within 30 minutes of complete ablation of neural activity (Granger and Guyton, 1969).

CNB IN VASCULAR PATIENTS

Vascular surgical patients have a high incidence of coronary artery disease and other medical problems. The vasodilatation produced by CNB may be beneficial to patients with impaired ventricular contractility by reducing preload and afterload as long as coronary perfusion is not compromised. In the patient whose cardiac output is dependent on a high preload (e.g. those with significant aortic stenosis and ventricular hypertrophy), CNB may be detrimental if not administered with great care. Decreased afterload may also be detrimental to the patient needing a high arterial pressure for coronary artery perfusion, or to maintain flow through other stenotic vessels.

Thoracic epidural anaesthesia (TEA), blocking segments Tl–T5, may favourably affect myocardial oxygen supply by decreasing preload and afterload while maintaining coronary blood flow, a favourable redistribution of blood flow from epicardial to endocardial vessels being postulated (Klassen et al., 1980). In the dog model, infarct size was smaller after coronary occlusion in the presence of TEA (Davis et al., 1986), and the luminal diameters of stenotic coronary arteries were increased in 64 per cent of patients while diameters of non-stenotic vessels were unchanged (Blomberg et al., 1990). Another study of patients with unstable angina pectoris, showed that those with TEA had reduced ST depression at similar workloads to those who did not (Blomberg et al., 1989). In terms of myocardial

preservation, TEA appears to offer more protection than lumbar block. The excellent review by Meibner and colleagues (1997) should be consulted on this point.

Combined general anaesthesia and CNB produces additive myocardial depression and vasodilatation, with resulting hypotension. If combined techniques are used, meticulous attention to haemodynamics is needed with judicious fluid loading and vasopressor administration as required.

SURVIVAL AND CARDIAC OUTCOME

There is much conflict over the effect of CNB on cardiac outcome. Yeager and colleagues (1987) showed improved survival and decreased cardiac complications in patients undergoing major surgery who received combined epidural and general anaesthesia. Epidural catheters were placed at high lumbar or low thoracic levels and were used throughout the perioperative period. The mortality in the general anaesthesia alone group was extraordinarily high at 16 per cent, but there were no deaths in the combined epidural and general anaesthetic group. The study groups were small and heterogeneous in their surgical procedure.

Tuman and colleagues (1991) randomized 80 patients undergoing major vascular surgery to combined TEA and general anaesthesia, or general anaesthetic alone, the epidural being continued into the post-operative period using low-dose local anaesthetics and opioids. Parenteral opioids were available as required for post-operative pain in both groups. There were no deaths, but cardiovascular complications, respiratory complications, hypercoagulability, graft occlusion, time to extubation, intensive-care unit (ICU) and hospital stay were all significantly reduced in the group who received TEA.

A prospective study by Rivers and colleagues (1991) compared lumbar epidural with general anaesthesia in 213 consecutive infra-inguinal bypass procedures. The 30-day mortality was 5 per cent after epidural anaesthesia and 3 per cent after general anaesthesia, and the incidences of cardiac complications were 20 and 25 per cent respectively. In a high risk subgroup (ASA grade IV and V) of 69 patients, there were no significant outcome differences.

In a prospective study, Bode and colleagues (1996) randomized 423 patients undergoing peripheral vascular procedures to one of three anaesthetic techniques: spinal, epidural or general. There were no statistically significant differences in peri-operative mortality or morbidity between the three groups, but it is interesting that there was an increased cardiac death rate associated with the failed regional requiring conversion to general anaesthesia.

Christopherson and colleagues (1993) looked at cardiac morbidity in a prospective randomized trial between lumbar epidural and general anaesthesia for lower-limb vascular surgery. The findings were that carefully conducted epidural and general anaesthesia had comparable rates of cardiac morbidity. The same group (Christopherson et al., 1996) examined the control of blood pressure and heart rate during epidural and general anaesthesia for lower-extremity vascular surgery. This study showed that patients randomized to general anaesthesia had greater blood pressure and heart rate lability than the epidural group. The general anaesthetic group had elevated catecholamine levels, while they remained at baseline levels in the epidural group.

These studies do not show consistent evidence for improved cardiac outcome by the use of CNB over general anaesthesia. It would be of interest to see prospective randomized studies using epidural blockade intra-operatively and into the post-operative period for 2–3 days compared to good parenteral analgesia such as a patient-controlled analgesia (PCA). Further studies comparing the use of CNB are needed, with documentation of the extent of block to conform adequacy of cover of the operative field.

From the cardiac aspect there is, at our current level of knowledge, no clear case for delaying surgery for correction of coagulation abnormalities to allow CNB. In addition, patient preference should be influential on the anaesthetic choice because there are no data which support a dogmatic position about choice of a specific technique.

The respiratory system

Epidural local anaesthetics may improve respiratory function in the post-operative period by decreasing diaphragmatic dysfunction resulting from the reflex inhibition of phrenic nerve activity produced by upper abdominal and thoracic surgery. In patients with severe pain, especially after body trunk surgery, epidural analgesia also improves vital capacity, functional respiratory capacity, the ability to cough and take a deep breath, as well as PaO_2 in the early post-operative period. TEA may result in paralysis of intercostal nerves, but this appears to be of little clinical significance. In healthy volunteers TEA causes a small reduction in ventilatory response to carbon dioxide (Kochi et al., 1989), but this does not appear to influence hypoxic drive, so TEA may be utilized on patients with chronic airway limitation who are dependent on such hypoxic drive. General anaesthesia results in atelectasis, impaired mucociliary function, residual muscle paralysis, a requirement for instrumentation of the airway, hypoventilation and shunting (Bendixen et al., 1963). Regional anaesthesia can avoid many of these problems, especially if associated with minimal sedation.

RESPIRATORY OUTCOME

Epidural analgesia has been shown to allow earlier extubation after coronary artery surgery (Stenseth et al., 1996), but there is still much controversy over its benefit in improving longer-term respiratory outcome. In high-risk patients, the greatest benefit might be expected if the block is used, with active mobilization and nutrition encouraged, to provide analgesia for at least 48 hours into the post-operative period. A meta-analysis (Ballantyne et al., 1998) showed a clear benefit of epidural over systemic opioids in decreasing post-operative pulmonary complications (see Fig. 9.2).

Stress response

Surgical trauma results in the stress response with increases in serum adrenaline, noradrenaline, prolactin, growth hormone, adrenocorticotrophic hormone (ACTH), antidiuretic hormone (ADH), cortical, aldosterone and renin. The intensity and duration of this response is dependent on the degree and location of the trauma and may last between a few days and weeks. A hypermetabolic state occurs with increases in cardiac output, catabolic hormones and protein breakdown, coagulation activated and fibrinolysis inhibited, salt and water retained and immunofunction inhibited.

It is uncertain whether a decrease in the stress response is beneficial; some studies suggest that it is important in survival after a surgical insult

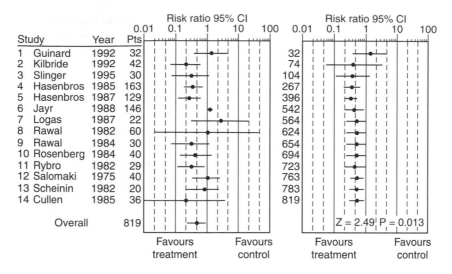

Figure 9.2 *Risk ratios and confidence intervals (CI) for post-operative pulmonary dysfunction in randomized controlled trials of epidural opioid versus intramuscular as-needed opioid, intravenous opioid by continuous infusion, or patient-controlled intravenous opioid bolus doses. Left: Results from individual trials. Right: Estimates obtained by stepwise accumulation of results from successive trials. (With permission from Ballantyne et al., 1998.)*

(Udelsman *et al.*, 1986). In high-risk patients, modifying the surgical stress response may limit the hypertension, tachycardia and the resultant increased myocardial oxygen consumption which is so detrimental to patients with coronary artery disease and which may result in cardiac ischaemia, cardiac failure and possible myocardial infarction.

The stress response can be reduced by high dose opioid administration (3 mg/kg morphine or 100 μg/kg fentanyl), but not by other forms of general anaesthesia. Epidural block can abolish the stress response after lower-limb or lower-abdominal surgery, but only results in minimal or varying degrees of modulation after upper abdominal or thoracic surgery. The effects include reduced protein catabolism, reduced activation of the coagulation system and reduced catecholamine release resulting in less tachycardia and hypertension, but the block needs to be continued for at least 48 hours after major surgery. Immunological function is better maintained after surgery performed under regional than general anaesthesia (Hale *et al.*, 1982). These features are obviously of theoretical benefit to the vascular surgical patient (Kehlet, 1998), but while many studies have demonstrated the ability of epidural block to decrease hormonal changes, few have demonstrated improved outcome.

Gut function

Post-operative ileus is a common complication of abdominal surgery which can be reduced by the use of epidural analgesia (Liu *et al.*, 1995a). This allows early enteral feeding which is known to decrease the surgical stress response, reduce septic complications and improve wound healing (Liu *et al.*, 1995b). To obtain maximal benefit the epidural should be utilized for several days post-operatively and combined with early removal of nasogastric tubes, early enteral feeding and early mobilization. The opioid dose should also be kept to a minimum. There is some concern that the increased peristalsis occurring with CNB may increase the risk of anastomotic dehiscence in colorectal surgery, but this of no relevance to vascular patients.

Blood coagulability

Surgery normally results in stimulation of clotting and inhibition of fibrinolysis. Epidural anaesthesia moderates these changes with reductions in antithrombin III catabolism, fibrinogen synthesis and serum plasminogen activator inhibitor levels (Modig *et al.*, 1980). In vascular patients these effects, together with the increase in lower limb blood flow produced by vasodilatation (Cousins and Wright, 1971), contribute to reductions in the risks of venous thromboembolism and arterial graft occlusion.

DEEP-VEIN THROMBOSIS

The accepted rate of deep vein thrombosis (DVT) (diagnosed by venography) after lower-limb joint replacement performed under general anaesthesia is around 70 per cent. About 5 per cent of these patients develop clinically significant pulmonary embolism, with a mortality rate of 0.5–2 per cent. The incidence of DVT can be reduced to 25 per cent by dense epidural block (0.5 per cent bupivacaine) continued for 24 hours (Modig et al., 1981). The use of a sequential calf compression device in addition to dense epidural block can reduce the DVT rate to 6 per cent (Lieberman et al., 1994). With lower-dose bupivacaine and fentanyl, the DVT rate is reduced from 70 per cent to only 40 per cent. For comparative purposes, it should be noted that low-molecular-weight heparin (LMWH) results in a DVT rate of about 30 per cent (Besgqvist et al., 1996).

In addition to the factors mentioned above, other mechanisms for the effect of epidural block on DVT rates are inhibition of leukocyte adhesion to blood vessel walls and possibly earlier mobilization. It is interesting that lidocaine (1 mg/kg bolus dose followed by 2 mg/min for 6 days) has been shown to reduce the DVT rate after hip surgery from 78 per cent to 21 per cent (Cook et al., 1977). This suggests that the reduction in DVT rate produced by CNB may be a result of systemic local anaesthetic action rather than secondary to the effects of nerve blockade.

GRAFT PATENCY

In peripheral vascular surgery epidural lumbar sympathetic block decreases peripheral resistance (Cousins and Wright, 1971). This increased blood flow improves peripheral circulation and, with the coagulation factors noted above, encourages maintenance of graft patency. Studies by Tuman and colleagues (1991) and Christopherson and colleagues (1993) showed improved graft patency with regional anaesthesia, but Pierce and colleagues (1997) found no improvement in early graft patency or limb salvage.

In a patient with a pre-existing vascular graft, hypotension in association with CNB may result in graft occlusion. This has been reported (Harris et al., 1987) in two patients whose aortofemoral grafts occluded during epidural anaesthesia for bowel surgery. Maintenance of an adequate blood pressure is thus essential.

Post-operative pain control

Post-operative pain is both unpleasant and a cause of deleterious effects which contribute to pulmonary complications, DVT, immobilization, hyperdynamic circulation and myocardial ischaemia. Thus good pain relief is important for both humanitarian and physiological reasons. Such pain relief may be achieved by well-administered parenteral opioids (e.g. by PCA) or by CNB with local anaesthetics and or opioids. Pain relief at rest and patient satisfaction are similar with these two techniques, but pain on movement is better relieved by CNB and so allows earlier mobilization (Sinatra, 1998).

The role of regional techniques in reducing the incidence of phantom limb after amputation is controversial. Bach and colleagues (1988) found that three days of epidural block prior to the amputation reduced the incidence of phantom-limb pain in the first year. However, this was not a controlled study and the result has not been reproduced by others. Central (spinal cord) sensitization produced by the noxious stimulation of surgery has been demonstrated in man, but only when no pre-emptive analgesia was provided (Pederson et al., 1996). The use of opioids, nitrous oxide or regional anaesthesia prevent significant central sensitization in the majority of patients.

COMPLICATIONS OF REGIONAL ANAESTHESIA

There are a number of potential complications of CNB of greater than average significance in the vascular surgical patient. Whatever the merits or demerits of CNB in these patients it is essential that the clinician is aware of the problems so that they can be managed or prevented as appropriate.

Hypotension

The major cardiovascular complication of CNB is severe hypotension, the degree being related to the extent of sympathetic block (Stanton-Hicks, 1975; Cousins and Veering, 1998) and the resultant vasodilatation. Block above T5 may also affect the cardiac sympathetic fibres, and result in more profound hypotension and bradycardia. Systemic absorption of a large dose of local anaesthetic may also contribute, and accidental intravascular or intrathecal injection of an epidural dose will have profound cardiovacular effects. Hypovolaemia and cardiac disease increase the rate and severity of hypotension, but this can be limited by adequate volume replacement, gradual extension of level of block, and the appropriate use of vasoconstrictors. Epidural block allows more time for cardiovascular compensation, but does result in higher systemic concentrations of local anaesthetic.

Vascular surgical patients often have widespread vascular disease and may have stenotic vessels unrelated to the operative site. The organs supplied by these stenotic vessels may be at risk of ischaemia if hypotension occurs. The combination with general anaesthesia increases the risk of significant hypotension (Cousins and Veering, 1998), and requires meticulous attention to haemodynamic control. Careful fluid management is needed because it is easy to overload patients, especially those with poor ventricular function. In patients with poor renal function, fluid overload may occur as the epidural wears off. Sympathetic tone returns and fluid is displaced from the previously dilated vessels, resulting in pulmonary congestion.

Sprung and colleagues (1996) have reported two disturbing cases of coronary artery spasm, one resulting in the death of the patient, during recovery from epidural anaesthesia after peripheral vascular surgery. It is possible that the coronary artery spasm occurred as a result of an altered balance between sympathetic and parasympathetic nervous system and emphasizes the importance of monitoring for myocardial ischaemia and cardiovascular stability during recovery from CNB.

Anterior spinal artery syndrome

The anterior spinal artery syndrome is caused by ischaemia of the region of the spinal cord supplied by the artery, and is characterized by painless flaccid paralysis of the legs. Both surgical (clamping of the abdominal aorta) and anaesthetic (trauma from a misplaced needle) factors may directly impair the

supply from the artery of Adamkiewicz, and flow will depend on spinal cord perfusion pressure (SCPP). This is the mean arterial blood pressure minus the venous or cerebrospinal fluid (CSF) pressure (whichever is the higher). Epidural bolus injection may increase CSF pressure and therefore decrease SCPP. If the arterial supply is already compromised (i.e. vascular disease, aortic clamping or hypotension) the injection could lead to cord ischaemia. Thus bolus epidural injections should not be made while the aorta is cross-clamped or the patient is hypotensive.

Vertebral canal haematoma (VCH)

The fear of causing vertebral canal haematoma (VCH) prevents many anaesthetists from using CNB for vascular surgery. The condition has been reported in all age groups and at all levels of the spinal canal, but most frequently in the thoracic region in elderly patients. It may occur spontaneously without any apparent risk factor, or in association with anticoagulant or antiplatelet therapy, vertebral canal neoplasia or vascular abnormalities, blood dyscrasias, and the insertion of a needle and or catheter.

Any instrumentation of the canal must cause some bleeding, but an overtly 'bloody tap' occurs in around 3 per cent of spinal or epidural needle or catheter insertions. Withdrawal of an epidural catheter may dislodge any blood clot and cause further bleeding. The small amount of bleeding that usually occurs into the subarachnoid or epidural space is of little clinical significance, but if it continues the haematoma may compress the spinal cord, the cauda equina or their blood supply. Epidural haematoma usually occurs in the posterior part of the space. With ageing, the loose alveolar tissue around the intervertebral foramina becomes increasingly dense and may reduce the escape of blood, and make the elderly more susceptible to VCH.

Early recognition and treatment of VCH provide the best outcome. Patients who receive CNB, especially if in association with factors that affect coagulation, require regular neurological assessment. Severe back pain with a developing radicular component has usually been considered the first sign of VCH. This is then followed by neurological deficit, often with bladder and bowel symptoms. The time course may vary from hours to days. At the earliest indication of VCH, any anticoagulation should cease, the neurosurgical team should be consulted, and a spinal magnetic resonance image (MRI) scan performed urgently. If the latter is not available a computed tomography (CT) scan should be arranged, but it is not as reliable a method for this purpose. If a VCH is diagnosed, the coagulation state should be corrected rapidly, and a decompressive laminectomy performed urgently. Delay beyond 12 hours of the onset of symptoms usually results in permanent disability.

PREVENTATIVE STRATEGIES

Although VCH is rare, it is a catastrophic complication and the vascular anaesthetist who uses regional techniques must have a defined position on the risk. A growing number of patients presenting for vascular surgery are taking aspirin or non-steroidal anti-inflammatory drugs (NSAIDs). Low-dose aspirin is used to reduce the risk of thrombotic complications, and many elderly patients take NSAIDs for joint pain. In addition, prophylaxis of thromboembolism is essential after major surgery, and may be provided by low-dose unfractionated heparin (UH), low-molecular-weight heparin (LMWH) or oral anticoagulants, as well as by physical methods.

The question of whether performing CNB in a patient receiving one or more of these drugs increases the risk of VCH causes much anxiety amongst anaesthetists. Theoretically, there is a greater risk of all haemorrhagic complications, but neurological sequelae of CNB are exceedingly rare. The exact incidence of VCH may never be known because of its rarity, and this makes prospective randomized trials impossible. However, information from case reports and large surveys is available and can be used to guide practice. It is important to remember that VCH may occur spontaneously in anticoagulated patients not undergoing CNB.

Low-dose-unfractionated heparin prophylaxis
There are two reports of VCH occurring in association with low dose (5000 units b.d.) UH prophylaxis (Metzger et al., 1991). Thus the incidence is so low that the possible coincidence with a spontaneous haematoma should be considered. However, some patients may have therapeutic plasma concentrations of heparin between 2 and 4 hours after a subcutaneous dose. The half-life of UH given by this route is

3 hours, so it may be wise to avoid insertion or removal of an epidural within 4–6 hours of injection. In addition, at least 1 hour should elapse after CNB or catheter removal before the next dose of UH.

Low-molecular-weight heparin
LMWH has been shown to be as effective and safe as UH in the prophylaxis of DVT. The agents have higher and more predictable bioavailabilities, longer half lives (needing administration only once daily) and less influence on platelet function and lipolysis than UH. These factors all imply that the risk should be even less than with UH, and in a review of 9000 patients receiving both LMWH prophylaxis and CNB there were no neurological complications (Bergqvist et al., 1993). Because of longer bioavailability, it is advisable to avoid insertion or removal of an epidural catheter for 10–12 hours after LMWH. However, the agents are as effective if given the night before as on the morning of surgery so this requirement is easily complied with. One hour should elapse after insertion or removal of an epidural catheter and the next dose of LMWH.

Unfortunately this reasonably reassuring view of the position has been shaken by a large number of cases of VCH after CNB in patients receiving enoxaparin in the USA. Analysis suggests that the problem was multi-factorial (Checketts and Wildsmith, 1999).

Aspirin and NSAIDs
It is unknown whether the use of NSAIDs increases the risk of epidural bleeding. A few cases of spontaneous VCH have been reported in patients taking aspirin, but the incidence in patients taking NSAIDs is extremely low. Horlocker and colleagues (1990; 1995) conducted both a retrospective and a prospective study to ascertain if NSAIDs caused more haemorrhagic complications in association with CNB. There was a slightly higher incidence of blood being aspirated from the epidural needle, but no increased incidence of VCH.

Trying to assess the risk of VCH in patients taking these drugs by performing a bleeding time is controversial. The test is difficult to perform reproducibly, is painful, leaves a scar and lacks both sensitivity and specificity. The bleeding time may return to normal within 72 hours of aspirin ingestion although it may take 7–10 days for in vitro platelet aggregation tests to return to normal. However, the bleeding time is the only presently feasible bedside test that gives any information about the aggregating capabilities of platelets. If a bleeding time is performed, the limitations must be recognized. Some propose an upper limit of 8–10 minutes for proceeding with CNB although there are no data to support this figure. However, it may be a useful guide to the trainee to seek further advice.

Systemic heparinization

The incidence of VCH after CNB in vascular surgical patients receiving systemic heparinization is unknown. Rao and El-Etr (1981) reviewed 3164 patients receiving continuous subarachnoid or epidural anaesthesia for lower-limb vascular surgery. Heparin was given, at least 1 hour after the block, to produce twice the baseline activated clotting time. If blood was aspirated during CNB the procedure was deferred and the patient given a general anaesthetic the next day. Baron and colleagues (1987) reviewed retrospectively 912 patients who underwent lower-limb vascular surgery under epidural anaesthesia and who received 75 units/kg of heparin and a further 1000 units/hour after 2 hours. No patient in either study developed a VCH.

OVERVIEW

The incidence of VCH is extremely low even in patients heparinized for vascular surgery. It seems that CNB can be used safely in these patients if instituted by experienced personnel at least 1 hour prior to heparinization. It is as important to ensure that catheters are removed when coagulation is normal. If fibrinolytic agents or prolonged anticoagulation are to be employed, the balance of risk changes and requires greater consideration. The use of CNB in patients exposed to antiplatelet or anticoagulant medication is meant to be 'atraumatic'. Thus, it would seem wise to avoid CNB in patients who may be technically difficult, such as those with severe scoliosis, ankylosing spondylitis and severe osteoporosis, unless the risk–benefit analysis for the individual patient warrants the increased risk of a potentially more traumatic CNB. Other precautions that may help to reduce the likelihood of a traumatic CNB are:

- insertion of the catheter only 3–5 cm into the epidural space;
- use of the midline approach to the vertebral canal because fewer epidural vessels are encountered than with the lateral approach;
- use of the smallest diameter needle that is practical; and
- careful consideration of published guidelines when LMWHs are in use (Horlocker and Wedel, 1998; Checketts and Wildsmith, 1999).

CNB should obviously be avoided in patients with blood dyscrasia, raised intracranial pressure (ICP) and coagulopathy.

ASPECTS OF BLOCK TECHNIQUE

Intrathecal morphine

A single dose of intrathecal morphine can provide analgesia for approximately 24 hours after surgery. It is a useful technique when one wishes to avoid using a catheter or where there are no facilities to run an epidural post-operatively. For major abdominal or thoracic vascular surgery the dose of intrathecal morphine is 0.4–0.6 mg in patients under 65 years of age and 0.2–0.4 mg for older patients. The patient should have respiratory monitoring for at least 16 hours after the injection and supplementary pain relief may be allowed if needed, as long as such monitoring is in place. An advantage is the reduced requirement for subsequent PCA, something that may extend to the entire post-operative period (Sinatra, 1998). It is likely that the urinary catheter can be removed approximately 24 hours after surgery and this makes some vascular surgeons less anxious about infection of the vascular graft. Respiratory depression, which may be late in onset but rarely beyond 16 hours, is the main concern. Nausea and vomiting, sedation and urinary retention can occur, but they all respond to a small dose of naloxone without reversal of the analgesic effect.

Continuous spinal anaesthesia

An intrathecal catheter has the advantage of allowing a titratable, dense and rapid onset CNB with minimum drug dosage so avoiding the risk of systemic effect. The major disadvantage is the risk of dural puncture headache and fine-gauge catheters were developed to minimize this. These catheters are technically demanding to use and have been associated with cauda equina syndrome when used with concentrated solutions of local anaesthetic (De Jong, 1994). However, the incidence of headache is low in the elderly population presenting for vascular surgery so fine-gauge catheters are not needed, and the technique may be a useful option in this population.

Regional anaesthesia for carotid endarterectomy

Regional anaesthesia for carotid endarterectomy (CEA) allows continuous neurological assessment, avoids any detrimental effect of general anaesthesia (but misses any neurological protection provided by general anaesthesia) and avoids endotracheal intubation in a high-risk population (Stoneham and Knighton, 1999). There is also decreased requirement for vascular shunting, even in high-risk patients (Benjamin et al., 1983), and a lower incidence of post-operative hypotension and hypertension compared to general anaesthesia (Jopling et al., 1983). Tangkanakul and colleagues (1997) looked at the safety of CEA under regional or general anaesthesia by reviewing 17 non-randomized (5970 operations) and three randomized studies (143 operations). The data in the non-randomized trials suggested that the use of regional anaesthesia resulted in approximately half the incidence of stroke, myocardial infarct and pulmonary complications than general anaesthesia. There were insufficient data in the randomized trials to confirm or refute these findings.

Carotid endarterectomy under regional block requires a co-operative patient who can be communicated with, and an anaesthetist and surgeon skilled in the techniques required. Sedation to allow the patient to tolerate the surgery must be administered very cautiously to allow cerebral monitoring and the patient to respond to commands. Small increments of opioids and benzodiazepines produce appropriate sedation that can be readily reversed with naloxone and flumazenil if required.

Cervical plexus block

Most of the area of the operation is supplied by the cervical plexus (C2 to C4), but some supplementary infiltration by the surgeon may be needed to pro-

vide complete anaesthesia for CEA. The clavicular end of the incision may be supplied by the second thoracic nerve, and the mandibular end by the mandibular branch of the trigeminal nerve. Anteriorly, there may be overlap from the contralateral cervical nerves. The structures within the carotid sheath are innervated from the ninth and tenth cranial nerves.

DEEP CERVICAL PLEXUS BLOCK

Deep cervical plexus block (Fig. 9.3) can be performed using a single or three-needle technique. A 22-g 5-cm needle is directed medially and caudally to avoid inadvertent entry into the intervertebral foramen. It should contact the transverse process and be 'walked' anteriorly or posteriorly until paraesthesiae are produced. With a three-needle technique 3–4 mL of 0.375 per cent bupivacaine is injected at each site. For a single-injection technique, 8 mL of 0.375 per cent bupivacaine is injected at the transverse process of C4, and distal compression is used to encourage upward spread of the local anaesthetic.

SUPERFICIAL CERVICAL PLEXUS BLOCK

Superficial cervical plexus block (Fig. 9.4) anaesthetizes the cutaneous component of the plexus which supplies sensation to the anterolateral neck. Bupivacaine 0.375 per cent (5–7 mL) is injected along the middle third of the posterior border of the sternomastoid muscle. If accessory nerve block is desired for paralysis of the trapezius muscle, a second injection (4 mL 0.375 per cent bupivacaine) is made deep to the deep fascia of the neck.

There are three specific complications:

- The vertebral artery lies near the needle tip during deep cervical plexus block. If only a minute amount of local anaesthetic is injected into this artery, severe neurological toxicity will occur because of its direct transport to the brain. Frequent aspiration tests should be performed to reduce the risk, and close contact maintained with the patient to allow early detection of any toxicity.
- Subdural injection may occur if the needle enters the dural sheath around the nerve roots. Subarachnoid block is possible, with loss of

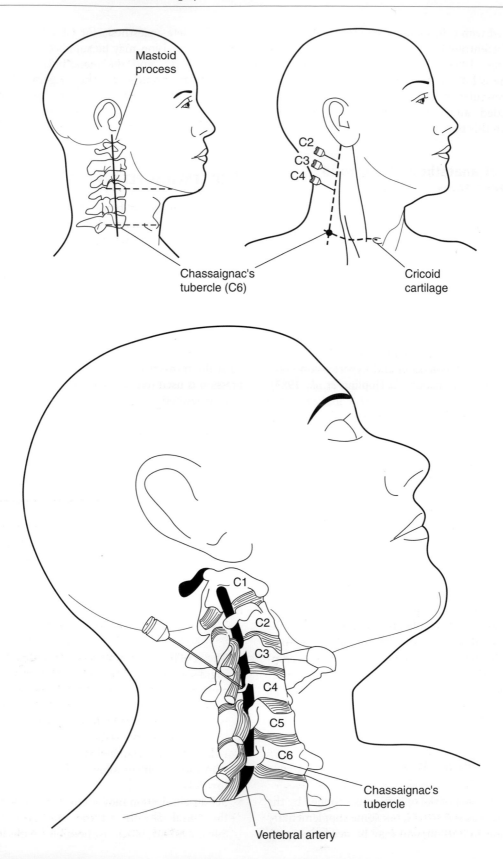

Mastoid process

Chassaignac's tubercle (C6)

C2
C3
C4

Cricoid cartilage

C1
C2
C3
C4
C5
C6

Chassaignac's tubercle

Vertebral artery

Figure 9.3 *Deep cervical plexus block. A line is drawn from mastoid process to Chassaignac's tubercle (C6). The latter lies on a line extended laterally from the cricoid cartilage. This line lies over the 'gutters' in the superior surface of the transverse processes upon which the cervical nerve roots pass laterally. The C4 nerve root is located at the junction of the vertical line and a line horizontally drawn to the lower border of the mandible, with the head in a neutral position. The C3 and C2 nerve roots can be located by dividing the distance between the mastoid and horizontal line into thirds (see upper right panel). The C5 nerve root lies midway between the 'C6 line' and the line above. Individual cervical nerve roots may be blocked by injecting small volumes of local anaesthetics, as shown in the upper right. Single injection block of cervical plexus can be obtained by a technique similar to interscalene brachial plexus block, since the cervical nerve roots are contained in a continuous space between the scalene muscles. A single needle is inserted on the vertical line at the C4 level, and directed medially and slightly caudad to contact the 'gutter' of the transverse process (lower panel). Note that the caudad direction is essential to avoid penetration of an intervertebral foramen, with possible injection into epidural space or dural sleeve (and thus direct entry to CSF). Note also the proximity of the vertebral artery passing through the foramina transversaria of the transverse processes. (With permission from M. Cousins and P. Bridenbaugh,* Neural blockade, *1998: 508.)*

consciousness and hypotension. Proper needle angulation is essential to avoid this.

- Phrenic nerve block is common and usually of little clinical significance, but it is wise to avoid deep plexus block in patients with limited respiratory reserve. Bilateral deep cervical plexus block should be avoided because not even normal patients can tolerate bilateral phrenic block.

Nerve block for lower-limb surgery

Vascular procedures on the lower limb may be performed after femoral, obturator, sciatic and lateral cutaneous nerve of the thigh block. Large volumes of local anaesthetic are required and there may be significant vascular absorption. The sympathetic block is limited to one limb and it may be a useful technique in the occasional patient in whom there may be contraindications to both CNB and general anaesthesia. Giordano and colleagues (1986) reviewed 13 patients who received peripheral blocks for femoropopliteal and tibial surgery. Analgesia was adequate except in one patient who required supplementary nitrous oxide. Another patient died on the sixth day post-operatively from

cardiac complications which commenced intra-operatively.

CONCLUSION

No one anaesthetic technique can be recommended for vascular surgery. The choice needs to be made on the basis of the type of surgery, its expected duration, individual patient risk–benefit analysis, patient preference, surgical tolerance, anaesthetic expertise and the hospital resources available.

The risk–benefit analysis has to be made for each patient in the light of the available research data, but patient preference and psychological state must be taken into account. Good operating conditions (a still, calm patient) need to be provided to give the surgeon maximum assistance in the performance of often technically difficult procedures. The anaesthetist must be skilled in the technique chosen and adequate resources must be available to support its use during and after the operation. A review (Kehlet, 1997) of the multimodal approach to controlling post-operative physiology emphasizes the importance of optimizing the beneficial effects of regional techniques by using minimally invasive surgery where feasible, continuing

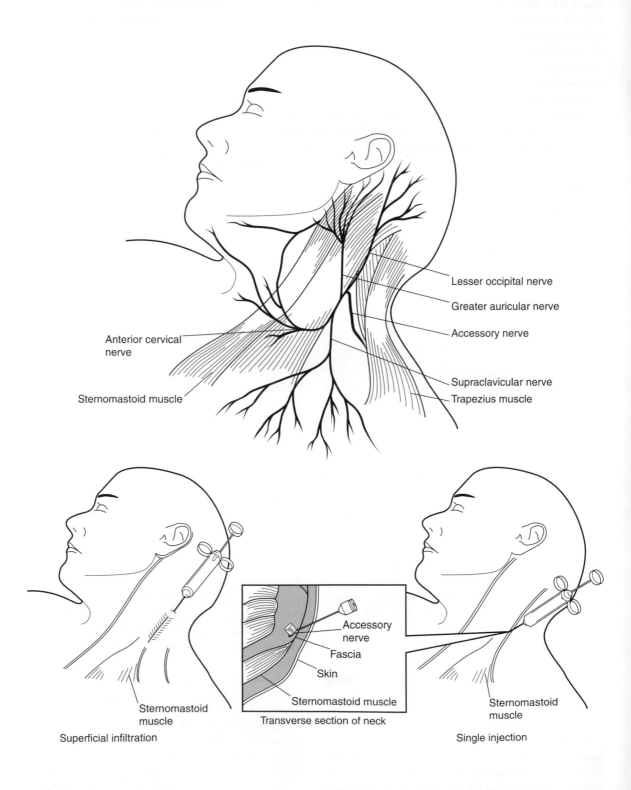

Lesser occipital nerve

Greater auricular nerve

Accessory nerve

Supraclavicular nerve

Trapezius muscle

Anterior cervical nerve

Sternomastoid muscle

Accessory nerve

Fascia

Skin

Sternomastoid muscle

Transverse section of neck

Sternomastoid muscle

Superficial infiltration

Sternomastoid muscle

Single injection

Figure 9.4 *The superficial cervical plexus, which is blocked in the posterior triangle of the neck as it emerges adjacent to the midpoint of the posterior border of the sternomastoid muscle. Superficial infiltration is extended along the middle third of the posterior border of the sternomastoid muscle. Note the close relationship of the accessory nerve as it emerges from the posterior border of the sternomastoid muscle at the junction of its middle and upper third, that is, just above the emerging superficial cervical plexus. Single-injection technique for accessory nerve block. Note that the accessory nerve lies deep to the deep fascia of the neck and that this needs to be pierced as shown in the 'single injection', which is sometimes used as an adjunct to produce muscle paralysis of the trapezius muscle in shoulder operations. Successful block of the superficial cervical plexus results in analgesia corresponding to the C2, C3, and C4 dermatomes. (With permission from M. Cousins and P. Bridenbaugh,* Neural blockade, *1998: 506.)*

analgesia into the post-operative period, and feeding and mobilizing the patient as soon as possible after surgery.

ACKNOWLEDGEMENTS

The authors are grateful to Dr Stephen Barratt for his advice in preparing this chapter and to Mrs Susan Ulstrup for her secretarial assistance.

REFERENCES

Bach, S., Noren, M. and Tjellan, N.V. 1988. Phantom limb pain in amputees during the first 12 months following limb amputation after preoperative lumbar epidural block. *Pain* **33**, 297–301.

Ballantyne, J.C., Carr, D.B., Chalmers, T.C. *et al.* 1998. Comparative effects of postoperative analgesic therapies upon respiratory function: meta-analyses of initial randomised control trials. *Anesthesia and Analgesia* **86**, 598–606.

Baron, H., La Raja, R., Rossi, G. and Atkinson, D. 1987. Continuous epidural analgesia in the heparinised vascular surgical patient. A retrospective review of 912 patients. *Journal of Vascular Surgery* **6**, 144–146.

Bendixen, H., Hedley-Whyte, J. and Chir, B. 1963. Impaired oxygenation in surgical patients during general anaesthesia with controlled ventilation. *New England Journal of Medicine* **269**, 991–996.

Benjamin, M., Silva, M. and Watt, C. *et al.* 1993. Awake patient monitoring to determine the need for shunting during carotid endarterectomy. *Surgery* **114**, 673–679

Bergqvist, D., Benoni, G. and Bjorgell, O. 1996. Low molecular weight heparin (enoxaparin) as prophylaxis against venous thromboembolism after total hip replacement. *New England Journal of Medicine* **335**, 696–700.

Bergqvist, D., Lindblad, B. and Matzsch, T. 1993. Risks of combining low molecular weight heparin from thromboprophylaxis and epidural or spinal anaesthesia. *Seminars in Thrombosis and Hemostasis* **19**, 147.

Blomberg, S., Curelaru, J., Emanueisson, H. *et al.* 1989. Thoracic epidural anaesthesia in patients with unstable angina pectoris. *European Heart Journal* **10**, 437–444.

Blomberg, S., Emanuelson, H., Kvist, H. *et al.* 1990. Effects of thoracic epidural anaesthesia on coronary arteries and arterioles in patients with coronary artery disease. *Anesthesiology* **73**, 840–847.

Bode, R., Lewis, K., Zarich, S. *et al.* 1996. Cardiac outcome after peripheral vascular surgery comparison of general and regional anaesthesia. *Anesthesiology* **84**, 3–13.

Checketts, M.R. and Wildsmith, J.A.W. 1999. Editorial: Central nerve block and thromboprophylaxis–is there a problem? *British Journal of Anaesthesia* **82**, 164–167.

Christopherson, R., Beattie, C., Frank, S. *et al.* 1993. Perioperative morbidity in patients randomised to epidural or general anaesthesia for lower extremity vascular surgery. *Anesthesiology* **79**, 442–434.

Christopherson, M., Glauen, J., Norris, E. *et al.* 1996. Control of blood pressure and heart rate in patients randomised to epidural or general anaesthesia for lower extremity vascular surgery. *Journal of Clinical Anesthesia* **8**, 578–584.

Cook, E.D., Lloyd, M., Bowcock, S. and Pilcher, M. 1977. Intravenous lignocaine in the prevention of deep venous thrombosis after elective hip surgery. *Lancet* **1**, 797–799.

Cousins, M. and Wright, C. 1971. Graft muscle skin blood flow after epidural block in vascular surgical procedures. *Surgery, Gynecology and Obstetrics* **133**, 59–64.

Cousins, M.J. and Veering, B.T. 1998. Epidural neural blockade. In Cousins, M.J. and Bridenbaugh, P.O. (eds), *Neural blockade in clinical anesthesia and management of pain*, 3rd edn. Philadelphia: Lippincott Raven, 243–322.

Davis, R, Deboer, L. and Maroko P. 1986. Thoracic epidural anaesthesia reduces myocardial infarct size after coronary artery occlusion in dogs. *Anaesthesia and Analgesia* **65**, 711–717.

De Jong, R. 1994. Last round for a heavy weight. *Anaesthesia and Analgesia* **7**, 3–4.

Giordano, J., Morales, G., Trout, H. and DePalma, R. 1986. Regional nerve block for femoropopliteal and tibial artery reconstructions. *Journal of Vascular Surgery* **4**, 351–354.

Granger, H. and Guyton, A. 1969. Autoregulation of the total systemic circulation following destruction of the central nervous system in the dog. *Circulation Research* **25**, 379–388.

Jopling, W., de Sanctis, C. and McDowell, D. 1983. Anaesthesia for carotid endarterectomy: A comparison of regional and general techniques. *Anesthesiology*, **59**, 217–221.

Hale, A., Vansgaard, G. and Breivik, H. 1982. Monocyte functions are depressed during and after surgery under general anaesthesia but not under epidural anaesthesia. *Acta Anaesthesia* **26**, 301–307.

Harris, K. and Provan, J. 1987. Hazards of epidural anaesthesia in patients with previous vascular grafts. *Canadian Journal of Surgery* **30**, 124.

Horlocker, T.T. and Wedel, D.J. 1998. Spinal and epidural blockade and perioperative low molecular weight heparin: smooth sailing on the Titanic. *Anesthesia and Analgesia* **86**, 1153–1156.

Horlocker, T., Wedel, D. and Offord, K. 1990. Does preoperative antiplatelet therapy increase the risk of haemorrhagic complications associated with regional anesthesia? *Anaesthesia and Analgesia* **70**, 631–634.

Horlocker, T., Wedel, .D. and Offord, K. 1995. Preoperative antiplatelet drugs do not increase the risk of spinal cord haematoma associated with regional anaesthesia. *Anaesthesia and Analgesia* **80**, 303–309.

Kehlet, J. 1997. Multimodal approach to control postoperative pathophysiology and rehabilitation. *British Journal of Anaesthesia* **78**, 606–617.

Kehlet, H. 1998. Modifications of responses to surgery by neural blockade: clinical implications. In Cousins, M. and Bridenbaugh, P. (eds), *Neural blockade in clinical anaesthesia and management of pain*. Philadelphia: Lippincott Raven, 129–175.

Klassen, G., Bramwell, R., Bromage, P. and Zborowska-Sluis, D. 1980. Effect of acute sympathectomy by epidural anesthesia on the canine coronary circulation. *Anesthesiology* **52**, 8–15.

Kochi, T., Sako, S., Nishina, T. and Mizuguchi, T. 1989. Effects of high thoracic extradural anaesthesia on ventilatory response to hypercapnia in normal volunteers. *British Journal of Anaesthesia* **62**, 362–367.

Liu, S., Carpenter, R. and Mackey, D. et al. (1995a) Effects of perioperative analgesic techniques on rate of recovery after colon surgery: *Anesthesiology* **83**, 757–765.

Liu, S., Carpenter, R. and Neal, J. (1995b) Epidural anesthesia and analgesia: their role in postoperative outcome. *Anesthesiology* **82**, 1474–1506.

Lieberman, J., Huo, M. and Hanway, J. 1994. The prevalence of deep venous thrombosis after total hip arthroplasty with hypotensive epidural anaesthesia. *Journal of Bone and Joint Surgery* **76A**, 341–348.

Meibner, A., Rolf, N. and Van Aken, H. 1997. Thoracic epidural anaesthesia and the patient with heart disease: Benefits, risks and controversies. *Anaesthesia and Analgesia* **85**, 517–528.

Metzger, G. and Singbar, IG. 1991. Spinal epidural haematoma following epidural anaesthesia versus spontaneous spinal subdural haematoma. Two case reports. *Acta Anaesthesiologica Scandinavica* **35**, 105–107.

Modig, J., Hjelmstedti, A., Sahistedi, B. and Maripuu, E. 1981. Comparative influences of epidural and general anaesthesia on deep venous thrombosis and pulmonary embolism after total hip replacement. *Acta Anaesthesiologica Scandinavica* **147**, 125–130.

Modig, J., Maimberg, P. and Saideen, T. 1980. Comparative effects of epidural and general anaesthesia on fibrinolysis function lower limb rheology and thrombembolism after total hip replacement. *Anesthesiology* **53**, S34.

Pederson, J., Crawford, M. and Brennum, J. 1996. Effects of preemptic nerve block on inflammation and hyperalgesia after human thermal injury. *Anesthesiology* **84**, 1020–1026.

Pierce, E., Pomposelli, F., Stanley, G. *et al*. 1997. Anesthesia type does not influence early graft patency or limb salvage rates of lower extremity arterial bypass. *Journal of Vascular Surgery* **25**, 226–232.

Rao, T. and El-Etr, A. 1981. Anticoagulants following placement of epidural and subarachnoid catheters. *Anesthesiology* **55**, 618–20.

Rivers, P., Scher, L., Sheehan, E. and Veith, F. 1991. Epidural versus general anesthesia for infrainguinal arterial reconstruction. *Journal of Vascular Surgery* **14**, 764–70.

Sinatra, R.S. 1998. Acute pain management and acute pain services. In Cousins, M.J. and Bridenbaugh, P.O. (eds), *Neural blockade in clinical anesthesia and management of pain*, 3rd edn. Philadelphia: Lippincott Raven, 793–836.

Sprung, J., Lesitsky, M., Jaqetia, A. *et al*. 1996. Cardiac arrest caused by coronary spasm in two patients during recovery from epidural anaesthesia. *Regional Anaesthesia* **21**(3), 253–260.

Stanton-Hicks, M.A. 1975. Cardiovascular effects of extradural anaesthesia. *British Journal of Anaesthesia* **47**, 253–261.

Stenseth, R., Bjelia, L., Berg, E. *et al*. 1996. Effects of thoracic epidural analgesia on pulmonary function after coronary artery bypass surgery. *European Journal of Cardiothoracic Surgery* **10**, 859–865.

Stoneham, M.D. and Knighton, J.D. 1999. Regional anaesthesia for carotid endarterectomy. *British Journal of Anaesthesia* **82**, 910–919.

Tangkanakul, C., Cousell, C. and Warlow, C. 1997. Local versus general anaesthesia in carotid endarterectomy; a systematic review of the evidence. *European Journal of Vascular and Endovascular Surgery* **13**(5), 491–494.

Tuman, K., McCarthy, R., March, R. *et al*. 1991. Effects of epidural anesthesia and analgesia on coagulation and outcome after major vascular surgery. *Anesthesia and Analgesia* **73**, 696–704.

Udelsman, R., Ramp, J. and Gallucci, W. 1986. Adaption during surgical stress. A re-evaluation of the role of glucocorticoids. *Journal of Clinical Investigation* **77**, 1377–1381.

Yeager, M., Glass, D., Neff, R. and Brinck-Johnsen, T. 1987. Epidural anaesthesia and analgesia in high risk surgical patients. *Anesthesiology* **66**, 729–736.

10

Anaesthesia for surgery on the descending thoracic aorta

CHRISTOPHER J O'CONNOR AND KENNETH J TUMAN

INTRODUCTION

Surgery on the descending thoracic aorta involves dramatic alterations in cardiovascular and cerebral haemodynamic variables, and may be the most challenging vascular procedure for both surgeon and anaesthetist. This chapter will review the pathophysiological events occurring during thoracic aortic surgery and, using information based on current clinical and experimental data, provide practical guidelines on the management of these complex procedures.

PRE-OPERATIVE CONSIDERATIONS

Disease of the descending thoracic aorta is due to either aneurysmal dilatation or dissection of the aortic media (Crawford, 1990). The aneurysms are usually secondary to atherosclerosis, connective-tissue disease or trauma (Crawford, 1990). In contrast,

aortic dissections occur when the wall has been split and contains extraluminal blood; an aneurysm may or may not be present.

Although many classification systems exist for thoracic aortic disease, the most commonly recognized is that applied to aortic dissections. Debakey type I dissections are those extending from the ascending aorta into the descending aorta, whereas type II lesions are confined to the ascending aorta (Fig. 10.1). Type III lesions begin in the descending aorta and extend from the left subclavian artery to the diaphragm (IIIa) or beyond (Svensson and Crawford, 1992a). In contrast, the Daily classification designates dissections that involve the ascending aorta as type A, regardless of their extent, and all other dissections as type B (Fig. 10.1). These classifications have therapeutic importance because acute distal dissections are initially treated medically, while proximal lesions are surgical emergencies (Svensson and Crawford, 1992b). Thoraco-abdominal aneurysms are also subdivided according to the origin of the aneurysm and the degree of involvement of the distal thoracic and abdominal aorta (Fig.

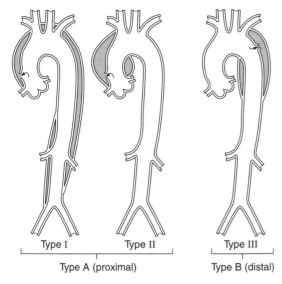

Type I   Type II   Type III

Type A (proximal)   Type B (distal)

Figure 10.1 *Classification schemes for aortic dissections. See text for discussion. (Redrawn with permission from Larson, E.W. and Edwards, W.D. 1984. Risk factors for aortic dissection: a necropsy study of 101 cases.* American Journal of Cardiology *53, 850.)*

INTRA-OPERATIVE MANAGEMENT

Monitoring

Rapid and profound changes in arterial pressure occur frequently during thoracic aortic surgery, and necessitate the use of continuous invasive blood-pressure monitoring. Pre-operatively, blood pressure should be assessed in each arm since clinically significant differences related to atherosclerotic occlusive disease or dissection may involve the subclavian or innominate arteries and result in false interpretation (Frank *et al.*, 1983). During procedures involving the descending thoracic aorta, placement of clamps between the left subclavian and common carotid arteries precludes use of the left arm and mandates use of the right for monitoring arterial pressure. Both the right radial and brachial arteries are available, and studies have demonstrated the safety of cannulation of both for peri-operative pressure monitoring (Slogoff *et al.*, 1983; Bazaral *et al.*, 1990). Finally, femoral artery pressure is also monitored frequently if a shunt or extracorporeal support is employed in order to assess distal perfusion pressure.

PULMONARY ARTERY CATHETERIZATION

The marked haemodynamic changes that occur during thoracic aortic clamping and unclamping, coupled with a relatively large intra-operative blood loss and the frequent need for titration of vasoactive

10.2) (Crawford, 1990). Pre-operative identification of type I and II thoraco-abdominal aneurysms is essential, because these require the most extensive surgical resection and are associated with the highest incidence of post-operative paraplegia. Awareness of the anticipated complexity of a specific type of aneurysm resection will permit appropriate anaesthetic preparation.

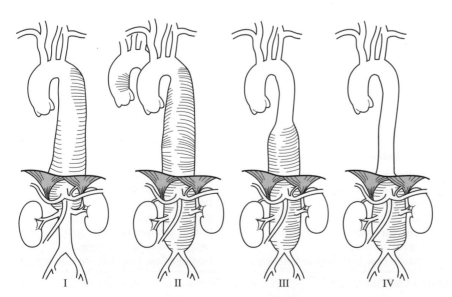

I   II   III   IV

Figure 10.2 *Crawford classification of thoraco-abdominal aneurysms. Type I extends from the proximal descending to the upper abdominal aorta, but terminates before the renal arteries. Type II extends below the renal arteries. Type III begins in the distal half of the descending aorta and extends for a variable length into the abdomen. Type IV involves most of the abdominal aorta. (Redrawn with permission from Svensson and Crawford, 1992b.)*

drugs, necessitate the intra-operative use of pulmonary artery catheterization. In addition to providing information about acute haemodynamic events, the pulmonary artery catheter facilitates fluid management as well as titration of both anaesthetic and non-anaesthetic drugs to manipulate preload, afterload and myocardial contractility.

However, accurate interpretation of pulmonary artery catheter data can be difficult during surgical procedures involving the descending thoracic aorta. If the tip of the pulmonary artery catheter is in the left pulmonary artery when the left lung is collapsed, the measured occlusion pressure (PAOP) will overestimate left atrial pressure and left ventricular end-diastolic pressure (LVEDP), primarily because of Starling resistor forces (venocompression) (Banistor and Torrance, 1960). Decreases in left lung blood flow during one-lung ventilation effectively 'insulate' the thermistor at the tip of a catheter lying in the left lung and may result in spurious overestimation of cardiac output. In addition, *in vivo* measurement of pulmonary artery oxygen saturation is often confounded by measurement artifact related to excessive light reflectance from vessel walls whenever a fibre-optic oximetry catheter tip lies in a small branch of the pulmonary artery. This commonly occurs when a pulmonary artery catheter tip is in the upper lung (with or without one-lung ventilation) and pulmonary blood volume is decreased, especially if the catheter tip is in a distal branch rather than the main pulmonary artery. Fortunately, the pulmonary artery catheter enters the right pulmonary artery in the majority of patients, and these potential inaccuracies become less significant.

Pulmonary artery catheter-derived data must therefore be interpreted carefully during thoracic aortic procedures, because conditions frequently exist which potentially invalidate the assessment of left ventricular preload and cardiac output. Not surprisingly, even continuous mixed venous oximetry may not reflect changes in cardiac output, especially during aortic cross-clamping and unclamping (Shenaq *et al.*, 1987). Nonetheless, with careful attention to detail, the pulmonary artery catheter can provide useful information during, and especially after, surgical procedures on the thoracic aorta.

TRANSOESOPHAGEAL ECHOCARDIOGRAPHY (TOE)

Transoesophageal echocardiography is considered by many to be the diagnostic procedure of choice for suspected acute aortic dissection (Cigarroa *et al.*, 1993; Erbel, 1993). Although its role in the initial evaluation of aortic dissections is well accepted, TOE also has many valuable applications as an intra-operative monitor. These include evaluation of left ventricular function after aortic cross-clamping, monitoring for myocardial ischaemia, estimating the adequacy of left ventricular filling and retrograde aortic perfusion during distal circulatory support, and assessment of the quality and completeness of surgical repair (Imagawa *et al.*, 1993; Connelly *et al.*, 1995a,b; Hanowell *et al.*, 1996).

Confirmation of the pre-operative diagnosis, as well as identification of false and true lumens and the site of intimal tears, are essential components of intra-operative TOE monitoring during aortic dissection repair. Differentiating between true and false lumens may be difficult, however, and careful evaluation with two-dimensional and colour and pulsed Doppler analysis is necessary to distinguish the two lumens and the sites of intimal tears. Table 10.1 summarizes the transoesophageal echocardiographic features of aortic dissections.

Table 10.1 *Aortic dissection: transoesophageal echocardiographic differentiation between true and false lumens*

Parameter	True lumen	False lumen
Size	Reduced, compressed	Longer than true lumen
Pulsation	Systolic lumen increase	Systolic lumen decrease
Spontaneous echo contrast	Rare, low	Dense, regular
Thrombus	Rare	Regular, progressive
Localization	Inner curvature of aortic arch	Outer curvature of aortic arch
Aortic arch flow	Systolic forward	Delayed, reversed, or none
Entry tear	Systolic flow from true-to-false lumen	Diastolic flow from false-to-true lumen

Reprinted with permission from Erbel, 1993.

One-lung ventilation

Surgical exposure of the descending thoracic aorta is best accomplished through a left thoracotomy. Because exposure of the aneurysm is greatly facilitated by collapse of the left lung, a double-lumen endobronchial tube (DLT) is used routinely. Lung collapse and isolation improves exposure and protects the non-dependent lung from the trauma of surgical retraction. In addition, the dependent lung is protected from blood entering the left main stem bronchus because of left intrapulmonary haemorrhage, especially during procedures requiring systemic heparinization or when the left lung is adherent to the aneurysm.

Left-sided DLTs are typically recommended because of the potential for right upper-lobe obstruction with right-sided tubes (Benumof, 1995). However, special considerations apply during insertion of a left-sided DLT in the presence of very large descending aneurysms, where endobronchial placement may be technically difficult and hazardous due to distortion or compression of the left mainstem bronchus or distal trachea by the aneurysm (Verdant, 1984; Cohen et al., 1986; Campos et al., 1990; Gorman et al., 1993; Mora et al., 1993). Compression occurs because of the close relationship of the aorta to the tracheobronchial tree and pulmonary artery (Mora et al., 1993). Prolonged tracheobronchial compression by a large thoracic aneurysm may also produce tracheomalacia, which may increase the risk of tracheobronchial disruption with DLT placement. To avoid these complications in high-risk patients (i.e. those with very large aneurysms or respiratory symptoms suggesting airway compromise), left DLT placement is best accomplished by visualizing the anatomy of the distal trachea and left mainstem bronchus with a fibreoptic bronchoscope prior to intubation. Pulsatile extrinsic compression of the left mainstem bronchus or bronchial erosion by the aneurysm contraindicates placement of a left-sided DLT. In this situation, a right-sided DLT can be used, although compression of the right mainstem bronchus by a large thoraco-abdominal aneurysm may occur rarely (Gorman et al., 1993). Ideally, correct positioning of a DLT should be confirmed using a paediatric bronchoscope, particularly with a right-sided tube where proper apposition of the slotted bronchial cuff over the right upper lobe orifice is necessary for adequate ventilation of the right upper lobe.

Anaesthetic technique

Coronary artery disease and a history of hypertension are prevalent in patients undergoing surgery of the descending thoracic aorta. Consequently, intra-operative management of haemodynamic changes is important to avoid myocardial ischaemia as well as impairment of ventricular function. Both afterload and LVEDP can increase significantly as a result of thoracic aortic clamping and result in myocardial oxygen supply/demand imbalance and the risk of ventricular failure or myocardial infarction. Reduction of myocardial work during proximal aortic clamping involves reduction of both preload and afterload, controlling heart rate and potentially decreasing contractility. While all of these factors can be manipulated pharmacologically using non-anaesthetic drugs (e.g. nitroglycerine, nitroprusside, esmolol), the choice of anaesthetic technique and drugs also significantly affects these parameters.

Many sound approaches to the induction and maintenance of anaesthesia can be utilized, but all have the central features of maintaining adequate myocardial and vital organ perfusion while reducing ventricular stress. A common determinant of the choice of anaesthetic technique is the extent of pre-operative ventricular dysfunction. Patients with significant underlying ventricular dysfunction typically undergo induction of anaesthesia with small amounts of a sedative–hypnotic agent (such as etomidate or a benzodiazepine), followed by the addition of moderate doses of fentanyl (10–20 μg/kg) or sufentanil (2–5 μg/kg). Anaesthesia may be safely induced in patients with intact ventricular function using a variety of other techniques, with the common goal of controlling adrenergic responses during laryngoscopy and intubation. This will avoid increases in aortic shear forces that may precipitate aneurysm rupture or dissection or increase the risk of adverse cardiac events. Since use of even very high doses of potent opioids does not consistently control hypertensive and/or tachycardic responses to intense noxious stimuli, intravenous esmolol and vasodilators are often necessary to attenuate haemodynamic sequelae of laryngoscopy and intubation. Inhalational anaesthetics can also be administered, especially when pre-operative ventricular function is intact, to help control haemodynamic responses while ensuring adequate depth of anaesthesia. Under these circumstances, inhalational anaesthetics may also be useful to reduce myocardial work during aortic clamping, although intravenous vasodilators may be necessary in patients with severely compromised myocardial function who cannot tolerate even small reductions in contractility. At the present time, there are no well controlled, randomized studies addressing whether choice of anaesthetic alters outcome for thoracic aortic surgery.

Management of haemostasis and intra-operative blood loss

Despite modern surgical techniques, intra-operative haemorrhage remains a major cause of early mortality after thoracic aortic surgery. Haemorrhage alone may contribute to 23 per cent of early deaths from acute aortic dissections (Jex et al., 1986). Severe intra-operative blood loss is secondary to multiple factors including surgical bleeding from numerous vascular interruptions and anastomoses, dilutional thrombocytopaenia and factor deficiencies, heparinization, hypothermia, acidosis, and disseminated intravascular coagulation from prolonged hypotension and hypoperfusion. The median intra-operative blood-product requirement during descending thoracic aortic surgery in 336 patients was seven autotransfusion red cell units, six packed red blood cells (RCC), 12 units of fresh frozen plasma (FFP), 20 units of platelets, and 4 units of cryoprecipitate (Svensson et al., 1993b). In high-risk patients, however, transfusion requirements frequently exceed these values. Haemorrhage is most pronounced with extensive thoraco-abdominal aneurysm resections, with traumatic aneurysm repairs when systemic heparinization is used, during acute dissection repair, and with prolonged aortic cross-clamping without distal circulatory support (von Seggeser et al., 1993; von Oppell et al., 1994).

Initial pre-operative preparation for surgery of the thoracic aorta typically includes type and cross-matching for at least 10 units each of RCC, FFP and platelets. Additional blood products are obtained in advance of continued haemorrhage. In addition to a pulmonary artery catheter and two large bore (14-gauge) peripheral venous catheters, it is useful to place an 8.5 French gauge sheath in an internal jugular vein. A rapid infusion device, such as the Rapid Infusion System (Haemonetics Corp., Braintree, MA, USA) or Level One (Level One Technologies Inc., Rockland, MA, USA) blood-warming systems,

facilitates rapid infusion of large volumes of warmed blood products. This will minimize intra-operative hypothermia and hypovolaemia. In addition, blood scavenging devices are recommended to salvage blood lost into the operative field. Finally, intraoperative monitoring of coagulation function with frequent assessment of platelet count, prothrombin and partial thromboplastin times (PT, PTT), and fibrinogen levels, along with the use of thromboelastography (TEG), will guide appropriate blood component replacement therapy.

PHYSIOLOGICAL EFFECTS OF CROSS-CLAMPING THE THORACIC AORTA

Haemodynamic changes

The pathophysiology of cross-clamping of the thoracic aorta is complex and incompletely defined, despite abundant experimental work examining both the mechanism and the magnitude of the haemodynamic changes associated with it. In both animal and clinical models, severe proximal hypertension is the most consistent and dramatic response to proximal aortic occlusion (Kouchoukos et al., 1979; Normann et al., 1983; Gelman et al., 1983, 1988a, b, 1990, 1994; Mutch et al., 1990; Gelman, 1995). The aetiology of this hypertensive response has traditionally been attributed to an increase in systemic vascular resistance and a sudden impedance to aortic outflow (Silverstein et al., 1979; Gelman, 1995). However, considerable data suggest that other factors may contribute to the observed hypertension. During thoracic aortic occlusion, increased plasma concentrations of catecholamines, angiotensin and renin have been demonstrated (Normann et al., 1983; Symbas et al., 1983; Joob et al., 1986; Gelman et al., 1989). These substances, as well as other humoral factors released from tissues below the cross-clamp, may influence vascular tone in vessels proximal to it (Berkowitz and Shetty, 1974; Normann et al., 1983; Symbas et al., 1983; Joob et al., 1986; Gelman et al., 1990). In addition, Gelman and others have noted a significant increase in blood volume in organs and tissues above the level of the aortic cross-clamp, as well as increased upper body and superior vena caval (SVC) blood flow (Barcroft and Samaan, 1935; Gregoretti et al., 1990; Gelman et al., 1994). Presumably, blood is diverted from splanch-

Table 10.2 *Haemodynamic response to aortic clamping and to decompression with a temporary shunt in eight patients undergoing repair of the descending thoracic aorta*

Parameter	Baseline (Period I)	Aorta clamped (Period II)	Shunt opened (Period III)
MAP (mmHg)	90.3 ± 4.0	122.1 ± 4.1*	86.8 ± 4.4
MPAP (mmHg)	21.3 ± 2.1	30.5 ± 3.1*	19.9 ± 1.7
CVP (mmHg)	7.0 ± 0.5	11.5 ± 2.2*	7.8 ± 1.5
PAOP (mmHg)	9.6 ± 1.9	17.6 ± 2.4*	10.4 ± 1.9
CI (L/min/m^2)	2.7 ± 0.3	1.9 ± 0.3*	2.2 ± 0.2†
HR (bpm)	85.2 ± 7.6	89.8 ± 11.8	86.6 ± 4.5
SVI (mL/beat/m^2)	34.0 ± 6.4	23.0 ± 3.8	26.0 ± 3.0
LVSWI (g/m/m^2)	35.6 ± 4.9	31.8 ± 4.6	25.8 ± 2.4†

Abbreviations: MAP, mean arterial pressure; MPAP, mean pulmonary arterial pressure; CVP, central venous pressure; PAOP, pulmonary artery occlusion pressure; CI, cardiac index; HR, heart rate; SVI, stroke volume index; LVSWI, left ventricular stroke work index.
All values given are mean ± standard error. *$P < 0.05$ (I vs. II). †$P < 0.05$ (I vs. III).
Reprinted with permission from Kouchoukos *et al.*, 1979.

nic venous capacitance beds, which collapse during thoracic aortic cross-clamping, to the central venous compartment (Gelman, 1995). Blood volume redistribution from the lower to upper body produces an increase in preload, which may represent the mechanism whereby central venous pressures (CVP) and left ventricular end-diastolic volumes increase after high aortic cross-clamping (Roizen *et al.*, 1984; Gelman *et al.*, 1994). It is argued that proximal hypertension is, in part, caused by changes in cardiac output as a consequence of the preload-augmenting effect of blood transferred from lower-body venous capacitance vessels to the SVC. Left ventricular function is then augmented via the Frank–Starling mechanism (Barcroft and Samaan, 1935; Stockland *et al.*, 1980; Gelman *et al.*, 1994).

In addition, increases in myocardial contractility during thoracic aortic occlusion are also believed to be secondary to augmentation of endocardial blood flow, a physiological process termed the 'Anrep effect' (Gelman, 1995). Consistent with this theory are several animal models of aortic occlusion that have demonstrated an increase or no change in cardiac output with thoracic aortic cross-clamping (Barcroft and Samman, 1935; Longo *et al.*, 1969; Brusoni *et al.*, 1978; Gelman *et al.*, 1983, 1988a; Stockland *et al.*, 1980; Symbas *et al.*, 1983; Gregoretti *et al.*, 1990; Aakhus *et al.*, 1995).

Clinical assessment of patients undergoing thoracic and supracoeliac aortic cross-clamping has not, however, uniformly confirmed the results of these animal experiments. Kouchoukous and colleagues (1979) assessed the haemodynamic effects of clamping the proximal thoracic aorta in eight patients, and

of opening a Gott shunt 2 minutes later. Mean arterial pressure (MAP), CVP, mean pulmonary artery pressure (PAP) and PAOP increased by 35, 56, 43, and 90 per cent, respectively. In contrast, cardiac output decreased by an average of 29 per cent (Table 10.2). All figures returned to baseline after the shunt was opened, except cardiac index which remained below baseline. Roizen and colleagues (1984) provided more definitive evidence of cross-clamp-induced ventricular dysfunction in a study of 12 patients undergoing aortic surgery involving cross-clamping at infrarenal, suprarenal, and supracoeliac levels using TOE analysis of left ventricular dimensions and ejection fraction.

Supracoeliac cross-clamping produced substantial increases in left ventricular end-systolic and end-diastolic areas and decreased ejection fraction, despite the administration of vasodilators and anaesthetics to maintain preclamp haemodynamic variables (Table 10.3). In addition, a high incidence of regional wall motion abnormalities was observed, suggesting the potential for myocardial ischaemia with proximal aortic occlusion. Cardiac output and stroke volume were maintained by increased end-diastolic and end-systolic volumes, an observation consistent with other experimental findings (Gelman *et al.*, 1994). Although Roizen and colleagues (1984) failed to characterize the precise type of wall motion abnormalities observed, myocardial ischaemia may have accounted, in part, for the decline in ejection fraction. More recent use of TOE-derived parameters of ventricular function during proximal aortic cross-clamping have also demonstrated significant increases in end-systolic wall stress that accompany substantial decreases

Table 10.3 *Percentage change in cardiovascular variables on initiation of aortic occlusion*

Level of aortic occlusion	Percentage change after occlusion at		
	Supracoeliac	Suprarenal–infracoeliac	Infrarenal
Mean arterial blood pressure	+54	+5*	+2*
Pulmonary capillary wedge pressure	+38	+10*	0*
End-diastolic area	+28	+2*	+9*
End-systolic area	+69	+10*	+11*
Ejection fraction	−38	−10*	−8*
Patients with wall-motion abnormalities	+92	+33	0
New myocardial infarctions	+8⁻	+0	0

* Statistically different ($P < 0.05$) from group undergoing supracoeliac aortic occlusion.
Reprinted with permission from Roizen *et al.*, 1984.

in fractional area shortening, suggesting global impairment of left ventricular systolic function (Connelly *et al.*, 1995a).

Experimentally, coronary blood flow increases with thoracic aortic occlusion, presumably due to increased perfusion pressure or coronary blood flow autoregulation induced by increases in myocardial oxygen demand and consumption (Longo *et al.*, 1969; Brusoni *et al.*, 1978; Gelman, 1995). However, an increase in left ventricular end-diastolic pressure may reduce the effective coronary perfusion pressure gradient. This is not uncommon in patients with underlying coronary artery disease and left ventricular hypertrophy, which may produce an imbalance of myocardial oxygen supply and demand (Brusoni *et al.*, 1978). Although myocardial ischaemia may contribute to a reduction in ejection fraction, inadequate control of proximal hypertension may also precipitate deterioration in ventricular function, especially in patients with impaired contractility who are intolerant of increases in afterload.

Decrements in cardiac output after proximal aortic clamping may not only occur because of ischaemia or altered loading conditions, but may also represent an appropriate response to a decrease in total body oxygen consumption. Evidence suggests that thoracic aortic clamping is accompanied by a 43 to 57 per cent reduction in oxygen consumption caused by exclusion from the circulation of a substantial amount of metabolically active tissue below the cross-clamp (Gelman *et al.*, 1988b; Gregoretti *et al.*, 1990). Thus, some fraction of the reduction in cardiac output may be in response to a decrease in oxygen consumption rather than from myocardial dysfunction.

Arterial pressure distal to the aortic cross-clamp decreases substantially (to 20–40 mmHg) and is strongly dependent on proximal aortic pressure (Gelman *et al.*, 1983; Gelman, 1995). Blood flow to vascular beds below the level of the cross-clamp is by collateral vessels and is dependent primarily on perfusion pressure rather than cardiac output, suggesting that proximal aortic pressures should be maintained as high as possible to ensure distal perfusion (Gelman, 1995). TOE can be used to monitor the left ventricular response to aortic clamping and serve as a guide to the degree of proximal hypertension that can be safely tolerated.

Simple cross-clamping of the thoracic aorta also leads to intracranial hypertension and increased cerebrospinal fluid (CSF) pressure (Hantler and Knight, 1982; D'Ambra *et al.*, 1988). The precise mechanism of the rise in intracranial pressure (ICP) is unknown, although proximal hypertension causing cerebral vasodilatation and engorgement of the intracranial compartment (Kazama *et al.*, 1994), increased cerebral blood flow (Saether *et al.*, 1996) and blood-volume redistribution into cerebral venous capacitance vessels (Gelman, 1995) are all postulated. Increases in CSF pressure, along with profound decreases in distal aortic pressure, dramatically reduce spinal cord perfusion pressure. Data indicate that a minimum perfusion pressure of 50 mmHg must be maintained to protect against spinal cord injury (Kazama *et al.*, 1994). Spinal cord perfusion is considered further later on. Table 10.4 summarizes the major pathophysiological sequelae of thoracic aortic cross-clamping.

Metabolic effects

Thoracic aortic cross-clamping results in anaerobic metabolism and lactic acid production in tissues below the cross-clamp. By reducing hepatic blood flow, simple aortic cross-clamping also decreases

Table 10.4 *Major pathophysiological effects of thoracic aortic cross-clamping*

- Proximal arterial hypertension
- Distal arterial hypotension
- Decreased ejection fraction
- Increased LVEDA, pulmonary artery and pulmonary artery occlusion pressures, and central venous pressure
- Increased CSFP and ICP
- Decreased SCPP
- Decreased renal and splanchnic blood flow

Abbreviations: LVEDA, left ventricular end-diastolic area; CSFP, cerebrospinal fluid pressure; ICP, intracranial pressure; SCPP, spinal cord perfusion pressure.

hepatic clearance of lactate and further contributes to metabolic acidosis. O'Rourke and colleagues (1985) observed a threefold elevation in serum lactate levels in 11 patients undergoing supracoeliac occlusion for abdominal aortic aneurysm repair. With higher thoracic clamping, a more profound metabolic acidosis should be anticipated, especially with prolonged clamp times. Von Segesser and colleagues (1983) documented an average pH of 7.29 after thoracic aortic cross-clamp release.

MANAGEMENT OF AORTIC CROSS-CLAMPING

Management of the haemodynamic and metabolic consequences of aortic cross-clamping depends, in part, on the surgical technique employed. With simple aortic cross-clamping, haemodynamic changes will be sudden and profound and require active intervention. The control of proximal hypertension must therefore begin *before* the aortic cross-clamp is applied, and vasodilators are titrated to reduce the preclamp systolic blood pressure to approximately 90 mmHg. This, in conjunction with gradual cross-clamp application by the surgeon, will attenuate the marked increase in blood pressure.

Pharmacological control of proximal hypertension

Pharmacological control of clamp-induced hypertension associated with simple clamp and sew techniques is commonly and effectively achieved by vasodilata-

tion with a combination of sodium nitroprusside and isoflurane. In addition, judicious titration of short-acting intravenous beta-adrenergic antagonists such as esmolol or labetalol can control heart rate and lower the dose requirements for nitroprusside. Data suggest that nitroprusside may reduce distal perfusion pressure and accentuate the already profound decrease in renal and spinal cord blood flow that accompanies high aortic occlusion (Gelman *et al.*, 1983; Marini *et al.*, 1989; Shine and Nugent, 1990; Woloszyn *et al.*, 1990; Cernaianu *et al.*, 1993; Simpson *et al.*, 1994; 1995; Gelman, 1995). In addition, nitroprusside can also increase cerebral blood flow and intracranial and intraspinal pressures, further compromising spinal cord perfusion (Clark *et al.*, 1992; D'Ambra *et al.*, 1988; Gelman, 1995; Shine *et al.*, 1990; Ryan *et al.*, 1993). For these reasons, avoidance of large doses of nitroprusside has been advocated (Gelman, 1995).

In a canine model of thoracic aortic cross-clamping, isoflurane produced a higher spinal cord perfusion pressure and was associated with a lower incidence of neurological injury than nitroprusside. At end-expired concentrations of up to 2.5 per cent, isoflurane can adequately control proximal hypertension during thoracic aortic cross-clamping, although not as effectively as nitroprusside (Godet *et al.*, 1990). Moreover, the negative inotropic effects of isoflurane in these concentrations may be undesirable in patients with depressed left ventricular function. Intravenous calcium channel blockers, such as nicardipine, are appealing antihypertensive agents since they have been shown to be neuroprotective during experimental spinal cord ischaemia (Schittek *et al.*, 1992). Unfortunately, they have not been evaluated clinically during thoracic aortic surgery.

Nitroglycerine is an attractive agent since coronary vasodilatation and preload reduction accompany its antihypertensive effects. Unfortunately, nitroglycerine is a weak vasodilator and is often inadequate as a sole agent to control proximal hypertension. One reasonable approach is a combination of nitroprusside and nitroglycerine, with a background of low concentrations of isoflurane. This combination allows for the rapid termination of pharmacologic vasodilatation before aortic unclamping.

Distal perfusion techniques

The rationale behind distal perfusion is twofold: the attenuation of proximal hypertension and adequate

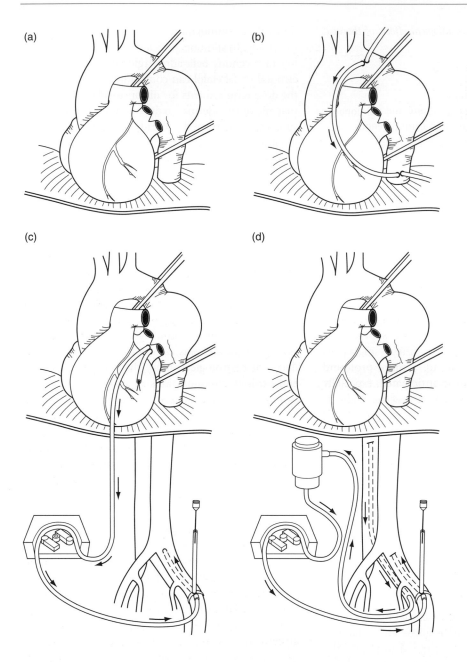

(a)

(b)

(c)

(d)

Figure 10.3 *(a) Simple cross-clamping of the descending aorta; (b) aneurysm exclusion with a passive Gott shunt from the aortic arch to the distal thoracic aorta. (c) Left atriofemoral bypass with pump. (d) Femoral–femoral bypass using a pump oxygenator. (Reprinted with permission from Ochsner, J. and Ancalmo, N. 1992. Descending thoracic aortic aneurysm. Chest Surgery Clinics of North America **2**, 291–309.)*

perfusion of tissues below the aortic cross-clamp. By providing blood flow to the lower body, bypass and shunt strategies diminish the incidence of renal failure and paraplegia (Jex *et al.*, 1986; Svensson and Crawford, 1992a,b; Najafi, 1993; Read *et al.*, 1993; Coselli, 1994; Forbes and Ashbaugh, 1994; Lawrie *et al.*, 1994; Safi *et al.*, 1994; von Oppell *et al.*, 1994; Bavaria *et al.*, 1995; Biglioli *et al.*, 1995; Verdant *et al.*, 1995; Nicolosi *et al.*, 1996) and prevent the metabolic acidosis and dramatic hypotension char-

acteristic of clamp removal (Janusz, 1994). The manner in which bypass and shunts control hypertension differs according to the type of bypass technique chosen (Fig. 10.3). Shunting blood from proximal ventricular or aortic sites to the distal aorta primarily reduces afterload. In contrast, femoral veno-arterial cardiopulmonary bypass (CPB) and atriofemoral bypass using centrifugal pumps reduce venous pressure by a reduction in preload and cardiac output.

Table 10.5 *Advantages and disadvantages of distal perfusion techniques*

Advantages	Disadvantages
Control of proximal hypertension	Possible atrial, ventricular, aortic or femoral artery injury
Reduction of visceral and renal ischaemia	Air emboli/embolic stroke
Prevention of acidosis and declamping shock	Interference with the operative field
Ability to rapidly warm patients	Increased operative time
Access for rapid volume infusion	Potential for excess haemorrhage with anticoagulation
Potential reduction in the incidence of DIC	Bleeding from cannulation sites
Supplementary oxygenation with extracorporeal oxygenators	Difficult proximal exposure for atrial/proximal aortic cannulation
Reduced incidence of paraplegia	Shunt dislodgement

DIC, disseminated intravascular coagulation.

The issue of distal support for surgery on the thoracic aorta continues to be controversial, with some authors advocating that chronic localized aneurysms of the descending aorta that are amenable to expeditious reconstruction within 30 minutes be managed with simple cross-clamping (Najafi, 1993). More complex repairs, including extensive thoracoabdominal aneurysms that are likely to require prolonged clamp times, should be managed with some form of distal circulatory support (Najafi, 1993; Svensson and Crawford, 1993a; Safi *et al.*, 1994). A summary of the advantages and disadvantages of distal circulatory support is presented in Table 10.5, and a detailed discussion of the currently available techniques follows.

SHUNTS

Gott shunts from the proximal to the distal aorta are passive methods of aortic bypass and distal perfusion (Fig. 10.3b). The shunt is a transparent, heparin-coated conduit that eliminates the need for systemic anticoagulation (Verdant, 1992; Verdant *et al.*, 1995). The proximal end of the cannula is typically placed in the ascending aorta, although the aortic arch, the left subclavian artery and the proximal descending aorta are acceptable proximal cannulation sites. The distal end is placed in the descending aorta or femoral artery and the femoral artery pressure monitored (Lee and Jihayel, 1991). Verdant and colleagues (1995) reported their experience with 366 consecutive patients undergoing descending thoracic aortic repair using a Gott shunt and noted mean femoral artery pressures of 64.5 mmHg and mean shunt flows of 2.5 L/min, with flows greater than 2 L/min in 85 per cent of patients. Shunt flow, which is directly related to proximal pressure and

inversely related to peripheral resistance, was highest with the proximal cannulation in the ascending aorta and least with cannulation in the proximal descending aorta. They also employ a flow probe to monitor shunt flow and optimize shunt function (e.g. decreased flow may represent malposition or kinking of the conduit) (Kopman and Ferguson, 1977). An interesting, albeit complex alternative to standard Gott shunting, is decompression of the proximal circulation and perfusion of the distal vasculature by construction of an axillofemoral bypass graft immediately prior to resection of the aneurysm (Stuhmeier *et al.*, 1993; Comerota and White, 1995). The additional operative time and the creation of two surgical wounds are, however, substantial disadvantages of this approach.

ATRIOFEMORAL BYPASS

With this form of left heart bypass, the left atrium is cannulated and oxygenated blood is diverted to the femoral artery by a centrifugal pump (Fig. 10.3c). In contrast to systems incorporating a reservoir, centrifugal pump bypass requires either no or minimal heparin to maintain an activated clotting time of 200 s (Lee and Jihayel, 1991). The use of heparin-coated circuits has, in some reports, completely eliminated the need for heparin (Contino *et al.*, 1994; Sander-Jensen *et al.*, 1995).

Experimental work suggests that shunt flows of 35 mL/kg/min improve ventricular function to near control levels (Mandelbaum and Webb, 1963) (Fig. 10.4). However, Hug and Taber (1969) found that flow rates approaching 60–90 mL/kg/min were necessary to effectively decompress the left heart. These values actually approximate *normal* blood flow in the descending aorta and are not practically obtainable

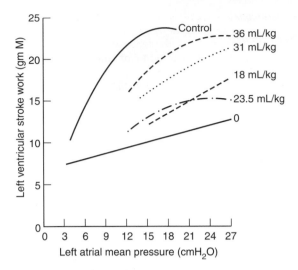

Figure 10.4 *Left ventricular function curves during occlusion of the proximal thoracic aorta and the effect of left atrial–femoral bypass at varying shunt flow rates. A shunt flow of 36 mL/kg/min permitted near-normal left ventricular function. (Reprinted with permission from Mandlebaum and Webb, 1963.)*

in humans. Clinically, bypass flow rates of 25–40 mL/kg/min appear sufficient to normalize proximal pressures and maintain adequate distal perfusion (Wakabayashi *et al.*, 1975; Ergin *et al.*, 1991; Ataka *et al.*, 1993; Egener *et al.*, 1993; Fehrenbacher *et al.*, 1993; von Segesser *et al.*, 1993; Borst *et al.*, 1994; Sander-Jensen *et al.*, 1995). Careful monitoring of PAOP and left ventricular end-diastolic area will detect hypovolaemia if excess blood is pumped from the left atrium, and proximal hypotension will be evident if this occurs.

FEMORAL VENO-ARTERIAL CARDIOPULMONARY BYPASS

Femoral veno-arterial CPB (Fig. 10.3d) is an increasingly popular method of distal perfusion because it offers several advantages over shunts and left heart bypass: the shunt does not clutter the operative field, supplementary oxygenation is provided, the CPB circuit may be used for resuscitation and complete CPB if necessary, and distal perfusion is independent of cardiac output (Reed and Stratford, 1989; Ergin *et al.*, 1991). However, it does require an oxygenator, a roller pump, and complete systemic heparinization. Heparinization may be responsible for excess bleeding and probably accounts for the increased mortal-

ity noted during repair of traumatic lesions (von Oppell *et al.*, 1994). As discussed above for left heart bypass, flow rates of 25–40 mL/kg/min and distal pressures of 40–60 mmHg appear adequate and obtainable in most patients (Kazui *et al.*, 1987).

To ensure satisfactory venous return, a 28–32 French gauge femoral venous cannula is inserted and advanced as far as possible into the inferior vena cava. An adjustable clamp on the line controls gravity induced venous return. Clamp removal and collection of blood in the venous reservoir reduces venous return to the heart and cardiac output, and effectively decreases proximal aortic blood pressure. Conversely, clamping of the venous line increases flow and proximal pressure. Careful control of venous return becomes critical in maintaining stable haemodynamics because individual patients may demonstrate marked changes in proximal pressures with translocation of as little as 100–200 mL of blood into the central circulation (Reed and Stratford, 1989). Factors such as small venous cannula size and suboptimal cannula positioning will limit venous return and, hence, bypass flow rates. In addition, if venous return to the reservoir is suboptimal because of technical factors, any increase in pump flow will augment central venous return and potentially increase cardiac output and, therefore, proximal pressure, because blood preferentially flows into the inferior vena cava (IVC) rather than into the venous reservoir. Of course, increasing pump flow in the face of inadequate venous return will rapidly deplete the venous reservoir, necessitating either a reduction in pump flow or addition of fluid to the venous reservoir.

In summary, technical problems with cannula size and placement that alter venous return not only impair distal perfusion, but also reduce the effectiveness of the bypass circuit to control proximal blood pressure and unload the left ventricle. Table 10.6 provides guidelines for haemodynamic management during aortic surgery when femoral veno-arterial CPB is used.

PHYSIOLOGICAL SEQUELAE AND MANAGEMENT OF AORTIC UNCLAMPING

In those instances where distal circulatory support is not employed, thoracic aortic cross-clamp release results in profound haemodynamic and metabolic

Table 10.6 *Haemodynamic management during femoral veno-arterial cardiopulmonary bypass for repair of the descending thoracic aorta*

Proximal aortic pressure*	Femoral artery pressure**	PAOP/LVEDA	Diagnosis	Intervention
Normal	Normal	Low	Optimal haemodynamics and proximal decompression	None
High	Low	Normal	Inadequate decompression vs. primary HTN	↑ VR to pump, ↑ Pump flows,*** vasodilators
Low	Low	Very low	Hypovolaemia	↓ VR to pump, volume replacement
Low	Low	High	Rule out LVF	↑CO/contractility, inotropes, ↑VR to pump, ↑pump flows
Low	Normal	Very low	Excess VR to pump, ± hypovolaemia	Clamp venous line and ↓ VR to pump, volume replacement if reservoir volumes low

Abbreviations: VR, venous return (to pump); HTN, hypertension; PAOP, pulmonary artery occlusion pressure; LVF, left ventricular failure; CO, cardiac output; LVEDA, left ventricular end-diastolic area by transoesophageal echocardiography.

* Proximal pressures are considered 'normal' when at or slightly above baseline, i.e. proximal pressures are frequently maintained above the normal range to ensure distal perfusion. 'High' proximal pressures are those well above desired or baseline values.

** Femoral pressures are considered 'normal' if flows and pressures are adequate (i.e. 25–35 mL/kg/min and 40–60 mmHg), and low if below these values. The highest distal flows compatible with normal proximal pressure and PAOP should be maintained. Femoral pressures are presumed to reflect flow, although this agreement is not absolute.

*** Increased pump flows must be accompanied by an increase in venous return to the pump, i.e. equilibrium between VR and arterial pump flow.

changes that have been termed 'declamping shock' (Brant *et al.*, 1970). The severity of these changes will vary with the duration of visceral and lower extremity ischaemia, the blood pressure and cardiac filling volumes before cross-clamp release, and the continued influence of vasodilators, beta-adrenergic antagonists and inhaled anaesthetics. The typical changes encountered are substantial (up to 50 per cent) decreases in arterial blood pressure and calculated vascular resistance (Longo *et al.*, 1969; Roberts *et al.*, 1983; Symbas *et al.*, 1983; Livesay *et al.*, 1985). In addition, there are increases in pulmonary artery pressure, end-tidal carbon dioxide, arterial P_{CO_2}, and serum lactate, accompanied by a concomitant decline in arterial pH (von Segesser *et al.*, 1993; Biglioli *et al.*, 1995). Although initially the PAOP and CVP decrease, the cardiac output and stroke volume may increase, presumably owing to the marked decrease in afterload. The pulmonary hypertension seen with unclamping is probably caused by the effects on the pulmonary vasculature of lactic acidosis, hypercarbia, and vasoactive mediators released from ischaemic vascular beds (Beattie and Frank, 1993). Although the primary cause of arterial hypotension appears to be related to peripheral

vasodilatation and central hypovolaemia (Gelman, 1995), other mechanisms invoked include reactive hyperaemia in previously underperfused vascular beds (Lee and Jihayel, 1991; Gelman, 1995), redistribution of blood from the upper to the lower body, sequestration of blood in venous capacitance vessels (Normann *et al.*, 1983), the systemic effects of ischaemic metabolites released from unperfused tissues, and myocardial depression (Brant *et al.*, 1970). Vasodilatation may occur secondary to the effects of ischaemia on arterial resistance and venous capacitance vessels or to the influence of as yet unidentified vasoactive substances released from tissues below the cross-clamp (Brant *et al.*, 1970; Normann *et al.*, 1983). Cohen and colleagues (1992) documented increases in intestinal permeability with supracoeliac cross-clamping in dogs. These alterations in gut mucosal integrity may allow translocation of endotoxin and intestinal bacteria into the portal circulation and may account for some of the haemodynamic instability after aortic unclamping.

Preventing or minimizing declamping hypotension is achieved by aggressive intravascular volume administration before cross-clamp removal, discontinuation of vasodilators, beta-adrenergic

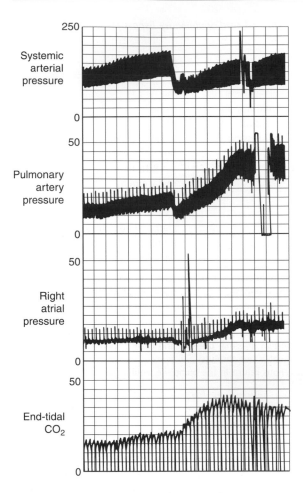

Figure 10.5 *Continuous recording of arterial, pulmonary artery, and right atrial pressures and end-tidal carbon dioxide before and after release of a supracoeliac cross-clamp (arrow). Pressures increase before cross-clamp release caused by the discontinuation of vasodilators and the administration of volume. A dramatic decrease in arterial blood pressure is seen with cross-clamp release. Vasopressor and volume administration then return blood pressure to preclamp values. (Reprinted with permission from Beattie and Frank, 1993.)*

antagonists and anaesthetics well in advance of cross-clamp release, increased minute ventilation during the period of cross-clamping, and release of the cross-clamp by the surgeon over 2–4 min. Gradual cross-clamp release may limit the impact of vasodepressant substances released from ischaemic tissues (Gelman, 1995) and may also attenuate reperfusion-associated injury of organs below the aortic cross-clamp. Some authors advocate the

administration of a sodium bicarbonate infusion during the period of aortic cross-clamping to minimize the acidosis observed with unclamping (Saleh *et al.*, 1982; Van Norman *et al.*, 1989). Despite these prophylactic manoeuvres, hypotension is commonly profound and usually requires brief administration of vasopressors such as phenylephrine, norepinephrine, or epinephrine. However, vasopressors should be administered cautiously and in small doses, as even transient hypertension may precipitate bleeding. In addition, should a distal aortic anastomotic leak require re-application of the aortic cross-clamp, inappropriate vasopressor use may produce severe hypertension and jeopardize the integrity of the proximal anastomosis.

With appropriate volume loading and vasopressor use, hypotension is usually transient and well tolerated. Pulmonary artery pressure eventually returns to normal as the effects of lactic acidosis, hypercarbia, prior volume loading and previous vasopressor administration dissipate (Fig. 10.5).

SPINAL CORD PERFUSION AND NEUROLOGICAL INJURY

The most feared complication of descending thoracic aortic surgery is post-operative paraplegia/paresis secondary to spinal cord ischaemia. The nature of this injury is related to the degree and duration of inadequate spinal cord blood flow during both thoracic aortic cross-clamping and periods of post-operative hypotension in patients in whom spinal cord perfusion depends on collateral blood flow (Laschinger *et al.*, 1983; Kouchoukos and Rokkas, 1993; Svensson and Crawford, 1993; Svensson *et al.*, 1993a; Livesay *et al.*, 1985; Gharagozloo *et al.*, 1996).

Incidence

The incidence of spinal cord injury ranges from 0.4 to 40 per cent, with the lowest figures observed in children undergoing repair of co-arctation of the aorta (<2 per cent), spinal cord blood flow being maintained through extensive collateral radicular branches of the upper intercostal arteries (Lerberg *et al.*, 1982; Marini and Cunningham, 1993). Similarly, the incidence of spinal cord injury is also low (1.4

per cent) after elective repair of chronic traumatic aneurysms (Kouchoukos and Rokkas, 1993). In contrast, the incidence approaches 40 per cent after repair of extensive dissecting thoraco-abdominal aneurysms. Approximately 50 per cent of patients with immediate spinal cord injury will never recover neurologically (Gelman, 1995).

Two patterns of injury are observed: immediate onset paraplegia that is related to intra-operative interruption of spinal cord perfusion; and delayed paraplegia, an event that occurs in about one-third of cases between 1 and 30 days after surgery (Crawford, 1990; Crawford et al., 1990; Kouchoukos and Rokkas, 1993; Marini and Cunningham, 1993; Svensson and Crawford, 1993a; Svensson et al., 1993b). Delayed neurological injury appears to be due to spinal cord hypoperfusion from significant post-operative hypotension (Svensson et al., 1993a,b; Marini and Cunningham, 1993), especially when critical intercostal arteries are interrupted surgically, because the collateral circulation becomes tenuous (Coselli, 1994). Other factors such as spinal cord oedema, reperfusion injury and thromboembolic occlusion of re-attached vessels may also be responsible (Svensson et al., 1993a,b).

Anatomy of spinal cord blood supply

Understanding the complex and often unpredictable anatomy of the spinal cord's blood supply is important in recognizing the mechanisms by which spinal cord injury occurs. The spinal cord is supplied by three arteries: one that supplies the anterior two-thirds of the cord and two posterior vessels that supply the posterior one-third (Svensson et al., 1986a). Unfortunately, the anterior spinal artery may become very small below the level of C_3 to C_5. The middle section usually depends on one or probably two intercostal artery branches and is, therefore, extremely vulnerable. Blood supply to the lower section is almost entirely supplied by the arteria radicularis magna, the so-called artery of Adamkiewicz. Although this artery may originate from between the T9 and L3 levels, it arises from between T9 and T12 in 75 per cent of the population (Shenaq and Svensson, 1993). It is this portion of the spinal cord (where collateral blood supply is minimal and dependent on the artery of Adamkiewicz) that is at greatest risk of ischaemia from prolonged aortic cross-clamping or sustained profound hypotension

Table 10.7 *Factors influencing the incidence of spinal cord injury after surgery of the descending thoracic aorta*

- Duration of aortic cross-clamping
- Failure to re-implant critical intercostal/lumbar arteries
- Aneurysm location and type
- Presence of rupture/dissection
- Peri-operative hypotension
- Patient age
- ? Use of sodium nitroprusside, ? peri-operative hyperglycaemia

(Wadouh et al., 1984; Livesay et al., 1985; Svensson et al., 1986b).

Aetiology of spinal cord injury

The factors influencing the incidence of spinal cord injury after surgery of the descending thoracic aorta are listed in Table 10.7. The vast majority of studies conclude that the duration of aortic cross-clamping is a critical determinant of this injury (Crawford and Rubio, 1973; Najafi et al., 1980; Katz et al., 1981; Laschinger et al., 1983; Lawrie et al., 1994; Livesay et al., 1985; Jex et al., 1986; Svensson et al., 1993a; von Oppell et al., 1994; Nicolosi et al., 1996). Several authors have established that the risk increases in a sigmoid fashion after 30 min of aortic occlusion without distal circulatory support, with the risk increasing dramatically when cross-clamp times exceed 45 min (Katz et al., 1981; Jex et al., 1986; Svensson et al., 1993a; Lawrie et al., 1994). The risk then levels off after 60 min, with current data suggesting the absolute safe ischaemic interval to be as short as 18 min (Marini and Cunningham, 1993).

Patients sustaining acute rupture or dissection of the thoracic aorta are also at increased risk of paraplegia, because collateral blood flow to the spinal cord may be either inadequately developed (rupture) or disrupted (dissection) (Kouchoukos and Rokkas, 1993). In addition, the location and extent of the aneurysm both directly influence the incidence of spinal cord injury. Table 10.8 illustrates the significant impact of the extent of thoraco-abdominal aneurysms and the presence of dissection on the incidence of post-operative paraplegia/paresis.

Distal hypotension reduces spinal cord perfusion pressure and, unless blood flow is provided by circulatory support or collaterals, the cord will become

Table 10.8 *Frequency of post-operative spinal cord injury after descending thoracic artery surgery*

Location of surgery	Incidence of paraparesis/paraplegia	
	Without dissection	With dissection
Descending aorta to renal arteries (Crawford type I)	8–10%	21%
Entire thoracic and abdominal aorta (Crawford type II)	21%	40%
Distal descending aorta and varying segments of abdominal aorta (Crawford type III)	2–3%	14%

Adapted with permission from Crawford *et al.* 1986. Thoracoabdominal aortic aneurysms: preoperative and intraoperative factors determining intermediate and long-term results of operations in 605 patients. *Journal of Vascular Surgery* **3**, 389–404.

ischaemic. Experimental data indicate that nitroprusside, as well as nitroglycerine, may increase the risk of paraplegia by decreasing proximal and distal aortic pressures and increasing CSF pressure, thus lowering perfusion pressure (Marini *et al.*, 1989; Shine and Nugent, 1990; Cernaianu *et al.*, 1993; Ryan *et al.*, 1993; Simpson *et al.*, 1994, 1995; Gelman, 1995). The reduction in proximal blood pressure may shunt blood away from high-resistance collateral vessels that supply the distal vasculature to low-resistance proximal vascular beds dilated by nitroprusside (Marini and Cunningham, 1993). While contrary experimental evidence exists regarding the potentially deleterious effects of this agent (Wadouh *et al.*, 1984; Clark *et al.*, 1992), Svensson and colleagues (1993a) believe that the essential issue is not whether nitroprusside (or any other hypotensive agent) should be used, but rather the degree of proximal hypertension that can be safely tolerated by the heart and aorta, because uncontrolled hypertension jeopardizes myocardial function and the integrity of fragile aortic wall above the cross-clamp. For these reasons, lower proximal pressures must often be tolerated (or distal support used) at the expense of potentially impaired spinal cord perfusion (Cernaianu *et al.*, 1993). Despite these reservations, nitroprusside continues to be a commonly used vasodilator and no clinical data exist to contraindicate its use in this setting.

Severe prolonged post-operative hypotension, anterior spinal artery occlusion, and occlusion of a re-implanted intercostal artery have also been implicated as risk factors for delayed onset paraplegia (Najafi *et al.*, 1980; Coselli, 1994), although experimental models have failed to confirm these theories (Moore and Hollier, 1991). In addition, collateral blood flow to the spinal cord influences the degree of spinal cord ischaemia (Livesay *et al.*, 1985), and in the event of traumatic rupture or dissection, collateral flow may be underdeveloped or disrupted.

Failure to re-implant critical intercostal arteries is often cited as a cause of spinal cord injury

(Fehrenbacher *et al.*, 1993; Borst *et al.*, 1994; Coselli, 1994; Safi *et al.*, 1994; Comerota and White, 1995), although the inability to reliably identify the important intercostal vessels (Kouchoukos and Rokkas, 1993; Svensson *et al.*, 1993a, b), the time required for selective re-implantation (Crawford *et al.*, 1990; Verdant *et al.*, 1995), early occlusion of re-attached vessels (Kouchoukos and Rokkas, 1993) and the lack of a proven benefit of this approach (Crawford *et al.*, 1990) have led to considerable debate. Svensson and colleagues (1991) demonstrated a lower incidence of spinal cord injury when lower intercostal and lumbar arteries were re-implanted. Unfortunately, identification of the artery of Adamkiewicz by pre-operative angiography itself carries a small risk of paraplegia (Kieffer *et al.*, 1989; Svensson *et al.*, 1991) and intra-operative identification of critical intercostal arteries using hydrogen-saturated saline has not been validated (Svensson *et al.*, 1990b).

Despite these controversies, re-implantation of intercostal and lumbar arteries may be important and many authors recommend re-implantation of all patent large lower intercostal and lumbar arteries (Svensson *et al.*, 1991, 1993a; Kouchoukos and Rokkas, 1993; Coselli, 1994; Comerota and White, 1995). In addition, once the aorta is opened, Fogarty balloon occlusion catheters are often used to minimize retrograde bleeding from intercostal arteries into the open aortic lumen (Kouchoukos and Rokkas, 1993). This may prevent further reduction of spinal cord blood flow by a steal phenomenon (i.e. reverse flow *out of* rather than *into* the intercostal arteries). Ultimately, the benefit of re-implanting critical intercostal arteries must be weighed against the additional period of aortic cross-clamping required to identify and re-attach these vessels (Kouchoukos and Rokkas, 1993).

Finally, experimental data suggest an association between hyperglycaemia and the risk of ischaemic neuronal injury. During aortic cross-clamping, glucose provides the spinal cord with a substrate that,

when metabolized, may result in an increased production of oxygen free radicals (LeMay *et al.*, 1987;
Drummond and Moore, 1989). Although supportive human data are inconclusive, it appears prudent
to monitor serum glucose levels in the peri-operative
period and avoid hyperglycaemia.

Monitoring spinal cord function

The primary method available for monitoring spinal
cord function during aortic surgery is measurement
of evoked potentials. Recording of somatosensory-
evoked potentials (SEP) has been the standard form
of evoked-potential monitoring during thoracic aortic surgery, but conflicting results have been reported (Laschinger *et al.*, 1982, 1987a, b; de Mol *et al.*,
1990; Kaplan *et al.*, 1986). In a small study,
Cunningham and colleagues (1987) showed that loss
of the SEP signal for longer than 30 minutes resulted in a 71 per cent incidence of paraplegia. Others
have used SEP to guide intercostal re-implantation
and to assess the adequacy of distal perfusion when
shunt or bypass support is utilized, and have reported satisfactory results (Galla *et al.*, 1994; Schepens *et
al.*, 1994; Guerit *et al.*, 1996). Unfortunately, there
have been reports of the failure of SEP monitoring to
detect or predict post-operative paraplegia
(Ginsburg *et al.*, 1985; Takaki and Okumura, 1985;
Crawford *et al.*, 1988) and the reported incidence of
false-positive SEP is as high as 67 per cent (Crawford
et al., 1988). These limitations, plus the associated
technical difficulties associated with SEP monitoring
(e.g. effects of anaesthetics, temperature and peripheral nerve ischaemia) (McNulty *et al.*, 1991;
Stühmeier *et al.*, 1993) have prompted interest in
motor-evoked (Coles *et al.*, 1982; North *et al.*, 1991;
Mongan *et al.*, 1994) and spinal cord-evoked potentials (Stühmeier *et al.*, 1993; Matsui *et al.*, 1994;
Yamamoto *et al.*, 1994; Shiiya *et al.*, 1995) as methods of improving early detection of spinal cord
ischaemia. Preliminary results of these investigations
have not resolved the role of evoked-potential monitoring during thoracic aortic surgery.

Methods of spinal cord protection

Optimizing spinal cord perfusion by limiting aortic
cross-clamp time and providing adequate distal perfusion are important elements of spinal cord protec-

Table 10.9 *Manoeuvres to reduce spinal cord
ischaemia during surgery of the descending thoracic
aorta*

- Minimize aortic cross-clamp time
- Distal circulatory support
- Re-implantation of critical intercostal and lumbar
  arteries
- CSF drainage
- Hypothermia (systemic, regional aortic, epidural)
- Pharmacotherapy
    Systemic agents (steroids, opioid antagonists,
    barbiturates, calcium-channel antagonists, oxygen
    free-radical scavengers, NMDA antagonists,
    perfluorochemical emulsions)
    Intrathecal agents (papaverine, magnesium,
    tetracaine, perfluorochemical emulsions)

tion during aortic surgery. Although no one method
has been shown to prevent post-operative neurological injury, a number of techniques and pharmacological interventions have been attempted in an
effort to preserve spinal cord function (Table 10.9).

DISTAL CIRCULATORY SUPPORT

The impact of distal circulatory support on the incidence of spinal cord injury after thoracic aortic
surgery remains controversial, because no randomized, controlled study has been performed to resolve
this complex issue.

Verdant and colleagues (1995), employing a Gott
shunt for distal perfusion during 366 consecutive
thoracic aortic aneurysm resections, reported a zero
incidence of paraplegia. While it was a non-randomized study, this represents an impressive argument
for the use of distal perfusion. In a larger yet similar
retrospective, non-randomized evaluation, Lawrie
and colleagues (1994) reported that atriofemoral
bypass reduced the incidence of paresis in 659
patients undergoing descending thoracic aneurysm
resection. Similarly, Svensson and colleagues (1993)
demonstrated that atriofemoral bypass reduced the
risk of spinal cord injury in 832 patients when aortic
cross-clamp times exceeded 40 min. Finally, a meta-
analysis of repair of traumatic aortic rupture
revealed a 19.2 per cent incidence of paraplegia with
simple aortic cross-clamping compared to 6.1 per
cent if distal perfusion was used (von Oppell *et al.*,
1994). In summary, distal circulatory support may
provide perfusion when adequate collateral blood
flow is absent, and it may prolong the safe period of

aortic occlusion for repair of extensive aneurysms and re-attachment of important intercostal arteries.

CSF DRAINAGE

The role of CSF drainage in spinal cord protection is controversial, with experimental studies reporting conflicting results (Wadouh et al., 1984; Bower et al., 1988; Dasmahapatra et al., 1988; Elmore et al., 1991; Nugent, 1992; Kazama et al., 1994; McCullogh et al., 1988; Wisselink et al., 1994; Kaplan et al., 1995). Theoretically, CSF drainage decreases CSF pressure, thereby improving spinal cord perfusion pressure. Despite favourable results in a number of animal models, Crawford and colleagues (1990) failed to show a decrease in the incidence of paraplegia in a prospective, randomized trial of CSF drainage in 98 patients undergoing thoraco-abdominal aneurysm repair. Murray and colleagues (1993) noted similar results in a retrospective clinical analysis. Critics of Crawford's study claim that limiting CSF drainage to a volume of 50 mL may have failed to decrease CSF pressure adequately (Schoenwald et al., 1992; Wisselink et al., 1994), and that in some patients, large volumes of CSF may need to be removed to achieve a beneficial effect (Hollier et al., 1992; Hill et al., 1994; Wisselink et al., 1994). However, the protective effect of CSF drainage alone is said to be limited because it increases perfusion pressure by only 8–10 mmHg, a degree that is unlikely to prevent ischaemia (Kazama et al., 1994). CSF drainage may more effectively augment perfusion when distal circulatory support is used, because distal perfusion controls both determinants of spinal cord perfusion pressure (Kaplan et al., 1995). Data also suggest that CSF removal may have a beneficial effect on spinal cord protection when used in conjunction with methylprednisolone (Woloszyn et al., 1990), naloxone (Acher et al., 1990, 1994; Wynn et al., 1993), or intrathecal papaverine (Svensson et al., 1990a). Finally, large-volume CSF removal has been suggested as an effective treatment for delayed-onset paraplegia (Hill et al., 1994). Despite the controversial evidence, CSF drainage may still prove to be an important adjunct for the prevention of spinal cord injury.

HYPOTHERMIA

Hypothermic reduction of spinal cord metabolism may have a protective effect on spinal cord function by prolonging the period of spinal cord ischaemia that can be tolerated (Vacanti and Ames, 1983; Kouchoukos et al., 1995). It can be accomplished by several different methods: profound systemic hypothermia with circulatory arrest, regional cooling of aortic segments isolated between the cross-clamp, and epidural and intrathecal cooling. Hypothermic circulatory arrest has been associated with a low risk of spinal cord injury in patients undergoing high-risk thoracic aneurysm repair (Grabenwoger et al., 1994; Kieffer et al., 1994; Kouchoukos et al., 1995). Moderate hypothermia (34°C) with atriofemoral bypass has also been used successfully (Frank et al., 1994), while infusion of cold crystalloid solution directly into the excluded segment of the thoracic aorta has also been reported to safely protect vulnerable spinal cord segments (Fehrenbacher et al., 1993). Finally, epidural cooling has been performed in both experimental and clinical studies with favourable preliminary results (Tabayashi et al., 1993; Davison et al., 1994).

PHARMACOLOGICAL METHODS

Many drugs have been used to ameliorate the degree of spinal cord ischaemia, although their clinical efficacy has yet to be demonstrated. Corticosteroids reduce the incidence of experimental spinal cord injury, possibly related to membrane stabilization and prevention of release of chemical mediators, as well as free-radical oxygen scavenging (Laschinger et al., 1984). Opiate receptor antagonists such as naloxone and nalmefene have been used both experimentally and in clinical studies, and act by blocking neuronal activity and reducing tissue metabolism (Yum and Faden, 1990; Acher et al., 1994). Thiopentone was protective in a canine model of spinal cord ischaemia (Nylander et al., 1982), but has not been employed in man. Calcium-channel antagonists such as flunarizine and nimodipine, and oxygen free-radical scavengers such as allopurinol and superoxide dismutase, have all been employed, although with minimal success (Qayumi et al., 1992; Schittek et al., 1992). Neuronal cell death after proximal aortic occlusion may be mediated by extracellular glutamate, a neurotoxin that stimulates the N-methyl-D-aspartate (NMDA) channel, causing the intracellular influx of calcium and subsequent cell death (Choi and Rothman, 1990). NMDA-receptor antagonists that block this channel may thus prove to be an effective way to reduce the incidence of neurological injury during thoracic aorta surgery (Follis *et al.*, 1994). Systemic and intrathecal magnesium may also improve neurological outcome, possibly by antagonism of this receptor (Altura and Altura, 1984; Simpson *et al.*, 1994). Finally, a number of agents including magnesium, papaverine, and tetracaine may be administered intrathecally for spinal cord protection (Breckwoldt *et al.*, 1991; Simpson *et al.*, 1994). As with all of the other agents mentioned above, none has been proven clinically effective.

In summary, spinal cord injury during thoracic aortic surgery is a multifactorial event that is not completely preventable. However, a combination of measures including distal circulatory support, maintenance of modest degrees of proximal hypertension and hypothermia, CSF drainage, re-implantation of critical intercostal arteries, certain drugs, and most importantly, limiting the duration of aortic cross-clamping, may be the most promising and sensible approach to reduce the incidence of this feared complication.

POST-OPERATIVE CONSIDERATIONS

Post-operative renal insufficiency occurs in about 5 per cent of patients after thoracic aortic surgery and in approximately 10–15 per cent of patients after thoraco-abdominal aortic surgery, and is associated with a high mortality rate (37 per cent in-hospital survival) (Svensson *et al.*, 1989). Significant risk factors include the aortic clamp time (and renal ischaemia time), the presence of aortic dissection, advanced age and primary renal dysfunction. Post-operative and intra-operative use of low-dose dopamine to augment mesenteric and renal blood flow often results in increased urine production, but preservation of renal function has not been proven. The possibility of renal artery thrombosis or dissection should be considered in any patient when urinary output ceases abruptly after any operation involving the thoracic or thoraco-abdominal aorta, especially if the patient is well hydrated and does not respond to diuretics.

Coagulopathy is a frequent occurrence and is related to the degree and duration of visceral ischaemia as well as total blood volume loss. Coagulation parameters should be monitored frequently, with coagulation factors and platelets replaced accordingly. Fibrinolysis is typically treated with continuous infusion of synthetic antifibrinolytics such as ϵ-aminocaproic acid or tranexamic acid.

Pulmonary complications including atelectasis, pneumonia, adult respiratory distress syndrome (ARDS) and pulmonary insufficiency are common after surgery of the thoracic aorta. Pulmonary insufficiency, defined as the need for ventilatory support for more than three days post-operatively, occurs in as many as 25 per cent of patients. Aetiological factors include pre-operative pulmonary dysfunction related to smoking or chronic obstructive pulmonary disease (COPD), as well as the presence of a thoracotomy incision and division of the diaphragm during the operation. Clinically significant pleural effusions are common post-operatively and compound the problem. Judicious administration of fluid, pulmonary toilet and use of bronchodilators when indicated, as well as adequate post-operative analgesia, are important aspects of post-operative care.

Controversy currently exists over the use of epidural anaesthesia and analgesia for this type of surgery. A number of studies have demonstrated the beneficial effects of both thoracic and high lumbar epidural block, not only on post-operative pain, but also in attenuating the adrenal cortical stress response, protein catabolism, the hypercoagulable state and immunosuppression, as well as pulmonary and myocardial morbidity (Liu *et al.*, 1995). Unfortunately, there are no randomized trials evaluating the effects of epidural anaesthesia and analgesia on outcome after thoracic aortic surgery. Clinical experience suggests that the benefits are most apparent in patients who require thoracic or thoraco-abdominal incisions. Improved outcome in terms of decreased frequency of post-operative pulmonary complications after these procedures requires continued epidural analgesia well into the post-operative period. Nonetheless, until outcome studies are performed to compare combined epidural–general anaesthesia with general anaesthesia alone for thoracic aortic surgery, the use of epidural block remains a decision for individual anaesthetists and surgeons to make between them.

REFERENCES

Aakhus, S., Aadahl, P., Strömholm, T. and Myhre, H.O. 1995. Increased left ventricular contractility during cross-clamping of the descending thoracic aorta. *Journal of Cardiothoracic and Vascular Anesthesia* **9**, 497–502.

Acher, C.W., Wynn, M.M. and Archibald, J. 1990. Naloxone and spinal fluid drainage as adjuncts in the surgical treatment of thoracoabdominal and thoracic aneurysms. *Surgery* **108**, 755–762.

Acher, C.W., Wynn, M.M., Hoch, J.R. *et al.* 1994. Combined use of cerebral spinal fluid drainage and naloxone reduces the risk of paraplegia in thoracoabdominal aneurysm repair. *Journal of Vascular Surgery* **19**, 236–248.

Altura, B.T. and Altura, B.M. 1984. Interactions of magnesium and potassium on cerebral vessels. Aspects in view of stroke. *Magnesium* **3**, 195–211.

Ataka, K., Okada, M., Yoshimura, N. *et al.* 1993. Surgical treatment for aneurysms of the descending aorta using temporary perfusion by a centrifugal pump: clinical analysis of 33 cases. *Artificial Organs* **17**, 901–905.

Banistor, J. and Torrance, R.W. 1960. The effect of tracheal pressure upon flow: pressure relations in the vascular bed of isolated lungs. *Quarterly Journal of Experimental Physiology* **45**, 352–637.

Barcroft, H. and Samaan, A. 1935. The explanation of the increase in systemic flow caused by occluding the descending thoracic aorta. *American Journal of Physiology* **85**, 47–61.

Bavaria, J.E., Woo, J., Hall, R.A. *et al.* 1995. Retrograde cerebral and distal aortic perfusion during ascending and thoracoabdominal aortic operations. *Annals of Thoracic Surgery* **60**, 345–353.

Bazaral, M.G., Welch, M., Golding, L.A.R. and Badhwar, K. 1990. Comparison of brachial and radial arterial pressure monitoring in patients undergoing coronary artery bypass surgery. *Anesthesiology* **73**, 38–45.

Beattie, C. and Frank, S.M. 1993. Anesthesia for major vascular surgery. In Rogers, M., Tinker, T. and Covino, B. (eds) *Principles and practice of anesthesiology*. St Louis, MO: Mosby, 1931–1967.

Benumof, J.L. 1995. *Anesthesia for thoracic surgery*. Philadelphia: W.B. Saunders, 386.

Berkowitz, H.D. and Shetty, S. 1974. Renin release and renal cortical ischemia following aortic cross-clamping. *Archives of Surgery* **109**, 612–617.

Biglioli, P., Spirito, R., Pompilio, G. *et al.* 1995. Descending thoracic aorta aneurysmectomy: left-left centrifugal pump *versus* simple clamping technique. *Cardiovascular Surgery* **3**, 511–518.

Borst, H.G., Jurmann, M., Bühner, B. and Laas, J. 1994.

Risk of replacement of descending aorta with a standardized left heart bypass technique. *Journal of Thoracic and Cardiovascular Surgery* **107**, 126–133.

Bower, T.C., Murray, M.J. and Gloviczki, P. 1988. Effects of thoracic aortic occlusion and cerebrospinal fluid drainage on regional spinal cord blood flow in dogs: correlation with neurologic outcome. *Journal of Vascular Surgery* **9**, 135–144.

Brant, B., Armstrong, R. and Vetto, R.M. 1970. Vasodepressor factor in declamp shock production. *Surgery* **67**, 650.

Breckwoldt, W.L., Genco, C.M. and Connolly, R.J. 1991. Spinal cord protection during aortic occlusion: Efficacy of intrathecal tetracaine. *Annals of Thoracic Surgery* **51**, 959–963.

Brusoni, B., Colombo, A., Merlo, L. *et al.* 1978. Hemodynamic and metabolic changes induced by temporary clamping of thoracic aorta. *European Surgical Research* **10**, 206–216.

Campos, J.H., Ajax, T.J., Knutson, R.M. *et al.* 1990. Case conference 5–1990. A 76–year-old man undergoing an emergency descending thoracic aortic aneurysm repair has multiple intraoperative and postoperative complications. *Journal of Cardiothoracic Anesthesia* **4**, 631–645.

Cernaianu, A.C., Olah, A., Cilley, Jr. *et al.* 1993. Effect of sodium nitroprusside on paraplegia during cross-clamping of the thoracic aorta. *Annals of Thoracic Surgery* **56**, 1035–1038.

Choi, D.W. and Rothman, S.M. 1990. The role of glutamate neurotoxicity in hypoxic–ischemic neuronal death. *Annual Review of Neuroscience* **13**, 171–183.

Cigarroa, J.E., Isselbacher, E.M., DeSanctis, R.W. and Eagle, K.A. 1993. Diagnostic imaging in the evaluation of suspected aortic dissection. Old standards and new directions. *New England Journal of Medicine* **328**, 1637–1638.

Clark, F.J.S., Mutch, W.A.C., Sutton, I.R. *et al.* 1992. Treatment of proximal aortic hypertension after thoracic aortic cross-clamping in dogs: phlebotomy versus sodium nitroprusside/isoflurane. *Anesthesiology* **77**, 357–364.

Cohen, J.A., Denisco, R.A., Richards, T.S. *et al.* 1986. Hazardous placement of a Robertshaw-type endobronchial tube. *Anesthesia and Analgesia* **65**, 100–101.

Cohen, J.R., Sardari, F., Paul, J. *et al.* 1992. Increased intestinal permeability: implications for thoracoabdominal aneurysm repair. *Annals of Vascular Surgery* **6**, 433–437.

Coles, J.G., Wilson, G.J., Sima, A.F. *et al.* 1982. Intraoperative detection of spinal cord ischemia using somatosensory cortical evoked potentials during thoracic aortic occlusion. *Annals of Thoracic Surgery* **34**, 299–306.

Comerota, A.J. and White, J.V. 1995. Reducing morbidity of thoracoabdominal aneurysm repair by preliminary axillofemoral bypass. *American Journal of Surgery* **170**, 218–222.

Connelly, G.P., Arkoff, H., McKenney, P.A. and Davidoff, R. 1995a. Left ventricular function during proximal aortic crossclamping and left atrial–femoral bypass. *Anesthesiology* **83**, A56.

Connelly, G.P., Arkoff, H., McKenney, P.A. and Davidoff, R. 1995b. Pressure-flow data does not reflect left ventricular function during proximal aortic crossclamping and left atrial–femoral bypass. *Anesthesiology* **83**, A57.

Contino, J.P., Follette, D.M., Berkoff, H.A. *et al.* 1994. Use of carmeda-coated femoral-femoral bypass during repair of traumatic aortic pseudoaneurysms. *Archives of Surgery* **129**, 933–939.

Coselli, J.S. 1994. Thoracoabdominal aortic aneurysms: experience with 372 patients. *Journal of Cardiac Surgery* **9**, 638–647.

Crawford, E.S. 1990. The diagnosis and management of aortic dissection. *Journal of the American Medical Association* **264**, 2537–2541.

Crawford, E.S. and Rubio, P.A. 1973. Reappraisal of adjuncts to avoid ischemia in the treatment of aneurysms of descending thoracic aorta. *Journal of Thoracic and Cardiovascular Surgery* **66**, 693–704.

Crawford, E.S., Mizrahi, E.M. and Hess, K.R. 1988. The impact of distal aortic perfusion and somatosensory evoked potential monitoring on prevention of paraplegia after aortic aneurysm operation. *Journal of Thoracic and Cardiovascular Surgery* **95**, 357–367.

Crawford, E.S., Svensson, LG., Hess, K.R. *et al.* 1990. A prospective randomized study of cerebrospinal fluid drainage to prevent paraplegia after high-risk surgery on the thoracoabdominal aorta. *Journal of Vascular Surgery* **13**, 36–46.

Cunningham, J.N., Laschinger, J.C. and Spencer, F.C. 1987. Monitoring of somatosensory evoked potentials during surgical procedures on the thoracoabdominal aorta, Part IV. *Journal of Thoracic and Cardiovascular Surgery* **94**, 275–285.

D'Ambra, M.N., Dewhirst, W., Jacobs, M. *et al.* 1988. Cross-clamping the thoracic aorta: effect on intracranial pressure. *Circulation* **78** (Suppl. 3), 198–202.

Dasmahapatra, H.K., Coles, J.G. and Wilson, G.J. 1988. Relationship between cerebrospinal fluid dynamics and reversible spinal cord ischemia during experimental thoracic aortic occlusion. *Journal of Thoracic and Cardiovascular Surgery* **95**, 920–923.

Davison, J.K., Cambria, R.P., Vierra, D.J. *et al.* 1994. Epidural cooling for regional spinal cord hypothermia during thoracoabdominal aneurysm repair. *Journal of Vascular Surgery* **20**, 304–310.

de Mol, B.A.J.M, Boezeman, E.H.J.F. and Hamerlijnck, R.P.H.M. 1990. Experimental and clinical use of somatosensory evoked potentials in surgery of aneurysms of the descending thoracic aorta. *Thoracic and Cardiovascular Surgeon* **38**, 146–150.

Drummond, J.C. and Moore, S.S. 1989. The influence of dextrose administration on neurologic outcome after temporary spinal cord ischemia in the rabbit. *Anesthesiology* **70**, 64–70.

Egener, T.H., O'Connor, B. and Leckie, R.S. 1993. Temperature maintenance during prolonged thoracoabdominal aneurysm repair by a simple heat exchanger in a centrifugal perfusion circuit. *Anesthesia and Analgesia* **76**, 1359–1362.

Elmore, J.R., Glovickzi, P. and Harper, M. 1991. Failure of motor evoked potentials to predict neurologic outcome in experimental thoracic aortic occlusion. *Journal of Vascular Surgery* **14**, 131–139.

Erbel, R. 1993. Role of transesophageal echocardiography in dissection of the aorta and evaluation of degenerative aortic disease. *Cardiology Clinics* **11**, 461–472.

Ergin, M.A., Galla, J.D., Lansman, S.L. *et al.* 1991. Distal perfusion methods for surgery on the descending aorta. *Seminars in Thoracic and Cardiovascular Surgery* **3**, 293–299.

Fehrenbacher, J.W., McCready, R.A., Hormuth, D.A. *et al.* 1993. One-stage segmental resection of extensive thoracoabdominal aneurysms with left-sided heart bypass. *Journal of Vascular Surgery* **18**, 366–371.

Follis, F., Miller, K., Scremin, O.U. *et al.* 1994. NMDA receptor blockade and spinal cord ischemia due to aortic crossclamping in the rat model. *Canadian Journal of Neurological Science* **21**, 227–232.

Forbes, A.D. and Ashbaugh, D.G. 1994. Mechanical circulatory support during repair of thoracic aortic injuries improves morbidity and prevents spinal cord injury. *Archives of Surgery* **129**, 494–498.

Frank, S.M., Norris, E. and Crawley, H. 1983. Right and left arm blood pressure discrepancies in vascular surgery patients. *Anesthesiology* **73**, A105.

Frank, S.M., Parker, S.D., Rock, P. *et al*. 1994. Moderate hypothermia, with partial bypass and segmental sequential repair for thoracoabdominal aortic aneurysm. *Journal of Vascular Surgery* **19**, 687–697.

Galla, J.D., Ergin, M.A., Sadeghi, A.M. *et al*. 1994. A new technique using somatosensory evoked potential guidance during descending and thoracoabdominal aortic repairs. *Journal of Cardiac Surgery* **9**, 662–672.

Gelman, S. 1995. The pathophysiology of aortic cross-clamping and unclamping. *Anesthesiology* **82**, 1026–1060.

Gelman, S., Bredle, D.L., Bradley, W.E. and Cain, S.M. 1990. Angiotensin and α-adrenoreceptor activation play a role in hemodynamic response to aortic cross-clamping. *American Journal of Physiology* **259**, H68–H73.

Gelman, S., Khazalei, M.B., Orr, R. and Henderson, T. 1994. Blood volume redistribution during cross-clamping of the descending aorta. *Anesthesia & Analgesia* **78**, 219–224.

Gelman, S., Rabbani, S. and Bradley, E.L. 1988a. Inferior and superior vena caval blood flows during cross-clamping of the thoracic aorta in pigs. *Journal of Thoracic and Cardiovascular Surgery* **96**, 387–392.

Gelman, S., McDowell, H., Varner, P.D. *et al*. 1988b. The reason for cardiac output reduction following aortic crossclamping. *American Journal of Surgery* **155**, 578–5786.

Gelman, S., Reves, J.G., Fowler, K. *et al*. 1983. Regional blood flow during cross-clamping of the thoracic aorta and infusion of sodium nitroprusside. *Journal of Thoracic and Cardiovascular Surgery* **85**, 287–291.

Gelman, S., Roytblat, L., Henderson, T. and Bradley, E.L. 1989. Arterial hypertension and humoral factors during crossclamping of the thoracic aorta. *Anesthesiology* **71**, 3A.

Gharagozloo, F., Larson, J., Dausmann, M.J. *et al*. 1996. Spinal cord protection during surgical procedures on the descending thoracic and thoracoabdominal aorta. *Chest* **109**, 799–809.

Ginsburg, H.H., Shetter, A.G. and Raudzens, P.A. 1985. Postoperative paraplegia with preserved intraoperative somatosensory evoked potentials. *Journal of Neurosurgery* **63**, 296–300.

Godet, G., Bertrand, M., Coriat, P. *et al*. 1990. Comparison of isoflurane with sodium nitroprusside for controlling hypertension during thoracic aortic cross-clamping. *Journal of Cardiothoracic Anesthesia* **4**, 177–184.

Gorman, R.B., Merritt, W.T., Greenspun, H. *et al*. 1993. Aneurysmal compression of the trachea and right mainstem bronchus complicating thoracoabdominal aneurysm repair. *Anesthesiology* **79**, 1424–1427.

Grabenwöger, M., Ehrlich, M., Simon, P. *et al*. 1994. Thoracoabdominal aneurysm repair: spinal cord protection using profound hypothermia and circulatory arrest. *Journal of Cardiovascular Surgery* **9**, 679–684.

Gregoretti, S., Gelman, S., Henderson, T. and Bradley, E.L. 1990. Hemodynamics and oxygen uptake below and above aortic occlusion during crossclamping of the thoracic aorta and sodium nitroprusside infusion. *Journal of Thoracic and Cardiovascular Surgery* **100**, 830–836.

Guerit, JM. Verhelst, R. Rubay, J. *et al*. 1996. Multilevel somatosensory evoked potentials (SEPs) for spinal cord monitoring in descending thoracic and thoraco-abdominal aortic surgery. *European Journal of Cardiothoracic Surgery* **10**, 93–103.

Hanowell, L.H., Siegel, L.C., Frank, R. and Allen, R.H. 1996. Leftward deviation of the interatrial septum during left heart bypass for repair of a thoracic aortic aneurysm. *Journal of Cardiothoracic and Vascular Anesthesia* **10**, 251–252.

Hantler, C.B. and Knight, P.R. 1982. Intracranial hypertension following cross-clamping of the thoracic aorta. *Anesthesiology* **1982**, 146–147.

Hill, A.B., Kalman, P.G., Johnston, K.W. and Vosu, H.A. 1994. Reversal of delayed-onset paraplegia after thoracic aortic surgery with cerebrospinal fluid drainage. *Journal of Vascular Surgery* **20**, 315–317.

Hollier, L.H., Money, S.R., Naslund, T.C. *et al*. 1992. Risk of spinal cord dysfunction in patients undergoing thoracoabdominal aortic replacement. *American Journal of Surgery* **164**, 210–213.

Hug, H.R. and Taber, R.E. 1969. Bypass flow requirements during thoracic aneurysmectomy with particular attention to the prevention of left heart failure. *Journal of Thoracic and Cardiovascular Surgery* **57**, 203–213.

Imagawa, H., Takano, H., Kato, M. *et al*. 1993. Evaluation of left ventricular function utilizing transesophageal echocardiography during and after thoracic aortic aneurysm repair. *European Journal of Cardiothoracic Surgery* **7**, 371–375.

Janusz, M.T. 1994. Experience with thoracoabdominal aortic aneurysm resection. *The American Journal of Surgery* **167**, 501–504.

Jex, R.K., Schaff, H.V., Piehler, J.M. *et al*. 1986. Early and late results following repair of dissections of the descending thoracic aorta. *Journal of Vascular Surgery* **3**, 226–237.

Joob, A.W., Harman, P.K., Kaiser, D.L. and Kron, I.L. 1986. The effect of renin-angiotensin system blockade on visceral blood flow during and after thoracic aortic cross-clamping. *Journal of Thoracic and Cardiovascular Surgery* **91**, 411–418.

Kaplan, B.J., Friedman, W.A. and Alexander, J.A. 1986. Somatosensory evoked potential monitoring of spinal cord ischemia during aortic operations. *Neurosurgery* **19**, 82–90.

Kaplan, D.K., Atsumi, N., D'Ambra, M.N. and Vlahakes, G.J. 1995. Distal circulatory support for thoracic aortic operations: effects on intracranial pressure. *Annals of Thoracic Surgery* **59**, 448–452.

Katz, N.M., Blackstone, E.H. and Kirklin, J.W. 1981. Incremental risk factors for spinal cord injury following operation for acute traumatic aortic transection. *Journal of Thoracic and Cardiovascular Surgery* **81**, 669–674.

Kazama, S., Masaki, Y., Maruyama, S. and Ishihara, A. 1994. Effect of altering cerebrospinal fluid pressure on spinal cord blood flow. *Annals of Thoracic Surgery* **58**, 112–115.

Kazui, T., Komatsu, S. and Yokoyama, H. 1987. Surgical treatment of aneurysms of the thoracic aorta with the aid of partial cardiopulmonary bypass: an analysis of 95 patients. *Annals of Thoracic Surgery* **43**, 622–627.

Kieffer, E., Koskas, F., Walden, R. *et al.* 1994. Hypothermic circulatory arrest for thoracic aneurysmectomy through left-sided thoracotomy. *Journal of Vascular Surgery* **19**, 457–464.

Kieffer, E., Thierry, R. and Chiras, J. 1989. Preoperative spinal cord arteriography in aneurysmal disease of the descending thoracic and thoracoabdominal aorta: Preliminary results in 45 patients. *Annals of Vascular Surgery* **3**, 34–26.

Kouchoukos, N.T., Daily, B.B., Rokkas, C.K. *et al.* 1995. Hypothermic bypass and circulatory arrest for operations on the descending thoracic and thoracoabdominal aorta. *Annals of Thoracic Surgery* **60**, 67–77.

Kouchoukos, N.T., Lell, W.A., Karp, R.B. and Samuelson, P.N. 1979. Hemodynamic effects of aortic clamping and decompression with a temporary shunt for resection of the descending thoracic aorta. *Surgery* **85**, 25–30.

Kouchoukos, N.T. and Rokkas, C.K. 1993. Descending thoracic and thoracoabdominal aortic surgery for aneurysm or dissection: How do we minimize the risk of spinal cord injury? *Seminars in Thoracic and Cardiovascular Surgery* **5**, 47–54.

Kopman, E.A. and Ferguson, T.B. 1977. Intraoperative monitoring of femoral artery pressure during replacement of aneurysm of descending thoracic aorta. *Anesthesia and Analgesia* **56**, 603–605.

Laschinger, J.C., Cunningham, N.J. and Catinella, FP. 1982. Detection and prevention of intraoperative spinal cord ischemia after cross-clamping of the thoracic aorta: Use of somatosensory evoked potentials. *Surgery* **92**, 1109–1117.

Laschinger, J.C., Cunningham, J.N. and Baumann, F.G. 1987a. Monitoring of somatosensory evoked potentials during surgical procedures on the thoracoabdominal aorta, Part III. *Journal of Thoracic and Cardiovascular Surgery* **94**, 271–274.

Laschinger, J.C., Cunningham, J.N. and Cooper, M.M. 1987b. Monitoring of somatosensory evoked potentials during surgical procedures on the thoracoabdominal aorta, Part I. *Journal of Thoracic and Cardiovascular Surgery* **94**, 260–265.

Laschinger, J.C., Cunningham, J.N. and Cooper, M.M. 1984. Prevention of ischemic spinal cord injury following aortic cross-clamping: Use of corticosteroids. *Annals of Thoracic Surgery* **38**, 500–507.

Laschinger, J.C., Cunningham, J.N. and Nathan, I.M. 1983. Experimental and clinical assessment of the adequacy of partial bypass in maintenance of spinal cord blood flow during operations on the thoracic aorta. *Annals of Thoracic Surgery* **36**, 417–426.

Lawrie, G.M., Earle, N. and De Bakey, M.E. 1994. Evolution of surgical techniques for aneurysms of the descending thoracic aorta: twenty-nine years experience with 659 patients. *Journal of Cardiac Surgery* **9**, 648–661.

Lee, Y. and Jihayel, A. 1991. Thoracic aortic aneurysm repair: Hemodynamic changes and complications. In Casthely, P.A. and Bregman, D. (eds), *Cardiopulmonary bypass: physiology, related complications, and pharmacology*. New York: Futura, 489–507.

LeMay, D.R., Neal, S. and Neal, S. 1987. Paraplegia in the rat induced by aortic cross-clamping: Model characterization and glucose exacerbation of neurologic deficit. *Journal of Vascular Surgery* **6**, 383–390.

Lerberg, D.B., Hardesty, R.I. and Siewers, R.D. 1982. Coarctation of the aorta in infants and children: 25 years of experience. *Annals of Thoracic Surgery* **33**, 159–170.

Liu, S., Carpenter, R.L. and Neal, J.M. 1995. Epidural anesthesia and analgesia: Their role in postoperative outcome. *Anesthesiology* **82**, 1474–1506.

Livesay, J.J., Cooley, D.A., Ventemiglia, R.A. *et al*. 1985. Surgical experience in descending thoracic aneurysmectomy with and without adjuncts to avoid ischemia. *Annals of Thoracic Surgery* **39**, 37–46.

Longo, T., Marchetti, G. and Vercellio, G. 1969. Coronary hemodynamic changes induced by aortic cross-clamping. *Journal of Cardiovascular Surgery* **10**, 36–42.

Mandelbaum, I. and Webb, M.K. 1963. Left ventricular function during cross-clamping of the descending thoracic aorta. *Journal of the American Medical Association* **186**, 229–231.

Marini, C.P. and Cunningham, Jr. J.N. 1993. Issues surrounding spinal cord protection. In R. Karp *et al*. (eds). *Advances in Cardiac Surgery*. Vol 4, St Louis, MO: Mosby-Year Book, Inc, 89–107.

Marini, C.P., Grubbs, P.E., Toporoff, B. *et al*. 1989. Effect of sodium nitroprusside on spinal cord perfusion and paraplegia during aortic cross-clamping. *Annals of Thoracic Surgery* **47**, 379–383.

Matsui, Y., Goh, K., Shiiya, N. *et al*. 1994. Clinical application of evoked spinal cord potentials elicited by direct stimulation of the cord during temporary occlusion of the thoracic aorta. *Journal of Thoracic and Cardiovascular Surgery* **107**, 1519–1527.

McCullough, J.L., Hollier, L.H. and Nugent, M. 1988. Paraplegia after thoracic aortic occlusion: Influence of cerebrospinal fluid drainage. *Journal of Vascular Surgery* **7**, 153–160.

McNulty, S., Arkoosh, V. and Goldberg, M. 1991. The relevance of somatosensory evoked potentials during thoracic aorta aneurysm repair. *Journal of Cardiothoracic and Vascular Anesthesia* **5**, 262–265.

Mongan, P.D., Peterson, R.E. and Williams, D. 1994. Spinal evoked potentials are predictive of neurologic function in a porcine model of aortic occlusion. *Anesthesia and Analgesia* **78**, 257–266.

Mora, M., Chuma, R., Kiichi, Y. *et al*. 1993. The anesthetic management of patient with a thoracic aortic aneurysm that caused compression of the left mainstem bronchus and the right pulmonary artery. *Journal of Cardiothoracic and Vascular Anesthesia* **7**, 579–584.

Moore, W.M. and Hollier, L.H. 1991. The influence of severity of spinal cord ischemia in the etiology of delayed-onset paraplegia. *Annals of Surgery* **213**, 427–432.

Murray, M.J., Bower, T.C., Oliver, W.C. *et al*. 1993. Effects of cerebrospinal fluid drainage in patients undergoing thoracic and thoracoabdominal aortic surgery. *Journal of Cardiothoracic and Vascular Anesthesia* **7**, 266–272.

Mutch, W.A.C., Thomson, I.R., Teskey, J. *et al*. 1990. Phlebotomy reverses the hemodynamic consequences of thoracic aortic cross-clamping. *Anesthesiology* **73**, A630.

Najafi, H. 1993. Descending aortic aneurysmectomy without adjuncts to avoid ischemia – 1993 update. *Annals of Thoracic Surgery* **55**, 1042–5104.

Najafi, H., Javid, H., Hunter, J. and Serry, C. 1980. Descending aortic aneurysmectomy without adjuncts to avoid ischemia. *Annals of Thoracic Surgery* **30**, 326–335.

Nicolosi, A.C., Almassi, G.H., Bousamra, M. *et al*. 1996. Mortality and neurologic morbidity after repair of traumatic aortic disruption. *Annals of Thoracic Surgery* **61**, 875–878.

Normann, N.A., Taylor, A.A., Crawford, E.S. *et al*. 1983. Catecholamine release during and after cross clamping of descending thoracic aorta. *Journal of Surgical Research* **34**, 97–103.

North, R.B., Drenger, B. and Beattie, C. 1991. Monitoring of spinal cord stimulation evoked potentials during thoracoabdominal aneurysm surgery. *Neurosurgery* **28**, 325–330.

Nugent, M. 1992. Pro: Cerebrospinal fluid drainage prevents paraplegia. *Journal of Cardiothoracic and Vascular Anesthesia* **6**, 366–368.

Nylander, W.A., Plunkett, R.J. and Hammon, J.W. 1982. Thiopental modification of spinal cord injury in the dog. *Annals of Thoracic Surgery* **33**, 64–68.

O'Rourke, K., Beattie, C. and Walman, A.T. 1985. Acidosis during high cross-clamp surgery. *Anesthesiology* **63**, A266.

Qayumi, A.K., Janusz, M.T., Jamieson, W.R.E. and Lyster, D.M. 1992. Pharmacologic interventions for prevention of spinal cord injury caused by aortic crossclamping. *Journal of Thoracic and Cardiovascular Surgery* **104**, 256–261.

Read, R.A., Moore, E.E., Moore, F.A. and Haenel, J.B. 1993. Partial left heart bypass for thoracic aorta repair. *Archives of Surgery* **128**, 746–752.

Reed, C.C. and Stratford, T.B. 1989. *Cardiopulmonary bypass*. Houston, TX.: Surgimedics. 452–460.

Roberts, A.J., Nora, J.D., Hughes, W.A. *et al*. 1983. Cardiac and renal responses to cross-clamping of the descending thoracic aorta. *Journal of Thoracic and Cardiovascular Surgery* **86**, 732–741.

Roizen, M.F., Beaupre, P.N., Albert, R.A. *et al*. 1984. Monitoring with two-dimensional transesophageal echocardiography. Comparison of myocardial function in patients undergoing supraceliac, suprarenal-infraceliac, or infrarenal aortic occlusion. *Journal of Vascular Surgery* **1**, 300–305.

Ryan, T., Mannion, D., O'Brien, W. *et al*. 1993. Spinal cord perfusion pressure in dogs after control of proximal aortic hypertension during thoracic aortic cross-clamping with esmolol or sodium nitroprusside. *Anesthesiology* **78**, 317–325.

Sæther, O.D., Juul, R.M , Aadahl P. *et al*. 1996. Cerebral haemodynamics during thoracic and thoracoabdominal aortic aneurysm repair. *European Journal of Vascular and Endovascular Surgery* **12**, 81–85.

Safi, H.J., Bartoli, S., Hess, K.R. *et al*. 1994. Neurologic deficit in patients at high risk with thoracoabdominal aortic aneurysms: the role of cerebral spinal fluid drainage and distal aortic perfusion. *Journal of Vascular Surgery* **20**, 434–443.

Saleh, S.A., Crawford, E.S. and Bomberger, R.A. 1982. Intraoperative acid-base management for the resection of thoracoabdominal aneurysms: A comparison of continuous infusion of sodium bicarbonate versus the bolus. *Anesthesia and Analgesia* **61**, A213.

Sander-Jensen, K., Krogager, G. and Pettersson, G. 1995. Left atrial-aortic/femoral bypass with a centrifugal pump without systemic heparin during surgery on the descending aorta. *Artificial Organs* **19**, 774–776.

Schepens, M.A.A.M., Boezeman, E.H.J.F., Hamerlijnck, R.P.H.M. *et al*. 1994. Somatosensory evoked potentials during exclusion and reperfusion of critical aortic segments in thoracoabdominal aortic aneurysm surgery. *Journal of Cardiac Surgery* **9**, 692–702.

Schittek, A., Bennink, G.B.W.E., Cooley, D.A. and Langford, L.A. 1992. Spinal cord protection with intravenous nimodipine. *Journal of Thoracic and Cardiovascular Surgery* **104**, 1100–1105.

Schoenwald, P., Gottlieb, A., Lewis, B. and O'Hara, P. 1992. Cerebrospinal fluid pressure (CSFP) during aortic cross-clamp (XC) as a predictor of neurologic outcome during thoracoabdominal aneurysm repair. *Anesthesiology* **77**, A71.

Shenaq, S.A., Casar, G., Chelly, J.E. *et al*. 1987. Continuous monitoring of mixed venous oxygen saturation during aortic surgery. *Chest* **92**, 796–799.

Shenaq, S.A. and Svensson, L.G. 1993. Paraplegia following aortic surgery. *Journal of Cardiothoracic and Vascular Anesthesia* **7**, 81–94.

Shiiya, N., Yasuda, K., Matsui, Y. *et al*. 1995. Spinal cord protection during thoracoabdominal aortic aneurysm repair: Results of selective reconstruction of the critical segmental arteries guided by evoked spinal cord potential monitoring. *Journal of Vascular Surgery* **21**, 970–975.

Shine, T. and Nugent, M. 1990. Sodium nitroprusside decreases spinal cord perfusion pressure during descending thoracic aortic cross-clamping in the dog. *Journal of Cardiothoracic Anesthesia* **4**, 185–193.

Silverstein, P.R., Caldera, D.L., Cullen, D.J. *et al*. 1979. Avoiding the hemodynamic consequences of aortic cross-clamping and unclamping. *Anesthesiology* **50**, 462–466.

Simpson, J.I., Eide, T.R., Schiff, G.A. *et al*. 1994. Intrathecal magnesium sulfate protects the spinal cord from ischemic injury during thoracic aortic cross-clamping. *Anesthesiology* **81**, 1493–1499.

Simpson, J.I., Eide, T.R., Schiff, G.A. *et al*. 1995. Isoflurane versus sodium nitroprusside for the control of proximal hypertension during thoracic aortic cross-clamping: effects on spinal cord ischemia. *Journal of Cardiothoracic and Vascular Anesthesia* **9**, 491–496.

Slogoff, S., Keats, A.S. and Arlund, C. 1983. On the safety of radial artery cannulation. *Anesthesiology* **59**, 42–47.

Stockland, O., Miller, M.M., Ilebekk, A. and Kiil, F. 1980. Mechanism of hemodynamic responses to occlusion of the descending thoracic aorta. *American Journal of Physiology* **238**, H423–429.

Stühmeier, K.D., Grabitz, K., Mainzer, B. *et al*. 1993. Use of the electrospinogram for predicting harmful spinal cord ischemia during repair of thoracic or thoracoabdominal aortic aneurysms. *Anesthesiology* **79**, 1170–1176.

Svensson, L.G., Klepp, P. and Hinder, R.A. 1986a. Spinal cord anatomy of the baboon: Comparison with man and implications for spinal cord blood flow during thoracic aortic cross-clamping. *South African Journal of Surgery* **24**, 32–34.

Svensson, L.G., Von Ritter, C.M. and Groeneveld, H.T. 1986b. Cross-clamping of the thoracic aorta. *Annals of Surgery* **204**, 38–47.

Svensson, L.G., Cosselli, J.S., Safi, H.J. *et al*. 1989. Appraisal of adjuncts to prevent acute renal failure after surgery on the thoracic and thoracoabdominal aorta. *Journal of Vascular Surgery* **10**, 230–239.

Svensson, L.G., Grum, D.F. and Bednarski, M. 1990a. Appraisal of cerebrospinal fluid alterations during aortic surgery with intrathecal papaverine administration and cerebrospinal fluid drainage. *Journal of Vascular Surgery* **11**, 423–429.

Svensson, L.G., Patel, V. and Coselli, J.S. 1990b. Preliminary report of localization of spinal cord blood supply by hydrogen during aortic operations.

Annals of Thoracic Surgery **49**, 528–535.

Svensson, L.G., Patel, V. and Robinson, M.F. 1991. Influence of preservation or perfusion of intraoperatively identified spinal cord blood supply on spinal motor evoked potentials and paraplegia after aortic surgery. *Journal of Vascular Surgery* **13**, 355–365.

Svensson, L.G. and Crawford, E.S. 1992a. Aortic dissection and aortic aneurysm surgery: Clinical observations, experimental investigations, and statistical analyses, Part I. *Current Problems in Surgery* **November**, 826–909.

Svensson, L.G. and Crawford, E.S. 1992b. Aortic dissection and aortic aneurysm surgery: Clinical observations, experimental investigations, and statistical analyses, Part II. *Current Problems in Surgery* **December**, 922–1011.

Svensson, L.G. and Crawford, E.S. 1993. Aortic dissection and aortic aneurysm surgery: Clinical observations, experimental investigations, and statistical analyses, Part III. *Current Problems in Surgery* **January**, 10–163.

Svensson, L.G., Crawford, E.S., Hess, K.R. *et al*. 1993a. Experience with 1509 patients undergoing thoracoabdominal aortic operations. *Journal of Vascular Surgery* **17**, 357–370.

Svensson, L.G., Crawford, E.S., Hess, K.R. *et al*. 1993b. Variables predictive of outcome in 832 patients undergoing repairs of the descending thoracic aorta. *Chest* **104**, 1248–1253.

Symbas, P.N., Pfaender, L.M., Drucker, M.H. *et al*. 1983. Cross-clamping of the descending aorta. *Journal of Thoracic and Cardiovascular Surgery* **85**, 300–305.

Tabayashi, K., Niibori, K., Konno, H. and Mohri, H. 1993. Protection from postischemic spinal cord injury by perfusion cooling of the epidural space. *Annals of Thoracic Surgery* **56**, 494–498.

Takaki, O. and Okumura, F. 1985. Application and limitation of somatosensory evoked potential monitoring during thoracic aortic aneurysm surgery: A case report. *Anesthesiology* **63**, 700–3.

Vacanti, F.X. and Ames, A.A. 1983. Mild hypothermia and Mg^{2+} protect against irreversible damage during CNS ischemia. *Stroke* **15**, 695–698.

Van Norman, G., Pavlin, E. and Pavlin, J. 1989. Hemodynamic and metabolic changes after thoracic aortic unclamping. *Anesthesiology* **71**, A59.

Verdant, A. 1984. Chronic traumatic aneurysm of the descending thoracic aorta with compression of the tracheobronchial tree. *Canadian Journal of Surgery* **27**, 278–279.

Verdant, A., Cossette, R., Pagé, A. *et al*. 1995. Aneurysms of the descending thoracic aorta: Three hundred sixty-six consecutive cases resected without paraplegia. *Journal of Vascular Surgery* **21**, 385–391.

Verdant, A. 1992. Descending thoracic aortic aneurysms: Surgical treatment with the Gott shunt. *Canadian Journal of Surgery* **35**, 493–496.

Von Oppell, U.O., Dunne, T.T., De Groot, K.M. and Zilla, P. 1994. Spinal cord protection in the absence of collateral circulation: meta-analysis of mortality and paraplegia. *Journal of Cardiovascular Surgery* **9**, 685–691.

Von Segesser, L.K., Killer, I., Jenni, R. *et al*. 1993. Improved distal circulatory support for repair of descending thoracic aortic aneurysms. *Annals of Thoracic Surgery* **56**, 1373–1380.

Wadouh, F., Lindemann, E.M., Arndt, C.F. *et al*. 1984. The arteria radicularis magna anterior as a decisive factor influencing spinal cord damage during aortic occlusion. *Journal of Thoracic and Cardiovascular Surgery* **88**, 1–10.

Wakabayashi, A., Connolly, J.E., Stemmer, E.A. *et al*. 1975. Heparinless left heart bypass for resection of thoracic aortic aneurysms. *The American Journal of Surgery* **130**, 212–218.

Wisselink, W., Becker, M.O., Nguyen, J.H. *et al*. 1994. Protecting the ischemic spinal cord during aortic clamping: the influence of selective hypothermia and spinal cord perfusion pressure. *Journal of Vascular Surgery* **19**, 788–796.

Woloszyn, T.T., Marini, C.P. and Coons, M.S. 1990. Cerebrospinal fluid drainage and steroids provide better spinal cord protection during aortic cross-clamping than does either treatment alone. *Annals of Thoracic Surgery* **49**, 78–83.

Wynn, M.M., Acher, C.W. and Popic, P.M. 1993. Combined use of spinal fluid drainage and naloxone reduces the risk of neurologic deficit in thoracoabdominal aneurysm repair. *Anesthesiology* **79**, A165.

Yamamoto, N., Takano, H., Kitagawa, H. *et al*. 1994. Monitoring for spinal cord ischemia by use of the evoked spinal cord potentials during aortic aneurysm surgery. *Journal of Vascular Surgery* **20**, 826–833.

Yum, S.W. and Faden, A.I. 1990. Comparison of the neuroprotective effects of the N-Methyl-D-Aspartate antagonist MK-801 and the opiate-receptor antagonist nalmefene in experimental spinal cord ischemia. *Archives of Neurology* **47**, 277–281.

11

Anaesthesia for abdominal aortic surgery

N B SCOTT

INTRODUCTION

As a result of an increase in the numbers of people living well into their eighties, diseases of the aorta are an increasing problem. Although frequently asymptomatic they may have either disastrous or debilitating complications, but many patients have significant disease of other major organs that increases the risk of surgery. In recent years, the rapid expansion of computerized technology within medicine has led to interventional non-surgical techniques, such as stenting, being used as a primary treatment modality for such patients. Where available, such techniques reduce the need for operative intervention. In addition, laparoscopic vascular bypass procedures are becoming feasible so that the advantage of reduced morbidity may be extended to patients undergoing vascular procedures. It is hoped that, following appropriate evaluation, these techniques will gain further and more widespread acceptance, so reducing the need for, and risk of, surgical intervention.

However, many of the patients do come to surgery and of these, the majority have severe widespread atherosclerosis and concomitant disease. Elective and emergency aortic aneurysm surgery

can be performed with excellent survival and a good quality of life, and therefore should not be denied to any patient on the basis of age alone. Improvements in the operative mortality and morbidity rates of elective aorto-iliac replacement, which are largely a result of refinements in surgical technique and perioperative management, have allowed a more aggressive approach to surgical treatment. Despite the obvious merit in operating on such patients, surgery, as with any form of trauma, stimulates a complex series of integrated pathways and networks which have largely deleterious effects on peri-operative organ function and reserve. The greater the trauma the greater the magnitude of these responses and the greater the risk of peri-operative mortality and morbidity (Kehlet, 1993). As a result of these changes, patients who come through surgery successfully may still take many months to convalesce fully.

Typically, one in three patients has hypertension, with associated renal pathology, and two out of three patients have ischaemic heart disease. Mortality is higher in both these risk groups. Smoking ages the arteries and increases the risk of surgery and is prevalent in 70 per cent of patients presenting with peripheral vascular disease. The mortality for elective abdominal aortic surgery is between 1.5 and 8 per cent, with myocardial infarction, multi-organ failure (MOF) and pulmonary atelectasis and infection the major causes of post-operative morbidity and mortality. Coronary artery disease is responsible for 50–60 per cent of early and late mortality in patients with peripheral vascular disease. For each death, there are eight patients who suffer myocardial ischaemia or infarction.

Anaesthetists therefore, have an increasing role to play in the overall peri-operative management of these patients because of their involvement in the intensive-care unit and, more recently, in the management of acute pain. These should lead to improvements in patient care resulting in reductions in mortality and morbidity and earlier ambulation of the patient with reduced in-hospital stay. At present, the *intra*-operative use of any single anaesthetic agent or technique has no established direct benefit on post-operative outcome (Kehlet, 1993). In addition, many of the controversies in the literature concerning various specialized techniques at certain points during abdominal vascular surgery, e.g. cross-clamping of the aorta, have not been resolved. Therefore, if overall morbidity is to be reduced, it is important to focus on the main therapeutic steps required: first to allow surgery to be performed in a safe and controlled environment; second, to maintain organ function during and after surgery.

GENERAL FACTORS

Incision

There are several approaches to the abdominal aorta and surgeons will continue to debate the relative merits of these. However, it does appear that, compared to a midline approach, incisions such as the retroperitoneal, transverse or paramedian avoid bilateral disruption of the respiratory apparatus, and minimize both pain and the metabolic response to trauma. They also result in fewer post-operative complications, shorter hospital and intensive care stay, and lower overall cost (Rosenbaum *et al.*, 1994; Sicard *et al.*, 1995). In addition, modern methods of post-operative pain control seem to decrease the incidence of pulmonary complications associated with abdominal surgery (Major *et al.*, 1996).

Suprarenal surgery

There are two major concerns with this type of surgery: first, the end organ ischaemia that results from aortic clamp application – particularly the kidneys, spinal cord and in the mesenteric vessel distribution; second, intra-operative and post-operative haemorrhage which may either lead to or arise from coagulation disorders. Access is difficult and a high level of surgical skill is required for such procedures.

Renal artery stenosis

Stenosis of either or both renal arteries results in ischaemia which activates the renin–angiotensin–aldosterone system and leads to systemic hypertension. This is often severe, requiring high-dose long-term drug therapy. Most of these lesions are due to proximal atheroma or fibromuscular hyperplasia in the renal arteries. They are increasingly being treated by angioplasty and stenting because the results of surgery are disappointing. However, corrective surgery may be indicated when medical management is producing serious side effects. Such surgery obviously necessitates suprarenal aortic cross-clamping. By itself, this may lead to high cardiovascular morbidity (Gelman, 1995). Moreover, many of these patients have left ventricular hypertrophy and ischaemia and a low intravascular volume. The younger patients with fibromuscular hyperplasia alone, and without atherosclerosis, usually have excellent results, but the operation still has an overall mortality of about 5 per cent, usually secondary to myocardial infarction.

Mesenteric surgery

Visceral ischaemia may be secondary to a variety of conditions including atherosclerosis, fibromuscular hyperplasia, arteritis and extrinsic compression (Wilkie's syndrome). Diagnosis of these conditions may prove difficult because they are far less common than other visceral pathologies and symptoms are non-specific. Atheroma is usually confined to the proximal segments of the coeliac and superior mesenteric arteries. When the superior mesenteric artery and the coeliac artery are diseased, the major mesenteric supply is from the inferior mesenteric artery via the marginal artery. Because of the rich supply from collateral vessels, two of these three vessels usually have to be affected before symptoms develop.

The long-term results of elective surgery for both acute and chronic visceral ischaemia are disappointing with high recurrence rates. The main concerns are to prevent graft kinking due to the mobility of the mesentery and to ensure antegrade flow from the aorta using a supracoeliac graft and end-to-end anastomosis.

PATIENT CONSIDERATIONS

Surgical trauma stimulates a complex series of integrated networks and pathways. These include the autonomic nervous system, neuroendocrine activation, acute phase response, immunosuppression, hypercoagulation, hypercatabolism and pain. The net effect of these changes is major disruption in organ function post-operatively, the severity of which is proportional to the magnitude of surgery. Since major organ dysfunction is responsible for post-operative morbidity and mortality, it seems worthwhile to attempt to block these responses to surgery in order to maintain peri-operative homeostasis. When given in combination with neuromuscular blockade, both intravenous and inhalational anaesthesia provide good operating conditions for the vascular surgeon, but they have no significant ability to prevent the body's response to surgery. At present, only regional anaesthesia has the ability to do so, but only for procedures below the umbilicus and infrarenal aortic surgery. However, the existing data show only moderate reductions in morbidity and morbidity with regional anaesthesia possibly because the changes that occur following surgical trauma continue beyond the duration of the block (Kehlet, 1993).

Monitoring

Bed availability in the intensive-care unit is a continuing worldwide problem, but monitoring and optimization of organ blood flow appears to be the cornerstone of peri-operative and post-operative care. In the ideal situation, a high-risk patient should be admitted to the intensive-care unit the evening before surgery and have all lines inserted at that time.

This strategy will also allow direct correction of any biochemical disturbances, especially hypokalaemia, hypocalcaemia and hypomagnesaemia. Although direct evidence is available for only small numbers of patients (Grounds, 1997), it does appear that such a strategy does lead to reductions in the incidence of post-operative complications.

Furthermore, established tissue hypoperfusion for more than 24 hours significantly increases mortality and morbidity (Shoemaker et al., 1992). All patients undergoing major abdominal vascular reconstruction should have baseline blood glucose and arterial blood gas estimation prior to induction and invasive monitoring of arterial pressure, typically using the radial artery of the arm with the highest pressure. Because renal function is easily compromised during vascular procedures, the bladder should be catheterized and urine output recorded hourly. In addition, a central venous catheter should be inserted and venous pressure monitored routinely.

Temperature

Inadvertent hypothermia after prolonged major thoracic or abdominal procedures is more severe as age increases. It is associated with marked catabolism, increased energy expenditure and may lead to increased cardiovascular stress and hypoxaemia. After major surgery, recovery is quicker and complications are reduced if the intra-operative core temperature is maintained (Bush et al., 1995; Kurz et al., 1996). Core temperature should be monitored and maintained above 35.5°C. Anaesthetic gases should be delivered through heat and moisture exchangers which are simple to insert into the circuit and extremely effective. Heating blankets are available which cover and heat the non-operated surfaces of the body, with the head being covered with a heat-reflecting cap. The small bowel has a very large surface area, and should be wrapped to reduce heat loss. Intravenous fluids should be administered through a blood-warming set.

Occasionally, if there is additional concern about the risk of spinal cord ischaemia, it may be appropriate to reduce core temperature to provide mild hypothermia (32–34°C) to reduce spinal cord oxygen consumption. The operating theatre is cooled to an ambient temperature of 15°C and the anaesthetist should remember to wear thermal underwear before coming to work that morning!

Pulmonary artery flow catheters

The routine insertion of the Swan–Ganz or pulmonary artery flow catheter (PAFC) has been questioned in recent years and some studies suggest that they may even increase overall morbidity (Connors *et al.*, 1996). However, because left ventricular dilatation will result in cardiovascular instability and failure and is to be avoided, a PAFC may be appropriate for the high-risk patient undergoing major vascular surgery to prevent excessive fluid administration. Once inserted, careful monitoring should ensure patient safety. Continuous cardiac output catheters are available which provide real-time analysis and management of central venous pressure, pulmonary capillary wedge pressure, cardiac index, systemic vascular resistance and mixed venous oxygen saturation. As a rule cardiac index (CI), which equals cardiac output divided by body surface area, is best maintained between 3 and 4 by inotropic support, maintaining pulmonary capillary wedge pressure (PCWP) at 12–15 mmHg and systemic vascular resistance on the low side of normal at between 800 and 1000 units. Thus preload, inotropy and afterload can be optimized for each patient. In those with severely reduced ventricular ejection fractions (i.e. less than 35 per cent), a CI of 3.5 may not be achievable without causing a tachycardia. Since diastolic filling is reduced this is potentially detrimental and in these patients a moderate increase in CI above the baseline figure is all that is required.

Maintenance of blood volume

In any form of vascular surgery the most serious intra-operative complication is the sudden loss of a large volume of blood. Therefore, if massive haemorrhage is anticipated, rapid infusion devices should be available. Several of these are now in clinical use. The use of a rapid autotransfusion device may not be necessary in every patient undergoing routine aortic surgery, but it is a very useful adjunct to the anaesthetic technique and should be available for more complicated procedures such as suprarenal and revisional surgery. It is always desirable to be able to accelerate away from impending disaster and with these machines the anaesthetist can feel much more in control when managing severe haemorrhage.

Devices range from a simple high-pressure infusion system to sophisticated machines which can provide metered infusion flow rates between 10 and 1500 mL/min, with selectable infusate pressure limits and precise temperature control at all flow rates. Pre-connected disposables allow for quick and easy set-up and air can be detected at several points in the circuit. Thus, they can provide the anaesthetist with a rapid continuous infusion while at the same time minimizing the risks of air embolism, hypovolaemic shock, hypothermia and overpressurization.

PRESERVATION OF ORGAN FUNCTION AND BLOOD FLOW

Heart

The most important causes of mortality and morbidity after all forms of vascular surgery are pre-existing coronary artery disease and hypertension which are present in at least 60 per cent of these patients (Clark and Stanley, 1994). The major pre-clinical findings which will determine severity of operative risk are previous myocardial infarction, hypertension, congestive cardiac failure and pre-existing arrhythmias such as atrial fibrillation (Goldman *et al.*, 1977; Clark and Stanley, 1994). Further, patients with aortic valve disease do not tolerate aortic cross-clamping well, and they should have echocardiography performed to assess their left ventricular function. It is now clear that correction of myocardial ischaemia prior to abdominal surgery, either by angioplasty or surgery, does improve post-operative outcome (Henderson and Effeney, 1995).

During surgery, ischaemia, infarction and the development of arrhythmias are the direct consequences of changes in autonomic activity and alterations in oxygen delivery and consumption. More than in any other type of surgery, avoidance of tachycardias and large swings in blood pressure are desirable because these have been shown to increase the risk to the myocardium. Such lability is most probably a result of pre-existing hypertension which leads to a decrease in intravascular volume. In addition, hypoxaemia may induce cardiovascular instability. The routine use of magnesium sulphate reduces the incidence of peri-operative conduction disturbances (James, 1992).

It is important to observe the surgical field regularly because there may be physical reasons for the sudden onset of an arrhythmia such as direct contact with the diaphragm below the pericardium or the use of cold fluid for peritoneal lavage.

CNS

Damage to the brain or spinal cord may occur as a result of ischaemia or reperfusion, the development of oxygen free radicals, and any disturbance of electrolyte balance, particularly sodium, magnesium and calcium. Thus, sodium, magnesium, calcium and blood glucose should be maintained within normal limits throughout the peri-operative period. Mannitol, ketamine and magnesium may be of benefit prophylactically as free-radical scavengers. In patients who develop reperfusion injury with cerebral oedema, steroids, barbiturates, ketamine and calcium antagonists may also have a place in reducing neurological deficits which occur (Naslund et al., 1992; Gajraj and White, 1994). Reducing cerebral metabolic rate also reduces damage.

Spinal cord damage following procedures on the aorta is an unpredictable and dreadful complication of multifactorial origin. Lower aortic surgery results in an incidence of less than 1 per cent, but as the clamp level rises so does the incidence of spinal cord injury. The incidence for thoraco-abdominal aneurysms has been quoted as high as 40 per cent (Naslund et al., 1992), and it is vital to provide as much protection as possible. Paraplegia may be transient, immediate or delayed (Naslund and Hollier, 1993).

Transient lower limb paralysis can occasionally be seen in some patients on awakening in the intensive-care unit and may last 24–48 hours before recovery is evident. It appears that the major causes of *immediate paraplegia* are surgical, i.e. the depth and duration of ischaemia during the period of aortic cross-clamping and failure to identify and re-implant critical vessels that supply blood to the spinal cord. The critical vessel is the radicular artery of Adamkiewicz which comes off the aorta between T8 and T12 in 75 per cent of subjects, but may be at any level from T1 to L1. If the level of aortic clamping is above this artery and/or causes hypoperfusion of the artery, then spinal cord ischaemia with resultant flaccid paralysis is likely. *Delayed paraplegia*, which has been reported to occur from 1 to 21 days after

surgery, is most likely to be secondary to prolonged periods of post-operative hypotension.

Prevention of paraplegia after procedures on the thoracic and supra-renal aorta is probably best achieved by a surgical technique that ensures oxygenation of the spinal cord during aortic cross-clamping, along with a method that can uniformly depict critical vessels that must be re-implanted at the time of surgery (Hollier and Money, 1992).

Although the primary concern for the anaesthetist is to maintain proximal aortic pressures throughout surgery, a variety of drugs and techniques have been advocated to further reduce the incidence. None has been shown to provide conclusive evidence of effect, but intensive efforts must be made to avoid the problem. These include surface hypothermia, somatosensory and motor evoked potential recording, steroids and magnesium (James, 1992). Spinal cord drainage and cooling is popular at present. Drainage of CSF for 24–48 hours is performed because raised CSF pressures do increase the degree of spinal cord injury (Hollier and Money, 1992). The technique involves inserting a silastic catheter at L3/L4 and connecting it to a manometer which is level with the right atrium. A limit of 15 cmH$_2$O is set and if pressures exceed this then CSF will overflow into a reservoir. The volume of CSF varies greatly and care must be taken to avoid coning. Spinal cord cooling is achieved by inserting a 4F catheter at T12 and a thermistor at L3 and injecting cold perfusate through the catheter for the duration of surgery to achieve regional temperatures of 23–25°C.

Gut

Stress ulceration is a well-recognized risk of major cardiovascular surgery (Martin, 1994) and routine prophylaxis is used in many centres. H$_2$-receptor antagonists such as ranitidine or a chelating agent such as sucralfate are recommended to prevent stress-induced changes in the stomach and duodenum and also to reduce the risk of aspiration of gastric content.

In the majority of abdominal aortic aneurysm resections, the inferior mesenteric artery is sacrificed by the surgeon and collateral flow to the descending colon, sigmoid colon and rectum is maintained by the mid-colic artery, a branch of the superior mesenteric artery. However, ischaemic colitis is a recognized complication of the procedure with an incidence as high as 7 per cent (Panneton and Hollier, 1995).

Colonic and gastric tonometry have been used to try to ensure earlier detection of ischaemia. Following aortic reconstruction, not only did a low intramural pH (pH_i) predict subsequent ischaemic colitis, but also the cross-clamp time and the duration of sigmoid ischaemia correlated with the incidence of post-operative septic complications (Schiedler et al., 1987). A colonic pH_i below 6.86 predicted endoscopically detectable ischaemic colitis. A gastric pH_i below 7.20 predicted major complications with a sensitivity of 100 per cent and specificity of 81 per cent (Bjorck and Hedberg, 1994). Gastric and colonic pH tonometers are becoming more widely available and both procedures are easy to perform. Data from large series are now required to establish their place in the perioperative period.

Kidneys

Pre-operative renal insufficiency is seen in approximately 5–10 per cent of patients and may result from atherosclerosis, diabetes mellitus, hypertension or poor myocardial function. Pre-existing renal disease is one of the main determinants of post-operative outcome and up to 70 per cent of patients with renal artery disease will have a prolonged hospital stay after aortic surgery (Martin et al., 1994). Further, the kidneys may be damaged by radiological dyes during pre-operative assessment either by a direct toxic effect or by reducing intravascular volume through an osmotic diuretic effect. It is therefore imperative to identify at-risk patients and plan their peri-operative care carefully. It is prudent to postpone surgery for at least a week if the urea and creatinine increase after angiography.

Aortic cross-clamping results in raised systemic vascular resistance (SVR), systolic pressure and left ventricular pressure and these impair left ventricular performance. As a result, peripheral blood flow is impaired and the kidneys in particular are damaged. Although cortical blood flow is three- to fourfold that of medullary blood flow, the renal medulla is particularly sensitive to hypoperfusion since it extracts more oxygen from blood. Ischaemia results in cell membrane and microsomal disruption with rises in intracellular calcium, all of which are worsened on reperfusion.

The importance of maintenance of intravascular volume and a stable cardiac output cannot be overstressed for the maintenance of renal blood flow. In addition, the surgeon must give careful consideration to the route of exposure, location of the proximal aortic clamp and duration of cross-clamp time. High sodium loads should be avoided. The renal protective effects of dopamine and mannitol are probably overstated, but most centres advocate one or other agent or a combination of the two. Low-dose dopamine does increase overall renal blood flow and glomerular filtration (Moss and Craigo, 1993) while mannitol is a free-radical scavenger as well as an osmotic diuretic, providing, in theory at least, some degree of renal protection. In the presence of an adequate intravascular volume (i.e. central venous pressures of 8–12 mmHg or PCWP of 12–15 mmHg) prior to clamping the combination of these increases renal blood flow and urine output. The addition of frusemide at this point will further increase urine output.

Lungs

Routine pre-operative pulmonary function tests and arterial blood gases cannot predict respiratory complications after abdominal aortic surgery (Durand et al., 1995). However they provide important baseline information in individual patients with pre-existing pulmonary disease and should be performed on them.

The diaphragm accounts for 70 per cent of the work involved during normal respiration, while the rectus muscles above the umbilicus play an important role in quiet breathing and forced respiration. Disruption of either of these muscle groups is a direct consequence of upper abdominal surgery. In addition to the physical and mechanical effects of the incision and the pain it causes, bulbosplanchnic reflexes are stimulated that inhibit respiration (Albano and Garnier, 1983). The use of systemic opioids increases intra-abdominal wall muscle tension (Duggan and Drummond, 1987; 1989), but no parallel data exist for regional techniques. Thoracic epidural anaesthesia (TEA) appears to diminish the alterations in lung volumes seen with upper abdominal surgery, by an effect that is independent of the analgesia it provides. TEA produces an increase in diaphragmatic activity, via inhibition of afferent pathways that produce an inhibitory effect on diaphragmatic activity.

Recently, the use of nitrous oxide and high inspired oxygen concentrations (FiO_2) have been shown to result in absorption atelectasis (Benumof, 1994). Positive end-expiratory pressure (PEEP) should also be used to further minimize basal atelectasis (Hedenstierna *et al.*, 1984). Thus oxygen-enriched air with an FiO_2 of less than 40 per cent and 5 mmHg of PEEP is the best mixture for initial ventilation under anaesthesia. Arterial blood gases can be monitored regularly and the FiO_2 increased if the PaO_2 falls below 10 kPa.

Some anaesthetists advocate the use of ketamine instead of opioids in conjunction with a thoracic epidural for the high-risk respiratory patient since this combination provides good analgesia and does not further depress ventilation. There is merit in using this drug, but upper airway secretions may be profuse in the intubated patient and the incidence of CNS side effects following emergence is in the region of 30 per cent. Administering the ketamine from a target controlled-infusion (TCI) pump can reduce the side effects (see below).

Post-operatively, nursing patients in the supine position results in upward pressure from the abdominal viscera, further inhibiting respiratory effort. Nursing them semi-sitting at 60° as soon as the blood pressure permits and avoiding any unnecessary pain easily prevents such impairment of a patient's ability to breathe. Regular physiotherapy with instruction in the use of incentive spirometry pre-operatively will encourage deep breathing and coughing and further reduce complications.

Coagulation and blood loss

After surgery, there are large increases in the procoagulants fibrinogen, factor VIII coagulant, factor VIIIRag, von Willebrand factor and α_1-antitrypsin. These changes are a result of the surgical trauma and are greatest between the second and fourth post-operative days. At the same time, there are marked decreases in the naturally occurring anticoagulants protein C and antithrombin III, and in α_2-macroglobulin. Post-operative changes in thrombelastographic patterns confirm that hypercoagulability occurs in whole blood following abdominal aortic bypass surgery. Thus, patients are 'hypercoagulable' in the post-operative period. This may contribute to the development of coronary artery thrombosis since the time course of these changes coincides with that of peri-operative myocardial infarction. Further studies are warranted to determine whether modification of post-operative hypercoagulability reduces the incidence of thrombotic complications in this group of patients.

Complicating this, severe blood loss requiring large volumes of transfused blood, i.e. more than 1500 mL, which is a relatively frequent occurrence for suprarenal aortic surgery, can result in disseminated intravascular coagulation (DIC) and/or fibrinolysis (Hollier and Money, 1992). Bleeding may occur from multiple sites. These problems are usually easy to anticipate and correct with fresh frozen plasma and platelets, which should be made available at the start of surgery and given with each 6 units of concentrated red blood cells. Secondary haemorrhage may occur as a result of fibrinolysis, especially after supracoeliac surgery. There is some evidence that this is secondary to visceral ischaemia and may occur with ischaemic times of less than 30 minutes. Prolonged visceral ischaemia may be prevented by restoring visceral blood flow immediately after the proximal aortic anastomosis using a Dacron side graft (Hollier and Money, 1992).

For patients undergoing complex or revisional surgery, or in patients with a pre-existing bleeding abnormality, the routine use of aprotinin or ε-aminocaproic acid intra-operatively and continued for 24 hours is recommended. However there are case reports of myocardial ischaemia and infarction secondary to coronary thrombosis associated with the use of aprotinin. Standardized infusion regimes for this drug do not exist, but our regime is 200 mL in the first hour, followed by 50 mL/h for 4 hours and then 50 mL every 4 hours for 24 hours.

CARDIOVASCULAR MANAGEMENT

Avoidance of pressor responses

Both intubation *and* extubation of the trachea may be associated with a marked vasopressor response that is neither desirable nor beneficial to the patient. These effects are largely obtunded by a smooth induction and equally careful management of recovery from anaesthesia.

Application and release of the aortic clamp are the two major stresses during elective surgery, their severity increasing with the level of the clamp. The physiology of cross-clamping has been carefully elucidated in many laboratory and clinical studies.

Regardless of the anaesthetic technique, the critical period for the patient is aortic unclamping (Gelman, 1995).

CROSS-CLAMPING OF THE AORTA

In essence, clamping decreases blood flow to the tissues below the level of the clamp and increases blood pressure and left ventricular afterload above it. The main determinants of afterload are end-diastolic myocardial tension and systolic pressure. On cross-clamping, as systolic load increases, myocardial contractility decreases, resulting in reduced stroke volume, ejection fraction and cardiac output. These decrease between 15 and 40 per cent with infrarenal cross-clamping. If intravascular volume is low at the time then the cardiovascular effects of cross-clamping will be more profound. As mentioned before, at greatest risk from these alterations are the myocardium, kidneys, gastrointestinal tract and spinal cord. Overall effects on organ function, especially the myocardium will depend additionally on the pre-operative state and the choice of anaesthetic. In the absence of ischaemic heart disease, the changes seen are far less dramatic than in its presence. It is important therefore to plan meticulously and increase clinical awareness in the high-risk patient.

Patients with ischaemic heart disease, particularly those with reduced ventricular contractility, are likely to develop ischaemic changes on the ECG associated with left ventricular failure and a significant incidence of arrhythmias. Transoesophageal echocardiography has also shown that, following supracoeliac clamping, these changes are even more pronounced and associated with segmental wall motion abnormalities. When the clamp is applied, reduction in aortic pressure is best achieved by increasing the depth of anaesthesia and commencing sodium nitroprusside or glyceryl trinitrate infusions. Not infrequently, both may have to be given to maintain satisfactory pressures. In addition an inotropic agent such as dobutamine can enhance ventricular performance. Again, the phosphodiesterase inhibitors such as enoximone or milrinone may have beneficial effects by reducing afterload and increasing inotropy.

Unclamping

On cross-clamping, the resulting decrease in organ blood flow will lead to vasoactive paralysis and ischaemic vasodilatation in the lower limbs and pelvic organs resulting in anaerobic metabolism and accumulation of lactate and hydrogen ions and other vasoactive metabolites (Gelman, 1995). Subsequent release of the clamp opens up the distal vascular tree, releasing these metabolites into the circulation, leading to reductions in systemic vascular resistance. The changes in cardiac output are dependent on the left ventricular filling pressure and this must be maintained above normal baseline values prior to release of the clamp, as assessed by central venous pressure or, where indicated, by pulmonary capillary wedge pressure and continuous cardiac output monitoring.

Blood pooling may also result from a reactive hyperaemia in the freshly revascularized areas and as a result systemic vascular resistance, venous return and cardiac output will decrease. If excessive, then further reductions in myocardial, splanchnic, renal and spinal cord blood flow are to be expected via an internal 'steal' mechanism. If the decrease in cardiac output and systemic vascular resistance are concomitant and profound, severe hypotension will result. This is known as 'declamping shock'. However, provided increased central venous pressure (or PCWP) and cardiac output are ensured prior to clamping and throughout the grafting period, declamping 'shock' is thankfully uncommon. The surgeon and anaesthetist must also be aware of sources of hidden bleeding at the time of unclamping.

Vasopressors

The vasopressors in common use are methoxamine, phenylephrine (alpha-1 agonists), ephedrine (a mixed action sympathomimetic) and metaraminol (an alpha-1 and beta-1 agonist). In considering which to use, it is important to remember that the main requirement is to raise blood pressure, but to avoid tachycardia, particularly in patients with a history of overt ischaemic heart disease. This is in contrast to obstetric use where the main caveat when using a vasopressor is to preserve uterine blood flow. Each drug has its advocates, but metaraminol (either by bolus of between 0.25 and 0.5 mg or by infusion) increases inotropy and cardiac output within 20–30s following administration. It does not increase heart rate, but care must be taken with its administration to avoid excessive hypertension. Occasionally, phenylephrine may be preferred for patients who develop declamping shock because it is a pure vaso-constrictor, twice as potent as metaraminol, and it has no effect on the myocardium.

Vasodilators

The two main vasodilators used to treat hypertension are sodium nitroprusside, which acts mainly on the arterial side and reduces myocardial work, and glyceryl trinitrate which is predominantly a veno-dilator. Glyceryl trinitrate also improves coronary blood flow and therefore is arguably the best individual agent for this type of surgery. However, not infrequently, they are used in combination if the patient's blood pressure is not responding to either by itself. The attenuation of clamp-induced hypertension by nitroprusside may be associated with a dramatic increase in cardiac output and cardiac work.

Inotropic agents

The debate over which inotropic agent to use will probably continue for many years and, again, the main issue is to determine the need for myocardial support. Epinephrine is probably still the best inotropic agent available (and is also one hundred times less expensive than the others) when given by infusion. As already mentioned, the renal protective effects of dopamine are overstated and in addition heart rates of 120–140 per minute are not unusual with this agent. Dobutamine will also induce similar heart rates. For high-risk cardiac patients, in order to optimize cardiac output prior to induction of anaesthesia, gentle introduction of one or other of these three drugs by infusion will prevent such tachycardia. However, care must be taken with dobutamine because it causes a reduction in SVR which the anaesthetist must be aware of following release of the aortic clamp. In contrast, norepinephrine dramatically increases SVR and may be needed following release of the cross-clamp if vasodilatation is severe. The author has only limited experience with milrinone and enoximone, the phosphodiesterase inhibitors, which increase myocardial contractility and produce arterial dilatation, thereby reducing afterload. This dual effect may prove to be beneficial in some patients, but great care must be taken since

hypotension secondary to the arterial dilatation may be severe.

ANAESTHETIC CONSIDERATIONS

Choice of anaesthetic technique

As with any specialist area, it is fair to say that no single agent, technique (or, indeed, anaesthetist) affords ideal conditions for the surgeon, anaesthetist or patient 100 per cent of the time. In one study comparing a neuroleptic technique with TEA, the latter was characterized by greater haemodynamic stability during surgery, while patients in the neurolept anaesthesia group had significant lability of blood pressure, heart rate and cardiac index (Bonnet et al., 1989).

The relative merits of intravenous and inhalational anaesthesia are very topical. Protagonists of either an intravenous or inhalational technique usually focus on the demerit of the other rather than true benefits but evidence is accumulating that total intravenous anaesthesia (TIVA) is indeed as safe as inhalational anaesthesia. Furthermore, it may offer more to the patient in terms of post-operative recovery, since the drugs used have such rapid pharmacokinetics allowing rapid offset of both effects and side effects. If this is so, then it may offset the concern in some quarters over the higher cost of administering TIVA since there are potential savings to be made in preventing and treating side effects of surgery such as nausea and vomiting and poor pain management.

Inhalational anaesthesia

Inhalational anaesthesia remains the more widely practised technique because, over many decades, sophisticated delivery systems have been developed. These are simple and cheap to use and allow the anaesthetist a fine degree of control over the concentration administered to the patient. The three most widely used agents, halothane, enflurane and isoflurane have been joined by two newer agents, desflurane and sevoflurane. All of these drugs have a negative inotropic effect on the myocardium, and in vascular patients, great care must be taken to minimize this effect. In addition, once experience is achieved, their use reduces the requirement for muscle relaxants. These agents all lower systemic vascular resistance by a direct effect on blood vessels (Pavlin and Su, 1994). Thus they are often used as an adjunct to glyceryl trinitrate or sodium nitroprusside, thereby reducing the dose requirements of each. This allows additional filling of the intravascular space which, provided excessive amounts of crystalloid are avoided and care is taken with filling pressures, will help to maintain organ blood flow without the risk of fluid overload and pulmonary oedema as the anaesthetic wears off.

With the older drugs, if surgery is prolonged, when the volatile agent is switched off, the effects may continue well into the recovery period, resulting in undesirable effects such as post-operative shivering, hangover and nausea and vomiting. On the other hand, this technique provides a gradual wake-up which may allow prompt control of pain management with narcotics before the patient is fully conscious. Isoflurane is regarded by some as the volatile anaesthetic of choice because it is the most potent vasodilator and has the least inotropic effect. Desflurane and sevoflurane have similar cardiovascular profiles to isoflurane at equivalent minimum alveolar concentration (MAC), but are expensive and probably do not provide any additional beneficial effect over isoflurane for anaesthesia *for major surgery*.

Intravenous anaesthesia

Until recently, the intravenous drugs and delivery equipment available to the anaesthetist meant that TIVA was only practised by enthusiasts. It is only in the last decade with the introduction of new intravenous agents, our knowledge of their pharmacokinetics and the development of sophisticated but 'user-friendly' computerized delivery systems that TIVA has been able to rival traditional techniques in terms of simplicity and efficacy.

Propofol is increasing in popularity as the hypnotic component for TIVA because of its short elimination half-life and high clearance which lead to a rapid onset and offset. It may also possess an intrinsic anti-emetic effect (Borgeat *et al.*, 1992). Care must be taken at induction for vascular procedures because hypotension secondary to reduced systemic vascular resistance and to a lesser degree decreased left ventricular function, may occur. Propofol may also lead to respiratory depression (Fragen, 1994).

The recent development of computer software enabling use of target-controlled infusions of propofol

(TCI) can minimize side effects of the drug (Sutcliffe *et al.*, 1995). TCI infusions incorporate the pharmacokinetic parameters describing the distribution and elimination of a drug and are designed to maintain a predetermined blood concentration appropriate for any individual patient and level of surgical stimulation at any time. Although the mathematical formulae within the software are complex, the practical administration of the anaesthetic is simple. The anaesthetist needs only to enter the weight and age of the patient and the desired concentration. The system then calculates and delivers a bolus designed to achieve this concentration, followed by a continuously adjusting infusion to maintain this level. The target can be adjusted at any stage and if a lower level is chosen the machine will stop until it has calculated that the new level has been achieved and recommence at a lower rate.

TCI propofol is particularly suited for vascular procedures, especially those requiring post-operative sedation in the intensive-care unit because, at the end of surgery the anaesthetist chooses a level of propofol suitable for sedation. The infusion can be finely controlled until the patient is ready for extubation and on cessation of the infusion recovery is rapid allowing removal of the tube within 30 minutes in most patients. Other drugs have been programmed for TCI and these include alfentanil, midazolam, etomidate and ketamine. The most recent of the short-acting opioids, remifentanil, has also been added to this list and may afford even smoother control during the peri-operative period.

NEUROMUSCULAR BLOCKING AGENTS

Surgeons have traditionally required profound neuromuscular blockade to gain access to the abdominal aorta and its branches and the viscera. It is important to note, however, that provided adequate levels of anaesthesia are being administered throughout the procedure, additional muscle relaxation is only necessary for intubation and at opening and closure of the wound. If TIVA or inhalational anaesthesia are to be used, then the anaesthetist will be required to provide suitable relaxation, but the degree of relaxation previously employed is quite unnecessary. There is little to choose between atracurium, cis-atracurium, vecuronium and mivacurium with regard to clinical profiles. In theory at least, atracurium (which is metabolized via Hoffman degradation and does not accumulate in liver and renal failure) and mivacurium, (metabolized by plasma cholinesterase), may have an advantage in patients with pre-existing renal or hepatic impairment. Continuous infusions, although theoretically attractive, are not necessary and minimal use of relaxant techniques will avoid the risk of awareness under anaesthesia, which is no less of a problem with the newer agents. The use of long-acting drugs such as pancuronium or *d*-tubocurarine is not to be encouraged as these have been shown to increase post-operative pulmonary complications (Berg *et al.*, 1997).

REGIONAL ANAESTHESIA

The topic is discussed more fully elsewhere. However, when addressing the specific needs of the individual patient undergoing major vascular surgery, several points are worthy of mention.

Firstly, every one of the many controlled clinical trials on the topic of post-operative pain relief has demonstrated that opioid analgesia is far inferior to regional analgesia as an analgesic regime for major surgery (Scott, 1991).

Secondly, regional analgesia is often accused of being an inherently more dangerous technique than conventional analgesia. Paradoxically, 30 per cent of the published studies that have investigated post-operative morbidity comparing regional techniques with conventional regimens demonstrate an actual reduction in morbidity with regional analgesia (Kehlet, 1993). Not one of these studies has managed to demonstrate opioid analgesia by whatever technique to have less intrinsic morbidity than regional analgesia, which one would expect if regional techniques are truly more dangerous (Scott, 1991).

Thirdly, the incidence of pulmonary complications, thromboembolism and vascular occlusion rates, blood loss (requiring transfusion) and pain following abdominal surgery range from 5 to 100 per cent. The quoted incidence for lower-limb paralysis as a direct consequence of the surgery following extensive supracoeliac aortic surgery is as high as 70 per cent. All of these complications should be mentioned to the patient by the surgeon prior to consent for surgery. The risk of each is reduced by regional anaesthesia (Kehlet, 1993) resulting in a smoother post-operative recovery for a given patient. The overwhelming reason proffered for the avoidance of regional anaesthesia is the development of epidural abscess or haematoma. The highest quoted incidence of this admittedly dire complication is 1 in 15 000, i.e. 0.006 per cent.

Therefore, for major abdominal vascular surgery, which carries such an enormous risk of surgical complications at an increased overall cost, there is little clinical or theoretical justification for avoiding regional anaesthesia. Prior to surgery and following administration of antibiotic prophylaxis which thus covers both the catheter insertion as well as the procedure, a thoracic epidural catheter is inserted allowing a block suitable for the incision to be established in a methodical way using small boluses of 0.5 or 0.75 per cent bupivacaine. This leads to precise control of the required block while at the same time decreasing the incidence of hypotension and/or bradycardia. More importantly, it also reduces motor weakness in the lower limbs and therefore patients are not confined to bed and can be actively mobilized in the presence of superb analgesia and the absence of narcotics.

However, the technique is not, by itself, a panacea and used only intra-operatively does not lead to subsequent reductions in post-operative morbidity (Baron *et al.*, 1995). All patients will spend the first 24–48 hours in the intensive-care or high-dependency units and thoracic epidural infusions can be used safely in these areas. Following transfer back to the general ward, provided that appropriate nurse education and monitoring of the patient is available, infusions may be safely continued for several days and further reductions in post-operative morbidity can be achieved.

Finally, the current medico-legal 'need' for patients with thoracic epidurals to remain in a high-dependency or intensive-care unit is dependent again on respiratory complications associated with the use of opioid analgesics in the epidural regime. Equivalent analgesia can be provided by a multi-modal approach. Continuous infusions substituting opioids with an alpha-agonist such as clonidine gives an effective and safer alternative regimen which obviates the need for high dependency for the technique, unless surgical complications exist or ensue.

Studies that have examined current techniques and regimes of regional anaesthesia have produced only small reductions in peri-operative morbidity (Kehlet, 1993). However, it is possible for patients who have had major abdominal vascular surgery employing a thoracic epidural technique to be walking and eating the following day (personal data). Much research and audit is required to establish the theoretical benefit of regional anaesthesia at the same time improving its safety in order that the technique may be practised more widely.

Whichever technique is chosen for the surgery by an experienced anaesthetist, provided that haemodynamic stability has been sustained throughout the procedure, this will result in the smooth transfer of a stable patient back to the intensive-care unit in the majority of cases. However, the key to the peri-operative management of the vascular patient is to sustain the intra-operative strategy into the post-operative period. TIVA plus thoracic epidural anaesthesia provides superb operating conditions for the surgeon without the need for relaxant or large doses of a long-acting opioid. This, in turn, results in rapid awakening and recovery of a pain-free patient and minimal post-operative morbidity.

REFERENCES

Albano, J. P. and Garniers, L. 1983. Bulbo-spinal respiratory affects originating from the splanchnic afferents. *Respiration Physiology* **51**, 229–239.

Baron, J. F., Bertrand, M., Barre, E. *et al*. 1995. Combined epidural and general anesthesia versus general anesthesia for abdominal aortic surgery. *Anesthesiology* **75**(4), 611–618.

Berg, H., Viby-Mogensen, J., Roed, J. *et al*. 1997. Residual neuromuscular block is a risk factor for postoperative pulmonary complications. A prospective randomised and blinded study of postoperative pulmonary complications after atracurium, vecuronium and pancuronium. *Acta Anaesthesiologica Scandinavica* **41**, 1095–1103.

Benumof, J.L. 1994. Respiratory physiology and respiratory function during surgery. In Miller, R.D. (ed.) *Anesthesia*, 4th edn. Edinburgh: Churchill Livingstone.

Bjork, M. and Heberg, B. 1994. Early detection of major postoperative complications after abdominal aortic surgery: predictive value of sigmoid colon and gastric intramuscular pH monitoring. *British Journal of Surgery* **81**, 25–30.

Bonnet, F., Touboul, C., Picard, A.M. *et al*. 1989. Neuroleptanesthesia versus thoracic epidural anesthesia for abdominal aortic surgery. *Annals of Vascular Surgery* **3**, 214–219.

Borgeat, A., Wilder-Smith, O.H. Saiah, M., and Rifat, K. 1992. Subhypnotic doses of propofol possess direct anti-emetic properties. *Anesthesia and Analgesia* **74**, 539.

Bush, H.J., Hydo, L.J., Fischer, E. *et al*. 1995. Hypothermia during elective abdominal aortic aneurysm repair: the high price of avoidable morbidity. *Journal of Vascular Surgery* **21**, 392–402.

Clark, N.J. and Stanley, T.H. 1994. Anesthesia for vascular surgery. In Miller, R.D. (ed.) *Anesthesia*, 4th edn. Edinburgh: Churchill Livingstone.

Connors, A.F., Speroff, T., Dawson, N.V. *et al*. 1996. The effectiveness of right heart catheterisation in the initial care of critically ill patients. *Journal of the American Medical Association* **276**(11), 889–897.

Duggan, J.E. and Drummond, G.B. 1987. Activity of lower intercostal and abdominal muscle after upper abdominal surgery. *Anesthesia and Analgesia* **66**, 852–855.

Duggan, J.E. and Drummond, G.B. 1989. Abdominal muscle activity and intraabdominal pressure after upper abdominal surgery. *Anesthesia and Analgesia* **69**, 598–603.

Durand, M., Combes, P., Briot, R. *et al*. 1995. Prediction of respiratory complications after surgery of the abdominal aorta. *Canadian Journal of Anaesthesia* **42**, 1101–1107.

Fragen, R.J. 1994. Clinical pharmacology and applications of intravenous induction agents. In Bowdle, T.A., Horita, A. and Kharasch, E.D. (eds) *The pharmacological basis of anesthesiology*. London: Churchill Livingstone.

Gajraj, N. and White, P.F. 1994. Clinical pharmacology and applications of ketamine. In Bowdle, T.A., Horita, A. and Kharasch, E.D. (eds) *The pharmacological basis of anesthesiology*. London: Churchill Livingstone.

Gelman, S.G. 1995. The pathophysiology of aortic cross-clamping and unclamping. *Anesthesiology* **82**, 1026–1060.

Goldman, L., Caldera, D.L. and Nusscaum, S.R. 1977. Multifactorial index of cardiac risk in non-cardiac surgical patients. *New England Journal of Medicine* **297**, 845.

Grounds, R.M. 1997. Peroperative cardiovascular optimisation of high-risk surgical patients. *Current Opinions in Anaesthesiology* **10**, 72–76.

Hedenstiema, G., Baehrendtz, S., Klingskedt, C. *et al*. 1994. Ventilation and perfusion of each lung during differential ventilation with selective PEEP. *Anesthesiology* **461**, 369–376.

Henderson, A. and Effeney, D. 1995. Morbidity and mortality after abdominal aortic surgery in a population of patients with high cardiovascular risk. *Australian and New Zealand Journal of Surgery* **65**(6), 417–420.

Hollier, L.H. and Money, S.R. 1992. Technical modifications and adjunctive therapy for surgical problems in suprarenal aortic surgery. *Seminars in Vascular Surgery* **5**, 192–197.

James, M.F.M. 1992. Clinical use of magnesium infusions in anesthesia. *Anesthesia and Analgesia* **74**, 129–136.

Kehlet, H. 1993. General versus regional anaesthesia. In Rogers, M.C., Tinker, J.H., Covina, B.G. and Longnecker, D.E. (eds) *Principles and practice of anesthesiology*. London: Mosby Year Book.

Kurz, A., Sessler, D.L. and Lenhardt, R. 1996. Perioperative normothermia to reduce the incidence of surgical wound infection and shorten hospital stay. *New England Journal of Medicine* **334**, 1209–1215.

Major, C.P., Greer, M.S., Russell, W.L. and Rose, S.M. 1996. Postoperative pulmonary complications and morbidity after abdominal aneurysmectomy: a comparison of postoperative epidural versus parenteral opioid analgesia. *American Surgeon* **62**, 45–51.

Martin, L.F. 1994. Stress ulcers are common after aortic surgery. Endoscopic evaluation of prophylactic therapy. *American Surgeon* **60**(3), 169–174.

Martin, L.F., Atnip, R.G., Holmes, P.A. *et al*. 1994. Prediction of postoperative complications after elective aortic surgery using stepwise logistic regression. *American Surgeon* **60**, 163–168.

Moss, J. and Craigo, P.A. 1993. The autonomic nervous system. In Rogers, M.C., Tinker, J.H., Covino, B.G. and Longnecker, D.E. (eds) *Principles and practice of anesthesiology*. London: Mosby Year Book.

Naslund, T.C. and Hollier, L.H. 1993. Reducing the risk of spinal cord injury during thoracoabdominal aortic aneurysm surgery. *Advances in vascular surgery*. Boston, MA: Mosby Year Book.

Naslund, N.C., Hollier, L.H., Money, S.R. *et al*. 1992. Protecting the ichemic spinal cord during aortic cross-clamping. *Annals of Surgery* **215**, 409–415.

Panneton, J.M. and Hollier, L.H. 1995. Nondissecting thoracoabdominal aortic aneurysms: Part 1. *Annals of Vascular Surgery* **9**, 503–514.

Pavlin, E.G. and Su, J.T. 1994. Cardiopulmonary pharmacology. In Miller, R.D. (ed.) *Anesthesia*, 4th edn. London: Churchill Livingstone.

Rosenbaum, G.J., Arroyo, P.J. and Sivina, M. 1994. Retroperitonial approach used exclusively with epidural anesthesia for infrarenal aortic disease. *American Journal of Surgery* **162**, 136–139.

Schiedler, M.G., Cutler, B.S. and Fiddian-Green, R.G. 1987. Sigmoid intramural pH for prediction of ischaemic colitis during aortic surgery. *Archives of Surgery* **122**, 881–886.

Scott, N.B. 1991. The effects of pain and its relief. In Wildsmith, J.A.W. and McClure, J. (eds) *Conduction blockade in postoperative analgesia*. London: Edward Arnold.

Shoemaker, W.C., Appel, P.L. and Kram, H.B. 1992. Role of oxygen debt in the development of organ failure, sepsis and death in high-risk surgical patients. *Chest* **102**, 208–215.

Sicard, J.A., Reilly, J.M., Rubin, B.G. *et al*. 1995. Transabdominal versus retroperitoneal incision for abdominal aortic surgery: a report of a prospective randomised trial. *Journal of Vascular Surgery* **21**(2), 174–183.

Sutcliffe, N.P., Akthar, T.M. and Kenny, G.N.C. 1995. Infusion techniques in anaesthesia. In Kaufmann, L. and Ginsburg, R. (eds) *Anaesthesia Review*, Vol. 12. Edinburgh: Churchill Livingstone.

Turfrey, D.J., Ray, D.A.A., Sutcliffe, N.P. *et al*. 1997. Thoracic epidural anaesthesia for coronary artery by-pass graft surgery. Effects on postoperative complications. *Anaesthesia* **52**, 1090–1113.

12

Anaesthesia for renovascular surgery and renal transplantation

J W SEAR

RENAL ANATOMY AND PHYSIOLOGY

The main blood supply to each kidney is a single renal artery, which divides sequentially into interlobar, arcuate and interlobular arteries, with the afferent glomerular arterioles arising from the last named. The renal venous architecture follows that of the arterial tree branches. Most of the nephrons arise from the superficial cortical region of the kidney, although about 15 per cent originate in the juxtaglomerular region.

Renal blood flow far exceeds the metabolic needs of the kidney, and hence the arteriovenous oxygen difference is small (about 1.7 mL/dL compared with a systemic difference of 5 mL/dL). The utilization of oxygen varies linearly with blood flow, because as flow increases so does the glomerular filtration rate (GFR), and hence the rate at which solutes (e.g. sodium) are re-absorbed. However blood flow is not uniform throughout the kidney, with the cortex receiving 75–80 per cent of total flow. There is maintenance of renal blood flow over a wide arterial pressure range (about 60–160 mmHg) by autoregulation.

This property is an intrinsic phenomenon which occurs even in the denervated kidney, and the underlying mechanism is still controversial (Knox and Spielman, 1983).

Solute and xenobiotic removal is the resultant of three separate processes (glomerular filtration, tubular transport and tubular re-absorption) related by the following equation:

Excretion = Filtration + Secretion - Reabsorption.

Filtration

This occurs in the glomerulus and is limited by the physicochemical properties of the solute molecule. Filtration is a non-selective process and results in the passage of all molecules with a molecular weight < 60–70 000 daltons (this is related to the size of the pores being 75 Å in diameter). Filtration is the main excretory route for uncharged molecules; charged ions are handled by other pathways (see later). Glomerular filtration is a passive process which occurs at a rate of about 180 L/day, with net

Table 12.1 *Transport carrier systems present for the secretion of endogenous substances by the renal tubules*

Anions	Cations
Ascorbate	Choline
Pantothenic acid	N-Methyl nicotinamide
Biliary salts	Acetylcholine
cAMP; cGMP	Dopamine
Conjugates of drugs and	Histamine
steroids	Adrenaline
Oxalate	Noradrenaline
Prostaglandins	Serotonin
Urate	Riboflavin

re-absorption of all except about 1.5–2.0 L. The GFR is best measured using inulin or ^{51}Cr-EDTA (ethylenediaminetetraacetic acid) clearance; creatinine clearance being inaccurate because of the influence of tubular secretion, which leads to overestimations especially at low GFRs.

Although the GFR is normally maintained over a wide range of systemic arterial blood pressures by renal autoregulation (see earlier), variations may occur to alter the rate of drug elimination. An important drug interaction is the reduction in GFR by non-steroidal anti-flammatory drugs (NSAIDs) (because the decrease in vasodilatation by the reduction in prostaglandin synthesis will allow a greater vasoconstrictor effect by angiotensin II). GFR also decreases with age; the creatinine clearance falls from around 140 mL/min/1.73 m^2 at age 20 years to 100 mL/min/1.73 m^2 at age 80 years.

Tubular secretion

There are two different general tubular mechanisms for handling the ions (Table 12.1). In renal failure, reduction in amine secretion will lead to their accumulation in the plasma, and to some of the clinical features of uraemia. The acidic and basic transport mechanisms have some common features and some which separate one from the other. Both systems are located exclusively in the proximal tubular region of the nephron. They are non-selective, and involve a transporter protein which binds the ion or drug and carries it from the blood into the nephron lumen against an electrochemical or concentration gradient. The transporter proteins exist in a finite quantity and hence saturation kinetics apply. Substrates may also compete for the transporter proteins if

secretion occurs by the same systems. The distribution of the transporter proteins within the proximal tubule is heterogeneous and species-dependent; both cation and anion systems are ATP (adenosine triphosphate) dependent.

Tubular re-absorption

This may be an active and/or passive process. Some passive reabsorption occurs for nearly all substances that are filtered.

PASSIVE RE-ABSORPTION

Normal nephron function involves re-absorption of water and electrolytes from the glomerular filtrate mainly in the proximal convoluted tubule, although it occurs throughout the tubule length. As a result, only about 10 per cent of the filtered sodium reaches the distal convoluted tubule.

ACTIVE RE-ABSORPTION

This is mainly the route of elimination for endogenous substances (e.g. electrolytes, glucose, amino acids and vitamins).

The final volume and composition of urine is influenced in the main by the tubular transport of sodium and water. The former occurs as an active process throughout the length of the nephron tubule except for the thin descending limb of the loop of Henle; water is re-absorbed as a passive process that parallels that of sodium. The filtrate from the glomerulus undergoes 65 per cent re-absorption in the proximal convoluted tubule – sodium being co-transported with glucose or amino acids, or exchanged for hydrogen ions which are then re-absorbed with bicarbonate ions.

In the loop of Henle and distal convoluted tubule, the absorption of water and sodium are influenced by the countercurrent multiplier system, and by three hormones – antidiuretic hormone (ADH), aldosterone and atrial natriuretic factor (ANF):

- ADH is produced in the posterior pituitary. Its release is controlled by stimulation of the osmoreceptors in the hypothalamus, and inhibited by stimulation of the atrial cardiac volume receptors. It acts in two ways: to increase the permeability of the cells of the collecting tubules, and to cause cortical arteriolar constriction with shunting of blood to the juxtaglomerular nephrons, which are able to produce highly concentrated urine.

• Aldosterone is secreted from the adrenal cortex following the release of renin from the juxtaglomerular cells of the kidney. There are three main stimuli to its release:

— The afferent arteriolar baroreceptor mechanism: decreased wall tension in the afferent arteriole caused by decreased perfusion;

— Sympathetic innervation of the granular cells: a systemic baroreceptor reflex activated by a reduction in effective circulating blood volume (and consequent blood pressure);

— The macula densa, which responds to decreased sodium delivery to the distal tubule.

The messenger for the release of aldosterone is angiotensin II, which is itself also a powerful vasoconstrictor. Aldosterone release can also be stimulated by high circulating levels of ACTH, or high extracellular potassium concentrations. Aldosterone increases sodium re-absorption and potassium secretion in the distal convoluted tubule, where water re-absorption occurs in parallel.

• ANF is a peptide produced in the cardiac atria released via the coronary sinus as a result of increased right- or left-atrial pressures or atrial distension. It is a powerful arterial vasodilator including the renal artery, so its effects increase renal blood flow and the glomerular filtration rate, and hence urine output and sodium excretion.

The action of these three hormonal systems is normally integrated to maintain intravascular and extracellular fluid volumes, and sodium and potassium homeostasis. However, in patients with renal artery stenosis in a single functional kidney (native or transplanted) or bilateral renal artery stenosis, there is loss of vasoconstrictor effect of angiotensin II which maintains the efferent arterial tone. As a result the GFR falls.

RENOVASCULAR HYPERTENSION

In the classical experiments of Goldblatt and colleagues (1934), partial occlusion of one renal artery in the dog caused systemic hypertension. It has now

been established that the reduction in renal perfusion causes an increase in the release of renin from the affected kidney (Fig. 12.1). In the initial stages, the increased blood pressure is probably the result of the vasoconstrictor action of angiotensin II. Salt and water are retained by the other kidney due to the enhanced effects of aldosterone. Later, the persistent hypertension may lead to the other kidney becoming damaged, and then the ability to excrete excesses of sodium and water is lost. Then the arterial hypertension becomes the resultant of the increased circulating concentrations of angiotensin II and the increased intravascular fluid volume. Thus, in the early phase, there is excretion of high levels of renin by the ischaemic kidney and its production by the other kidney is suppressed. Later, the retention of salt and water further suppresses renin production by both kidneys.

Causes of renovascular hypertension

In 70 per cent of cases, the main aetiological factor is atherosclerosis. This is seen particularly in the elderly male patient, and may be associated with other manifestations of ischaemic heart disease and peripheral vascular disease. The other 30 per cent of cases arise from a variety of causes and include medial fibromuscular dysplasia (seen in about 20 per cent) which affects the distal two-thirds of the main renal artery and its primary branches. It is common in young women, and may also affect both renal arteries as well as the carotids and iliac vessels. Other causes of renovascular hypertension include trauma, renal artery aneurysms, arteriovenous fistulae, Takayasu's disease (an arteritis causing stenosis of arteries arising from the aorta and found mainly in young adults and children of Asian origin) and renal artery hypoplasia.

Renovascular hypertension only becomes significant when stenosis is such as to reduce renal blood flow by 70 per cent. In general hypertensive populations, renovascular hypertension is the causative factor in about 1–5 per cent, although in patients with peripheral vascular disease, the overall prevalence of renal artery stenosis is about 30 per cent with 12 per cent of cases having bilateral disease.

In patients with severe hypertension (diastolic pressure >120 mmHg), there is a likely prevalence of renovascular hypertension of about 30 per cent; in cases of accelerated hypertension and accompanying

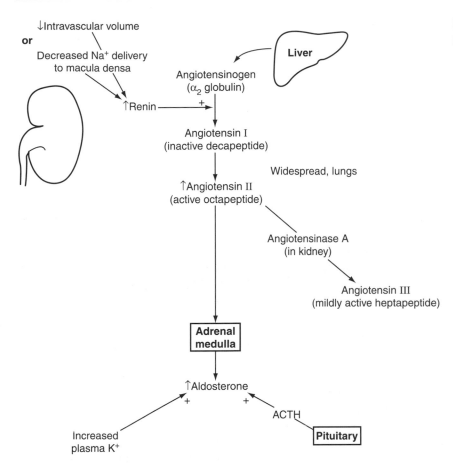

Figure 12.1   *The renin–angiotensin system.*

renal failure, the prevalence is about 45 per cent. If a patient is older than 50 years when they develop significant arterial hypertension (defined as a diastolic pressure >105 mmHg), then they too should be investigated for probable renovascular hypertension, as should the elderly patient with hypertension who develops associated renal failure.

The progress of renovascular disease is not the same in all patients; about 50 per cent of atherosclerotic patients will progress over a four- to five-year period, this pattern is less commonly seen in those patients with fibromuscular dysplasias. If stenosis reduces the diameter of the renal artery by 75 per cent or more, then 12–40 per cent of those patients with atherosclerotic disease will go on to complete renal artery occlusion over one year. One-third of these patients will also present with bilateral disease, and of those with initial unilateral disease at presentation, 40 per cent will subsequently develop contralateral stenosis within the following four years.

In renal artery stenosis, the kidney shrinks with loss of functional nephrons. This is initially a reversible change. Furthermore about 25 per cent of patients also develop acute pulmonary oedema which can similarly be reversed by revascularization of the affected kidney(s).

Pharmacological management

The main line of medical treatment has been β-adrenoceptor blocking drugs because they have several actions which decrease cardiac output: decreasing myocardial contractility, blocking peripheral adrenoceptors, and possibly decreasing plasma renin activity. More recently, other therapies (calcium-entry blockade and angiotensin-converting enzyme (ACE) inhibitors) have also been used, often in combination. However, in patients with reduced renal function, the introduction of the latter drugs may lead to a further reduction in the glomerular filtration rate by removing the vasoconstrictor effects of angiotensin II on the efferent arterioles, and so precipitate renal failure.

Surgical approaches to renal artery stenosis

Those patients subjected to surgery will usually undergo a midline laparotomy followed by extensive retroperitoneal dissection, temporary aortic cross-clamping, and a variable period of total renal ischaemia. The application of a suprarenal aortic clamp is often necessary, and the accompanying increase in afterload to a compromised myocardium may precipitate myocardial ischaemia and/or left ventricular failure (Roizen et al., 1984).

Possible operative procedures include

• Renal endarterectomy
• Aortorenal bypass grafting using saphenous vein or synthetic material
• Aortic bifurcation grafting with a separate 'jump' graft to the kidney
• Ilio- or viscerorenal reconstruction
• Autotransplantation to the iliac fossa with anastomosis of the kidney to the iliac vessels
• Nephrectomy: the treatment of choice in cases where there is a shrunken kidney, poor renal function, and arterial hypertension with accompanying high renin output.

The results of surgery are variable. About 15 per cent of patients with atherosclerotic renovascular disease progress to dialysis-dependent renal failure; in contrast, this is only seen in about 2 per cent of those with renal artery stenosis due to fibromuscular dysplasia. Overall, surgical treatment will improve renal function in 50 per cent of patients, stabilize function in 40 per cent and cause worsening in the remaining 10 per cent of patients. The operative mortality is not insignificant (between 1 and 6 per cent), and is usually the result of peri-operative myocardial infarction (Stanley and Fry, 1977).

Anaesthesia for correction of renovascular hypertension

The major intra-operative anaesthetic problems are those of optimal control of blood pressure and correction of intravascular fluid volume depletion. Suprarenal clamping of the aorta can result in significant increases in vascular resistance leading to myocardial ischaemia and ventricular failure, and the accompanying large fluid shifts seen on release of the clamp need to be adequately redressed in order to avoid severe post-clamping hypotension.

Invasive monitoring should be instituted before induction of anaesthesia. Arterial and central venous lines are routine, with a Swan–Ganz pulmonary artery catheter being inserted in patients with significant left ventricular hypertrophy, a past history of left ventricular failure or severe associated coronary arterial disease.

High doses of β-adrenoceptor blocking drugs do not appear, in the absence of heart failure, to affect intra-operative myocardial performance or ventricular ejection. Prys-Roberts (1982) showed that (in renovascular hypertensive patients with mean daily doses of propranolol of 21 mg/kg/day) induction of anaesthesia with an opioid and a small dose of hypnotic agent did not significantly affect arterial blood pressure or aortic dP/dt, and the pressor and chronotropic responses to laryngoscopy and intubation were obtunded. Despite the combination of direct and indirect myocardial depressant effects of the propranolol and the direct depressant effects of nitrous oxide–opioid anaesthesia, there occurred no evidence of intra-operative ventricular failure as had been previously described by Attia and colleagues (1976).

In a separate study, Ponten and colleagues (1982) have shown that abrupt withdrawal of β-adrenoceptor blocking drugs may result in a significant incidence of peri-operative myocardial ischaemia, which is not seen in patients where therapy is maintained. Furthermore in the presence of inhalation anaesthesia and coronary artery stenosis, β-adrenoceptor blockade leads to improved cardiovascular stability and myocardial protection (Foex et al., 1982). Thus, overall, the picture is supportive of the maintenance of the β-adrenoceptor blocking therapy.

However, there is controversy over the advisability of maintaining ACE-inhibitor therapy in surgical patients. Colson and colleagues (1992b) have studied the haemodynamic effects of neurolept anaesthesia in hypertensive patients maintained on a variety of ACE inhibitors. Induction of anaesthesia with fentanyl and flunitrazepam caused a greater reduction in arterial pressure, cardiac output and pulmonary capillary wedge pressure (when compared with hypertensive controls), requiring fluid loading and phenylephrine. When the ACE inhibitors (either captopril or enalapril) were stopped the evening before surgery, the incidence of induction-associated hypotension was reduced (20 per cent as compared with 78 per cent) (Coriat *et al.*, 1994). Intravascular volume regulation may be difficult to manage in patients on ACE inhibitors, especially in those patients with poor ventricular compliance; again use of the Swan–Ganz catheter may help.

However, data from patients with mild to moderate hypertension (mean pre-operative blood pressure 155/88 mmHg) treated by one of four monotherapies failed to show a larger arterial pressure or systemic vascular resistance reduction in patients on ACE inhibitors compared with β-adrenoceptor blockade, calcium-entry blockade or diuretics (Sear *et al.*, 1994).

The combination of calcium entry-blocking (CEB) drugs and anaesthesia leads to myocardial depression and delayed atrioventricular conduction, with enflurane showing a greater interaction than either halothane or isoflurane (Gorven *et al.*, 1986). There is no potentiation, however, of the depressant effects of the halogenated agents on intraventricular conduction. Opioid-based anaesthetic techniques are generally well tolerated in these patients (Durand *et al.*, 1991). While barbiturate–CEB interactions at induction of anaesthesia are similar to those with other antihypertensive agents, there is a tendency to higher post-induction heart rates compared with β-adrenoceptor blockade (Sear *et al.*, 1994).

Thus, the optimum anaesthetic approach in the patient with renovascular disease is one of an opioid-based technique with controlled ventilation, and the facility to continue ventilation into the post-operative period. Minute-by-minute control of blood pressure is best achieved by titration of the volatile agent, and infusions of esmolol or glyceryl trinitrate, and an α-adrenoceptor agonist such as phenylephrine.

RENAL PROTECTION DURING MAJOR VASCULAR SURGERY

In the healthy patient, the kidney receives about 20 per cent of the total cardiac output. However, the distribution of blood flow within the kidney varies. The cortex receives >90 per cent of total blood flow, and extracts about 18 per cent of total oxygen delivered. In contrast, the medulla extracts 79 per cent of delivered oxygen and has a very low tissue oxygen tension (about 8 mmHg; 1–2 kPa). Acute tubular

necrosis can be induced by a 40–50 per cent decrease in renal blood flow.

Medullary hypoxic injury is characterized by necrosis of renal tubules that are the farthest away from the blood vessels. The main determinant of medullary oxygen requirement is the rate of active re-absorption of salt and water in the thick ascending loop of Henle (mTAL) region. Where this process is inhibited by loop diuretics, there occurs an increase in the medullary oxygen partial pressure from 2 to 4 kPa. There are a number of mediators which can alter medullary blood flow, and hence the magnitude of ischaemic injury. These include:

- Vasodilators: nitric oxide, PGE_2, adenosine, dopamine and urodilantin (an analogue of atrial natriuretic hormone).
- Vasoconstrictors: endothelin, angiotensin II and ADH (vasopressin).
- Tubuloglomerular feedback: a reflex mechanism which causes glomerular afferent constriction when there is insufficient re-absorption of sodium by the renal tubules. This reduces filtration and hence the delivery and re-absorption of tubular solute.
- Medullary tubular growth factors. These include: insulin-like growth factor I; epidermal growth factor; and tumour necrosis factor (TNF). They may all accelerate the rate of recovery after experimental acute renal failure.

Because the work associated with salt and water re-absorption predisposes to medullary hypoxic damage, a major therapeutic advantage would seem to occur when there is volume- and salt-loading. This will reduce the work associated with urine concentration and thus medullary oxygen utilization. By the reverse, injury will be made worse by factors that counter this, such as some antibiotics, renal hypertrophy, NSAIDs, angiotensin II, calcium ions, myoglobin and contrast media.

Under a variety of different clinical situations, the glomerular filtration rate may be only 10 per cent of normal and it will remain low, despite a restoration of renal blood flow, because of tubular obstruction and backleak. Tubuloglomerular feedback and excessive stimulation of the renin–angiotensin system will often lead to profound and prolonged acute renal failure.

The kidney is largely devoid of β_2-receptors, and so any increase in circulating catecholamines (especially epinephrine) will cause vasoconstriction via α_1-receptors and renin–angiotensin system activation. As a result, intramedullary ischaemia will occur, despite a normal total renal blood flow especially in the mTAL region where the sodium–potassium ATPase enzymes are very sensitive to the effects of ischaemia. These increases in sympathomimetic hormones lead to renal cortical vasoconstriction, which is a compensatory attempt by the body to redistribute blood flow to the renal medulla, but in fact, it causes cortical ischaemia. As a result, there is reduced chloride re-absorption by the mTAL, leading to tubuloglomerular feedback via the macula densa with activation of the renin–angiotensin system and glomerular mesangial constriction.

Effects of aortic surgery on renal function

Breckwoldt and colleagues (1992) studied 205 patients undergoing surgery involving either infra- or suprarenal aortic clamping. In the infrarenal population, there was a 10 per cent incidence of transient renal dysfunction, compared with 28 per cent after supra-renal clamping. However there was no difference in the percentage of patients (2–3 per cent) in the two groups who required long-term haemodialysis.

Infrarenal aortic cross-clamping can cause a reduction in renal blood flow of up to 40 per cent, due to an increase in renal vascular resistance of up to 75 per cent (Gamulin *et al.*, 1986) (Fig. 12.2). The reduction in renal blood flow in turn reduces the GFR and hence the rate of urine formation. The mechanism underlying this increased resistance is uncertain but may be due, in part, to the associated decrease in cardiac output during aortic cross-clamping, as well as due to humoral mechanisms which lead to increased release of renin. After declamping, there is a maldistribution of renal blood flow away from the cortex for at least 60 min, and the deterioration in both renal blood flow (RBF) and GFR (compared to pre-operative values) persists for some time after the period of hospitalization. Awad and colleagues (1992) have found evidence of impairment up to six months later.

The aim of the anaesthetist, therefore, should be to maintain urine flow at 40–60 mL/h peri-operatively. Some routinely give pharmacological support to help achieve this, either intravenous mannitol

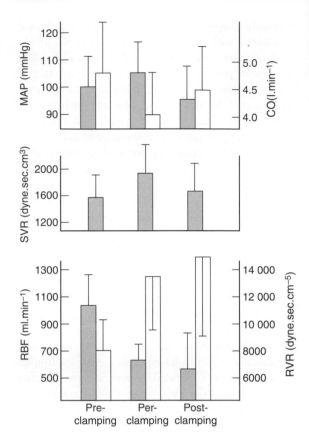

Figure 12.2 *Changes in mean arterial pressure (shaded columns) and cardiac output (open columns); systemic vascular resistance (shaded columns); renal blood flow (shaded columns) and renal vascular resistance (open columns) associated with aortic cross-clamping. (Adapted from Gamulin* et al.*, 1984; data shown as mean ± SD for 12 patients.)*

(25–50 g), frusemide or dopamine by infusion (1–3 µg/kg/min).

- Mannitol acts by two separate mechanisms. Firstly, as an osmotic diuretic it causes renal vasodilatation and thereby promotes renal tubular urine flow. It is also a free-radical scavenger, so reducing the effects of hydroxyl and other free radicals to cause ischaemic re-perfusion injury. It is essential that the mannitol is given prior to the ischaemic episode. However, mannitol can be injurious in large doses, because the osmotic diuresis may aggravate pre-existing medullary hypoxia.

- Frusemide also acts as a renal vasodilator.

- Dopamine increases sodium, potassium and urine output and creatinine clearance during infusion due to its effect on DA_1 receptors.

The influence of dopamine on renal function is controversial because it is not clear whether it can alleviate the decline in function that follows infrarenal aortic clamping. A number of studies have addressed this issue. Salem and colleagues (1988) showed a positive advantage of low-dose dopamine (2 µg/kg/min) when given in combination with fluid loading using Hartmann's solution (15 mL/kg/h) during aortic cross-clamping. There were post-operative increases in urine volume, creatinine clearance, and sodium and potassium output. However, a separate study by Paul and colleagues (1986) suggests that the effects of dopamine and mannitol are no different to those of extravascular volume expansion alone if the pulmonary artery wedge pressure is maintained at 12–15 mmHg. At lower wedge pressures (10 mmHg), Gamelin and colleagues (1984) were only able to maintain a urine output of 3 mL/min. A further study of 37 patients compared low-dose (3 µg/kg/min) dopamine and placebo on renal function after elective vascular surgery (Baldwin et al., 1994). Sufficient crystalloid was given to achieve normovolaemia, and to maintain a urine output of more than 1 mL/kg/h for the first 24 hours after surgery. Dopamine had no effect on post-operative plasma creatinine concentrations, creatinine clearance, or total urine output at 24 hours and five days.

More recent findings by Girbes and colleagues (1996) suggest that low-dose infusion of dopamine (2–4 µg/kg/min) will increase RBF and GFR (up to 20 and 21 per cent respectively) in patients undergoing aneurysmectomy under general anaesthesia supplemented by extradural analgesia. From this uncontrolled study of seven haemodynamically stable patients, the authors conclude that dopamine at 4 µg/kg/min is the optimum regimen. However, how does it produce its effects at this dose? At lower doses (0.5–3 µg/kg/min) dopamine augments RBF by DA_1-receptor-mediated intrarenal vasodilatation, and possibly the contributory engagement of DA_2-receptors on presynaptic sympathetic nerve terminals leading to inhibition of noradrenaline release. At intermediate doses of dopamine (3–10 µg/kg/min), dopamine augments renal perfusion by improving cardiac output via α_1-adrenoceptor stimulation.

However, these findings were made in normovolaemic subjects. What about the patient who may be hypovolaemic and hypothermic? In the study by Girbes and colleagues, the effect of low-dose dopamine in increasing renal blood flow was secondary to an increase in cardiac output. Plasma renin activity was unaltered, but plasma aldosterone concentrations were decreased. Thus, overall, these findings are at variance with the studies cited (Baldwin et al., 1994; Paul et al., 1986). The low doses of dopamine used by Girbes and colleagues (1996) probably act to increase urine output by a diuretic effect with an accompanying natriuresis and kaliuresis through a combination of some inotropic activity and renal vasodilator properties.

In a separate study, Joob and colleagues (1986) showed that increase in renal vascular resistance associated with cross-clamping can be prevented by pre-treatment with angiotensin-converting enzyme inhibitors; further double-blind controlled studies are needed to support these data.

MANAGEMENT OF RENAL ISCHAEMIC DAMAGE

If re-perfusion injury occurs, there are no clearly proven effective treatments. However, a number of approaches may be helpful, and there are also new treatments under evaluation.

In some centres, sodium bicarbonate may be routinely administered after infrarenal aortic clamping. The developing alkalosis may obtund the ischaemic damage. Secondly, there is usually a reflux of acid metabolites from the periphery after the release of the aortic clamp, and these may cause severe depression of myocardial contractility leading to hypotension.

To date there are two studies evaluating the effects of infusions of atrial natriuretic factor (ANF). Rahman and colleagues (1994) gave an infusion of ANF to 53 patients with ischaemic acute renal failure in a randomized controlled trial. Fewer patients in the treatment group required dialysis (23 vs. 52 per cent). However in a second study in patients receiving a cadaveric renal transplant, there was no advantage seen in those patients receiving an infusion of ANF commenced after revascularization (Sands et al., 1991).

Future advances in the treatment of renal ischaemic damage after aortic surgery may be made in the areas of nitric oxide homeostasis and endothelin antagonism. If nitric oxide synthase is inhibited by L-NAME, Booke and colleagues (1995) have shown an improvement in urine output and GFR in an awake sheep model of septic shock by returning systemic haemodynamics to the pre-septic state.

Several authors have found high concentrations of endothelin-1 in the plasma of patients with acute renal failure, with restoration to normal values after correction of the renal dysfunction (Tomita et al., 1989). Furthermore cross-clamping can increase plasma endothelin concentrations; the resulting renal vasoconstriction is preventable by nifedipine (Antonucci et al., 1990). Hence either endothelin receptor antagonists or endothelin antibodies might offer amelioration of hypoxic renal injury (Mino et al., 1992).

Effect of sympathetic block on renal function

Where there is effective autonomic sympathetic denervation due to central neuraxial blockade, and the unopposed effects of enhanced vagal activity, there will be both arterial and arteriolar denervation. However, there always remains some residual autonomic tone, such that the systemic vascular resistance falls by only 15–18 per cent. However, both spinal and epidural anaesthesia lead to a reduction in renal blood flow and glomerular filtration rate in the presence of a fall in mean arterial blood pressure. However, if correction is made for this fall in pressure, then there is no change in renal haemodynamics (Sivarajan et al., 1976).

If the fall in renal perfusion following cross-clamping is due to sympathetic overactivity, then interruption of the renal sympathetic inflow should obtund these changes. This was examined by Sivarajan and colleagues (1976) who measured systemic and regional blood flow changes during epidural anaesthesia in rhesus monkeys. They found that the decrease in renal blood flow was related to the height of the blockade. That is, if the block was up to T5, the blood flow fell by 25 per cent, and in the case of blockade to T1, by 31–37 per cent.

However, Gamulin and colleagues (1986) were unable to obtund the increase in renal vascular resistance after infrarenal clamping in patients undergoing aortic aneurysmectomy when epidural anaesthesia to T6 or above was established prior to induction of general anaesthesia.

Renal function after suprarenal aortic clamping

After vascular surgery involving suprarenal cross-clamping of the aorta, or thoracic or thoraco-abdominal aortic surgery, there is a high incidence of acute tubular necrosis. Svensson and colleagues (1989) found an overall hospital incidence of dialysis-requiring acute renal failure (ARF) of 5.5 per cent, with an in-hospital mortality of 63 per cent. The most important predictor of ARF was haemodynamic instability, while renal endarterectomy provided significant protection in patients with pre-existing renal dysfunction.

Following cross-clamping of the aorta above the renal arteries, even in the presence of mannitol protection, there is still a period of acute tubular necrosis with the GFR 2 h after clamp release being only 39 per cent of figures seen after infrarenal clamping (23 vs. 60 mL/min) (Myers et al., 1984). This lesion takes about 48 hours to correct.

Overall studies in patients undergoing aortic clamping show that the decrease in RBF does *not* correlate well with any measured decrease in cardiac output or change in mean arterial pressure, and the decrease in urine output does nor correlate with the degree of reduction in GFR. Neither does the magnitude of the decrease in urine output predict the occurrence or not of post-operative renal dysfunction.

ASSESSMENT OF PATIENTS UNDERGOING RENAL TRANSPLANTATION

As with any patient undergoing peripheral vascular surgery, the renal transplant recipient is at risk of peri-operative complications related to the various underlying intercurrent problems that they manifest. Patient survival after renal transplantation may appear superior to that associated with long-term dialysis, but until recently the older (>55 years) and sicker patients were less likely to be transplanted. However, survival following living related transplantation is certainly greater than in the patient maintained on dialysis (Burton and Walls, 1987).

Of greatest importance to the peri-operative well-being of the transplant recipient is a proper assessment of the cardiovascular and other systematic problems of end-stage renal failure. The former (which include arterial hypertension, atherosclerosis and hyperlipidaemia, and pericarditis) represent the commonest cause of death in these patients. In most centres, the one-year graft survival for a first cadaveric graft is greater than 80 per cent, with a peri-operative mortality of <1 per cent.

Hypertension, ischaemic heart disease and pericarditis

These represent the common intercurrent problems in patients presenting with end-stage renal disease. The incidence of pre-operative hypertension varies between 68 and 94 per cent in patients undergoing renal transplantation, while the incidence of ischaemic heart disease is also high: about 1 in 20 of recipients aged < 55 years and higher in the elderly.

The aetiology of hypertension of chronic renal failure is often a consequence of volume expansion secondary to salt and water retention (Brown et al., 1971). In patients in whom the hypertension cannot be controlled by dialysis alone, it is suggested that an abnormal relationship exists between plasma renin activity, intravascular fluid volume and blood pressure. There may also be an inappropriate level of sympathetic activity (Converse et al., 1992). However, improvements in dialysis technology have led to a significant reduction in the numbers of patients receiving antihypertensive therapy. Those needing treatment (about 10–15 per cent) often show high plasma renin activities and are refractory to single agents requiring large doses of combinations of antihypertensive drugs (e.g. β-adrenoceptor blocking drugs, calcium-channel blockers, vasodilators and angiotensin-converting enzyme inhibitors). As a result, there may be significant drug interactions with volatile and intravenous anaesthetic agents (Jenkins and Scoates, 1985; Durand et al., 1990; Colson et al., 1992a; Coriat et al., 1994; Sear et al., 1994).

About 50–70 per cent of patients receiving a renal transplant will suffer marked swings in blood pressure during surgery (± 30 per cent shifts from the awake pre-induction value), and will also show exaggerated vascular responses to induction of anaesthesia, laryngoscopy and intubation, and extubation, as seen in the patient with hypertension due to other non-renal causes. Similarly, postural hypotension may also occur – especially following dialysis – due to the combination of excess fluid removal, over treatment with antihypertensive therapy, or accompanying coincidental diabetic autonomic neuropathy. In order to optimize the patient, current antihypertensive or anti-anginal treatment should normally be given as part of the premedication. Poorly controlled hypertension may be treated by additional intravenous β-adrenoceptor blockade (Prys-Roberts et al., 1973). Stone and colleagues (1988) have also demonstrated the efficacy of pre-operative oral β-adrenoceptor blockade in reducing haemodynamic lability in response to surgical stress, and the associated incidence of myocardial ischaemia. The association of pre-existing hypertension and post-operative mortality in elective general surgical practice has been recently shown in a case–control study from Howell and colleagues (1996), and there is no reason to question the same association in the high-risk patient with renal failure, although this was not factor defined by Solomonson and colleagues (1996) in a retrospective analysis of patients having an arteriovenous fistula created.

Pulmonary oedema (secondary to congestive failure) is common in patients with end-stage renal disease and may be due to fluid overload, or as a consequence of peri-operative myocardial ischaemia or infarction. The incidence of infarction is about ten times more common for age- and sex-matched patients in the presence of end-stage renal disease. Rarer causes include excessive flow through an arteriovenous shunt, or a hyperdynamic circulation in the presence of severe anaemia.

Patients with renal failure, especially those on dialysis, are prone to develop accelerated atherosclerosis and peripheral vascular disease. The increase in triglyceride levels in renal failure correlates significantly with the incidence of occlusive coronary artery disease and peripheral vascular disease. Uraemic cardiomyopathy and pericarditis and effusions also occur in patients with renal failure, resulting in further decreases in contractility and cardiac output.

In the diabetic uraemic patient, about 33 per cent will have accompanying peripheral vascular disease, as well as a degree of gastroparesis and autonomic neuropathy, which may lead to post-operative cardiovascular instability.

Respiratory consequences of uraemia

Uraemic lung is the radiological entity of perihilar pulmonary venous congestion secondary to fluid retention. Excessive fluid administration may therefore result in the development of right heart failure.

Anaemia

Anaemia is one of the major problems in the anaesthetic management of patients with renal failure. Haemoglobin concentrations in patients on haemodialysis are often 6–8 mg/100 mL with haematocrits of 20–25 per cent. The clinical presentation is a normochromic, normocytic anaemia of complex aetiology. The various factors include impaired erythropoiesis due to decreased erythropoietin synthesis and release, bone-marrow depression to uraemia, decreased red cell lifespan, increased haemolysis and bleeding, repeated blood loss during haemodialysis, and aluminium toxicity. Other causative factors include iron, folate and vitamin B_6 and B_{12} deficiencies.

Introduction of biosynthetic erythropoietin (EPO) to increase haemoglobin concentrations has improved the picture in many patients (Winnearls et al., 1986). However, its use is accompanied by significant side effects if the haematocrit is raised above 35 per cent. These include hypertension, cerebrovascular accidents, thrombosis of fistulae and epileptiform activity (Eschbach et al., 1987). The positive advantage is the reduction in the need for repeated top-up blood transfusions, and the likely development of anti-HLA (human leukocyte antigen) cytotoxic antibodies.

Coagulation

Some patients show persistent heparinization after haemodialysis before transplantation (Hampers et al., 1966). In addition, a small percentage of uraemic patients, normally those inadequately dialysed or transplanted before requiring dialysis, exhibit a separate haemorrhagic diathesis. Several coagulation factor abnormalities have been described (platelet dysfunction, decreased levels of platelet factor III resulting in poor adhesiveness and thrombocytopaenia). Laboratory investigations show no alteration in prothrombin or partial thromboplastin time, but the bleeding time is prolonged. The decrease in platelet factor III occurs through accumulation of toxic endogenous waste products including guanininosuccinate, phenol and phenolic acid. If these products are removed by adequate dialysis, there is return to normal platelet function (Weir and Chung, 1984).

Other methods of treatment of uraemic coagulopathy include platelet transfusion, cryoprecipitate and infusions of desamino-8-D-AVP (DDAVP), the last acting to increase the activity of coagulation factors VIII, XII, von Willebrand's factor, and high-molecular-weight kininogen (Mannucci et al., 1983). After a dose of 0.3 µg/kg, platelet function improves for up to 4 h.

Acid–base and electrolyte abnormalities

Increases in plasma creatinine and urea occur when more than 70 per cent of glomerular mass is lost. Patients with renal failure have an inability to excrete water, electrolytes and free acids. The presence of a metabolic acidosis with its associated electrolyte disturbances (hyponatraemia, hyperchloraemia and hyperkalaemia) may cause problems with respect to the adequacy of reversal of residual neuromuscular blockade at the end of anaesthesia. However, this has become less important with the routine dialysis of all patients before transplantation.

The main electrolyte abnormality relates to the pre-operative serum potassium concentration. At concentrations greater than 6.5 mmol/L, abnormal electrocardiographic (ECG) changes are common, so high potassium levels should be avoided. There is, however, some evidence that uraemic patients can tolerate mild-to-moderate degrees of hyperkalaemia, and it is probably safe to conduct anaesthesia in the presence of higher than normal potassium concentrations, unless there are ECG changes associated with hyperkalaemia (high-peaked T-waves, decreased amplitude of the R-wave, widened QRS complexes and progressive diminution of P-wave amplitude). In this case, treatment includes glucose–insulin therapy, intravenous calcium gluconate or chloride, calcium resonium enema (30–60 g) or continuous haemofiltration or haemodialysis.

Hypokalaemia is unusual in end-stage renal disease, but may occur in the fluid overloaded anephric patient, or in the patient on loop diuretics. Potentiation of neuromuscular blockade may be seen unless the potassium depletion is corrected.

Central nervous system symptomatology

The central nervous system features of uraemia are initially malaise and reduced mental ability, but may proceed to myoclonus, grand mal convulsions, then to coma and death. Patients complain of pruritus, which tends to be severe at night and at rest, and is relieved by movement. Peripheral neuropathies are commonly seen in the lower limbs, and may involve the autonomic nervous system leading to postural hypotension.

Excessive dialysis can lead to a 'dysequilibration syndrome' with shrinkage of the extracellular fluid volume and cerebral oedema. An alternative presentation is one of progressive dementia (perhaps related to aluminium toxicity).

Endocrine effects of uraemia

Uraemic osteodystrophy encompasses a number of separate skeletal problems including osteomalacia, osteosclerosis and osteitis fibrosa cystica. The last develops as a result of secondary hyperparathyroidism. As renal function decreases, phosphate excretion falls and the resulting hyperphosphataemia leads to a reduced absorption of calcium and hyperactivity of the parathyroid glands in an attempt to maintain the serum calcium concentration.

Gastrointestinal symptoms

The uraemic patient will commonly complain of anorexia, nausea and vomiting, gut bleeding, diarrhoea and hiccups. Most of these problems will be attenuated by the introduction of dialysis prior to transplantation. All renal failure patients have delayed gastric emptying in addition to an increase in acidity and gastric volume. Hence patients will benefit from a histamine H_2 receptor antagonist as part of the premedication.

Problems associated with haemodialysis

The main sequelae are excessive or persistent heparinization, abnormal fluid shifts and transmission of viral infections (e.g. hepatitis A and B, human immunodeficiency virus (HIV), cytomegalovirus (CMV)). Residual heparinization presents as a bleeding diathesis occurring up to 10 hours after haemodialysis. It is readily corrected by protamine.

Protection of shunts and fistulae

Functional shunts or fistulae should be carefully protected during surgery, with the oscillometer cuff on the other arm. Venous lines should be restricted where possible to peripheral veins on the dorsum of the hand, with the preservation of all forearm and antecubital fossa veins. The monitoring of central venous pressure (CVP) is useful during transplantation as many patients come to surgery dehydrated following pre-operative dialysis and may need extensive volume replacement to maintain a normal CVP.

EFFECTS OF RENAL IMPAIRMENT ON ANAESTHETIC DRUG KINETICS

To provide appropriate anaesthesia, the clinician needs to have a clear understanding of the effects of renal dysfunction on drug disposition and elimination.

Premedicant drugs

Atropine and glycopyrrolate are 20–50 per cent eliminated via the kidney, but accumulation is unlikely to occur in renal failure because they are only administered as single doses. In contrast, only 1 per cent hyoscine is recoverable in the urine. Because glycopyrrolate has a lesser cardiac stimulant effect than atropine, it may be preferred in the patient with cardiac as well as end-stage renal disease.

The phenothiazines are cleared extensively by the liver and their disposition is not influenced by renal failure. However, their use may be associated with intra-operative cardiovascular instability through interaction of their α-adrenoceptor blocking effects with the hypovolaemia commonly seen post-dialysis.

Sedative and anxiolytic drugs

The disposition of several important benzodiazepines is altered in patients with acute or chronic renal impairment. For a given intravenous dose, the free concentration of diazepam is increased with an accompanying increased volume of distribution and systemic clearance (Ochs et al., 1981). Similar increases in the free fraction are seen with midazo-lam when given to patients with chronic renal failure (Vinik *et al.*, 1983). These changes are associated with greater total drug clearance and volumes of distribution.

More recently, the importance of the sedative properties of metabolites of midazolam have been recognized. The first step in the metabolism of the imidazolino-benzodiazepine is by hydroxylation involving cytochrome P450 IIIA4 to α-hydroxy-midazolam and 4-hydroxymidazolam. These are then both conjugated to the corresponding glucuronides, and eliminated by glomerular filtration and tubular secretion. In end-stage renal failure, high concentrations of α-hydroxymidazolam glucuronide accumulate, and in some patients may be responsible for prolonged sedation (Oldenhof *et al.*, 1988; Bauer *et al.*, 1995). Bauer and colleagues (1995) have shown there to be *in vitro* binding of the glucuronide to the cerebral benzodiazepine receptor, suggesting it may have substantial pharmacological activity.

The effects of end-stage renal disease on the disposition of other benzodiazepines used during anaesthesia are less clearly defined. Verbeeck and colleagues (1976) found the disposition of single doses of lorazepam to be unaltered in renal failure, although there was impaired clearance of the drug following chronic administration to two patients with uraemia.

Induction agents

BARBITURATES

Despite the increased sensitivity of patients in chronic renal failure to barbiturate drugs, thiopentone is still widely used for induction of anaesthesia. Normal doses of thiopentone induced prolonged unconsciousness, the duration being related to the blood urea concentration (Dundee and Richards, 1954). Various suggestions have been made as to the cause of this. These include increased blood–brain barrier permeability, increased unbound barbiturate in uraemic patients, qualitative plasma albumin abnormalities or abnormal cerebral uptake and metabolism of the barbiturate.

The disposition of thiopentone in patients with chronic renal failure has been studied by Burch and Stanski (1982), and Christensen and colleagues (1983) who found an unaltered total drug elimination half-life, but an increased free-drug fraction.

Unbound (free) drug kinetics were unaltered. However, the increased free-drug fraction will result in higher brain concentrations of thiopentone. If there is assumed to be no alteration in brain or cardiovascular sensitivity to thiopentone in the patient with chronic renal failure, then a decreased rate of administration rather than a decreased drug dosing should be used for induction of anaesthesia. There are presently no data on the disposition of methohexitone in patients with chronic renal failure.

ETOMIDATE

There are no formal studies on the disposition of the carboxylated imidazole, etomidate, in patients with renal failure, although Carlos and colleagues (1979) have shown a significant decrease in the plasma protein binding of etomidate in patients with uraemia. The dynamic properties of etomidate in patients with impaired cardiovascular function may be useful especially in the mildly hypovolaemic patient.

KETAMINE

Ketamine is probably best avoided for induction of anaesthesia for transplantation because it causes increases in both heart rate and blood pressure. These may be deleterious in the patient with pre-existing hypertension or coronary arterial disease.

PROPOFOL

Kinetic studies following induction of anaesthesia with diisopropyl phenol (propofol) show no significant effect of renal impairment on plasma protein binding (Costela *et al.*, 1996) or on the elimination half-life or systemic clearance (Kirvela *et al.*, 1992). These authors have also shown similar cardiovascular changes following propofol 2 mg/kg preceded by fentanyl 3 µg/kg in adequately volume-loaded uraemic patients to those in healthy subjects. There was significant vasodilatation in all patients, with falls in arterial blood pressure. Adequate antihypertensive therapy in the uraemic patients may have contributed to the cardiovascular stability.

Neuromuscular blocking drugs

Among the most used of the anaesthetic drugs to be affected by impaired renal function are the

Table 12.2 *Commonly used neuromuscular blocking drugs and their dependence on renal excretion for their elimination*

Extent of elimination by kidney (%)	Drugs
>95%	Gallamine
60–90	Pancuronium, *d*-methyl tubocurarine pipecuronium
25–60	*d*-tubocurarine, doxacurium
<25%	Vecuronium, atracurium, mivacurium, cis-atracurium, rocuronium, suxamethonium

neuromuscular blocking agents. Table 12.2 lists the extent of urinary excretion in the elimination of the various muscle relaxants.

DEPOLARIZING NEUROMUSCULAR RELAXANTS

One of the main areas of controversy relates to the use of suxamethonium in patients with end-stage renal disease. Wyant (1967) reported a decrease in the activity of the enzyme plasma pseudocholinesterase (and hence a decreased rate of degradation of suxamethonium) in patients on haemodialysis, but this does not appear to be a significant problem with current dialysis techniques. However there is undoubtedly prolongation of the action of suxamethonium in some patients with chronic renal failure. Although the exact incidence is unknown, Bastron and Deutsch (1976) quote a greater frequency than in the general surgical population.

A second problem is suxamethonium-induced increases in serum potassium concentrations. Way and colleagues (1972) have shown the increase in potassium in patients on haemodialysis to be comparable with that seen in normal healthy individuals. Pretreatment with non-depolarizing neuromuscular blocking drugs do not prevent this increase in plasma potassium concentrations.

NON-DEPOLARIZING (COMPETITIVE) NEUROMUSCULAR RELAXANTS

End-stage renal disease significantly affects the handling of some competitive neuromuscular blocking drugs (e.g. *d*-tubocurarine, *d*-methyl tubocurarine and pancuronium) which all undergo renal excretion to some extent (Table 12.3). With pancuronium and *d*-tubocurarine, some augmentation of biliary excretion may occur in patients with renal impairment. This allows these two relaxants to be used in patients with renal problems although the dose should be reduced.

Table 12.3 *Influence of chronic renal failure on the disposition of competitive neuromuscular blocking drugs*

	Patients with normal renal function			Patients with impaired renal function			
	$T_{1/2}$el	Cl_p	V_{ss}	$T_{1/2}$el	Cl_p	V_{ss}	
Tubocurarine	1.4	2.4	0.25	2.2*	1.5*	0.25	(Miller *et al.*, 1977)
Pancuronium	2.2	1.8	0.26	4.3*	0.9*	0.30	(Somogyi *et al.*, 1977)
	1.7	1.0	0.14	8.2*	0.3*	0.14	(McLeod *et al.*, 1978)
Gallamine	2.2	1.2	0.24	12.5*	0.2*	0.28	(Ramzan *et al.*, 1981)
d-Methyl tubocurarine	6.0	1.2	0.57	11.4*	0.4*	0.48	(Brotherton *et al.*, 1981)
Vecuronium	1.3	3.0	0.19	1.6	2.5	0.24	(Fahey *et al.*, 1981)
	0.88	5.3	0.20	1.36*	3.2*	0.24	(Lynam *et al.*, 1988)
Atracurium	0.35	6.1	0.18	0.40	6.7	0.22	(Fahey *et al.*, 1984)
	0.28	5.9	0.19	0.35	6.9	0.21	(deBros *et al.*, 1986)
	0.33	5.5	0.16	0.34	5.8	0.14	(Ward *et al.*, 1987)
Cisatracurium	0.50	4.2	0.13	0.57	3.6	0.13	(Eastwood *et al.*, 1996)
Pipecuronium	2.3	2.4	0.31	4.4*	1.6*	0.44	(Caldwell *et al.*, 1989)
Doxacurium	1.7	2.7	0.22	3.7	1.2*	0.27	(Cook *et al.*, 1991)

$T_{1/2}$el: elimination half-life (hours)
Cl_p: systemic clearance (mL/kg/min)
V_{ss}: apparent volume of distribution at steady state (L/kg)
*$P < 0.05$ vs. healthy subjects

d-Tubocurarine and *d*-methyl tubocurarine

Prolonged paralysis is seen only in the uraemic patient after use of large or repeated doses of *d*-tubocurarine. Normally, up to 70 per cent of an intravenous dose of *d*-tubocurarine is recovered in the urine. The renally excreted fraction of the methyl derivative is between 45 and 50 per cent in the healthy patient.

Pancuronium

In healthy patients, about 40 per cent of an intravenous dose is excreted in the urine, and another 10 per cent in the bile. Augmentation of biliary excretion occurs in renal failure, but there is still a decrease in systemic clearance of pancuronium (McLeod *et al.*, 1976; Somoygi *et al.*, 1977; Buzello and Agoston, 1978) coupled with prolonged neuromuscular blockade (Geha *et al.*, 1976).

Atracurium

Clinical studies by Hunter and colleagues (1982) have not shown any difference in the duration of neuromuscular blockade of an initial dose of atracurium, or from repeated doses, when the drug is administered to patients with normal function, compared to patients who were anephric. Similarly dynamic–kinetic studies (Fahey *et al.*, 1984; de Bros *et al.*, 1986) demonstrated that onset time, duration of action, recovery time (from 25 to 75 per cent initial twitch height) and disposition kinetics were unaltered in patients with renal failure.

Atracurium may also be administered by continuous infusion to maintain neuromuscular blockade, and rapid recovery has been reported with its use in this way in the patient with renal failure (Russo *et al.*, 1986; Richard *et al.*, 1986). However, Nguyen and colleagues (1985) observed a prolonged recovery rate and longer time to 90 per cent recovery of twitch height when administering atracurium by infusion to anephric patients.

Atracurium undergoes elimination by both Hofmann degradation and ester hydrolysis, although Fisher and colleagues (1985) have suggested that up to 50 per cent of total systemic clearance cannot be accounted for by either of these mechanisms. An important metabolite of atracurium, laudanosine, has been reported in animals to cause excitatory electroencephalogram (EEG) activity when administered in high doses.

A number of authors have investigated the relationship between renal function and plasma concentrations of laudanosine during anaesthesia and in the intensive-therapy unit (Yate *et al.*, 1987; Ward *et al.*, 1987; Parker *et al.*, 1988). After single doses of atracurium (up to 0.3 mg/kg), renal failure had no effect on the elimination of atracurium or its two metabolites, laudanosine and the associated monoquaternary alcohol. Peak laudanosine concentrations were not different from those in healthy patients. In intensive-therapy unit patients receiving an infusion of atracurium, maximum laudanosine concentrations have not exceeded about 5 μg/mL, even in the anephric patient. Similar values have been measured during infusions of atracurium to patients undergoing renal transplantation (Lepage *et al.*, 1987).

Cisatracurium

This is one of the ten stereoisomers of atracurium (the 1R-*cis*, 1R'-*cis* isomer), but unlike the parent compound, its metabolism is mainly by Hofmann degradation with no ester hydrolysis. Recent studies (Kisor *et al.*, 1996) confirm that the Hofmann pathway accounts for about 77 per cent of total body clearance, organ clearance 23 per cent and renal clearance 16 per cent. The drug has an elimination half-life of 23 min, and clearance in healthy subjects of about 5.2 mL/kg/min. The main metabolites are laudanosine and a monoquaternary acrylate.

Two recent studies have examined the dynamics and disposition of cisatracurium in renal failure. Boyd and colleagues (1995) showed that at a dose of $2 \times ED_{95}$ (0.1 mg/kg), onset times were longer in the renal failure group, but recovery was not affected. In these patients, the clearance of cisatracurium was decreased by 13 per cent and the half-life longer (34.2 vs. 30 min). Although plasma concentrations of laudanosine were elevated in patients with renal failure, the values were about one-tenth of those seen after atracurium (Eastwood *et al.*, 1995).

Vecuronium

Although initial studies (Fahey *et al.*, 1981) indicated that renal failure did not alter the duration of neuromuscular blockade or the kinetics of the drug, this study was limited by the sensitivity of the drug assay. A better evaluation of vecuronium kinetics has been carried out in patients receiving cadaveric renal allografts and a control group of healthy patients (Lynam *et al.*, 1988). Anaesthesia was maintained with nitrous oxide in oxygen and 1 per cent end-tidal isoflurane. The dynamics of the relaxant (duration of neuromuscular blockade and recovery indices) were prolonged in the renal failure group, but there were no kinetic differences.

A number of reports have suggested that there may be accumulation of vecuronium in the patient with renal failure (Bevan *et al.*, 1984; Lepage *et al.*, 1987; Cody and Dorman, 1987; Starsnic *et al.*, 1989). Because of the clinical importance of any dynamic interaction with renal failure, Beauvoir and colleagues (1993) conducted a meta-analysis of the available data. Based on six studies, they found a significant increase in the duration of effect (as assessed as the time from injection to 25 per cent recovery of twitch height) but no differences in onset time or 25–75 per cent recovery times.

This altered disposition of some neuromuscular blocking drugs in patients with renal failure therefore affects our clinical usage. If a small initial paralysing dose of a drug is given, its effect will be limited by distribution within the body. However, when drugs are given as larger doses or by multiple increments or by infusion, then recovery is influenced by the drug's terminal half-life. For all the competitive neuromuscular blocking agents, the clinician should aim to carefully titrate the dose so as to avoid high drug concentrations remaining in the blood at the completion of anaesthesia and surgery. Potentiation of neuromuscular blockade may also occur in patients with metabolic acidosis; the acidosis also opposes the reversal by neostigmine. In the uraemic patient undergoing renal transplant surgery, potentiation of blockade may also occur due to hypokalaemia, hypocalcaemia, hypermagnesaemia, parenteral or topical use of aminoglycoside antibiotics, frusemide, mannitol and methylprednisolone.

Newer neuromuscular blocking drugs

There are four new neuromuscular blocking agents which show different disposition profiles in renal failure.

Pipecuronium   This is a bisquaternary amino-steroid compound, which is mainly eliminated unchanged by the kidney. Renal failure causes a prolonged elimination half-life and reduced clearance (Caldwell *et al.*, 1989). There is also an increased apparent volume of distribution at steady state, suggesting a decrease in plasma protein binding.

Doxacurium   This is a long-acting drug with an elimination half-life of 99 min, and clearance of 2.7 mL/kg/min. It is mainly excreted unchanged (60 per cent) by the kidney, although esterase hydrolysis may contribute in part to the termination of drug effect. Clearance is reduced in patients with renal failure, with accompanying prolongation of effect (Cook *et al.*, 1991; Cashman *et al.*, 1992).

At present neither of these drugs appear likely to be available in the United Kingdom.

Mivacurium   This is a short-acting benzyliso-quinolinium compound which is metabolized by plasma esterases and presumably also in the liver. There is also about 10 per cent excretion via the kidney. In healthy subjects, De Bros and colleagues (1987) demonstrated an elimination half-life of 17 min, and a clearance of 54 mL/kg/min. The pharmacokinetics and duration of effect of bolus doses are not prolonged in renal failure (Cook *et al.*, 1992). However, when given by constant infusion (10 µg/kg/min), spontaneous recovery in anephric patients was slower than in healthy subjects (Phillips and Hunter, 1992), although this may reflect the reduction in plasma cholinesterase activity.

Mivacurium is formulated as three stereoisomers. The more potent are the *cis,trans* and *trans,trans* forms whose systemic clearance is inversely related to plasma cholinesterase activity. The least potent isomer (*cis,cis*) is probably eliminated via the kidneys. Head-Rapson and colleagues (1995) have shown reduced systemic clearance of the latter isomer (but not the other two) in patients with end-stage renal failure.

Rocuronium   This is another agent with a rapid onset of effect and intermediate duration of action. Being a steroid molecule, it is metabolized in the liver, with only 9 per cent of the injected dose being recoverable from the urine over the first 60 h after administration.

In a recent study comparing its kinetics and dynamics in both healthy anaesthetized subjects and patients undergoing cadaveric renal transplantation, Szenohradszky and colleagues (1992) have shown renal failure to alter drug distribution, but not systemic clearance. That drug dynamics are unaltered in end-stage renal failure has been confirmed (Khuenl-Brady *et al.*, 1993).

Thus, of these newer neuromuscular blocking drugs, both mivacurium and rocuronium would appear suitable alternatives to vecuronium, atracurium and cisatracurium in patients undergoing renal transplantation.

Table 12.4 *Influence of chronic renal failure on the disposition of anticholinesterases (adapted from Cronnelly and Morris, 1982)*

	Patients with normal renal function			Patients with impaired renal function		
	$T_{1/2}$el	Cl_p	V_{ss}	$T_{1/2}$el	Cl_p	V_{ss}
Neostigmine	80	9.0	0.7	183*	3.4*	0.8
Edrophonium	110	9.6	1.1	206*	2.7*	0.7
Pyridostigmine	112	8.6	1.1	379*	2.1*	1.0

$T_{1/2}$el: elimination half-life (min)
Cl_p: systemic clearance (mL/kg/min)
V_{ss}: apparent volume of distribution at steady state (L/kg)
*$P < 0.05$ vs. healthy subjects

Anticholinesterases

All these drugs are excreted by the combination of glomerular filtration and tubular secretion. A significant decrease in the clearance of all three anticholinesterases is seen in patients with renal failure (Cronnelly and Morris, 1982) (Table 12.4).

Opioid analgesic drugs

In the healthy patient, most opioid drugs are metabolized to inactive compounds which are then excreted in the urine or bile. For example, the metabolism of pethidine, alfentanil, fentanyl, sufentanil and morphine may be as high as 80–95 per cent. Phenoperidine differs from these other opioids in that about 50 per cent is normally eliminated in the urine in an unchanged form. Thus in renal failure, the action of phenoperidine is most likely to be prolonged.

FENTANYL, ALFENTANIL AND SUFENTANIL

In awake subjects with end-stage renal disease, the kinetics of fentanyl show an increased apparent volume of distribution, and an increased systemic clearance (Corall *et al.*, 1980). However, Bower (1982) found no change in the plasma protein binding of fentanyl in patients, such that the findings of Corall and colleagues (1980) require further confirmation. Most data from anaesthetized patients with uraemia indicate unaltered fentanyl disposition (Duthie, 1986; Koehntop and Rodman, 1997; Sear, 1986).

Studies evaluating alfentanil disposition indicate an increased free-drug fraction in anaesthetized uraemic patients (Chauvin *et al.*, 1987b; Bower and

Sear, 1989), resulting in greater total drug-clearance rates and volumes of distribution but no difference in free-drug kinetics.

Although not available for intravenous use in the United Kingdom, the disposition of sufentanil is similarly unaltered in end-stage renal disease (Fyman *et al.*, 1988; Davis *et al.*, 1988; Sear, 1989). There are, however, case reports of prolonged narcosis following administration of sufentanil to patients with chronic renal failure (Wiggum *et al.*, 1985; Fyman *et al.*, 1988), which are probably due to alterations in the dynamics of the opioid in the uraemic patient.

MORPHINE

Olsen and his colleagues (1975) have shown that the plasma protein binding of morphine in patients with uraemia was decreased, but the free fraction only increased from 65 to 70–75 per cent). There are several reports of prolonged or exaggerated clinical effects when intravenous morphine was given to patients with end-stage renal disease (Mostert *et al.*, 1971; Don *et al.* 1975; Stanley *et al.*, 1977).

Several authors have confirmed that renal failure *per se* has little effect on morphine parent-drug clearance, but does result in the accumulation of the analgesically active metabolite, morphine-6-glucuronide (Aitkenhead *et al.*, 1984; Sawe and Odar-Cederlof, 1987; Woolner *et al.*, 1986; Chauvin *et al.*, 1987a; Sear *et al.*, 1989) (Fig. 12.3). These higher concentrations of morphine-6-glucuronide may account for the profound analgesia and sedation seen in uraemic patients who receive large doses of morphine or papaveretum (Osborne *et al.*, 1986).

In uraemic patients undergoing transplantation who received 10 mg morphine i.v. as a supplement to nitrous oxide (67 per cent) in oxygen anaesthesia,

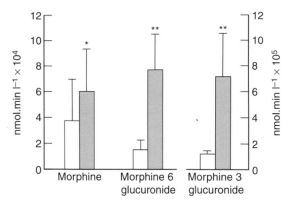

Figure 12.3 *Areas under the concentration versus time plots for morphine, morphine-3-glucuronide and morphine-6-glucuronide in anaesthetized patients with normal renal function (n = 5; open columns) and patients undergoing renal transplantation (n = 11; shaded columns). *P < 0.05; **P < 0.01. (Adapted from Sear et al., 1989.)*

elimination half-lives of morphine-6-glucuronide ranged between 220 and 900 min (compared with 100–200 min in the healthy anaesthetized patient) (Sear *et al.*, 1989). The influence of immediate graft function in transplanted patients was reflected by lower concentrations of morphine-6-glucuronide and a smaller AUC (area under the concentration–time curve) between 0 and 24 hours.

In the patients with chronic renal failure, there was also a larger AUC (between 0 and 24 hours) for morphine (Sear *et al.*, 1989). Together with other data (Mazoit *et al.*, 1990; Sloan *et al.*, 1991; Osborne *et al.*, 1993), this supports the view that the kidney may itself have a role in morphine metabolism. Whereas the papers of Mazoit and Sloan suggest that around 30–35 per cent morphine elimination may be by non-urinary excretion, non-hepatic degradation (i.e. potentially by renal parenchymal metabolism), the two studies in patients with renal failure offer another explanation. The increased plasma morphine concentrations (and larger AUC) could have occurred by hydrolysis of one or other of the accumulating glucuronides (probably the 3-glucuronide) back to the parent compound.

More recently, Milne and colleagues (1992) have examined the relationship between renal creatinine clearance and the renal clearances of morphine, morphine-3-glucuronide (M3G) and morphine-6-glucuronide (M6G) in intensive-care unit patients

with variable degrees of renal impairment. For all three compounds, there was a linear relationship between free drug clearance and creatinine clearance. The unbound clearance of morphine exceeded that of creatinine, whilst those of M3G and M6G were similar. The unbound fractions for morphine, M3G and M6G were 74, 85 and 89 per cent, respectively, the first figure being greater than that determined earlier (Olsen *et al.*, 1975).

Loetsch and colleagues (1996) have reported half-lives for M3G and M6G in healthy volunteers of the order of 2.8–3.2 h and 1.7–2.7 h respectively. The longer half-lives of M3G and M6G (41–141 h, and 89–136 h) reported (Osborne *et al.*, 1986; Sawe and Odar-Cederlof, 1987) in patients with impaired renal function may be clinically important in the prolonged effect of the parent drug. Sawe and Odar-Cederlof (1987) have shown a significant correlation between the M3G half-life and the plasma urea concentration while data from Sear and colleagues (1989) show a significant correlation between the half-lives of both M3G and M6G and the immediate post-operative 24 hour creatinine clearance in the patients undergoing transplantation ($r = 0.87$ and $r = 0.63$, respectively; $P < 0.01$ and $P < 0.05$). However, there are insufficient data at present to derive a nomogram relating plasma creatinine, predicted or measured creatinine clearance, and accumulation of the active M6G in the patient with renal impairment.

If infusions of morphine are administered to patients with impaired renal function, accumulation of M6G may occur to give a clinical picture of a persistently narcotized patient (Osborne *et al.*, 1986; Shelly *et al.*, 1986; Hasselstrom *et al.*, 1989). The importance of the 6-glucuronide can also be seen in the case reported by Covington and colleagues (1989), where severe respiratory depression was observed in a patient with end-stage renal disease receiving a morphine patient-controlled analgesia for post-cholecystectomy pain relief. The blood morphine concentration was 73 ng/mL (within the therapeutic range), but the 6-glucuronide level was significantly elevated at 415 ng/mL.

What is the contribution of M6G to the analgesic and depressant effects of morphine? In 14 patients with chronic pain (but normal renal function), Portenoy and colleagues (1992) assessed the contribution of the glucuronide to overall analgesia produced by a morphine infusion. Pain relief was greatest when the measured M6G/morphine molar ratio was >0.7 : 1; with a significant correlation between the molar ratio and pain relief.

There are also data to suggest increased concentrations of another morphine metabolite (normorphine) may be responsible for myoclonic activity, but this has not been confirmed by other researchers (Glare et al., 1990). Whether the altered kinetics of morphine and its surrogates are the sole explanation of their prolonged dynamic effect is uncertain. Uraemia is itself associated with CNS depression and the increased sensitivity to CNS depressant drugs may also be due to increased receptor responsiveness, or increased meningeal and/or cerebral permeability.

PETHIDINE

There are few kinetic data on the disposition of pethidine in patients with renal failure, the drug being mainly metabolized in the liver, with only 1–5 per cent excreted unchanged in the urine. However, Chan and colleagues (1987) have confirmed the importance of renal function for the excretion of the metabolite norpethidine. If repeated doses of pethidine are given to patients in chronic renal failure, there is accumulation of the N-demethylated metabolite, norpethidine. This compound has less analgesic, but greater convulsant activity than the parent drug, and Szeto and colleagues (1977) described two patients in renal failure where increased plasma ratios of norpethidine/pethidine were associated with excitatory signs.

INHALATIONAL ANAESTHETIC AGENTS

All inhalational agents are myocardial depressants, and may therefore reduce the cardiac output and blood flow to the transplanted kidney. Low concentrations of halothane (0.5–1.0 per cent) may be used to supplement to nitrous oxide–oxygen anaesthesia. However, it has no analgesic properties, and is liable to cause hypotension, especially if used in conjunction with d-tubocurarine or atracurium in patients currently receiving antihypertensive therapy, or following recent haemodialysis. Despite reports of halothane decreasing renal blood flow (Deutsch et al., 1966; Groves et al., 1990), this can be minimized by the maintenance of intra-operative normocapnia (Hunter et al., 1980).

Current practice in the United Kingdom is to provide anaesthesia with either enflurane or isoflurane to supplement nitrous oxide. However, use of the former may result in elevated serum fluoride concentrations. These ions are nephrotoxic, and the toxic threshold in man during methoxyflurane anaesthesia was a concentration of greater than 50 µmol/L.

In healthy patients, enflurane does not produce serum fluoride concentrations in excess of 50 µmol/L. Wickstrom (1981) studied the use of enflurane anaesthesia in patients undergoing living related donor renal transplantation. Administration of 2.4 minimum alveolar concentration (MAC)-hour enflurane (mean duration: 189 min) produced a peak fluoride concentration of 21 µmol/L. However, in one out of the ten patients, the serum fluoride concentration rose significantly to 40 µmol/L which presents a risk of nephrotoxicity. Because of this risk, enflurane is not used routinely as the sole anaesthetic for renal transplantation. However, there appears no contraindication to it supplementing a nitrous oxide–opioid technique. Choice of the three volatile agents does not appear to influence post-transplant renal function (Cronnelly et al., 1984) nor to influence intra-operative haemodynamics (Cronnelly et al., 1983).

There are few clinical data on the use of desflurane or sevoflurane to supplement nitrous oxide anaesthesia for renal transplantation. The former undergoes no significant metabolism, and in dogs has been shown to maintain renal blood flow at concentrations up to 2MAC (Merin et al., 1991). Sevoflurane similarly maintains renal blood flow at inspired concentrations up to 2MAC (Conzen et al., 1992). However its propensity to give rise to high fluoride concentrations (especially after prolonged anaesthesia) probably contraindicates its use for renal transplantation (Conzen et al., 1995).

INITIATION OF EARLY ALLOGRAFT FUNCTION

Both loop diuretics and/or mannitol may be used to promote a diuresis from the grafted kidney. Mannitol has the additional advantage that it may have a protective role as a free-radical scavenger, and its use reduces the incidence of impaired renal function immediately after transplantation from 55 to 14 per cent (Weimar et al., 1983). It has also been shown to improve renal blood flow by a greater percentage than can be accounted for by plasma volume expansion alone (Johnston et al., 1979).

Moote and Manninen (1987) examined the influence of mannitol on serum electrolytes in patients undergoing renal transplantation. Fifty grams of mannitol increased the central venous pressure, and reduced serum concentrations of sodium, chloride and bicarbonate. The rise in potassium was small, but this may assume clinical importance in patients also receiving a blood transfusion. The thiazide diuretics and frusemide are not open to the same criticism, although their use should be coupled with pre-loading of the patients with isotonic (0.154 M) saline.

Besides use of mannitol and diuretics to establish a brisk diuresis, adequate hydration to maintain the circulating volume is also of importance. Dawidson et al. (1987) showed that urine output is delayed after re-perfusion in patients when the intravascular volume was less than 70 mL/kg. Rehydration requirements can be estimated from the central venous pressure, using normal saline as the initial volume expander. If more than 40–90 mL/kg is required, then colloid solutions should be infused as well. The administration of this fluid load will also act as physiological stimulus to urine production.

Studies by Carlier and colleagues (1982, 1986) examined the concept of 'maximal hydration therapy' (up to 100 mL/kg normal saline) during anaesthesia, and its effect on early graft function. The stimulus to effectiveness is the release of ANF. Although the results were encouraging, fluid loads of this magnitude may precipitate pulmonary oedema in patients with poor myocardial function or poor respiratory reserve. If this approach is utilized, it is mandatory to insert a pulmonary artery catheter prior to anaesthesia and surgery.

Renal protection after transplantation

In cadaveric renal transplantation, there is much controversy over the use of agents to provide renal protection against ischaemia. Low-dose dopamine (2 µg/kg/min) has been shown in two studies to have no or little advantageous effects, and may be responsible for a greater incidence of fluid and electrolyte disturbances and associated arrhythmias (Grundmann et al., 1980; De los Angeles et al., 1985). However, a more recent study has demonstrated a significant protective role of the calcium

entry-blocking drug diltiazem (Wagner et al., 1987). Various mechanisms have been proposed for this effect (a reduction in the incidence of acute tubular necrosis from 41 to 10 per cent). These include: prevention of reflow-induced vasoconstriction after ischaemia; inhibition of the action of angiotensin II on the glomerulus; and a reduction in the accumulation of oxygen free radicals (Neumayer et al., 1993). Diltiazem and cyclosporin also appear to be metabolized by the same isoform of cytochrome P450, and the former may therefore also offer protection against cyclosporin-induced nephrotoxicity.

A RECOMMENDED TECHNIQUE FOR RENAL TRANSPLANTATION

The Nuffield department in Oxford has considerable experience with anaesthesia for renal transplantation, and the following represents the approach used since the mid-1970s.

Premedication is of great importance because many of the patients are understandably anxious at the time of transplantation, and suitable attenuation of anxiety may be achieved with one of the orally administered benzodiazepines. Intramuscular premedication is best avoided because of the tendency of the uraemic patient to bleeding disorders. Vagolytic drugs (e.g. atropine) are best given intravenously at the time of induction of anaesthesia if clinically indicated, for example, when suxamethonium is used to facilitate intubation, or when the combination of an opioid with one of the haemodynamically neutral muscle relaxants is administered. The avoidance of pronounced bradycardia is of particular importance in patients receiving chronic β-adrenoceptor blockade for the control of hypertension.

Routine prophylactic administration of antacids is advocated for patients with symptoms of peptic ulceration. A single dose of sodium citrate (30 mL) in the anaesthetic room is usual. Histamine H_2-receptor antagonists given with the premedication have also been used to reduce gastric hyperacidity. Care should be exercised with the administration of phenothiazine or choline alkaloid (e.g. metoclopramide) anti-emetics as they may cause prolonged sedation and extrapyramidal side effects in patients with renal failure.

Anaesthesia is induced with a sleep dose of thiopentone coupled with a loading dose of opioid (fentanyl 100–200 µg). With this technique, it is possible to minimize the haemodynamic responses to induction of anaesthesia, laryngoscopy and intubation. Neuromuscular blockade is achieved with atracurium or vecuronium, with additional increments given when indicated clinically. Neuromuscular transmission should always be monitored using a peripheral nerve stimulator. As an alternative technique, a continuous infusion of atracurium (6–8 µg/kg/min) may be employed. For the patient in whom there is the added problem of a difficult airway or an inadequate period of starvation before surgery, there is no contraindication to the use of suxamethonium; the roles of mivacurium and rocuronium in transplantation still need to be confirmed.

Maintenance of anaesthesia is best achieved with inhalational agents, which offer the advantages of non-renal elimination, and may be given with high inspired oxygen concentrations in the severely anaemic patient. The arterial blood carbon dioxide tension should be kept at normocapnia or mild hypocapnia, and monitored by end-tidal carbon dioxide sampling. Even short periods of hypoventilation can lead to haemoglobin desaturation, while excess hyperventilation with low arterial carbon dioxide tensions will cause a shift of the oxyhaemoglobin dissociation curve to the left.

At the end of surgery, anaesthesia is discontinued and residual muscular paralysis reversed with atropine or glycopyrrolate and neostigmine. The use of glycopyrrolate is preferred in patients with associated hypertensive or ischaemic heart disease to avoid excessive tachycardias. Once extubated, all patients should receive oxygen for 12–24 hours post-operatively.

Monitoring

The high incidence of ischaemic and hypertensive heart disease makes it essential to monitor the ECG and blood pressure continuously during induction of anaesthesia, the per-operative and the immediate post-operative period. The blood pressure may be satisfactorily measured using an automatic oscillometric apparatus. Because of the improvements in pre-operative preparation of kidney transplant recipients, and because excessive blood loss is the exception rather than the rule, arterial cannulation is only rarely needed. However, there is no contraindication if it is clinically indicated.

Measurement of the central venous pressure (CVP) is as important as that of the blood pressure in patients undergoing renal transplantation. Intra-operative fluids are given as physiological saline and colloid or blood (about 10 mL/kg/h), the aim being to raise the CVP to 7–10 cm by the time of revascularization. Use of sodium lactate (Ringer's) should be avoided as it contains potassium, and because lactate metabolism is decreased in uraemia.

Post-operative fluid requirements depend on early renal function, but should be aimed at keeping the CVP at its intra-operative level. In practice, this equates to a regimen of urine output plus 50–100 mL/h. Fluids should again be both crystalloid (equal volumes of 5 per cent dextrose and normal saline) and colloid in cases of a fall in CVP accompanied by arterial hypotension. Persistent hypotension in the presence of an adequate CVP (5–10 cmH$_2$O) will normally respond to dobutamine 1–20 µg/kg/min.

Although we would not routinely advocate the per-operative determination of electrolytes (and particularly potassium), there have been reports of sudden increases of plasma potassium levels leading to arrhythmias and cardiac arrest (Hirschmann and Edelstein, 1979). Several factors may be responsible: the administration of mannitol (Moreno et al., 1969) or stored blood; severe metabolic acidosis; and the hyperkalaemia of hyperglycaemia (Goldfarb et al., 1976). The aetiology of the latter mechanism is unknown. Prevention of this complication will assume greater significance in the diabetic patient undergoing renal transplantation.

Post-operative management

Because of the multiple pathology exhibited by the transplant patient, they should be nursed post-operatively in a high-dependency nursing unit, where controlled oxygen therapy and full monitoring can be provided. If controlled ventilation is needed, then admission to an intensive therapy unit is required. Strict monitoring of fluid input and output is essential. The major post-operative anaesthetic complications are: vomiting and pulmonary inhalation; cardiac arrhythmias, which can lead to cardiac arrest; pulmonary oedema; hypotension and hypertension; and delayed respiratory depression.

Analgesia in the post-operative period should be titrated according to patient demand. The choice of drugs (opioids and oral non-narcotic analgesics) must be carefully considered, as accumulation of active metabolites will occur in the patient with a non-functioning allograft. Excessive use of opioids may lead to delayed respiratory depression, sedation and convulsions (all relatable to both parent drug and active metabolite accumulation). The recent widespread awareness of the techniques of patient-controlled analgesia (PCA) may provide a more efficient method of drug dosing in the uraemic patient, although reports of excessive sedation and respiratory depression have been described (Covington *et al.*, 1989).

Although only a small percentage of NSAID drugs are eliminated unchanged via the kidney, there is evidence of reduced clearance of ketoprofen, fenoprofen, naproxen and carprofen in renal failure due to probable deconjugation of acyl glucuronide metabolites. NSAIDs may also cause reversible kidney damage, with reduction of renal blood flow and GFR, and oedema, interstitial nephritis and papillary necrosis in the kidney. These effects are probably caused by the action of the NSAIDs on prostaglandin synthesis, the latter being integral for renal blood flow and GFR autoregulation. Hence these drugs should be avoided in *all* patients with renal impairment.

Regional anaesthesia

There have been several reports of local anaesthesia being used for renal transplantation. After the initial report (Vandam *et al.*, 1962), Linke and Merin (1976) reviewed the use of spinal anaesthesia for renal transplantation. The advantages include: the avoidance of the use of neuromuscular blocking drugs; avoidance of endotracheal intubation; the reduced likelihood of regurgitation and inhalation in the patient with a full stomach; no interaction of acidosis and hyperkalaemia with anaesthetic and adjuvant drugs; and an awake and comfortable patient in the immediate post-operative period. Satisfactory operating conditions can be achieved using amethocaine (10–20 mg) in 5 per cent dextrose.

More recently, Pitkanen and colleagues (1985) and Orko and colleagues (1986) have investigated the duration of action of subarachnoid blockade with 0.75 per cent plain bupivacaine in uraemic and healthy patients undergoing lower abdominal surgery. In the chronic renal failure patients, there

was a faster onset of sensory analgesia, due to the combined effects of the acidosis causing a greater degree of ionization, and a reduced lumbar intrathecal space secondary to distension of the extradural and spinal veins by the hyperdynamic circulation. However, the duration of both sensory and motor blockades were shorter (20 per cent) in the patients with renal failure, the raised cardiac output causing a faster washout of the local anaesthetic from its site of action.

Subarachnoid anaesthesia in uraemic patients could technically produce an extradural haematoma, because of the tendency to bleeding. However, if the patient has been on an adequate dialysis programme, the primary platelet dysfunction is reversed (Weir and Chung, 1984). The incidence of other complications reported by Orko and colleagues (1986) was low. Post-dural puncture headache occurred in 2.5 per cent of patients, a rate similar to that described in the healthy patient by Scott and Thorburn (1975).

However, although regional analgesia has some theoretical advantage over the use of intravenous and inhalational agents (with the altered kinetics and dynamics of some opioids and neuromuscular blocking drugs), it is not widely used currently in the United Kingdom.

REFERENCES

Aitkenhead, A.R., Vater, M., Achola, K. *et al.* 1984. Pharmacokinetics of single-dose i.v. morphine in normal volunteers and patients with end-stage renal failure. *British Journal of Anaesthesia* **56**, 813–818.

Antonucci, F., Bertolissi, M. and Calo, L. 1990. Plasma endothelin and renal function during infrarenal aortic cross-clamping and nifedipine infusion. *Lancet* **336**, 1449.

Attia, R.R., Murphy, J.D., Snider, M. *et al.* 1976. Myocardial ischemia due to infra-renal aortic cross-clamping during aortic surgery in patients with severe coronary artery disease. *Circulation* **53**, 961–965.

Awad, R.W., Barnham, W.J., Taylor, D.N. *et al.* 1992. The effect of infrarenal aortic reconstruction on glomerular filtration rate and effective renal plasma flow. *European Journal of Vascular Surgery* **6**, 362–367.

Baldwin, L., Henderson, A. and Hideman, P. 1994. Effect of post-operative low-dose dopamine on renal function after elective major vascular surgery. *Annals of Internal Medicine* **120**, 744–747.

Bauer, T.M., Ritz, R., Haberthur, C. *et al*. 1995. Prolonged sedation due to accumulation of conjugated metabolites of midazolam. *Lancet* **346**, 145–147.

Bastron, R.D. and Deutsch, S. 1976. *Anesthesia and the kidney*. Orlando: Grune and Stratton.

Beauvoir, C., Peray, P., Daures, J.P. *et al*. 1993. Pharmacodynamics of vecuronium in patients with and without renal failure: a meta-analysis. *Canadian Journal of Anaesthesia* **40**, 696–702.

Bevan, D.R., Donati, F., Gyasi, H. and Williams, A. 1984. Vecuronium in renal failure. *Canadian Anaesthetists Society Journal* **31**, 491–496.

Booke, M., Meyer, J., Lingnau, W. *et al*. 1995. Use of nitric oxide synthase inhibitors in animal models of sepsis. *New Horizons* **3**, 123–138.

Bower, S. 1982. Plasma protein binding of fentanyl: the effect of hyperlipidaemia and chronic renal failure. *Journal of Pharmacy and Pharmacology* **34**, 102–106.

Bower, S. and Sear, J.W. 1989. Disposition of alfentanil in patients receiving a renal transplant. *Journal of Pharmacy and Pharmacology* **41**, 654–657.

Boyd, A.H., Eastwood, N.B., Parker, C.J.H. and Hunter, J.M. 1995. Pharmacodynamics of the 1R-*cis*,1R'-*cis* isomer of atracurium (51W89) in health and chronic renal failure. *British Journal of Anaesthesia* **74**, 400–404.

Breckwoldt, W.L., Mackey, W.C., Belkin, M. and O'Donnell, T.F. 1992. The effect of suprarenal cross-clamping on abdominal aortic aneurysm repair. *Archives of Surgery* **127**, 520–524.

Brotherton, W.D. and Matteo, R.S. 1981. Pharmacokinetics and pharmacodynamics of metocurine in humans with and without renal failure. *Anesthesiology* **55**, 273–276.

Brown, J.J., Duesterdieck, G. and Fraser, R. *et al*. 1971. Hypertension and chronic renal failure. *British Medical Bulletin* **27**, 128–135.

Burch, P.G. and Stanski, D.R. 1982. Decreased protein binding and thiopental kinetics. *Clinical Pharmacology and Therapeutics* **32**, 212–217.

Burton, P.R. and Walls, J. 1987. Selection-adjusted comparison of life expectancy of patients on continuous ambulatory peritoneal dialysis, haemodialysis and renal transplantation. *Lancet* **1**, 1115–1119.

Buzello, W. and Agoston, S. 1978. Pharmacokinetics of pancuronium in patients with normal and impaired renal function. *Der Anaesthesist* **27**, 291–297.

Caldwell, J.E., Canfell, P.C., Castagnoli, K.P. *et al*. 1989. The influence of renal failure on the pharmacokinetics and duration of action of pipecuronium bromide in patients anesthetized with halothane and nitrous oxide. *Anesthesiology* **70**, 7–12.

Carlier, M., Squifflet, J.P., Pirson, Y. *et al*. 1986. Anesthetic protocol in human renal transplantation: twenty two years of experience. *Acta Anaesthesiologica Belgica* **37**, 89–94.

Carlier, M., Squifflet, J.P., Pirson, Y. *et al*. 1982. Maximal hydration during anesthesia increases pulmonary arterial pressures and improves early function in human renal transplants. *Transplantation* **34**, 201–204.

Carlos, R., Calvo, R. and Erill, S. 1979. Plasma protein binding of etomidate in patients with renal failure or hepatic cirrhosis. *Clinical Pharmacokinetics* **4**, 144–148.

Cashman, J.N., Luke, J.J. and Jones, R.M. 1992. Neuromuscular block with doxacurium (BW A938U) in patients with normal or absent renal function. *British Journal of Anaesthesia* **64**, 186–192.

Chan, K., Tse, J., Jenning, F. and Orme, M.L. 1987. Pharmacokinetics of low-dose intravenous pethidine in patients with renal dysfunction. *Journal of Clinical Pharmacology* **27**, 516–522.

Chauvin, M., Lebrault, C., Levron, J.C. and Duvaldestin, P. 1987a. Pharmacokinetics of alfentanil in chronic renal failure. *Anesthesia and Analgesia* **66**, 53–56.

Chauvin, M., Sandouk, P., Scherrmann, J.M. *et al*. 1987b. Morphine pharmacokinetics in renal failure. *Anesthesiology* **66**, 327–331.

Christensen, J.H., Andreasen, F. and Jansen, J. 1983. Pharmacokinetics and pharmacodynamics of thiopental in patients undergoing renal transplantation. *Acta Anaesthesiologica Scandanivica* **27**, 513–518.

Cody, M.W. and Dormon, F.M. 1987. Recurarisation after vecuronium in a patient with renal failure. *Anaesthesia* **42**, 993–995.

Colson, P., Capdevilla, X., Cuchet, D. *et al*. 1992a. Does the choice of the anesthetic influence renal function during infrarenal aortic surgery? *Anesthesia and Analgesia* **74**, 481–485.

Colson, P., Saussine, M. and Seguin, J.R. *et al*. 1992b. Hemodynamic effects of anesthesia in patients chronically treated with angiotensin-converting enzyme inhibitors. *Anesthesia and Analgesia* **74**, 805–808.

Converse, R.L., Jacobsen, T.N., Toto, R.D. *et al.* 1992. Sympathetic overactivity in patients with chronic renal failure. *New England Journal of Medicine* **327**, 1912–1918.

Conzen, P.F., Nuscheler, M., Melotte, A. *et al.* 1995. Renal function and serum fluoride concentrations in patients with stable renal insufficiency after anesthesia with sevoflurane or enflurane. *Anesthesia and Analgesia* **81**, 569–575.

Conzen, P.F., Vollmar, B., Habazettl, H. *et al.* 1992. Systemic and regional hemodynamics of isoflurane and sevoflurane in rats. *Anesthesia and Analgesia* **74**, 79–88.

Cook, D.R., Freeman, J.A., Lai, A.A. *et al.* 1992. Pharmacokinetics of mivacurium in normal patients and in those with hepatic or renal failure. *British Journal of Anaesthesia* **69**, 580–585.

Cook, D.R., Freeman, J.A., Lai, A.A. *et al.* 1991. Pharmacokinetics and pharmacodynamics of doxacurium in normal patients and in those with hepatic or renal failure. *Anesthesia and Analgesia* **72**, 145–150.

Corall, I.M., Moore, A.R. and Strunin, L. 1980. Plasma concentrations of fentanyl in normal surgical patients and those with severe renal and hepatic disease. *British Journal of Anaesthesia* **52**, 101p (abstract).

Coriat, P., Richer, C., Douraki, T. *et al.* 1994. Influence of chronic angiotensin-converting enzyme inhibition on anesthetic induction. *Anesthesiology* **81**, 299–307.

Costela, J.L., Jimenez, R., Calvo, R. *et al.* 1996. Serum protein binding of propofol in patients with renal failure or hepatic cirrhosis. *Acta Anaesthesiologica Scandinavica* **40**, 741–745.

Covington, E.C., Gonsalves-Ebrahim, L., Currie, K.O. *et al.* 1989. Severe respiratory depression from patient-controlled analgesia in renal failure. *Psychosomatics* **30**, 226–228.

Cronnelly, R., Kremer, P.F., Beaupre, P.N. *et al.* 1983a. Hemodynamic response to anesthesia in patients with end-stage renal disease. *Anesthesiology* **59**, A47 (abstract).

Cronnelly, R. and Morris, R.B. 1982. Antagonism of neuromuscular blockade. *British Journal of Anaesthesia* **54**, 183–194.

Cronnelly, R., Salvatierra, O. and Feduska, N. 1984. Renal allograft function following halothane, enflurane or isoflurane anesthesia. *Anesthesia and Analgesia* **63**, 202 (abstract).

Davis, P.J., Stiller, R.L., Cook, D.R. *et al.* 1988. Pharmacokinetics of sufentanil in adolescent patients with chronic renal failure. *Anesthesia and Analgesia* **67**, 268–271.

Dawidson, I., Berglin, E., Brygner, H. and Reisch, J. 1987. Intravascular volumes and colloidal dynamics in relation to fluid management in living related kidney donors and recipients. *Critical Care Medicine* **15**, 631–636.

deBros, F., Basta, SJ., Ali, H.H. *et al.* 1987. Pharmacokinetics and pharmacodynamics of BW B1090U in healthy surgical patients receiving N2O/O2 isoflurane anesthesia. *Anesthesiology* **67**, A609 (abstract).

deBros, F.M., Lai, A., Scott, R. *et al.* 1986. Pharmacokinetics and pharmacodynamics of atracurium during isoflurane anesthesia in normal and anephric patients. *Anesthesia and Analgesia* **65**, 743–746.

De los Angeles, A., Baquero, A., Bannett, A. and Raja, A. 1985. Dopamine and furosemide infusion for prevention of post transplant oliguric renal failure. *Kidney International* **27**, 339 (abstract).

Deutsch, S., Goldberg, M., Stephen, G.M. and Wu, W.H. 1966. Effects of halothane anesthesia on renal function in normal man. *Anesthesiology* **27**, 793–804.

Don, H.F., Dieppa, R.A. and Taylor, P. 1975. Narcotic analgesics in anuric patients. *Anesthesiology* **42**, 745–747.

Dundee, J.W. and Richards, R.K. 1954. Effect of azotemia upon the action of barbiturate anesthesia. *Anesthesiology* **13**, 333–346.

Duthie, D.J.R. 1986. Renal failure, surgery and fentanyl pharmacokinetics. Proceedings of VII European Congress of Anaesthesiology, volume II. *Beitrage zur Anaesthesiologie und Intensivmedizin* **20**, 374–375.

Durand, P.G., Lehot, J.J. and Foex, P. 1991. Calcium-channel blockers and anaesthesia. *Canadian Journal of Anaesthesia* **38**, 75–89.

Eastwood, N.B., Boyd, A.H., Parker, C.J.H. and Hunter, J.M. 1995. Pharmacokinetics of 1R-cis 1R'-cis atracurium besylate (51W89) and plasma laudanosine concentrations in health and chronic renal failure. *British Journal of Anaesthesia* **75**, 431–435.

Eschbach, J.W., Egrie, J.C., Downing, M.R. *et al.* 1987. Correction of the anemia of end-stage renal disease with recombinant human erythropoietin. Results of a combined Phase I and II Clinical Trial. *New England Journal of Medicine* **316**, 73–78.

Fahey, M.R., Morris, R.B., Miller, R.D. *et al.* 1981. Pharmacokinetics of ORG NC45 (Norcuron) in patients with and without renal failure. *British Journal of Anaesthesia* **53**, 1049–1053.

Fahey, M.R., Rupp, S.M., Fisher, D.M. *et al*. 1984. The pharmacokinetics and pharmacodynamics of atracurium in patients with and without renal failure. *Anesthesiology* **61**, 699–702.

Fisher, D.M., Canfell, C., Fahey, M.R. *et al*. 1985. Elimination of atracurium in humans: contribution of Hofmann elimination and ester hydrolysis versus organ-bound elimination. *Anesthesiology* **65**, 6–12.

Foex, P., Francis, C.M. and Cutfield, G.R. 1982. The interactions between β-blockers and anaesthetics. Experimental observations. *Acta Anaesthesiologica Scandinavica* **26**, supplement 76. 38–46.

Fyman, P., Reynolds, J., Moser, F. *et al*. 1988. Pharmacokinetics of sufentanil in patients undergoing renal transplantation. *Canadian Journal of Anaesthesia* **35**, 312–315.

Gamulin, Z., Forster, A., Simonet, F. *et al*. 1986. Effects of renal sympathetic blockade on renal hemodynamics in patients undergoing major aortic abdominal surgery. *Anesthesiology* **65**, 688–692.

Gamelin, Z., Forster, A., Morel, D. *et al*. 1984. Effects of infra-renal aortic cross-clamping on renal hemodynamics in humans. *Anesthesiology* **61**, 394–399.

Geha, D.G., Blitt, C.D. and Moon, B.J. 1976. Prolonged neuromuscular blockade with pancuronium in the presence of acute renal failure: a case report. *Anesthesia and Analgesia* **55**, 343–345.

Girbes, A.R.J., Lieverse, A.G., Smit, A.J. *et al*. 1996. Lack of specific renal haemodynamic effects of different doses of dopamine after infrarenal aortic surgery. *British Journal of Anaesthesia* **77**, 753–757.

Glare, P.A., Walsh, T.D. and Pippenger, C.E. 1990. Normorphine, a neurotoxic metabolite? *Lancet* **335**, 725–726.

Goldfarb, S., Cox, M., Singer, I. and Goldberg, M. 1976. Acute hyperkalemia induced by hyperglycemia: hormonal mechanisms. *Annals of Internal Medicine* **84**, 426–432.

Goldblatt, H., Lynch, J., Hanzai, R.F. and Summerville, W.W. 1934. Studies on experimental hypertension – I: The production of persistent elevation of systolic pressure by means of renal ischaemia. *Journal of Experimental Medicine* **59**, 347–379.

Gorven, A.M., Cooper, G.M. and Prys-Roberts, C. 1986. Haemodynamic disturbances during anaesthesia in a patient receiving calcium channnel blockers. *British Journal of Anaesthesia* **58**, 357–360.

Groves, N.D., Leach, K.G. and Rosen, M. 1990. Effects of halothane, enflurane and isoflurane anaesthesia on renal plasma flow. *British Journal of Anaesthesia* **65**, 796–800.

Grundmann, R., Kindler, J., Meider, G. *et al*. 1980. Dopamine treatment of human cadaver kidney graft recipients: a prospectively randomised trial. *Klinische Wochenschrift* **ii**, 827–828.

Hampers, C.L., Balufox, M.D. and Merrill, J.P. 1966. Anticoagulation rebound after hemodialysis. *New England Journal of Medicine* **275**, 776–778.

Hasselstrom, J., Berg, U., Lofgren, A. and Sawe, J. 1989. Long lasting respiratory depression induced by morphine-6–glucuronide? *British Journal of Clinical Pharmacology* **27**, 515–518.

Head-Rapson, A.G., Devlin, J.C., Parker, C.J.R. and Hunter, J.M. 1995. Pharmacokinetics and pharmacodynamics of the three isomers of mivacurium in health, in end-stage renal failure and in patients with impaired renal function. *British Journal of Anaesthesia* **75**, 31–36.

Hirschmann, C.A. and Edelstein, G. 1979. Intra-operative hyperkalemia and cardiac arrest during renal transplantation in an insulin dependent diabetic patient. *Anesthesiology* **51**, 161–162.

Howell, S.J., Sear, Y.M., Yeates, D. *et al*. 1996. Hypertension, admission blood pressure and peri-operative cardiovascular risk. *Anaesthesia* **51**, 1000–1004.

Hunter, J.M., Jones, R.S. and Utting, J.E. 1980. Effects of hypocapnia on renal function in the dog artificially ventilated with nitrous oxide, oxygen and halothane. *British Journal of Anaesthesia* **52**, 197–198 (abstract).

Hunter, J.M., Jones, R.S. and Utting, J.E. 1982. Use of atracurium in patients with no renal function. *British Journal of Anaesthesia* **54**, 1251–1258.

Jenkins, L.C. and Scoates, P.J. 1985. Anaesthetic implications of calcium channel blockers. *Canadian Anaesthetists Society Journal* **32**, 436–447.

Johnston, P.A., Bernard, D.B., Donohoe, J.F. *et al*. 1979. Effect of volume expansion on hemodynamics of the hypoperfused rat kidney. *Journal of Clinical Investigation* **64**, 550–558.

Joob, A.W., Harman, P.K., Kaiser, D.L. and Kron, I.L. 1986. The effect of renin-angiotensin system blockade on visceral blood flow during and after thoracic aortic cross clamping. *Journal of Thoracic and Cardiovascular Surgery* **91**, 411–418.

Khuenl-Brady, K.S., Pomaroli, A., Puhringer, F. *et al*. 1993. The use of rocuronium (ORG 9426) in patients with chronic renal failure. *Anaesthesia* **48**, 873–875.

Kirvela, M., Olkkola, K.T., Rosenberg, P.H. *et al*. 1992. Pharmacokinetics of propofol and haemodynamic changes during induction of anaesthesia in uraemic patients. *British Journal of Anaesthesia* **68**, 178–182.

Kisor, D.F., Schmith, V.D., Wargin, W.A. *et al.* 1996. Importance of organ-independent elimination of cis-atracurium. *Anesthesia and Analgesia* **83**, 1065–1071.

Knox, F.G. and Spielman, W.S. 1983. Renal Circulation. In *Handbook of Physiology* Vol. 3, 183–217.

Koehntop, D.E. and Rodman, J.H. 1997. Fentanyl pharmacokinetics in patients undergoing renal transplantation. *Pharmacotherapy* **17**, 746–752.

LePage, J.Y., Malinge, M., Cozian, A. *et al.* 1987. Vecuronium and atracurium in patients with endstage renal failure. *British Journal of Anaesthesia* **59**, 1004–1010.

Linke, C.L. and Merin, R.G. 1976. A regional anesthetic approach for renal transplantation. *Anesthesia and Analgesia, Current Researches* **55**, 69–73.

Loetsch, J., Stockmann, A., Kobal, G. *et al.* 1996. Pharmacokinetics of morphine and its glucuronides after intravenous infusion of morphine and morphine-6–glucuronide in healthy volunteers. *Clinical Pharmacology and Therapeutics* **60**, 316–325.

Lynam, D.P., Cronnelly, R., Castagnoli, K.P. *et al.* 1988. The pharmacodynamics and pharmacokinetics of vecuronium in pateinets anesthetized with isoflurane with normal renal function or with renal failure. *Anesthesiology* **69**, 227–231.

McLeod, K., Watson, M.J. and Rawlins, M.D. 1976. Pharmacokinetics of pancuronium in patients with normal and impaired renal function. *British Journal of Anaesthesia* **48**, 341–345.

Mannucci, P.M., Remuzzi, C. and Pusineri, F. 1983. Desamino-8–D-arginine vasopressin shortens the bleeding time in uremia. *New England Journal of Medicine* **308**, 8–12.

Mazoit, J.X., Sandouk, P., Scherrmann, J-M. and Roche, A. 1990. Extrahepatic metabolism of morphine occurs in humans. *Clinical Pharmacology and Therapeutics* **48**, 613–618.

Merin, R.G., Bernard, J.M., Doursout, M.F. *et al.* 1991. Comparison of the effects of isoflurane and desflurane on cardiovascular dynamics and regional blood flow in the chronically instrumented dog. *Anesthesiology* **74**, 568–574.

Miller, R.D., Matteo, R.S., Benet, L.Z. and Sohn, T.I. 1977. The pharmacokinetics of d-tubocurarine in man with and without renal failure. *Journal of Pharmacology and Experimental Therapeutics* **202**, 1–7.

Milne, R.W., Nation, R.L., Somogyi, A.A. *et al.* 1992. The influence of renal function on the renal clearance of morphine and its glucuronide metabolites in intensive-care patients. *British Journal of Clinical Pharmacology* **34**, 53–59.

Mino, N., Kobayashi, M., Nakajima AAmano, H. *et al.* 1992. Protective effect of a selective endothelin receptor antagonist, BQ-123, in ischemic acute renal failure in rats. *European Journal of Pharmacology* **221**, 77–83.

Moote, C.A. and Manninen, P.H. 1987. Mannitol administered during renal transplantation produces profound changes in fluid and electrolyte balance. *Canadian Journal of Anaesthesia* **35**, s120 (abstract).

Moreno, M., Murphy, C. and Goldsmith, C. 1969. Increase in serum potassium resulting from the administration of hypertonic mannitol and other solutions. *Journal of Laboratory and Clinical Medicine* **73**, 291–298.

Mostert, J.W., Evers, J.L., Hobika, G.H. *et al.* 1971. Cardiorespiratory effects of anaesthesia with morphine or fentanyl in chronic renal failure and cerebral toxicity after morphine. *British Journal of Anaesthesia* **43**, 1053–1059.

Myers, B.D., Miller, D.C., Mehigand, T. *et al.* 1984. Nature of the renal injury following total renal ischemia in man. *Journal of Clinical Investigation* **73**, 329–341.

Neumayer, H.H., Gellert, J. and Luft, F.C. 1993. Calcium antagonists and renal protection. *Renal Failure* **15**, 353–358.

Nguyen, H.D., Kaplan, R., Nagashima, H. *et al.* 1985. The neuromuscular effect of atracurium in anephric patients. *Anesthesiology* **63**, A335 (abstract).

Ochs, H.R., Greenblatt, D.J., Kaschel, H.J. *et al.* 1981. Diazepam kinetics in patients with renal insufficiency or hyperthyroidism. *British Journal of Clinical Pharmacology* **12**, 829–832.

Oldenhof, H., De Jong, M., Steenhoek, A. and Janknegt, R. 1988. Clinical pharmacokinetics of midazolam in intensive care patients, a wide interpatient variability? *Clinical Pharmacology and Therapeutics* **43**, 263–269.

Olsen, G.D., Bennett, W.M. and Porter, G.A. 1975. Morphine and phenytoin binding to plasma proteins in renal and hepatic failure. *Clinical Pharmacology and Therapeutics* **17**, 677–684.

Orko, R., Pitkanen, M. and Rosenberg, P.H. 1986. Subarachnoid anaesthesia with 0.75 per cent bupivacaine in patients with chronic renal failure. *British Journal of Anaesthesia* **58**, 605–609.

Osborne, R., Joel, S., Grebenik, K.. *et al.* 1993. The pharmacokinetics of morphine and morphine glucuronides in kidney failure. *Clinical Pharmacology and Therapeutics* **54**, 158–167.

Osborne, R.J., Joel, S.P. and Slevin, M.L. 1986. Morphine intoxication in renal failure: the role of morphine-6–glucuronide. *British Medical Journal* **292**, 1548–1549.

Parker, C.J.R., Jones, J.E. and Hunter, J.M. 1988. Disposition of infusions of atracurium and its metabolite laudanosine in patients with renal and respiratory failure in an ITU. *British Journal of Anaesthesia* **61**, 531–540.

Paul, M.D., Mazer, C.D. and Byrick, R.J. *et al.* 1986. Influence of mannitol and dopamine on renal function during elective infra-renal aortic cross-clamping in man. *American Journal of Nephrology* **6**, 427–434.

Phillips, B. and Hunter, J.M. 1992. Use of mivacurium chloride by constant infusion in the anephric patient. *British Journal of Anaesthesia* **68**, 492–498.

Pitkanen, M., Tuominen, M. and Rosenberg, P.H. 1985. Bupivacaine spinal anesthesia compared with etidocaine epidural anesthesia in old and young patients. *Regional Anesthesia* **10**, 62–67.

Ponten, J., Biber, B., Bjuro, T. *et al.* 1982. β-receptor blocker withdrawal. A pre-operative problem in general surgery? *Acta Anaesthesiologica Scandinavica* **26** (Suppl. 76), 32–37.

Portenoy, R.K., Thaler, H.T., Inturrisi, C.E. *et al.* 1992. The metabolite morphine-6–glucuronide contributes to the analgesia produced by morphine infusion in patients with pain and normal renal function. *Clinical Pharmacology and Therapeutics* **51**, 422–431.

Prys-Roberts, C. 1982. Interaction of anaesthesia and high pre-operative doses of β-adrenoreceptor antagonists. *Acta Anaesthesiologica Scandinavica* **26** (Suppl. 76), 47–53.

Prys-Roberts, C., Meloche, R. and Foex, P. 1971. Studies of anaesthesia in relation to hypertension: I. Cardiovascular responses of treated and untreated patients. *British Journal of Anaesthesia* **43**, 122–137.

Prys-Roberts, C., Foex, P., Biro, G.P. and Roberts, J.G. 1973. Studies of anaesthesia in relation to hypertension. V. Adrenergic beta-receptor blockade. *British Journal of Anaesthesia* **45**, 671–681.

Rahman, S., Kim, G., Mathew, A. *et al.* 1994. Effects of atrial natriuretic peptide in clinical acute renal failure. *Kidney International* **45**, 1731–1738.

Ramzan, M.I., Shanks, C.A. and Triggs, E.J. 1981. Gallamine disposition in surgical patients with chronic renal failure. *British Journal of Clinical Pharmacology* **12**, 141–147.

Richard, J.P., Conil, J.P., Antonini, A. and Bareille, P. 1986. Utilisation du bromure de vecuronium administre a debit constant lors des transplantations renales. *Cahiers d'Anesthesiologie* **34**, 125–126.

Roizen, M.F., Beaupre, P.N., Alpert, R.A. *et al.* 1984. Monitoring of two dimensional transesophageal echocardiography. Comparison of myocardial function in patients undergoing supraceliac, infraceliac or infra-renal aortic occlusion. *Journal of Vascular Surgery* **1**, 300–305.

Russo, R., Ravagnan, R., Buzzetti, V. and Favini, P. 1986. Atracurium in patients with chronic renal failure. *British Journal of Anaesthesia* **58**, supplement 1, 63s (abstract).

Sawe, J. and Odar-Cederlof, I. 1987. Kinetics of morphine in patients with renal failure. *European Journal of Clinical Pharmacology* **32**, 337–342.

Salem, M.G., Crooke, J.W., Middle, J.G. *et al.* 1988. The effect of dopamine on renal function during aortic cross-clamping. *Annals of the Royal College of Surgeons of England* **70**, 9–12.

Sands, J., Neylan, J., Olson, R. *et al.* 1991. Atrial natriuretic factor does not improve the outcome of cadaveric renal transplantation. *Journal of the American Society of Nephrology* **1**, 1081–1086.

Scott, D.B. and Thorburn, J. 1975. Spinal anaesthesia. *British Journal of Anaesthesia* **47**, 421–422.

Sear, J.W. 1987. Disposition of fentanyl and alfentanil in patients undergoing renal transplantation. VII European Congress of Anaesthesiology, Proceedings I. *Beitrage zur Anaesthesiologie und Intensivmedizin* **19**, 53–58.

Sear, J.W. 1989. Sufentanil disposition in patients undergoing renal transplantation: influence of choice of kinetic model. *British Journal of Anaesthesia* **63**, 60–67.

Sear, J.W., Hand, C.W., Moore, R.A. and McQuay, H.J. 1989. Studies on morphine disposition: influence of renal failure on the kinetics of morphine and its metabolites. *British Journal of Anaesthesia* **62**, 28–32.

Sear, J.W., Jewkes, C., Tellez, J-C. and Foex, P. 1994. Does the choice of antihypertensive therapy influence haemodynamic responses to induction, laryngoscopy and intubation? *British Journal of Anaesthesia* **73**, 303–308.

Shelly, M.P., Cory, E.P. and Park, G.R. 1986. Pharmacokinetics of morphine in two children before and after liver transplantation. *British Journal of Anaesthesia* **58**, 1218–1223.

Sivarajan, M., Amory, D.W. and Lindbloom, L.E. 1976. Systemic and regional blood flow during epidural anesthesia without epinephrine in the rhesus monkey. *Anesthesiology* **45**, 300–310.

Sloan, P.A., Mather, L.E., McLean, C.F. *et al*. 1991. Physiological disposition of i.v. morphine in sheep. *British Journal of Anaesthesia* **67**, 378–386.

Solomonson, M.D., Johnson, M.E. and Ilstrup, D. 1996. Risk factors in patients having surgery to create an arteriovenous fistula. *Anesthesia and Analgesia* **79**, 694–700.

Somogyi, A.A., Shanks, C.A. and Triggs, E.J. 1977. The effect of renal failure on the disposition and neuromuscular blocking action of pancuronium bromide. *European Journal of Clinical Pharmacology* **12**, 23–29.

Stanley, J.C. and Fry, W.J. 1977. Surgical treatment of renovascular hypertension. *Archives of Surgery* **112**, 1291–1297.

Stanley, T.H. and Lathrop, G.D. 1977. Urinary excretion of morphine during and after valvular and coronary artery surgery. *Anesthesiology* **46**, 166–169.

Starsnic, M.A., Goldberg, M.E., Ritter, D.E. *et al*. 1989. Does vecuronium accumulate in the renal transplant patient? *Canadian Journal of Anaesthesia* **36**, 35–39.

Stone, J.G., Foex, P., Sear, J.W. *et al*. 1988. Myocardial ischemia in untreated hypertensive patients: Effect of a single small oral dose of a beta-adrenergic blocking agent. *Anesthesiology* **68**, 495–500.

Svensson, L.G., Coselli, J.S., Safi, H.J. *et al*. 1989. Appraisal of adjuncts to prevent acute renal failure after surgery on the thoracic or thoracoabdominal aorta. *Journal of Vascular Surgery* **10**, 230–239.

Szenohradszky, J., Fisher, D.M., Segredo, V. *et al*. 1992. Pharmacokinetics of rocuronium bromide (ORG 9426) in patients with normal renal function or patients undergoing cadaver renal transplantation. *Anesthesiology* **77**, 899–904.

Szeto, H.H., Inturrisi, C.E., Houde, R. *et al*. 1977. Accumulation of normeperidine, an active metabolite of meperidine in patients with renal failure or cancer. *Annals of Internal Medicine* **86**, 738–741.

Tomita, K., Ujiie, K., Nakanishi, T. *et al*. 1989. Plasma endothelin levels in patients with acute renal failure. *New England Journal of Medicine* **321**, 1127.

Vandam, L.D., Harrison, J.H., Murray, J.E. and Merrill, J.P. 1962. Anesthetic aspects of renal homo-transplantation in man. *Anesthesiology* **23**, 783–792.

Verbeeck, R., Tjandramanga, T.B., Verberckmoes, R. and de Schepper, P.J. 1976. Biotransformation and excretion of lorazepam in patients with chronic renal failure. *British Journal of Clinical Pharmacology* **3**, 1033–1039.

Vinik, H.R., Reves, J.G., Greenblatt, D.J. *et al*. 1983. The pharmacokinetics of midazolam in chronic renal failure patients. *Anesthesiology* **59**, 390–394.

Wagner, K., Albrecht, S. and Neumayer, H.H. 1987. Prevention of post-transplant acute tubular necrosis by the calcium antagonist diltiazem: a prospective, randomised study. *American Journal of Nephrology* **7**, 287–291.

Ward, S., Boheimer, N., Weatherley, B.C. *et al*. 1987. Pharmacokinetics of atracurium and its metabolites in patients with normal renal function, and in patients in renal failure. *British Journal of Anaesthesia* **59**, 697–706.

Way, W.L., Miller, R.D., Hamilton, W.K. and Layzer, R.B. 1972. Succinylcholine-induced hyperkalemia in patients with renal failure? *Anesthesiology* **36**, 138–141.

Weimer, W., Geerlings, S.W., Bijnen, A.B. *et al*. 1983. A controlled study on the effect of mannitol on immediate renal function after cadaver donor kidney transplantation. *Transplantation* **35**, 99–101.

Weir, P.H.C. and Chung, F.F. 1984. Anaesthesia for patients with chronic renal disease. *Canadian Anaesthetists Society Journal* **31**, 468–480.

Wickstrom, I. 1981. Enflurane anaesthesia in living donor renal transplantation. *Acta Anaesthesiologica Scandinavica* **25**, 263–269.

Wiggum, D.C., Cork, R.C., Weldon, S.T. *et al*. 1985. post-operative respiratory depression and elevated sufentanil levels in a patient with chronic renal failure. *Anesthesiology* **63**, 708–710.

Winnearls, C.G., Oliver, D.O., Pippard, M.J. *et al*. 1986. Effect of human erythropoietin derived from recombitant DNA on the anaemia of patients maintained by chronic haemodialysis. *Lancet* **ii**, 1175–1178.

Woolner, D.F., Winter, D., Frendin, T.J. *et al*. 1986. Renal failure does not impair the metabolism of morphine. *British Journal of Clinical Pharmacology* **22**, 55–59.

Wyant, G.M. 1967. The anaesthetist looks at tissue transplantation: three years' experience with kidney transplants. *Canadian Anaesthetists Society Journal* **14**, 255–275.

Yate, P.M., Flynn, P.J. and Arnold, R.W. 1987. Clinical experience and plasma laudanosine concentrations during the infusion of atracurium in the intensive therapy unit. *British Journal of Anaesthesia* **59**, 211–217.

13

Haematological considerations

SHIRLEY J FEARN AND ANDREW J MORTIMER

THE COAGULATION PROCESS

Coagulation pathways

A working knowledge of pathological states affecting blood coagulation and fibrinolysis are vital haematological considerations with which the anaesthetist must be familiar. The anaesthetist must maintain maximal oxygen carrying capacity by the blood to the tissues during surgery, and must therefore have a full working knowledge of blood replacement and substitution.

THE COAGULATION RESPONSE TO INJURY

Rudolph Virchow's concept of the pathogenesis of thrombosis comprises a triad of interaction between flowing blood, the vessel wall and blood constituents. The formation of clot after injury, or haemostasis, helps to preserve vascular integrity by the production of fibrin at the site of vessel damage. Removal of excess fibrin is achieved by fibrinolysis enabling blood to flow again after the breach in the vessel wall has healed.

The normal haemostatic mechanism therefore, is one of balance between coagulation and fibrinolysis, requiring normal vasculature and platelets, as well as normal coagulation and fibrinolysis. A defect in any one of these elements will result in abnormal bleed-ing or thrombosis. The primary response to injury involves local vasospasm, tissue swelling and adherence of platelets to the injured vessel wall and helps to reduce bleeding (Fischbach and Fagdall, 1981). In practice, however, the primary response occurs synchronously with coagulation.

Platelets produced from megakaryocytes in the bone marrow play a crucial role in blood clotting both by adhering to the vessel wall and aggregating together. There are normally $150–400 \times 10^9/L$ platelets circulating with a lifespan of 7–10 days. They do not normally adhere to vascular intima because the endothelial cell monolayer secretes prostacyclin (PGI_2), a powerful prostaglandin vasodilator which inhibits platelet aggregation through the cyclooxygenase pathway (Fig. 13.1). Platelet adhesion to an injured vessel wall is stimulated by exposure to elements of the vessel wall such as subendothelial collagen (Weiss, 1975), and is mediated by von Willebrand factor (vWF) secreted by both platelets and endothelial cells (Petrovitch, 1990).

Activation of the platelet membrane by the exposure of phospholipid causes release of intracytoplasmic granules containing adenosine diphosphate (ADP) and thromboxane A_2 (TxA_2), a prostaglandin and potent vasoconstrictor. A positive-feedback loop is created by ADP causing further platelet aggregation at the site of injury, and TxA_2 increasing the release of ADP. During the release of platelet

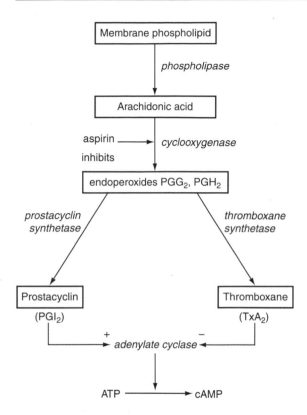

Figure 13.1 *The cyclooxygenase pathway. Thromboxane (TxA$_2$) and prostacyclin (PGI$_2$) are formed by the action of cyclooxygenase on membrane phospholipid. These compounds have opposing actions on platelet aggregation by controlling levels of cAMP.*

granules, arachidonate is liberated from the platelet membrane, increasing TxA$_2$ and platelet aggregation. These amplification loops culminate in the formation of a platelet plug at the site of injury.

The final common pathway in platelet aggregation results from a high concentration of free intracellular calcium which is controlled by the level of cyclic adenosine monophosphate (cAMP). In turn, the level of cAMP is controlled by the enzyme adenylate cyclase. TxA$_2$ and PGI$_2$ have opposing effects on adenylate cyclase; TxA$_2$ inhibits the adenylate cyclase necessary for the conversion of adenosine triphosphate (ATP) to cAMP and therefore promotes calcium release and platelet aggregation, whereas PGI$_2$ activates it, inhibiting calcium release and platelet aggregation. In this manner, PGI$_2$ secreted by normal endothelial cells, and TxA$_2$ secreted by activated platelets, limits the formation of a platelet plug to the area of injury (Gordon-Smith, 1995).

THE COAGULATION CASCADE

The coagulation process comprises a series of proteins which are sequentially activated to form activated clotting factors, the end result of which is the formation of insoluble fibrin from fibrinogen. Fibrin reinforces the more delicate platelet plug until the healing process can repair the injured vessel. Factors involved in the cascade are designated by Roman numerals which correspond to the order in which they were discovered. However, some factors are not referred to by a number, but by name: fibrinogen (I), prothrombin (II), calcium (IV) and tissue thromboplastin (III). Factor VI does not exist because it was found to be activated factor V. There are also several newly identified factors without numbers: prekallikrein and high-molecular-weight kininogen.

Most clotting factors circulate as proenzymes which are inactive. During the coagulation process, a portion of the molecule is cleaved off leaving an 'active clotting factor' designated by the suffix 'a' after the Roman numeral. Active clotting factors are enzymes that cleave the next factor in the chain, until fibrinogen is converted to fibrin. Some factors act as cofactors in the clotting cascade rather than becoming cleavage enzymes (Petrovitch, 1990).

The coagulation cascade has two discrete pathways (Fig. 13.2):

- *The intrinsic pathway* is so named because it is limited by the boundaries of the blood vessel. Initiation of coagulation occurs by exposure of platelet factor-3 (PF$_3$), a phospholipid surface exposed by activated platelets, which in turn activates factor XII. Sequential activation of factors XI, IX, X and prothrombin then follows (Furie, 1992). The function of this pathway is measured by the activated partial-thromboplastin time (aPTT), also known as the partial thromboplastin time with kaolin (PTTK).
- *The extrinsic pathway* is so named because it commences with the release of tissue thromboplastin from cell-surface membranes of tissues outside the blood vessel. This activates factor VII and prothrombin. The function of this pathway is measured by the prothrombin time (PT).

Both these pathways result in the formation of activated factor X (Xa) after which they merge to a final common pathway. Xa cleaves prothrombin (factor II) to thrombin in the presence of factor V.

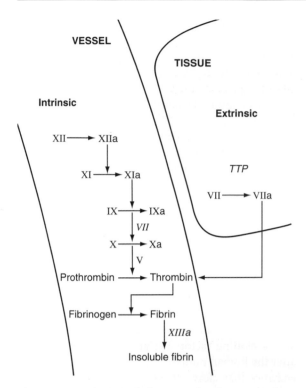

Figure 13.2 *The coagulation cascade. Tissue activation of factor VII via the extrinsic pathway and intraluminal activation of factor X convert prothrombin to thrombin. The conversion of fibrinogen to fibrin produces the end result of coagulation: the fibrin plug.*

Thrombin cleaves fibrinogen to produce fibrin monomers. These monomers subsequently aggregate to form a fibrin polymer or mesh which is stabilized by cross-links formed by factor XIII. Finally, the clot is consolidated by contraction of platelet actin and myosin fibres.

This simplified description does not take into account many other probable interactions between the intrinsic and extrinsic pathways. Thrombin, for example, has many other actions; in low concentrations it stimulates the intrinsic pathway, whereas in high concentrations it inhibits it. Thrombin also stimulates the release of ADP from platelets causing them to aggregate, as well as stimulating the release of PGI_2 from endothelial cells causing vessel relaxation.

Fibrinolysis

Platelets disaggregate after 24–48 hours leaving only the fibrin plug to maintain haemostasis (Fischbach

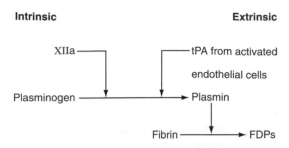

Figure 13.3 *Fibrinolysis. Intrinsic activated factor XII and extrinsic tissue plasminogen activator convert plasminogen to plasmin, a powerful protease enzyme which degrades fibrin clot into fibrin-degradation products.*

and Fagdall, 1981). To re-establish vascular patency, the fibrin meshwork is dissolved by fibrinolysis; the reverse of coagulation. As with the coagulation cascade, fibrinolysis occurs by two pathways (Fig. 13.3): the extrinsic pathway which is initiated by tissue plasminogen activator (tPA) from activated endothelial cells, and the intrinsic pathway which is initiated within the blood vessel by activated factor XII. Both pathways result in the formation of plasmin from its precursor plasminogen (Petrovitch, 1990).

Plasmin is a powerful protease enzyme which liquefies the clot by lysing fibrin to form degradation products (FDPs), which have half-lives of about 9 hours. The structure of FDPs varies according to whether plasmin is cleaving fibrinogen, cross-linked fibrin or fibrin that is not cross-linked (Petrovitch, 1990). Accumulation of FDPs inhibits coagulation, prevents cross-linking and alters platelet function. tPA binds strongly to fibrin, localizing the activity of plasmin to the site of thrombus (Gordon-Smith, 1995). If released systemically, plasmin will digest a number of coagulation factors including fibrinogen and factors V and VIII.

Regulation of coagulation and fibrinolysis

Coagulation and fibrinolysis are precisely regulated to prevent widespread clotting in the intact vasculature, whilst enabling haemostasis to occur rapidly at the site of injury. Primary haemostasis is controlled by the levels of two prostaglandins with opposing

Table 13.1   *Tests of haemostasis*

Test	Normal value	Factors assessed	Causes of prolongation
Bleeding time	3–8 min	Platelets	Inherited disorders of platelet function, drug-induced renal failure, von Willebrand's disease
Thrombin time	15–16 s	Fibrinogen, inhibitors of thrombin	Heparin therapy
Extrinsic path			
Prothrombin time	10–14 s	VII, V, X, prothrombin, fibrinogen	Liver disease, vitamin K deficiency, warfarin therapy, DIC
Intrinsic path			
Partial thromboplastin time with kaolin (PTTK)	30–40 s	VII, IX, XI, XII, V, X, prothrombin, fibrinogen	V, VIII deficiency (massive blood transfusion), haemophilias, heparin therapy
Activated partial thrombo-plastin time (aPTT)	<35 s		
Activated clotting time (ACT)	90–120 s		

actions (TxA_2 and PGI_2) as noted above. Artificial surfaces do not produce prostacyclin and therefore cannot confine or control platelet thrombus formation, so that once coagulation is initiated in a vascular graft, for example, the whole graft may thrombose (Fischbach and Fagdall, 1981). Most of the coagulation factors are present in the circulation in inactive forms and require a phospholipid surface or tissue thromboplastin for their activation and interaction.

Antithrombin III (AT-III) is a physiological inhibitor of the coagulation cascade. It binds thrombin and other activated factors, and its action is accelerated by heparin which occurs naturally on the surface of endothelial cells. High concentrations of thrombin act through a negative feedback loop to reduce thrombin synthesis by destroying the activity of factors V and VIIIC. Low levels of thrombin have the reverse effect, stimulating factor V and VIIIC activity. Protein C is a protease enzyme which destroys activated factor V and VIII. The activity of protein C is enhanced by protein S which facilitates binding of protein C to the platelet surface (see later).

Tests of coagulation and fibrinolysis

Screening tests for defects in clot formation and lysis usually assess several interactions rather than a single step in a chain of events (Table 13.1).

EXTRINSIC PATHWAY

The prothrombin time (PT) measures the function of the extrinsic pathway which includes factor VII as well as the common pathway factors V, X, prothrombin and fibrinogen. Thromboplastin is used to initiate the reaction and, because there is so much variation in thromboplastins, an International Normalization Ratio (INR) is used to aid control of oral anticoagulation. The normal value for PT is 10–14 s, INR 1.

INTRINSIC PATHWAY

There are three tests for the intrinsic and common pathways based on activating coagulation to accelerate simple clotting time.

* *The partial thromboplastin time* is a test in which platelet phospholipid or a substitute is added to the patient's blood and the time to form a fibrin clot is measured.
* *The activated partial thromboplastin time* (aPTT) is a modification in which factors XII and XI are added before the platelet phospholipid. Normal values are less than 35 s.
* *The activated clotting time* is determined by adding diatomaceous earth for surface activation of factors XII and XI. The patient's own blood provides platelet phospholipid and normal values are 90–120 s.

OTHER TESTS

Other tests include:

- *The thrombin time* is the time to form a clot when thrombin is added to the patient's blood, and assesses the conversion of fibrinogen to fibrin. The thrombin time will be prolonged if fibrinogen levels are reduced, e.g. disseminated intravascular coagulation (DIC), or if thrombin inhibitors are present, e.g. heparin or FDPs.
- *Platelet count and bleeding time*: A platelet count of less than 100 000/mm^3 may prolong the bleeding time, but platelet function is more important than their number. A formal test of bleeding time is indicated if a functional defect of platelets is suspected and the platelet count is normal. It measures the time to clot formation after cuts are made on the forearm under controlled conditions. Normal bleeding times are 3–8 min and may be prolonged in cases of reduced platelet numbers or function. It is a difficult test to perform and should therefore be carried out only by trained staff.
- *Fibrinogen and FDP levels*: fibrinogen levels (normally 150–300 mg/dL) are also a measure of the final common pathway. They may be low in liver disease or DIC. High levels are due either to primary fibrinolysis caused by a massive release of plasminogen activator, or secondary fibrinolysis initiated by DIC. The combination of a prolonged thrombin time and low fibrinogen levels is highly suggestive of DIC.

ABNORMALITIES OF HAEMOSTASIS

Bleeding disorders

Many disease states and drugs are associated with a bleeding tendency. The indications for regional anaesthesia, and spinal procedures in particular, must be carefully considered in these situations (Table 13.2).

CONGENITAL DISORDERS

Haemophilia
Haemophilia A has an incidence of 1 in 10 000 and is a sex-linked autosomal recessive trait, whereas

Table 13.2 *Causes of bleeding tendency*

Congenital	Acquired
Haemophilia A and B	Vitamin K deficiency
Christmas disease	Liver disease
Von Willebrand's disease	Heparin/warfarin therapy
Connective tissue disease	Platelet disorders/ abnormal consumption
	Antiplatelet therapy
	Thrombolysis
	Pentoxifylline
	Vascular purpuras

haemophilia B is an autosomal recessive trait. In haemophilia, the aPTT is prolonged, but the PT is normal. Peri-operative management should aim to replace relevant factors prior to surgery in close collaboration with a haematologist. Factor levels should be maintained near normal for up to 48 hours after surgery until the first stages of healing have occurred.

Von Willebrand's disease
This is caused by decreased activity of von Willebrand factor which has an important role both in platelet function and factor VIII activity. There are several forms of the disease, most of which are inherited as autosomal dominant traits, and the remainder as autosomal recessive traits. Defective platelet aggregation and reduced levels of factor VIII are manifest by a prolonged bleeding time and aPTT. Treatment with desmopressin acetate neutralizes defective platelet aggregation and increases levels of factor VIII.

Connective-tissue disorders
Although rare, many of these are associated with an increased risk of bleeding. Examples are Osler–Weber–Rendu disease (hereditary haemorrhagic telangiectasia) and Ehlers–Danlos syndrome.

ACQUIRED DISORDERS

Acquired disorders of haemostasis that cause bleeding are numerous. Among the commonest are vitamin K deficiency, liver disease and anticoagulant therapy.

Vitamin K deficiency
Vitamin K is required for the synthesis of factors II, VII, IX and X in the liver. Absorption of vitamin K

Table 13.3 *Platelet disorders*

Platelet disorder	Causes
Reduced production	Bone marrow infiltration
	Chemotherapy/radiotherapy
Increased destruction	Idiopathic thrombocytopenic
	purpura
	Massive blood transfusion
	Drugs
	Septicaemia
	Autoimmune disorders, e.g.
	rheumatoid arthritis, SLE
Excess sequestration	Hypersplenism
Platelet dysfunction	Uraemia
	Chronic liver disease
	Von Willebrand's disease
	DIC
	Drugs, e.g. antiplatelet
	therapy, ethanol,
	dipyridamole, dextran,
	propranolol, amitriptyline,
	phenothiazines,
	diphenhydramine

requires a normally functioning liver and gut. Mild deficiency prolongs the PT because factor VII is the most sensitive to vitamin K deficiency, but as levels decrease further, factors II, VII and X also become affected and the aPTT becomes prolonged. Oral anticoagulants (e.g. warfarin) block the vitamin K carboxylation of these factors, and can be reversed gradually by administration of intravenous vitamin K, or more rapidly by administration of fresh frozen plasma (FFP) which contains the factors in the intrinsic cascade.

Platelet disorders

Bleeding problems can result from a low platelet count or poor function. A reduction in numbers can result from:

- decreased production (e.g. after chemotherapy);
- increased destruction, which may be idiopathic or drug induced (see Table 13.3);
- excess sequestration of platelets as in hypersplenism; or
- increased consumption (e.g. DIC, sepsis).

Platelet dysfunction can result from drugs (Table 13.3), uraemia and chronic liver disease. If the underlying cause cannot be remedied pre-operatively platelets can be transfused.

Heparin therapy

Heparin may be administered pre-operatively to prevent thrombotic complications in patients at particular risk (e.g. the obese), those with a history of previous venous thromboembolism, those undergoing orthopaedic or pelvic surgery and those on long-term oral anticoagulation for artificial heart valves. Heparin is usually administered to vascular patients intra-operatively prior to cross-clamping a vessel.

Standard heparin consists of a wide range of mucopolysaccharides, but low-molecular-weight alternatives have been selected for better bioavailability and a longer half-life when administered subcutaneously. Heparin therapy may be reversed rapidly with protamine which prevents heparin complexing with AT-III, but can lead to profound hypotension. Rarely, patients may form heparin-dependent antiplatelet antibodies after 7–10 days of therapy leading to thrombocytopenia, but an increased tendency to thromboembolism.

Platelet consumption

A degree of platelet consumption occurs in patients who are critically ill, bleeding or who have been massively transfused. Packed red cells or whole blood stored for more than 24–48 hours do not contain platelets or significant amounts of factor VIII. Platelets and FFP can be transfused as replacement therapy.

Disseminated intravascular coagulation

DIC is associated with critical illness such as sepsis, shock, severe tissue injury, burns and transfusion reactions. Patients undergoing vascular surgery are more likely to develop DIC if shock has occurred, if the operation has been technically difficult or if vascular occlusion time has been prolonged. Low blood flow increases the tendency for platelet adhesion to occur and coagulation factors are not cleared from the blood so rapidly (Petrovitch, 1990).

Normally, the formation of clot is localized to the area of injury because clotting factors can only interact on phospholipid surfaces. If this mechanism breaks down widespread clotting may occur, as when circulating immune complexes or bacteria cause platelet aggregation and exposure of the phospholipid platelet factor-3 (Petrovitch, 1990). Tissue thromboplastin is released into the circulation in massive crush injuries, and haemolysed red cells release phospholipid after a transfusion reaction. Large areas of denuded vascular endothelium from burns or vasculitis also initiate diffuse coagulation.

Table 13.4 *Causes of hypercoagulable states*

Primary	Secondary
Antithrombin III deficiency	Malignancy
Protein C and S deficiency	Pregnancy
Activated protein C resistance	Oral contraceptive pill
Lupus anticoagulant	Hormone-replacement therapy
Anticardiolipin antibody	Diabetes mellitus
Fibrinolytic disorders e.g. abnormal plasminogen,	Artificial surfaces, e.g. haemodialysis/haemoperfusion,
defective tPA release, impaired activation of	cardiopulmonary bypass, prosthetic heart valves, vascular
plasminogen	grafts, intra-aortic balloon pumps, intravascular catheters
High-molecular-weight kininogen deficiency	Chronic occlusive arterial disease
Factor XII deficiency	Vasculitis
Prekallikrein deficiency	Smoking
Dysfibrinogenaemias	Surgery
Sickle cell disease	Trauma
	Immobilization
	Obesity
	Congestive cardiac failure
	Nephrotic syndrome

Initial laboratory investigation may be normal although a fall in platelet count is an early feature. Once established, DIC will result in falling fibrinogen levels, rising levels of FDPs and prolonged PT and aPTT. Treatment of the underlying cause is crucial. Replacing blood components consumed by coagulation, i.e. platelets, FFP and cryoprecipitates, is only required if abnormal bleeding is a clinical problem.

Antiplatelet therapy

Antiplatelet drugs are commonly prescribed for patients with vascular disease to prevent thrombosis. They include aspirin and non-steroidal anti-inflammatory agents (NSAIDs) such as dipyridamole. Aspirin inhibits cyclooxygenase which is involved in the conversion of arachidonic acid to TxA_2. Reduced levels of TxA_2 lead to reduced platelet aggregation and vasoconstriction, prolonging the bleeding time. This irreversible inhibition lasts the lifetime of those platelets affected therefore aspirin needs to be stopped a week prior to elective surgery. Dipyridamole has a synergistic effect with aspirin, but a different mechanism of action, that of increasing cAMP by inhibiting phosphodiesterase (Troianos and Ellison, 1991).

Thrombolysis

Thrombolytic therapy with agents such as tPA, streptokinase and urokinase, which promote fibrinolysis through the activation of plasminogen to plasmin, is used increasingly for acute vascular occlusion. tPA is selective and only acts on fibrin-bound plasmin, while streptokinase and urokinase activate free circulating plasmin as well. However, systemic fibrinolysis can occur after high-dose or prolonged use of tPA (Troianos and Ellison, 1991).

Emergency surgery may be required in patients who have recently received thrombolytic therapy, and certain precautions are needed. Vascular access sites are likely to bleed and therefore sites amenable to compression should be chosen. Intramuscular injections should be avoided, and FFP and cryoprecipitate (as an additional source of fibrinogen and factor VIII) can be used in uncontrollable bleeding.

Vascular disorders

Acquired disorders of vessels include the purpuras, which may be a result of ageing, steroid therapy, infection or associated with rheumatoid arthritis. In general, these conditions do not cause significant haemorrhage, but are usually only associated with bruising (Petrovitch, 1990).

Hypercoagulable states

Patients with hypercoagulable states are predisposed to thrombosis. Some states may have a detectable biochemical abnormality, but others may simply cause recurrent thrombosis without recognizable predisposing factors (Schafer, 1985). Primary disorders (Table 13.4) are usually inherited, but secondary or acquired disorders are associated with underlying systemic diseases such as malignancy, pregnancy, myeloproliferative disorders, hyperlipidaemias, diabetes mellitus and abnormalities of blood vessels and rheology. Drug therapy such as the oral contraceptive pill or hormone-replacement therapy may also increase the risk of thrombosis.

PRIMARY HYPERCOAGULABLE STATES

These are mostly congenital and familial, causing abnormalities that lead to thrombosis (usually venous) spontaneously, or at times of additional risk (e.g. during surgery, pregnancy or after immobilization) (Schafer, 1985).

Antithrombin III deficiency

Antithrombin III (AT-III) is the primary antagonist of thrombin and other activated clotting factors. The incidence of deficiency is about 1 in 2000, and the disease is inherited as an autosomal dominant trait. Homozygosity is incompatible with life; heterozygotes have AT-III levels between 25 and 60 per cent of normal. The condition usually manifests itself as recurrent venous thromboembolism which may occur at unusual anatomical sites. Most patients present in the second to third decade of life with thrombosis frequently triggered by events that may cause venous thromboembolism in the normal population. Treatment of thrombosis is with intravenous heparin and AT-III concentrates although higher doses may be required as heparin cannot work effectively without its natural cofactor AT-III. Lifelong anticoagulation is required for those patients in whom thrombosis recurs. Low levels of AT-III can occur in nephrotic syndrome (increased excretion of AT-III predisposing to renal vein thrombosis in particular), advanced liver disease (reduced synthesis of AT-III), extensive thrombosis and DIC (increased AT-III consumption), and women on the oral contraceptive pill.

Protein C and S deficiencies

Protein C deficiency has a similar mode of inheritance and clinical manifestation as AT-III deficiency. Protein C is vitamin K dependent so measurements will be difficult to interpret if the patient has liver disease or is taking oral anticoagulants. Protein S is a

cofactor for protein C activity. Deficiency also results in an increased risk of recurrent venous thromboembolism.

Activated protein C resistance (APCr)

More than 95 per cent of cases of APCr are thought to be due to a mutation of factor V (factor V Leiden) which was discovered only fairly recently (Dahlback et al., 1993). This is an inherited condition and may be responsible for thrombosis in patients in whom an underlying cause could not be found. The risk of thrombosis is increased if APCr coexists with protein C or S or AT-III deficiency, or use of the oral contraceptive pill (Rhodes, 1996).

Lupus anticoagulant and anticardiolipin antibody

Patients with systemic lupus erythematosus (SLE), other autoimmune disorders, malignancy or those on certain medications may spontaneously acquire antiphospholipid antibodies, such as lupus anticoagulant or anticardiolipin antibody, which can be associated with an increased risk of thrombosis.

Fibrinolytic disorders

These congenital or acquired disorders include abnormalities of plasminogen, defective plasminogen activator release and impaired activation of plasminogen.

Dysfibrinogenaemias

Abnormal fibrin can be resistant to lysis by plasmin, causing either a bleeding tendency or a hypercoagulable state.

Factor XII, prekallikrein and high-molecular-weight kininogen deficiency

These substances are all associated with contact activation of the coagulation cascade, enhancing blood fluidity by aiding activation of the fibrinolytic system, and generating vasodilators kinins. Depending on the balance between these conflicting actions, patients with such deficiencies may be predisposed to thromboembolic disease.

SECONDARY HYPERCOAGULABLE STATES

These are complex coagulopathies in which the exact pathophysiological basis for thrombosis is undefined. Management lies in treatment of the underlying cause (Schafer, 1985).

Malignancy

The association of malignancy with recurrent migratory thrombophlebitis was first noted by Trousseau (1865). The incidence of thrombosis is 5–15 per cent, but with some tumours (e.g. pancreatic carcinoma) the incidence is higher, up to 50 per cent. Episodes of thrombosis may predate the diagnosis of cancer by months or even years. Abnormalities of coagulation may be secondary to venous stasis from mediastinal or pelvic tumour invasion or compression although this is rare. However, several biochemical abnormalities have been recognized in malignancy, and reflect general activation of coagulation and chronic DIC with various degrees of compensation. Heparin therapy is better than warfarin in some instances.

Pregnancy

The risk of thrombosis increases with increasing age, parity, the presence of hypertension and the mode of delivery. Anatomical changes (e.g. raised intra-abdominal pressure and venous compression), physiological changes (e.g. relaxation of vascular smooth muscle) and biochemical changes (e.g. increased capacity for fibrin production and reduced ability for fibrin degradation) that occur in pregnancy and during the puerperium result in a low-grade and usually compensated intravascular coagulation.

Oral contraceptives (OCP)

Synthetic oestrogens increase the activity of several procoagulant factors and reduce the activity of AT-III and protein C. This increases the risk of venous thromboembolism in premenopausal women, and oestrogen-containing preparations are usually discontinued 4–6 weeks prior to elective surgery. Recent concerns have focussed on the increased risk of venous thrombosis with third-generation OCPs which contain the synthetic progestogens gestodene and desogestrel (Jick et al., 1995; Spitzer et al., 1996).

Hormone-replacement therapy (HRT)

HRT is being prescribed increasingly to postmenopausal women to prevent the effects of low oestrogens, in particular osteoporosis and coronary artery disease. Contrary to recent reviews, HRT is associated with an increased risk of venous thrombosis and should be discontinued prior to surgery. The usual prophylactic measures should be applied, namely graded compression stockings, peri-operative subcutaneous heparin and early mobilization.

Artificial surfaces

Haemodialysis, haemoperfusion, cardiopulmonary bypass, prosthetic heart valves, vascular grafts, intra-aortic balloon devices and catheters all activate platelets and contact coagulation factors. The resulting risk of localized thrombosis and systemic embolization may be reduced by platelet inhibitory therapy if indicated.

Chronic occlusive arterial disease

Peripheral arterial disease causes local thrombosis when plaque surfaces become irregular or rupture causing platelet adhesion and aggregation.

Surgery

Surgery, especially pelvic and orthopaedic surgery, is associated with an increased risk of venous thromboembolism. Increased levels of coagulation factors, reduced levels of coagulation inhibitors, enhanced in vitro platelet reactivity and impaired in vitro fibrinolysis have all been reported, suggesting a hypercoagulable state (Rosenfeld et al., 1993). These changes, which are a response to tissue injury, may increase the likelihood of arterial thrombotic events in patients with occlusive peripheral or coronary disease.

Two studies have shown a reduction in perioperative thrombosis if epidural anaesthesia and analgesia is used (Tuman et al., 1991; Rosenfeld et al., 1993). The use of this combination may attenuate the stress response and its resultant effects on the coagulation system. Other effects such as increased lower extremity blood flow, local anaesthetic-mediated reductions in platelet reactivity, limited postoperative rises in factor VIII and vWF and accelerated return of AT-III concentration to pre-operative levels, have also been implicated (Steele et al., 1991).

BLOOD TRANSFUSION

When the haemostatic mechanisms of vasoconstriction, platelet plugging and clot formation are overwhelmed by major injury or surgical trauma then blood is lost from the circulation (Table 13.5). Consequently, the circulating blood volume (CBV) is reduced leading to decreases in blood pressure and oxygen delivery, the development of stagnant hypoxia in the extremities and ultimately hypovolaemic shock which may result in the death of the patient.

Table 13.5   *The major categories of blood loss, the physiological response and the treatment*

Magnitude of blood loss (%)	Physiological compensatory mechanisms	Treatment required
Compensated		
0–20	Neural:	Crystalloid or colloid solutions only
	Vasoconstriction by sympathetic outflow	
(0–15 mL/kg)	Endocrine:	
	Vasopressin	
	Antidiuretic hormone	
	Atrial natriuretic peptide	
	Erythropoietin	
	Internal transfusion	
Uncompensated		
21–50	As above, with greater intensity plus tachycardia	As above, plus usually homologous blood
(16–35 mL/kg)		Autologous blood ideal
Massive		
51–100%	As above, with even greater intensity	Homologous blood essential
		Coagulation factors and platelets also
(36–70 mL/kg)		required

Blood loss

The normal total volume of blood in a 70-kg subject is approximately 5 L, thus there are 70 mL per kg of body weight. Knowledge of the body weight of a patient enables the estimated blood volume (EBV) to be calculated by multiplication of the body weight (kg) by the factor of 70 (mL).

COMPENSATED BLOOD LOSS

In the early stages of blood loss (up to 20 per cent CBV, 0–15 mL/kg) physiological compensatory mechanisms help to restore and maintain the CBV and the blood pressure. The stress response invoked by the blood loss includes neural and endocrine mechanisms. The neural response comprises massive sympathetic autonomic stimulation producing, in conjunction with the release of catecholamines from the adrenal medulla, widespread vasoconstriction. The endocrine response includes the release of hormones which also contribute to elevation of the blood pressure (vasopressin) and to restoration of the previous CBV (antidiuretic hormone and atrial natriuretic peptide). Replacement of red cell mass is stimulated by the release of erythropoietin. Up to 500 mL of intravascular volume is replaced by a transfer of extracellular fluid to the vascular compartment by

a change in perfusion pressure in the capillary beds: the process of internal transfusion.

The effects of these homeostatic mechanisms ensure that tissue oxygen delivery is not compromised. Blood loss up to 20 per cent of CBV is described as compensated because, in the absence of other adverse factors, no specific treatment is required. However, in any patient with an active haemorrhage, it would be normal practice to establish an intravenous infusion of crystalloid solution because at the outset, the magnitude of the haemorrhage will not be known.

UNCOMPENSATED BLOOD LOSS

Greater volumes of blood loss (21–50 per cent of CBV, 16–35 mL/kg) cannot be compensated for by the mechanisms described above and require replacement with either crystalloid or colloid solution, or a blood transfusion. Blood loss of this magnitude can be tolerated by a patient provided that the volume lost is adequately replaced and CBV maintained.

Hence blood loss down to a haemoglobin of 70 g/L can be accepted in clinical practice (National Institutes of Health Consensus Development Conference, 1989). Most authorities however, include a margin of safety and accept blood loss down to 90–100 g/L. The reason for this is that many of the surgical patients who will lose blood during an operation have coexisting diseases such as ischaemic heart disease and peripheral vascular disease.

MASSIVE BLOOD LOSS

Massive blood loss occurs when the blood loss exceeds 51 per cent of EBV (51–100 per cent CBV, 36–70 mL/kg). Unless treated with blood replacement, death from hypovolaemic shock invariably occurs within a few hours. Blood loss of this magnitude may be treated initially with crystalloid and colloid solutions, but will almost always require the administration of homologous (allogeneic) blood to restore CBV.

In current anaesthetic and surgical practice, the issues concerning the transfusion of small volumes of blood (2–5 units) are under scrutiny because of recognition of the potential hazards of blood transfusion. The remainder of this section is devoted to consideration of these hazards and the use of techniques which may minimize the need for the transfusion of homologous blood.

Blood groups

The features of the ABO blood group system are shown in Table 13.6. The salient feature is that donor blood of group O may be given to any recipient because of the absence of red cell antigens, hence the use of group O Rhesus D negative as the source of uncrossmatched blood for emergency use in the operating theatres, casualty and obstetric departments. All blood is characterized for the ABO and Rhesus D antigens on the red cell membrane to ensure that the donor's red cells are fully compatible with the recipient's plasma. Laboratory testing of these two factors ensures that up to 99.5 per cent of all blood transfusions will be compatible. There is a

Table 13.6 *The incidence and distribution of blood groups, red cell antigens and serum antibodies in the UK (modified from Contreras and Mollinson, 1998)*

Blood group	Incidence in UK (%)	Red cell (+ other cell) antigen	Antibodies in serum
O	47	Nil	Anti-A, Anti-B
A	42	A	Anti-B
B	8	B	Anti-A
AB	3	A + B	Nil

residual group of about 0.5 per cent in which other antibodies have been generated by previous blood transfusion. This requires further serological testing of donor and recipient blood (Contreras and Mollinson, 1998) to ensure compatibility.

Ideally, all blood components, such as platelets and white cells for transfusion should also be tested for the ABO and Rhesus D antigens. Packs of these products will be labelled appropriately. Failure to observe this guideline has resulted in complications after platelet transfusion (Serious Hazards of Transfusion Report, 1998).

Types of blood for transfusion

Blood lost through haemorrhage may be replaced using blood from one of two sources:

• other people (*homologous blood*); or
• the patient's own (*autologous blood*) collected before or during surgery. Regardless of the source, all blood and components collected prior to a surgical procedure, should undergo immunological compatibility testing. Autologous blood is tested in this way to minimize the risk of incorrect blood transfusion should the blood be transfused into a recipient other than the donor.

HOMOLOGOUS BLOOD

Homologous blood is the most widely used preparation for the treatment of blood loss throughout the world. Because it has the potential to stimulate antibody formation in the recipient, it is also called 'allogeneic blood'. It is collected from either volunteer or paid donors: paid donors predominate in the USA, but voluntary donation is usual in much of the rest of the world.

In the UK, a pack of donated whole blood has a volume of approximately 510 mL, consisting of 450 mL of blood and 63 mL of anticoagulant solution. This contains citrate (anticoagulant), phosphate (buffer), dextrose and adenine (both as red cell nutrients). This is designated as 'CPDA1 blood', and has a storage interval (shelf life) of 35 days, ensuring that approximately 70 per cent of the red cells are still viable at the expiry date assuming the life of a red cell to be 120 days. The haematocrit of collected homologous blood is between 35 and 45 per cent, being less than that of the donor because of dilution by the CPDA1 solution. There are no functional platelets or white cells in homologous blood because it is not usually available for transfusion within 48 hours of collection.

Fresh blood is the ideal for transfusion when required in the treatment of blood loss, because it is a valuable source of red cells, platelets and clotting factors. It is not usual to obtain this in the UK. More often the blood is towards the end of its shelf life and has had both plasma and platelets removed. Products from several donors are then pooled to produce fresh frozen plasma (FFP) for the treatment of coagulation defects, and platelet solutions for deficiency states. Thus the original diluted whole blood is usually supplied as red cell concentrate with a haematocrit ranging between 55 and 75 per cent. The absence of coagulation factors and platelets may need to be taken into account in the treatment of uncompensated blood loss. These other components will definitely be required in the treatment of massive haemorrhage.

Problems of homologous blood
The fact that homologous blood may be nearing the end of its shelf life when issued for use means that up to 30 per cent of the red cells will have died. In addition to providing as little as 70 per cent of effective blood transfusion, there are also recognized complications from the long-term storage of the blood, the potential for transmission of infection, incompatible transfusions and the introduction of human error in the handling, ordering and distribution of blood from the local blood bank.

Biochemical changes Donated blood is stored between 2 and 6°C. Massive transfusion may result in hypothermia in the recipient unless a blood-warming device is used. This is especially important in neonates and children. In addition, various deleterious changes occur during the possible storage time of up to 35 days, some producing theoretical problems, but others being of more practical relevance.

Progressive failure of the sodium–potassium pump in the red cell membrane allows potassium to leak from the red cells down the concentration gradient between intracellular fluid (150 mmol/L) and plasma (5 mmol/L). This may result in the administration of a high potassium load and resultant hyperkalaemia in a patient receiving a massive transfusion (10 units or more).

The anticoagulant effect of citrate in the storage medium is achieved by combination with the free ionized calcium in the plasma. Thus large transfusions require monitoring of the patient's plasma calcium concentration. The citrate is usually rapidly metabolized by the liver to bicarbonate, but may be a problem during operations such as liver transplantation because it may cause metabolic alkalosis.

Metabolic acidosis resulting from the production of lactic acid by red cells during several weeks of storage is again a theoretical hazard. However, resuscitation of the patient to minimize lactic acid formation in the extremities where there is stagnant blood flow overrides the administration of a small dose of lactate in transfused blood. Blood lactate monitoring is useful in this context.

Another metabolic change in stored red cells is the loss of 2,3-diphosphoglyceric acid (2,3-DPG). This causes the oxyhaemoglobin dissociation curve to move to the left. This means that oxygen is taken up effectively by the transfused red cells during passage through the lungs, but that it is not readily given up in the periphery.

Coagulation changes Normal function of the coagulation cascades described in the first section requires a minimum of 20 per cent of the normal concentration of each of the various factors. Factor V loses 50 per cent of activity within 14 days of storage whereas factor VIII (antihaemophilic factor) loses 50 per cent of activity within 24 hours, and 70 per cent within 5 days. Thus dilutional coagulopathy may need specific correction with factor VIII.

In addition to the rapid decline in activity of these two factors, platelets lose all activity after 48 hours refrigeration. This is why they are removed immediately from donor blood, then pooled and frozen for long-term storage.

Transmission of infection Potential blood donors undergo rigorous selection and screening procedures. Nevertheless, serious infections are occasionally transmitted by donated blood, despite testing (in the UK) for surface antigen to hepatitis B, and antibodies to hepatitis C, human immunodeficiency virus (HIV) and syphilis. During 1996 and 1997 there were eight confirmed cases of transfusion-transmitted infection in the UK (Serious Hazards of Transfusion Report, 1997, 1998) out of a total of approximately two million units of blood issued for transfusion each year (Table 13.7).

More recently, concern has been expressed about the potential for transmission of new variant

Table 13.7 *Transfusion-transmitted infection in the UK 1996–97*

Infection	Year of transfusion	
	1996	**1997**
Hepatitis		
A	1	–
B	1	–
C	1	–
HIV	1	
Bacteria	–	3
Malaria		1
Total	4	4

Creutzfeldt–Jakob disease (CJD) in the white cells of donor blood. By the end of 1999 all donated blood in the UK will have had the white cells removed to reduce this risk.

Immunological complications Immunological complications of homologous blood transfusion account for the majority of acute and delayed reactions. Almost 50 per cent of these are due to the transfusion of blood or a blood component (platelets, white cells) which was of the wrong group. This almost always results from human error occurring during the chain of events involved in sampling, ordering, labelling, storing, collecting and checking the donor blood against the recipient's details. Erroneous laboratory testing is very rare.

Acute haemolytic reactions Acute haemolytic reactions are most commonly caused by ABO incompatibility. The anti-A and anti-B factors in group O blood are potent IgM antibodies which may activate the full complement pathway and cause rapid intravascular lysis if blood other than group O is administered in error. Haemolysis may cause DIC and lead to free haemoglobin in the urine. Such reactions may be fatal.

Delayed haemolytic reactions These reactions occur in patients who have been previously sensitized to a foreign protein, but in whom the concentration of antibody in the serum is too low to be detected. Subsequent administration of the same antigen triggers a secondary immune response over 5–10 days, with features of fever, jaundice, haemoglobinuria and progressive anaemia. Reactions such as this occur in about 1 in 500 transfusions, but are rarely fatal.

Other reactions Various other reactions occur in response to blood transfusions. Acute and delayed haemolytic reactions occur with equal frequency, but there are other rarer conditions such as transfusion-related lung injury (TRALI), post-transfusion purpura (PTP) and graft-versus-host disease (GvHD).

*   *Transfusion-related lung injury* (TRALI) is defined as acute dyspnoea with hypoxia and bilateral pulmonary infiltrates occurring during, or in the 24 hours after, transfusion. Pyrexia, rigors and hypotension are associated features. The causative agent may be either red cells or platelets. The condition is fatal in about 25 per cent of patients, and treatment requires close monitoring and intense cardiorespiratory systems support.
*   *Post-transfusion purpura* (PTP) is thrombocytopenic purpura occurring 5–12 days after transfusion of red cells, and in association with pyrexia and the presence of antibodies against the human platelet antigen (HPA) systems. It is exclusively a condition of females who have been pregnant previously. The platelet count may fall below 10×10^9 L. Treatment is by transfusion of immunoglobulin.
*   Transfusion-associated *graft-versus-host disease* (GvHD) is defined as the development of rash, fever, liver dysfunction and pancytopenia up to six weeks after a blood transfusion without any other apparent cause. The condition is rare and invariably fatal.

Despite this extensive list of hazards and complications of the transfusion of blood and its components, their use, when necessary, is safe for most patients.

AUTOLOGOUS BLOOD

In an attempt to eliminate the hazards and complications of the transfusion of homologous blood, collection and re-infusion of the patient's own blood has assumed increasing importance in the last twenty years. Because it does not have the capacity to stimulate antibody formation, it is also called 'non-allogeneic blood'. The prime advantages of autologous blood relate to the avoidance of infectious and immunological side effects of allogeneic blood. Additionally, autologous blood collected immediately before or during surgery is fresh and has none of the deleterious biochemical and coagulation changes associated with storage. Furthermore, in the UK in particular, the supply of blood from volunteer donors is in decline, increasing the importance of autologous blood transfusion (ABT).

There are three main methods for ABT:

- pre-operative autologous donation (PAD);
- acute normovolaemic haemodilution (ANH); and
- intra-operative cell salvage (IS) (Consensus Statement on Autologous Transfusion, 1996).

These techniques are not mutually exclusive and may be used in combination.

Pre-operative autologous donation (PAD)

Pre-operative autologous donation was first used in 1921 in patients undergoing brain surgery. The technique developed rapidly in the USA during the 1980s in an attempt to minimize the transmission of the hepatitis B and HIV viruses, both of which were more prevalent in paid blood donors. Despite the popularity of the technique in the USA, it is not yet widely used in the UK.

Principle   Up to four units of whole blood may be donated, one per week, in the month before an elective operation. Obviously the method is dependent on the patient being given a guaranteed date for the proposed operation, and consent, separate to that for the procedure, is required (Gillon and Thomas, 1998).

Indications and eligibility   The indications for the use of PAD are broadly all operations where the hospital blood order schedule requires two units of blood be cross-matched. It is especially applicable to major joint surgery and prostatectomy.

There are no upper or lower age limits. If used in a child or an adult less than 50 kg in weight, then a paediatric blood collection bag should be used (250 mL) so as to reduce the volume of anticoagulant. No more than 12 per cent of the CBV should be removed at a single donation session, and the haemoglobin concentration should always exceed 110 g/L prior to each donation.

Contraindications   Exclusions to PAD include the presence of known infection, patients with epilepsy because of interference with plasma drug concentration, and severe cardiovascular conditions (e.g. uncontrolled hypertension, aortic stenosis, severe angina and cyanotic heart disease).

Process   Collection and storage of blood must be to the same standard as conventional blood donation, but a separate refrigerator is used for predonated blood to minimize errors. Iron supplements are given to the patients to optimize the recovery of the blood haemoglobin concentration. Blood collected pre-operatively in the UK is grouped, and tested for infectious agents, in the usual way just in case it is used erroneously. This is a real risk. Incorrect blood transfusions comprise 50 per cent of the incidents in the Serious Hazards of Transfusion haemovigilance reports. Any unused blood collected by pre-operative donation is discarded and not returned to the pool of blood in the blood bank. It is likely, in the UK at least, that this technique will be used more frequently to minimize the impact of reduced enthusiasm in the community to donate blood.

Acute normovolaemic haemodilution (ANH)

Principle   ANH involves the removal of the patient's own blood immediately prior to surgery. It requires that the CBV is maintained by the simultaneous administration of intravenous colloid or crystalloid solutions. There is no evidence of the superiority of one of these types of solution over the other, so either may be used.

Because normovolaemia is maintained, both haematocrit and blood viscosity are reduced with potential physiological advantages. First, the reduction in haematocrit results in an increase in cardiac output and systemic oxygen transport. Second, studies in dogs have shown that there is redistribution of blood flow between different parts of the circulation. There is increased flow to the heart and brain, but a decrease in flow to the liver, intestines, spleen and kidneys. Coronary artery blood flow increases (59 per cent) in excess of stroke volume (34 per cent). This is an important consideration because cardiac output is maintained by an increase in stroke volume as haematocrit decreases towards 25 per cent, whereas at lower haematocrits, heart rate also increases.

The final physiological advantage is conservation of red cell mass and provision of fresh red cells, platelets and coagulation factors at the end of the operation. Red cell mass is conserved because the blood which is lost during surgery has a haematocrit of about 75 per cent of normal. The blood which is collected is usually transfused to the patient at the end of surgery. It is best given rapidly (within one hour or so) so that the platelets and coagulation factors may contribute to surgical haemostasis.

Process Blood is collected passively from a venous cannula into a conventional blood collection bag after induction of anaesthesia, but prior to the surgical incision. This reduces the concentration of stress hormones in the collected sample. As with PAD, the haemoglobin concentration should exceed 110 g/L for the technique to be used. There is no universal end-point for the removal of the blood, but most authorities aim for the haemoglobin to be no lower than 90–110 g/L. This usually requires the removal of two to three units of whole blood.

Indications and eligibility The indications and contraindications for ANH are similar to those for PAD. There are no age or weight limits. The technique is especially useful in major procedures such as aortic reconstruction where the need for homologous blood can be reduced to one patient in three. It may also be useful in spinal surgery in young people and breast reconstruction after mastectomy.

Despite the enthusiasm of some surgical and anaesthetic teams for using ANH, evidence in favour of the technique is equivocal (Bryson *et al.*, 1997).

Intra-operative cell salvage

Principle IS involves the collection, temporary storage, washing and concentration of red cells which are aspirated into the surgical suction device during surgery. The shed blood is thus recycled as opposed to being discarded. To be cost effective the anticipated blood loss needs to exceed 500 mL because IS requires some system of sterile disposable tubing, reservoirs and collection bags plus, with some methods, the time of a skilled technician.

Indications and eligibility Any operation where the loss will exceed 500 mL (e.g. vascular, orthopaedic or urological surgery) is suitable for IS. It can be used in combination with either or both PAD and ANH. Contraindications are the presence of infection, bowel content, amniotic fluid or malignant disease at the site of the surgery because of the risk of contaminating the collected blood.

Principal techniques The simplest method of IS is collection of wound drainage fluid in the early post-operative period and its re-infusion after filtration to remove clots and other debris. This method is mostly applicable to knee surgery where a leg tourniquet has been used intra-operatively so that all the bleeding occurs in the post-operative period. It is also suitable for use in cardiothoracic surgery where there may be significant mediastinal drainage.

Automated cell-collection systems are gaining in popularity. These involve heparinization of the blood aspirated into the suction device, filtration to remove debris, washing and centrifugation to clean and concentrate the red cells and finally storage in a reservoir prior to re-infusion. Blood obtained in this way has a haematocrit of around 55 per cent. In the authors' experience, this is an excellent technique in combination with ANH during aortic reconstructive surgery.

Problems The major disadvantages of IS are the high initial capital cost of the equipment, the cost of disposables, and the cost of the technical assistant required to supervise the machine. However, now that leukodepletion of homologous blood has been introduced in the UK, the cost of processing homologous blood has increased by a significant margin (around 60 per cent), and IS is likely to become more cost effective. In this context, it should be pointed out that in the UK there is no charge for homologous blood other than the processing and storage costs (because it is freely donated).

Other strategies for reducing blood loss

The majority of this section has been concerned with homologous and autologous blood transfusion. However, there are additional strategies which can be employed to reduce the overall blood loss during a surgical procedure.

TOPICAL HAEMOSTATS

This involves the use of surgical swabs which help to promote blood clotting. There are currently two types available

- Medistat (made from porcine collagen).
- Kaltostat (made from calcium alginate fibres).

In the former, the collagen sponges act by activating platelets at the wound site thereby initiating platelet plugging, whereas the latter activates the clotting cascade by the exchange of calcium ions in the surgical swab with sodium ions in the plasma of the leaking blood. One consequence of the use of these swabs is a reduction in operating time.

PHARMACOLOGICAL AGENTS

Two drugs have been used to preserve platelet function during surgery and promote clotting, namely 1-desamino-8-D-arginine vasopressin (desmopressin) and aprotonin.

Desmopressin

This is a vasopressin analogue which works by releasing endothelial stores of von Willebrand's factor into the circulation thereby enhancing platelet function.

Aprotonin

This is a broad-based serine protease inhibitor which inhibits enzymes such as plasmin, trypsin, kallikrein, and the serine proteases involved in the coagulation cascade. It has mostly been used to prevent bleeding during high-risk surgical procedures such as revisional cardiac surgery.

Other groups of drugs which are antifibrinolytic (lysine analogues, ϵ-aminocaproic acid and tranexamic acid) have also been used to control excessive post-operative bleeding rather than intra-operative bleeding.

SURGICAL TECHNIQUE

Finally, every anaesthetist knows that surgeons vary in the amount of blood that is lost during a particular type of operation. Hopefully, a time will come when 'dry' surgeons can teach the 'wet' ones how they do it!

HAEMOGLOBIN SUBSTITUTES

Normal oxygen transport depends on respiratory function and an adequate circulation. Defects in any one component may result in tissue hypoxia and death. Complications of homologous transfusion, in particular viral transmission of HIV and hepatitis,

and increasing demands for stored blood have led to a rapid expansion in the search for an oxygen-carrying substitute (Tobias and Longnecker, 1995). Those that have already been developed can be grouped into either modified haemoglobin solutions (MHbs) or perfluorocarbon emulsions (PFCEs).

The saturation of haemoglobin (Hb) with oxygen depends on the partial pressure of oxygen available. Each Hb molecule weighing around 64 500 Da, comprises four monomers: two alpha (α) and two beta (β) subunits. The allosteric properties of these four monomers and the concentration of 2,3-DPG in each red blood cell result in a non-linear relationship between P_{O_2} and Hb saturation. MHbs and PFCEs cannot be regarded as blood substitutes because they have neither the encapsulated oxygen carrying capacity nor the regulatory, metabolic or host defence functions of blood. They are therefore only temporary compounds with limited clinical application.

An ideal Hb substitute would have the following properties:

- High oxygen-carrying capacity.
- Good oxygen delivery to the tissues.
- A similar P_{50} (partial pressure at which it is 50 per cent saturated) to Hb (3.6 kPa).
- Not react with oxygen or catalyse reactions between oxygen and other compounds.
- An adequate half-life.
- Similar viscosity, oncotic and osmotic pressure and rheological properties to blood.
- Be stable during sterilization and storage.
- Easy to obtain in large quantities and cost effective.

Modified Hb solutions and perfluorocarbon emulsions

MODIFIED Hb SOLUTIONS

When outside the erythrocyte, in the absence of 2,3-DPG, the affinity of Hb for oxygen is high and the ability to deliver oxygen to the tissues is lost (Lamy *et al.*, 1996). This leads to rapid formation of methaemoglobin. Free Hb also quickly dissociates into $\alpha\beta$ dimers which are cleared by the reticuloendothelial system and renal filtration, but when present in excess they can cause nephrotoxicity. In the extracellular compartment, free Hb can form free radicals. For these reasons MHb solutions have been prepared either from highly purified natural human or bovine Hb obtained by lysis of red blood cells and then modified, or genetically engineered by introducing normal or modified Hb genes into bacteria, yeasts or transgenic animals.

Modification of such natural Hb involves three processes:

1. Cross-linking internally between α or β dimers, or externally with a macromolecule. This process stabilizes the molecule, increases its half-life and oxygen delivery to the tissues, although it does not entirely block urinary excretion. Successful cross-linking to hydroxyethyl starch, polyethyleneglycol and Dextran 20 have been reported with half-lives of 2.5 days and a P_{50} of 2.2 kPa.
2. Polymerization, e.g. with glutaraldehyde or cyanates, can reduce renal elimination and oncotic pressure. Control of the degree of polymerization is a problem which results in a range of molecular weights being produced. Phase I clinical trials have been carried out with good tolerance to small doses.
3. Microencapsulation in liposomes made of cholesterol and natural lecithins or synthetic phospholipids rich in saturated fatty acids produces an artificial Hb with a high affinity for oxygen (P_{50} = 2.2 kPa), is stable during storage and has an acceptable half-life (up to 20 hours) without renal toxicity or antigenicity. However, massive trapping in the reticuloendothelial system leads to hepatic and splenic engorgement and may suppress immune function.

Side effects of modified MHb solutions include:

• Vasospasm, perhaps as a result of binding to nitric oxide (NO) preventing NO-mediated vascular relaxation.
• Nephrotoxicity.
• Reduction in macrophage phagocytosis for substances other than MHb.
• Antigenicity.
• Oxidation on storage.
• Activation of complement, kinin and coagulation.
• Histamine release.
• Iron deposition.

The production of large quantities of recombinant Hb remains expensive and there is a significant risk of endotoxin contamination. The use of human Hb for modification is not currently feasible as blood donors are in short supply. If bigger transgenic animals could be induced to produce genetically engineered human Hb variants, a large-scale source of optimized human Hb would be available (Jones, 1995).

PERFLUOROCARBON EMULSIONS (PFCEs)

PFCEs are a group of chemically stable and essentially inert compounds derived from hydrocarbons in which much of the hydrogen has been replaced with fluorine. The amount of oxygen and carbon dioxide which they carry is proportional to the surrounding partial pressure. These compounds transport and deliver oxygen by solubilization and not by binding to a carrier molecule. Linear molecules are better oxygen carriers than cyclic ones: they are virtually chemically and biochemically inert, are not metabolized (and therefore do not produce toxic degradation products), and are rapidly excreted by exhalation. They are administered intravascularly as an emulsion. Biocompatibility problems from surfactants used to stabilize the emulsion still exist (Lamy et al., 1996).

Various PFCs are being tested clinically for use as oxygen-carrier solutions (see Spence, 1995), and two blood-substitute products are in FDA-approved Phase III clinical trials (Winslow, 1997).

Potential clinical applications

RESUSCITATION AFTER BLOOD LOSS

Oxygen-carrying solutions are ideal for volume replacement and oxygen delivery with the advantage of a reduced blood viscosity. Instant availability without the need for cross-matching is an attractive alternative to banked blood (Jones, 1995). MHb solutions have been widely tested in animal models with excellent results but only cause short-term restoration of oxygen partial pressure, and more importantly can lead to significant vasoconstriction increasing mean arterial pressure for several hours. The first-generation PFCE, Fluosol® (Green Cross Corporation, Osaka, Japan) has been given to animal subjects and humans in surgical procedures, military situations and to members of

Jehovah's Witness. It contains a synthetic polymer as an emulsifying agent which caused anaphylactoid reactions amongst other side effects. Newer second-generation PFCEs contain egg-yolk phospholipids which have been used for many years in lipid emulsions for parenteral nutrition. Oxygent® (Alliance Pharmaceutical Corporation, San Diego, USA) contains the linear perfluorocarbon molecule perflubron, and has completed Phase I trials in normal healthy volunteers. Results of Phase II trials in patients with acute haemorrhage as a result of surgery are awaited. Because both MHb solutions and PFCEs are selectively taken up by the reticuloendothelial system, and large volumes may be required, there are several problems to be overcome before treatment with these agents is possible.

PERI-OPERATIVE HAEMODILUTION

Avoiding the side effects of homologous blood transfusion has become increasingly important. Autologous blood donation, acute pre-operative normovolaemic haemodilution and acceptance of lower haematocrits are possibilities, but MHb solutions and PFCEs are promising alternatives. Animal studies have been encouraging but adequate clinical trials are now essential.

OTHER USES

- Reperfusion after acute embolic or haemorrhagic stroke.
- Treatment of chronic anaemia.
- Prevention of myocardial ischaemia during coronary angioplasty.
- Reperfusion of the acutely ischaemic myocardium or limb.
- Preservation of organ and limb viability for transplantation and re-implantation.
- Liquid ventilation (PFCEs only).
- Intraluminal oxygenation of the gut (PFCEs only).
- Radiological imaging, in particular MRI and spectroscopy (Sakas et al., 1996).
- Improvement of tumour oxygenation and therefore susceptibility to radiation and chemotherapy.
- Decompression sickness and air embolism.
- Respiratory distress in pre-term infants (Biro, 1993).

REFERENCES

Biro, G.P. 1993 Perfluorocarbon-based red blood cell substitutes. *Transfusion Medicine Reviews* **VII** (2), 84–95.

Bryson, G.L., Laupacis, A. and Wells, G.A. 1998. Does acute normovolaemic hemodilution reduce perioperative allogeneic transfusion? A meta-analysis. *Anesthesia and Analgesia* **86**, 9–15.

Consensus Statement on Autologous Transfusion 1996. Proceedings on a Consensus Conference held at the Royal College of Physicians of Edinburgh, 4–6 October 1995. *British Journal of Anaesthesia* **76**, 470.

Contreras, M. and Mollinson, P.L. 1998. Testing before transfusion and blood ordering policies. In Contreras M (ed.), *ABC of transfusion*, 3rd edn. London: BMJ Books, 6–9.

Dahlback, B., Carlsson, M. and Svenson, P.J. 1993. Familial thrombophilia due to a previously unrecognised mechanism characterised by poor anticoagulant response to activated protein C. *Proceedings of the National Academy of Sciences (USA)* **90**, 1004–1008.

Fischbach, D.P. and Fogdall, R.P. 1981. *Coagulation: the essentials*. Baltimore: Williams & Wilkins.

Furie, B.C. 1992. Molecular and cellular biology of blood coagulation. *New England Journal of Medicine* **326**, 800–806.

Gillon, J. and Thomas, D.W. 1998. Autologous transfusion. In Contreras M (ed.), *ABC of transfusion*, 3rd edn. London: BMJ Books, 17–22.

Gordon-Smith, E.C. 1995. Haemostasis, haemoglobinopathies and anaesthesia. In Healy, T.E.J. and Cohen, P.J. (eds), *Wylie and Churchill-Davidson's A Practice of Anaesthesia,* Chapter 20, 6th edn. London: Edward Arnold.

Jick, H., Jick, S.S., Gurewich, V. *et al.* 1995. Risk of Idiopathic cardiovascular death and nonfatal venous thromboembolism in women using oral contraceptives with differing progestagen components. *Lancet* **346**,1589–1593.

Jones, J.A. 1995. Red cell substitutes: current status. *British Journal of Anaesthesia* **74**, 697–703.

Lamy, M., Remy, B. and Deby-Dupont, G. 1996. Modified haemoglobins and perfluorocarbons as oxygen-carrying solutions: characteristics and possible applications. *Bloodless Surgery International Symposium Paris.*

National Institutes of Health Consensus Development Conference 1989. Perioperative Red Cell Transfusion *Transfusion Medicine* **3**(I), 63–68.

Petrovitch, C.T. 1990. The bleeding patient. In Roizen MF (ed.), *Anesthesia for vascular surgery,* Chapter 4. New York: Churchill Livingstone.

Rhodes, E.G.H. 1996. Thrombophilia and the surgeon. *Annals of the Royal College of Surgeons of England* **78**, 331–335.

Rosenfeld, B.A., Beattie, C., Christopherson, R. *et al.* The Perioperative Ischemia Randomised Anesthesia Trial Study Group. 1993. The effect of different anesthetic regimens on fibrinolysis and the development of postoperative arterial thrombosis. *Anesthesiology* **79**, 435–443.

Sakas, D.E., Whittaker, K.W., Crowell, R.M. and Zervas, N.T. 1996. Perfluorocarbons: recent developments and implications for neurosurgery. *Journal of Neurosurgery* **85**, 248–254.

Schafer, A.I. 1985. The hypercoagulable states. *Annals of Internal Medicine* **102**, 814–828.

Serious Hazards of Transfusion (SHOT) Annual Report 1996–1997. SHOT Office, Manchester Blood Centre, Manchester.

Serious Hazards of Transfusion (SHOT) Annual Report 1997–1998. SHOT Office, Manchester Blood Centre, Manchester.

Spence, R.K. 1995. Perfluorocarbons in the 21st century: clinical applications as transfusion alternatives. *Artificial Cells, Blood Substitutes and Immobilisation Biotechnology* **23**(3), 367–380.

Spitzer, W.O., Lewis, M.A., Heineman, L.A.J. *et al.* on behalf of Transnational Research Group on Oral Contraceptives and the Health of Young Women. 1996. Third generation oral contraceptives and risk of venous thromboembolic disorders: an international case-control study. *British Medical Journal* **312**, 83–88.

Steele, S.M., Slaughter, T.F., Greenberg, C.S. and Reves, J.G. 1991. Epidural anaesthesia and analgesia: implications for perioperative coagulability. *Anesthesia and Analgesia* **73**, 683–685.

Tobias, M.D. and Longnecker, D.E. 1995. Recombinant haemoglobin and other blood substitutes. In Frink, E.J. and Brown, E.R. (eds), *Ballière's Clinical Anaesthesiology* **9**, 165–179. London: W.B. Saunders.

Troianos, C.A. and Ellison, N. 1991. Hematologic considerations in vascular surgery. In Kaplan, J.A. (ed.), *Vascular anesthesia,* Chapter 19. New York: Churchill Livingstone.

Trousseau, A. 1865. Phlegmasia alba dolens. *Clin Med Hotel Dieu de Paris* **3**, 94.

Tuman, K.J., McCarthy, R.J., Narch, R.J. *et al.* 1991. Effects of epidural anesthesia and analgesia on coagulation and outcome after major vascular surgery. *Anesthesia and Analgesia* **73**, 696–704.

Weiss, H.J. 1995. Flow-related platelet deposition on subendothelium. *Thrombosis and Haemostasis* **74** (1), 117–122.

Winslow, R.M. (1997) Progress on blood substitutes (letter). *Nature Medicine* **3**, 474.

14

Anaesthesia for carotid artery disease

LESLEY A DUNCAN

INTRODUCTION

The carotid artery may be affected by a number of disease processes, the commonest being atherosclerosis causing stenosis of the internal branch at its origin. Less commonly, aneurysmal dilatation of the extracranial portion of the carotid artery may occur and lead to symptoms due to embolization. Tumours of the carotid body can also present to vascular surgeons as pulsatile masses and require excision. This chapter will discuss anaesthesia for those patients undergoing carotid artery surgery with particular emphasis on those with occlusive disease.

CAROTID ENDARTERECTOMY

In certain circumstances, carotid endarterectomy (CEA) has been shown to be the treatment of choice for the prevention of ischaemic strokes due to ipsilateral stenosis. Both the European Carotid Surgery Trial (ECST, 1991) and the North American Symptomatic Carotid Endarterectomy Trial (NASCET, 1991) have shown that with severe (70–99 per cent) carotid stenosis and recent symptoms, the likelihood of ipsilateral disabling stroke and death is lower in patients receiving both CEA and medical treatment than in those given medical

treatment alone. The Asymptomatic Carotid Atherosclerosis Study (ACAS, 1995) has also shown a benefit for medical risk management and surgery in those with asymptomatic carotid stenoses of 60 per cent or greater, although the benefit appears to be less for females than males.

Because CEA is a prophylactic procedure, any benefit from surgery will be negated if there is high incidence of peri-operative complications related to patient, surgical or anaesthetic factors. For this reason, it has been suggested that CEA should be performed in a limited number of centres by surgeons and anaesthetists with a special interest in the procedure (Brown and Humphrey, 1992). It has also been recommended that units performing CEA have their results independently audited to ensure they maintain a low complication rate (AHA Ad Hoc Committee, 1995).

The anaesthetist has a major role to play in the management of patients undergoing CEA. As well as ensuring that the patient is pain free and that the surgeon has a satisfactory operative field, the anaesthetist must aim to minimize peri-operative cerebral and myocardial ischaemia. It is important to understand the risks of the procedure, the physiological changes that occur during surgery and the benefits and limitations of available techniques for monitoring cerebral function and providing cerebral protection.

Morbidity and mortality

The major cause of peri-operative morbidity after carotid surgery is cerebral ischaemic damage, while the commonest cause of both early and late mortality is myocardial infarction.

The incidence of peri-operative neurological morbidity is variable, with lower rates following surgery for asymptomatic lesions than for transient ischaemic attacks (TIA), or in those with residual deficits following stroke (Ruckley and Wildsmith, 1992, AHA Ad Hoc Committee, 1995). Sundt *et al.* (1975) attempted to devise a grading system to predict the likelihood of peri-operative cerebral and myocardial complications based on medical, angiographic and neurological risk factors. Patients who were healthy apart from symptomatic carotid artery disease had only a 1–2 per cent risk of significant peri-operative morbidity. However those with unstable neurological symptoms prior to surgery had a 10 per cent risk of morbidity, mainly in the form of stroke. In a recent meta-analysis, Rothwell *et al.* (1997) found an increased risk of operative stroke or death in women, and in patients of either sex with systolic hypertension or other peripheral vascular disease.

A number of factors have been implicated in the development of neurological deficits after carotid surgery. Steed *et al.* (1982) studied the aetiology of stroke and TIA after CEA performed under regional anaesthesia and found the majority of deficits were related to thromboembolic episodes, reperfusion phenomena or hypotension. In only one case could the deficit be attributed to cerebral ischaemia during the period of carotid cross-clamping. Towne and Bernhard (1980) showed an increased incidence of neurological deficit and mortality in patients who developed post-operative hypertension, and noted that this was most likely to occur in those who were hypertensive pre-operatively even if the blood pressure appeared to have been adequately treated. These findings, confirmed by Asiddao *et al.* (1982), illustrate the importance of ensuring hypertension is optimally treated prior to carotid surgery.

Most peri-operative strokes appear to be caused by thromboembolic rather than haemodynamic factors, and their incidence may be reduced by meticulous surgical technique (Wong, 1991). It has been suggested that acceptable rates of combined morbidity and mortality for this procedure are 3 per cent for asymptomatic patients, 5 per cent for those with transient ischaemic attacks and 7 per cent for those with previous stroke (Callow *et al.*, 1988). In many recent studies much lower complication rates have been recorded with peri-operative mortality less than 2 per cent and stroke rates of less than 4 per cent (Bernstein *et al.*, 1982; Ombrellaro *et al.*, 1996).

Myocardial ischaemia is the most important cause of both early and late mortality after CEA (Hertzer and Lees, 1981). In the series of Riles *et al.* (1979), the incidence of myocardial infarction after CEA was 14.9 per cent in those with a history of heart disease, but only 0.5 per cent in those with no previous cardiac history. The patients who died as a result of their infarcts were all in the group known to have heart disease pre-operatively. Hypertension did not appear to be a risk factor for the development of myocardial infarction except in the presence of heart disease. During this study, patients with ischaemic heart disease who required vasopressors during carotid cross-clamping to maintain blood pressure had an increased incidence of myocardial infarction (MI) compared with those with no history of heart disease who received vasopressors. Similar results regarding the use of vasopressors and an association with intra-operative myocardial ischaemia during CEA were also obtained by Smith *et al.* (1988), leading to the suggestion that these agents should be used with extreme caution especially in those with pre-existing heart disease.

Ombrellaro *et al.* (1996) compared the incidence of myocardial morbidity after CEA in patients receiving general or regional anaesthesia. Fourteen per cent of patients experienced an adverse cardiac event (angina, dysrhythmia, heart failure, MI). The overall incidence of MI was 1.5 per cent with no difference between the groups. A history of pre-operative heart disease was a significant predictor of an adverse cardiac outcome in this group.

The risks associated with CEA demonstrate the need for careful pre-operative assessment of the patient with cerebrovascular disease.

Pre-operative assessment

Assessment of the patient prior to vascular surgery is discussed in more detail elsewhere. Patients presenting for CEA, in common with other patients with vascular disease, tend to be elderly and frequently have coexisting medical problems. It is clear that particular attention should be paid to hypertension and ischaemic heart disease because of the increased incidence of peri-operative MI and neurological deficit.

Vascular patients frequently have a long history of smoking with associated chronic pulmonary disease and many suffer from diabetes mellitus. All medical problems should be optimally treated prior to surgery. Often these patients are on a variety of medications which in general should be continued up to and including the day of surgery. This is especially true for anti-anginal and antihypertensive therapies because rebound exacerbation of symptoms may occur if they are withdrawn suddenly. Patients on anticoagulants such as warfarin should have them discontinued about one week prior to surgery to enable clotting to normalize. If necessary intravenous heparin can be substituted until the morning of surgery. Some authors recommend that aspirin should also be withheld for up to a week before surgery (Moss, 1994) although others have shown a reduction in stroke rate with aspirin given peri-operatively (Edwards et al., 1984).

Premedication depends on the individual anaesthetist and patient. Pre-operative anxiety is associated with hypertension, tachycardia and increased myocardial oxygen consumption, all of which may be deleterious in this patient population. However, it is equally important to avoid oversedation with resultant hypotension, hypercapnia and detrimental effects on the cerebral circulation. If time is taken to establish a good rapport with the patient pharmacological anxiolysis may not be necessary, but some patients may benefit from light premedication, usually with a benzodiazepine.

Selection of anaesthetic technique

A variety of techniques have been used to provide anaesthesia for patients undergoing CEA. General anaesthesia and regional techniques each have their advocates, but at present there is no clear evidence that one technique is superior in reducing peri-operative complications (Tangkanakul et al., Cochrane Database, 1996).

REGIONAL ANAESTHESIA

Proponents of regional anaesthesia for CEA claim the ability to test for neurological complications throughout the period of carotid occlusion, coupled with a low incidence of myocardial complications, makes this the anaesthetic method of choice. Surgery can be performed under superficial and deep cervical plexus block, cervical extradural or local infiltration by the surgeon (Stoneham and Knighton, 1999).

Superficial and deep cervical plexus block for CEA has been associated with a high degree of patient satisfaction (Davies et al., 1990) and a low complication rate despite 55 per cent of patients developing tachycardia and 67 per cent hypertension. It can be expected that over a third of patients will require supplementation of the plexus blocks by the surgeon due to discomfort.

CEA may also be performed under cervical extradural block at either C6/7 or C7/T1. Bonnet et al. (1990) administered 15 mL of bupivacaine 0.37–0.5 per cent with or without the addition of fentanyl 50–100 µg. Most patients required additional sedation or intravenous analgesia during the procedure although patient satisfaction was reasonable (46 per cent). There were few complications in this series, but three patients with known respiratory disease required positive pressure ventilation due to progressive respiratory embarrassment. Hypotension affected only 10.9 per cent of patients and bradycardia 2.8 per cent.

A further advantage claimed for regional anaesthetic techniques is a reduction in costs due to shorter stays in intensive care and hospital. This reflects practice in the United States, not the United Kingdom, where few patients receive intensive care after carotid surgery. More detailed consideration of techniques of regional anaesthesia for carotid endarterectomy has been presented in Chapter 9.

GENERAL ANAESTHESIA

The use of a general anaesthetic technique for CEA allows the anaesthetist to control certain physiological variables which in turn may be used to improve cerebral blood flow (CBF), e.g. $PaCO_2$, PaO_2 and blood pressure (BP). Anaesthetic agents also affect CBF and cerebral metabolic rate for oxygen ($CMRO_2$), offering a potential mechanism by which to improve the brain's tolerance to ischaemia. If signs of ischaemia develop during anaesthesia, active physiological and pharmacological measures can be taken to minimize the risks.

The choice of specific anaesthetic agents is probably less important than ensuring peri-operative haemodynamic stability in order to optimize myocardial and cerebral blood flow.

Induction

Induction of anaesthesia is usually achieved with thiopentone, etomidate or propofol, all of which produce a dose-dependent reduction in $CMRo_2$. A non-depolarizing muscle relaxant is likely to be administered to facilitate endotracheal intubation and the sympathetic response to laryngoscopy may be obtunded by the use of an intravenous bolus of lignocaine, short-acting opioid or esmolol (Cucchiara *et al.*, 1990).

Maintenance

Although clinical evidence that general anaesthesia improves outcome after cerebral ischaemia is weak, some studies from the 1970s suggest that isoflurane may offer cerebral protection during periods of transient, incomplete ischaemia as seen during CEA. Messick *et al.* (1987) showed that critical CBF (below which signs of cerebral ischaemia were seen on electroencephalography) was 10 mL/100 g/min with isoflurane compared to 20 mL/100 g/min for halothane. In addition, fewer ischaemic electroencephalographic changes were seen with isoflurane than during halothane or enflurane anaesthesia (Michenfelder *et al.*, 1987) leading to suggestions that the brain is more tolerant to ischaemia during isoflurane anaesthesia. There are concerns that the use of isoflurane may adversely affect myocardial blood flow by producing 'coronary steal' in those patients with coronary artery disease, which includes many patients with carotid disease. However, Smith *et al.* (1988) observed fewer episodes of myocardial ischaemia in patients undergoing CEA with isoflurane compared to halothane. Thus there may be an advantage in the use of isoflurane in either air/oxygen or nitrous oxide/oxygen for maintenance of anaesthesia during CEA.

Propofol may be administered by infusion for maintenance of anaesthesia and will cause reduction of CBF and $CMRo_2$. Care is required because its effects on systemic vascular resistance may lead to a fall in cerebral perfusion pressure. Propofol may also have a further cerebral protective effect because it has been shown to possess free-radical scavenging activity (Murphy *et al.*, 1992). A further advantage of this technique is quick, clear-headed recovery allowing rapid neurological assessment.

Analgesia during surgery may be provided by short-acting opioids such as fentanyl, alfentanil or remifentanil as well as with superficial cervical plexus block. At the end of surgery, muscle relaxation should be reversed and anaesthesia discontinued to allow rapid, smooth and clear-headed awakening.

The anaesthetist must be prepared for the circulatory instability which can occur frequently during CEA. Carotid sinus baroreceptors lie in the bifurcation of the common carotid artery and respond to stretching of the vessel wall. Activity in these receptors is transmitted via the carotid sinus nerve to the vasomotor centre within the medulla oblongata, leading to a reduction in sympathetic tone and a decrease in heart rate and blood pressure. The opposite effect is seen when the baroreceptors are exposed to lower than normal pressures, leading to reduced activity and increased sympathetic tone. This can result in marked arterial hypertension at the time of carotid cross-clamping. After removal of the vascular clamps, blood pressure may decrease as the increased distensibility and diameter of the endarterectomized vessel lead to increased baroreceptor activity, reduced sympathetic tone and parasympathetic activation. Both hyper- and hypotension may be seen in the post-operative period. It has been postulated that hypertension may be related to damage to the carotid sinus nerves during surgery and that it is usually short-lived (Bove *et al.*, 1979). Post-operative hypotension is likely to be the result of abnormal activity in the carotid sinus nerve in response to increased diameter and distension of the carotid artery due to removal of plaque (Angell-James and Lumley, 1974). This effect may be attenuated by injection of local anaesthetic into the carotid sinus region thus temporarily blocking the sinus nerves (Pine *et al.*, 1983). However, blood pressure may remain labile due to loss of normal autoregulation.

Intra-operative monitoring

During CEA, the anaesthetist should aim to provide a pain-free, stable patient for the surgeon. With the use of appropriate monitoring equipment and its proper interpretation, the anaesthetist should help to minimize the risks of cerebral and myocardial ischaemia during the procedure.

Routine monitoring for CEA should include pulse oximetry and in the patient receiving general anaesthesia, capnography. This enables oxygenation to be optimized and normocarbia maintained. Continuous electrocardiographic (ECG) monitoring should also be employed, and on-line ST-segment analysis may be beneficial. Landesberg *et al.* (1993) have shown that the occurrence of ST-segment depression during carotid clamping, or soon after clamp removal, correlates well with the development of cardiac complications. Blood pressure should be measured using an indwelling arterial catheter, because changes occur suddenly and have to be dealt with quickly.

In addition to these routine monitors, a number of techniques can be employed to assess the adequacy of cerebral perfusion during anaesthesia and surgery. Even so, the only completely reliable way of ensuring continued adequate cerebral perfusion is with the patient fully conscious.

MONITORING CEREBRAL PERFUSION

Neurological deficits occurring peri-operatively have multiple aetiologies. The majority are related to embolic or thrombotic episodes and their incidence may be decreased by meticulous surgical technique (Naylor *et al.*, 1992). A significant number are haemodynamic in origin, related mainly to reduced cerebral perfusion after carotid cross-clamping, but also to problems with intra-arterial shunts.

Neurological monitoring of the awake patient

A number of centres carry out CEA under regional anaesthesia, usually combined superficial and deep cervical plexus block or cervical extradural blockade. During a test period of carotid clamping, the patient is assessed continuously for contralateral motor power, change in mental status and any speech abnormalities. Symptoms usually arise within 2 min although testing after this initial period is necessary because late symptoms can occur (Davies *et al.*, 1990). This technique may be useful in detecting ischaemia in patients with residual neurological deficits because new abnormalities may be difficult to interpret against a background of pre-existing ones (Rosenthal *et al.*, 1981).

Electroencephalograph and evoked potential monitoring.

The electroencephalograph (EEG) monitors activity on the surface of the cerebral cortex, the waveforms being the summation of post-synaptic potentials (both excitatory and inhibitory) arriving there. The

EEG is useful as a detector of cerebral ischaemia. Around 60 per cent of total brain oxygen consumption is used to generate the potentials responsible for EEG waveforms while 40 per cent is used to maintain cellular integrity (Jenkinson, 1994). As oxygen supply to the brain falls, EEG activity is depressed as energy is diverted to the maintenance of cellular integrity. As a result the EEG is altered before irreversible brain damage occurs. Cerebral blood flow is normally 50 mL/100 g/min and can decrease to 20 mL/100 g/min in the anaesthetized patient before EEG changes are seen. During anaesthesia, cerebral blood flow may decrease to as little as 10 mL/100 g/min before irreversible brain damage occurs. Thus there is a window of safety when the EEG alerts to reduced cerebral perfusion before permanent damage results.

The EEG has been used to predict the likelihood of cerebral ischaemia during CEA leading to post-operative neurological deficits (Rampil *et al.*, 1983). Ischaemic changes on the EEG lasting more than 10 min correlated with the occurrence of new deficits post-operatively. However, other studies have questioned the predictive value of the EEG. Many patients who develop changes indicative of ischaemia do not awake with deficits while some who show no evidence of ischaemic change do so (Green *et al.*, 1985). If EEG change is used as a criterion to insert an arterial shunt, many patients will be shunted unnecessarily and exposed to an increased risk of stroke due to technical problems. Morawetz *et al.* (1984) showed that EEG changes correlated with reductions in cerebral blood flow, but neither predicted the likelihood of post-operative neurological deficit.

Apart from false-positives and -negatives, other problems exist with the EEG as a predictor of cerebral ischaemia. It detects activity in the superficial layers of the cerebral cortex and may be normal in the presence of significant ischaemia in the deeper cortex and internal capsule (Green *et al.*, 1985). In patients with previous stroke, EEG abnormalities are likely to pre-exist and further changes may be difficult to interpret (Rosenthal *et al.*, 1981). The EEG waveform is itself influenced by anaesthetic agents, arterial P_{CO_2} and blood pressure, all of which should be kept stable during surgery. Interpretation of the EEG is difficult, requiring an experienced technician because most anaesthetists are not skilled in the technique. This has led to the development of monitors which process the raw EEG data and present it in a more easily understood form.

Somatosensory-evoked potentials (SSEP) monitor deeper sensory or motor pathways in brain or spinal cord. Recording electrodes placed over the sensory cortex pick up the EEG responses to sensory stimuli. The EEG is subtracted from the sensory-evoked response to leave a series of waves, the amplitude and latency of which reflect transmission of a stimulus (usually to the median nerve), centrally. As cerebral blood flow decreases to 20 mL/100 g/min, the amplitude of the waves decreases and the latencies increase, indicating reduced oxygen supply before critical levels are reached (Jenkinson, 1994). Measurement of SSEP during CEA has been found to reduce the use of arterial shunts when compared with measurement of internal carotid artery stump pressure (Markand et al., 1984). Lam et al. (1991) found SSEPs to be as useful a monitor as EEG during CEA and showed better predictive value from a reduction in waveform amplitude than from an increased latency. However, like the EEG, evoked potentials are affected by anaesthetic technique and blood pressure and also reflect integrity in only a small part of the central nervous system.

Cerebral blood flow

This can be measured intermittently during CEA using an injection of xenon-133 into the carotid artery before and after occlusion. A scintillation detector is placed over the scalp and from its reading cerebral blood flow is calculated. However the method gives only intermittent information and may not correlate with neurological outcome (Morawetz et al., 1984) or other methods of detecting cerebral ischaemia (Halsey et al., 1989). It has been shown that during CEA, cerebral blood flow of less than 18 mL/100 g/min measured using this technique is associated with EEG changes indicating ischaemia (Sundt et al., 1974).

Jugular venous oxygen saturation

It is possible to continuously measure jugular venous oxygen saturation (S_jO_2) using fibreoptic probes (Andrews et al., 1991). A fall in ipsilateral S_jO_2 may reflect global cerebral ischaemia although it may not be sensitive to regional ischaemia. The technique is, however, invasive and its place during CEA is not yet known.

Internal carotid artery stump pressure and backflow

Moore and Hall (1969) suggested that the pressure in the internal carotid artery distal to the arterial clamps would reflect the adequacy of the collateral circulation from the contralateral carotid artery and the vertebrobasilar system. After noticing that tolerance of carotid clamping was associated with brisk backbleeding from the internal carotid artery (ICA), they went on to measure the pressure in the ICA distal to the arterial clamps. They suggested a safe level of stump pressure of 25 mmHg above which patients would tolerate arterial clamping. Subsequently other studies have suggested different safe levels of stump pressure ranging from 25 to 70 mmHg. Although easy to carry out, assessment of backbleeding and stump pressure are single measurements and will not reflect changes in perfusion occurring throughout the period when the artery is clamped.

Kwaan et al. (1980) found great variability in the level of stump pressure associated with evidence of ischaemia in awake-patient testing, with many patients with pressures above 50 mmHg developing signs of reduced cerebral perfusion. There is a poor correlation between stump pressure and other techniques used to assess adequacy of cerebral perfusion including EEG and regional cerebral blood flow measurements (Mckay et al., 1976). Stump pressure is also affected by anaesthetic technique, systemic blood pressure and arterial P_{CO_2}. A high stump pressure may exist in the presence of inadequate cerebral blood flow if cerebrovascular resistance is high. If stump pressure is used as the sole criterion on which to base the decision of shunt insertion, then a number of patients will be shunted unnecessarily (McKay et al., 1976).

Transcranial Doppler monitoring

Velocity of blood flow in the middle cerebral artery can be measured by directing a low-frequency ultrasound beam through the relatively thin temporal bone (Aaslid et al., 1982). Positioning of the probe is critical and may not be possible in all patients. With the use of fixed-head probes it is possible to continuously monitor blood flow velocities during CEA. The transcranial Doppler (TCD) is able to predict reliably the changes in blood flow velocity which occur during CEA at the time of carotid clamping, shunt insertion and removal (Paydachee et al., 1986). As a continuous monitor of blood flow velocity, the TCD may produce valuable information during the period of carotid clamping and indicate problems with the arterial shunt (Naylor et al., 1991). However, velocity of blood flow does not necessarily equate with actual blood flow and Halsey et al. (1989) were only able to show a weak relationship between velocity of flow in the middle cerebral artery and regional cerebral blood flow, at blood flow <20 mL/100 g/min. The TCD is also useful for revealing potentially dangerous embolic events related to manipulation of the carotid artery and to shunt insertion (Naylor *et al.*, 1991). It may also have a role post-operatively in the differentiation of neurological deficits. If there is good flow velocity in the middle cerebral artery, it makes it unlikely that any deficit is the result of thrombosis at the operative site. A future role for transcranial Doppler monitoring may be the prediction of those patients at risk of developing thrombosis in the ICA post-operatively (Lennard *et al.*, 1997).

Cerebral oximetry

The cerebral oximeter uses principles of near-infrared spectroscopy similar to those used in peripheral pulse oximetry. However, the cerebral oximeter is unable to distinguish arterial haemoglobin oxygen saturation, measuring instead oxygen saturation in the total tissue bed, including capillaries, arteries and veins. Cerebral oximetry was first described in the early 1970s and was initially used to measure cerebral oxygen saturation in premature neonates (Jobsis, 1971). Modifications to the early equipment enabled use in adults to provide a continuous, non-invasive monitor of cerebral oxygen saturation (McCormick *et al.*, 1991).

The device consists of an adhesive sensor which incorporates a light source transmitting two different infrared wavelengths and two photodetectors. Light reflected from the tissues is scattered in parabolic curves and the detectors are positioned in order to be able to differentiate light received from superficial and deeper structures. A computer in the oximeter is then able to give a value for intracerebral oxygen saturation and this is displayed, numerically and as a continuous trace.

A number of investigators have evaluated cerebral oximetry during CEA, and compared this monitor with other methods of assessing adequacy of cerebral perfusion. Mason *et al.* (1994) found the oximeter responded appropriately to changes in cerebral perfusion related to arterial clamping and that this correlated closely with similar changes in middle cerebral artery velocity measured by TCD. In a different study comparing stump pressure, TCD and cerebral oximetry, Williams *et al.* (1994) showed that a fall in cerebral oxygen saturation of 5 per cent or more was associated with a decrease in middle cerebral artery velocity of at least 60 per cent, but there was no correlation with stump pressure. They suggested that using TCD in conjunction with cerebral oximetry may lead to a reduction in the number of patients having unnecessary shunt insertion during endarterectomy.

Changes in cerebral oxygen saturation at the time of application of arterial clamps have also been shown to correlate well with surgical assessment of backbleeding from the internal carotid artery, but not other methods of assessing cerebral perfusion (Duncan *et al.*, 1995). Samra *et al.* (1996) studied changes in cerebral oxygen saturation during carotid cross-clamping in awake patients undergoing endarterectomy. They found that the oximeter reliably responded to a reduction in oxygenation related to cross-clamping, but were unable to identify a critical level of cerebral oxygen saturation related to neurological dysfunction.

In summary, the cerebral oximeter appears to be a reliable indicator of cerebral oxygen saturation. However, wide variation is seen between patients in the absolute value of cerebral oxygen saturation and a critical level of saturation above which an arterial shunt would not be required cannot as yet be predicted. The cerebral oximeter may be useful in individual patients for demonstrating reduced saturation due to systemic hypotension or problems with arterial shunts (Duncan *et al.*, 1995).

Cerebral protection

THE PATHOPHYSIOLOGY OF CEREBRAL ISCHAEMIA

The events which precede neuronal cell death due to ischaemia have been elucidated (Toner and Stamford, 1996). Within a few minutes of the onset of ischaemia stores of adenosine triphosphate (ATP) are rapidly depleted. This results in failure of a number of homeostatic mechanisms, the most important of which is the sodium–potassium–ATPase pump, responsible for maintaining the extracellular–intracellular balance of sodium and potassium. There is an influx of sodium and chloride ions with water, and an efflux of potassium ions, ultimately leading to cellular oedema and depolarization. Depolarization is responsible for increasing the extracellular concentration of excitatory neurotransmitters, e.g. glutamate, and activation of voltage sensitive ion channels including the N-methyl-D-aspartate (NMDA) receptors. The NMDA receptors are linked to calcium ion channels and when activated allow influx of calcium. Elevation of the intracellular concentration of calcium in turn results in activation of a variety of enzyme systems, including phospholipases, which hydrolyse membrane phospholipids with accumulation of free fatty acids and arachidonic acid. These substances can be further converted to prostaglandins, leukotrienes and thromboxane, all of which can contribute to further cellular injury.

Cerebral protection implies the use of prophylactic measures, prior to the onset of ischaemia, with the aim of reducing the incidence of post-operative neurological deficit. Attempts at cerebral protection during CEA have largely depended on mechanical interventions aimed at rapidly restoring blood flow. Manipulation of physiological parameters and pharmacological methods have also been employed. Recent attention has been directed at trying to prevent the cascade of events leading to membrane depolarization, release of excitatory amino acids and activation of calcium ion channels.

INSERTION OF TEMPORARY INDWELLING BYPASS SHUNT

Temporary indwelling shunts may be used during CEA to maintain blood flow in the distal internal carotid artery, thus helping to restore perfusion and prevent cerebral hypoxia during the critical period of arterial clamping. A number of problems are associated with shunt use including difficulty with insertion, embolization of atheroma or air, intimal dissection, malfunction due to kinking, and thrombosis. Consequently, shunt use remains controversial with some surgeons claiming they increase the likelihood of complications. Practice therefore varies widely with some shunting routinely (Haynes and Dempsey, 1979), some never (Baker et al., 1977) and some selectively based on the results of neurological monitoring or pre-operative risk factors. Benjamin et al. (1993) showed that if empirical indications for shunting are used (contralateral carotid occlusion, previous stroke), a large number of patients will be shunted unnecessarily and perhaps exposed to increased neurological risk.

The criteria upon which the decision to insert a shunt are made vary widely. The use of EEG changes may overestimate the need for a shunt (Green et al., 1985), a safe level of ICA stump pressure has not been widely agreed (Kwaan et al., 1980) and even

patients having their surgery awake may still develop neurological deficits. It has been suggested that selective shunting for severe persistent ischaemia may help reduce complication rates, but that for mild ischaemia shunting may not be beneficial (Halsey, 1992). There is a widely held view that there is a need for randomized trials to evaluate the role of the shunt and the criteria upon which the decision to insert one is based (Naylor et al., 1992).

PHYSIOLOGICAL METHODS OF CEREBRAL PROTECTION

A number of simple physiological parameters can be manipulated during CEA in an attempt to improve neurological outcome.

Control of Pa_{CO_2}

Although the use of hypercapnia seems attractive, potentially leading to increased global cerebral blood flow due to vasodilatation, other problems arise making the technique undesirable. Intracerebral steal with diversion of blood away from already poorly perfused areas has been shown to occur in some patients during periods of hypercapnia (Boysen et al., 1971). Elevation of Pa_{CO_2} is also associated with increased myocardial work and a tendency to arrhythmias (Baker et al., 1976). In general, a policy of maintaining normocapnia during CEA is employed in most vascular units at present.

Induced hypertension

Blood vessels in ischaemic areas are thought to be maximally vasodilated and thus show pressure dependent alterations in blood flow. Those who advocate the use of induced hypertension argue that this will lead to a greater margin of safety in those areas of the brain with an already critical blood supply. Elevation of blood pressure has been shown to reverse ischaemic EEG changes associated with carotid clamping (Kresowik et al., 1991). However, artificial elevation of blood pressure with vasopressors increases myocardial work and may lead to an increased incidence of myocardial ischaemia in those with existing ischaemic heart disease (Riles et al., 1979). It has been shown that when light anaesthesia is used to produce an elevation in blood pressure there is a lower incidence of myocardial ischaemia than with techniques using vasopressors (Smith et al., 1988). Any benefits in neurological outcome associated with hypertensive techniques must be balanced against increased cardiac morbidity, which in many cases is the leading cause of peri-operative death.

Hypothermia

The brain uses energy to maintain cellular integrity as well as for electrical activity. Hypothermia reduces both these components of energy usage and can further reduce $CMRO_2$ even in the presence of an isoelectric EEG. $CMRO_2$ is reduced by approximately 7 per cent for every degree centigrade decrease in body temperature. Hypothermia may also confer a protective effect by leading to altered release of neurotransmitters (Busto et al., 1989). Although profound hypothermia, as produced during cardiopulmonary bypass, may not be of use (increasing risk and prolonging the duration of surgery), a mild degree of hypothermia is attainable and may confer some benefit during CEA (Nevin, 1994).

PHARMACOLOGICAL METHODS OF CEREBRAL PROTECTION

The use of general anaesthetic techniques during CEA allows close control of those physiological variables which affect cerebral blood flow and metabolism, e.g. arterial BP, PCO_2 and PO_2. In addition, many anaesthetic agents have a neuroprotective effect thought in large part to be related to their ability to modify cerebral metabolic rate for oxygen ($CMRO_2$). However, other related effects of these drugs may contribute to their neuroprotective activity, e.g. reduction in intracranial pressure (ICP), free-radical scavenging ability, anticonvulsant action and antagonism at voltage-sensitive ion channels.

Barbiturates

Thiopentone is the barbiturate most commonly used in the United Kingdom for intravenous induction of anaesthesia. Once consciousness is lost, it reduces $CMRO_2$ in a dose-dependent manner until the EEG becomes isoelectric, after which continued increases in tissue barbiturate concentration do not further reduce $CMRO_2$. The maximal reduction in $CMRO_2$ which can be obtained with barbiturates in this manner is approximately 50 per cent (Michenfelder, 1974). This effect differs from that produced by hypothermia where a continued reduction in temperature once the EEG becomes isoelectric leads to a further fall in $CMRO_2$. Steen et al. (1983) showed that $CMRO_2$ fell to 7 per cent of normal when hypothermia to 14°C was induced in dogs

and that the addition of barbiturate at this temperature was not associated with a further reduction. Barbiturates reduce cerebral blood flow, increase cerebrovascular resistance leading to a fall in intracranial pressure, and have membrane-stabilizing and free-radical scavenging activity, all of which may contribute to their cerebroprotective effect (Nevin, 1994).

There is, however, conflicting evidence regarding the usefulness of barbiturates in focal cerebral ischaemia. Some animal studies suggest that their administration reduces the extent of cerebral infarction prior to permanent middle cerebral artery (MCA) occlusion (Michenfelder et al., 1976). Other studies, in which a bolus dose of barbiturate was administered prior to temporary occlusion, thus mimicking the situation during CEA, failed to show a benefit (Gelb et al., 1986).

Clinical evidence for the use of barbiturates in focal cerebral ischaemia is limited and often anecdotal. Little information is available with regards to when, how much and for how long barbiturates should be administered. A single bolus dose of 4 mg/kg thiopentone administered prior to carotid occlusion has been shown to produce approximately 5 min of EEG burst suppression. This is much less than the time most surgeons require to carry out an endarterectomy (Moffat et al., 1983). If after a trial period of carotid occlusion during which ischaemic EEG changes occur and do not respond to shunt insertion or if a shunt cannot be sited, it has been suggested that administration of barbiturate may reduce the likelihood of neurological deficit (Shapiro, 1985). In this case, a bolus of thiopentone would be given prior to arterial clamping, to produce an isoelectric EEG, administration continuing for the duration of carotid occlusion. Use of barbiturates in this fashion can lead to profound cardiovascular depression which some believe is a greater risk to the patient than the small risk of a neurological deficit due to clamp ischaemia.

Barbiturate-induced coma has also been used to reverse new post-operative ischaemic deficits arising after CEA where the operated vessels have been shown to be patent (Markowitz et al., 1984).

Propofol

This relatively new intravenous anaesthetic reduces CBF and $CMRO_2$. It also causes a reduction in ICP, although overall cerebral perfusion pressure (CPP) may decrease because of hypotension. Propofol appears to have free-radical scavenging activity (Murphy *et al.*, 1992) similar to that of endogenous vitamin E and this may account for the improved neurological outcome after incomplete ischaemia in experimental rats (Kochs *et al.*, 1992). There is little evidence in humans for a neuroprotective effect although its pharmacokinetic profile makes it suitable for use by infusion for anaesthesia with the advantage of quick and clear-headed recovery.

Etomidate

This anaesthetic agent also produces reductions in CBF, $CMRo_2$ and ICP, but with perfusion pressure well maintained. There is little clinical data on the usefulness of etomidate as a neuroprotective agent and as it has detrimental effects on adrenocortical function, which may increase mortality in the critically ill, its use is likely to be limited (Watt and Ledingham, 1984).

Isoflurane

Isoflurane reduces $CMRo_2$, in similar degree to barbiturates, by reducing the component of $CMRo_2$ produced by electrical activity, and is capable of producing an isoelectric EEG at clinically relevant concentrations (Newberg *et al.*, 1983). It has therefore been suggested that isoflurane may have a cerebral protective effect similar to thiopentone, but with less hypotension and more rapid recovery. It is likely that any protective effect would be seen during incomplete ischaemia where there are zones of marginal perfusion with a gradual decrease in energy supply and membrane function. Michenfelder *et al.* (1987) showed that critical CBF during isoflurane anaesthesia for CEA was only 10 mL/100 g/min in comparison with 20 mL/100 g/min for halothane. The incidence of ischaemic EEG changes was less with isoflurane, but there were no differences in neurological outcome.

Despite these potential advantages of isoflurane, there is little evidence to suggest the existence of a significant neuroprotective effect during incomplete ischaemia. A number of studies have failed to show any difference in neurological outcome after temporary focal ischaemia in animals anaesthetized with isoflurane or halothane (Nehls *et al.*, 1987; Gelb *et al.*, 1989). Ruta *et al.* (1991) failed to show evidence of a reduction in histochemical dysfunction after focal ischaemia in rats anaesthetized with isoflurane rather than halothane. In an attempt to put into perspective the value of isoflurane as a cerebral protective agent,

Sano *et al.* (1992) studied the effect of isoflurane, halothane or mild hypothermia after temporary forebrain ischaemia in rats. They found no neuroprotective benefit of isoflurane over halothane in normothermic animals. However in those rats where cerebral temperature was allowed to fall by 3°C, the extent of ischaemic injury was significantly reduced, thus confirming other studies showing a neuroprotective effect with hypothermia, but not for isoflurane.

OTHER METHODS OF CEREBRAL PROTECTION

It has been suggested that the potential neuroprotective effects of hypothermia and anaesthetic agents cannot be explained solely by their ability to reduce $CMRo_2$ (Todd and Warner, 1992). They propose that it might be possible to intervene with neuroprotective agents at various stages in the cascade of events that occur after the onset of cerebral ischaemia. This has led to attempts to produce neuroprotective agents which act in ways other than simply reducing $CMRo_2$. After a decrease in CBF, anaesthetic agents and hypothermia slow the rate of energy utilization, and therefore time to depolarization, so delaying the onset of irreversible changes. If the ischaemic insult is very severe then the time gained by the use of these methods (a few minutes) becomes irrelevant.

Once depolarization has occurred, interventions may be aimed at the prevention of synthesis and release of detrimental substances such as excitatory neurotransmitters. Hypothermia has been shown to affect the release of neurotransmitters although a role for anaesthetic agents at this point in the cascade is less clear. There is also potential for the use of antagonists to these substances, e.g. the action of the neurotransmitter glutamate can be antagonized at both its NMDA and amino-3-hydroxy-5-methylisoxazole-4-propionic acid (AMPA) binding sites. During reperfusion, there is enhanced release of free radicals which cause further cell damage; some anaesthetic agents may have a free-radical scavenging effect but whether this is reflected in a neuroprotective effect is unclear.

A number of NMDA receptor antagonists exist and have been studied for their potential neuroprotective activity. Non-competitive NMDA antagonists which block the activated ion channel, have been shown to reduce infarct size in animal models of focal ischaemia when administered prior to the onset of the ischaemic episode (Muir and Lees, 1995). These agents appear to be concentrated within the ischaemic area and unlike competitive antagonists cannot be reversed by high concentrations of glutamate. Early competitive NMDA antagonists did not easily penetrate the blood–brain barrier although newer more lipid-soluble agents now exist. Antagonists at the glycine binding site on the NMDA receptor complex have also been studied for a potential neuroprotective role. The use of NMDA antagonists may be limited by their unwanted side effects which are common to all types. Psychomimetic disturbance may range from altered sensory perception to paranoia, hallucinations and, at very high doses, a catatonic state. Cardiovascular effects include hypertension and prolongation of the QTc interval on the ECG, possibly promoting arrhythmogenesis. Many older NMDA antagonists were too toxic to use clinically (MK801) or their side effects led to their use not being tolerated (phencyclidine). Some newer, better tolerated drugs are now entering clinical trials and may have a use in stroke and as prophylactic neuroprotective agents during short, high-risk procedures such as CEA.

The anti-oxidant and free-radical scavenger tirilazad, a 21-aminosteroid, has also been shown to reduce infarct size in experimental animals if given prophylactically and clinical trials are now ongoing (Fisher et al., 1994). Thus a number of avenues are being explored in the search for a neuroprotective agent for those undergoing short duration procedures which carry with them a high risk of cerebral ischaemia.

Post-operative considerations

In the immediate post-operative period the commonest potentially life-threatening emergencies to arise are haemorrhage with haematoma formation and stroke due to carotid occlusion.

Haemorrhage may be the result of a problem with closure of the arteriotomy site, but can also be due to bleeding from the wound surface, a complication more likely now that many patients receive aspirin pre-operatively. In the NASCET study the incidence of this complication was 5.5 per cent. Haemorrhage can present as rapid wound enlargement leading to respiratory obstruction as the haematoma and accompanying tissue oedema compress and distort the airway (Cox and Bannister,

1994). In this situation, the neck wound must be opened immediately and the patient transferred to theatre for re-exploration. The anaesthetist must be prepared for the likelihood of difficulty with tracheal intubation due to the airway distortion.

The incidence of peri-operative neurological deficit is variable depending on a number of patient and surgical factors, but in the ECST trial was 6.7 per cent although lower rates have been described. Approximately 67 per cent of deficits are the result of intra-operative problems, the majority of which relate to thrombosis, embolism or technical difficulties (Naylor and Ruckley, 1996). Only one-fifth of neurological deficits which arise intra-operatively are haemodynamic in origin. Neurological deficits present at the end of surgery are unlikely to be technically correctable and there is no indication for re-exploration of the artery. If progressive neurological changes develop in a patient who was initially well after surgery a technical problem may have arisen and most surgeons will decide to re-explore the carotid artery (Browse and Mansfield, 1997).

Cranial nerve injury is rarely mentioned in discussions of morbidity after carotid surgery, but during the NASCET study the incidence was 7.6 per cent. Damage to the mandibular branch of the facial nerve, recurrent laryngeal nerve and hypoglossal nerve have all been described. Most injuries are transient and are related to traction on the nerves during surgery.

Blood pressure lability is common in the early post-operative period, as well as during the surgery, and may lead to neurological and cardiac morbidity. A number of hypotheses exist to explain the mechanisms for the hypertension and hypotension seen. Hypertension may be the result of altered cerebral autoregulation, baroreceptor dysfunction, pre-operative hypertension, cerebral production of renin, noradrenaline and vasopressin or to intra-operative cerebral ischaemia (Ahn et al., 1989; Skydell et al., 1987; Archie, 1988). Careful monitoring and control of blood pressure are required in the post-operative period. Increases in systolic blood pressure may be self-limiting although treatment may decrease the likelihood of cardiac and neurological complications. Vasodilator drugs such as hydralazine or calcium-channel antagonists can be used to treat diastolic hypertension while beta-blockers help reduce systolic hypertension (Cucchiara et al., 1986).

Hypotension may be seen in up to 50 per cent of patients after carotid surgery. Removal of the atherosclerotic plaque exposes the carotid barore-ceptors to increased blood pressure which leads to increased baroreceptor activity and a subsequent reduction in sympathetic tone with vagal stimula-tion. In the first 24 hours after surgery, treatment with vagolytic or sympathomimetic drugs may be required although metaraminol should be avoided because it has been associated with an increased incidence of myocardial infarction (Riles *et al.*, 1979). Hypotension arising post-operatively may have a cardiac cause and this should be excluded or treated.

The hyperperfusion syndrome may occur in up to 30 per cent of cases after CEA, but is symptomatic in only 1–2 per cent. Impaired cerebral autoregulation in vessels previously maximally vasodilated in the presence of ischaemia, but now exposed to normal perfusion pressures, is thought to be the mechanism. Symptoms, including ipsilateral headache, cognitive impairment, seizures and haemorrhage, peak at around 6–12 hours post-operatively, but may last for up to 7 days. Diagnosis can be made and the condi-tion monitored by transcranial Doppler. Treatment includes elevation of the head and careful control of blood pressure (Naylor and Ruckley, 1996).

CAROTID BODY TUMOURS

These paraganglionomas usually present as painless swellings in the neck overlying the carotid artery. They are derived from neural crest cells which migrate in close association with autonomic gan-glion cells and some retain the capacity to secrete catecholamines. Functional tumours secreting nor-adrenaline can occur and present in much the same way as a phaeochromocytoma, with flushing, parox-ysmal hypertension and tachycardia. Although less than 10 per cent of carotid body tumours are malig-nant, they are locally invasive and can cause cranial nerve palsies. A family history is not uncommon and in these patients tumours are often bilateral or asso-ciated with other endocrine neoplasias such as phaeochromocytoma. These tumours can arise in any age group, being commonest between 30 and 50 years although one was described in a child of 12 years.

The aim of surgery is to excise the mass from around the carotid vessels through an avascular tis-sue plane thus avoiding the need for cross-clamping of the carotid artery. However, throughout surgery there is the potential for major haemorrhage as the tumours are highly vascular and locally invasive.

In general these patients are likely to have fewer systemic problems than those requiring surgery for occlusive arterial disease, but careful screening is still required. Patients with secretory tumours should be treated like any patient undergoing surgery for phaeochromocytoma. During surgery, cross-clamping of the carotid artery is usually not required therefore the risk of cerebral ischaemia is low. However, with large and highly invasive tumours it may be necessary to open or even excise a part of the carotid artery and repair it with graft, necessitating carotid cross-clamping with or without an intraluminal shunt. Manipulation of the carotid bifurcation during dissection of the mass can lead to episodes of hypotension and bradycardia even in those with non-functioning tumours, while in diseased arter-ies plaque rupture can lead to generation of thrombus and cerebral ischaemia.

General anaesthesia is usually employed using the same principles as discussed above for those under-going CEA. Standard monitoring including the use of continuous intra-arterial blood pressure analysis is required. A large-bore venous cannula should be placed because of the risk of brisk haemorrhage requiring rapid transfusion.

In the early post-operative period, the most com-mon complications are airway compromise due to the development of haematoma, tissue oedema or vocal cord paralysis. If severe a period of endo-tracheal intubation may be required. Disturbed baroreceptor function presenting as fluctuating pulse and blood pressure is common but usually does not require treatment. Cerebral ischaemia can arise if a graft thromboses and regular neurological observations should alert to this complication.

REFERENCES

Aaslid, R., Markwalder, T-M. and Nornes, H. 1982. Noninvasive transcranial doppler ultrasound recording of flow velocity in basal cerebral arteries. *Journal of Neurosurgery* **57**, 769–774.

Ahn, S.S., Marcus, D.R. and Moore, W.S. 1989. Post-carotid endarterectomy hypertension: association with elevated cranial norepinephrine. *Journal of Vascular Surgery* **9**, 351–360.

American Heart Association Ad Hoc Committee. 1995. Guidelines for carotid endarterectomy. *Stroke* **26**(1), 188–201.

Andrews, P.J.D., Dearden, N.M. and Miller, J.D. 1991. Jugular bulb cannulation: description of a cannulation technique and validation of a new continuous monitor. *British Journal of Anaesthesia* **67**, 553–558.

Angell-James, J.E. and Lumley, J.S.P. 1974. The effects of carotid endarterectomy on the mechanical properties of the carotid sinus and carotid sinus nerve activity in atherosclerotic patients. *British Journal of Surgery* **61**, 805–809.

Archie, J,P, Jr. 1988. The relationship of early hypertension following carotid endarterectomy to intraoperative cerebral ischaemia. *Annals of Vascular Surgery* **2**, 108–113.

Assidao, C.B., Donegan, J.H., Whitesell, R.C. and Kalbfleisch, J.H. 1982. Factors associated with perioperative complications during carotid endarterectomy. *Anesthesia and Analgesia* **61**, 631–637.

Baker, W.H., Dorner, D.B. and Barnes, R.W. 1977. Carotid endarterectomy: is an indwelling shunt necessary? *Surgery* **82**, 321–326.

Baker, W.H., Rodman, R.A., Barnes, R.W. and Hoyt, J.L. 1976. An evaluation of hypocarbia and hypercarbia during carotid endarterectomy. *Stroke* **7**, 451–4

Benjamin, M.E., Silva, M.B., Watt, C. *et al.* 1993. Awake patient monitoring to determine the need for shunting during carotid endarterectomy. *Surgery* **114**, 673–679.

Bernstein EF, Humber PB, Collins GM. *et al.* 1983. Life expectancy and late stroke following carotid endarterectomy. *Annals of Surgery* **198**, 80–86.

Bonnet F, Derosier JP, Pluskwa F. *et al.* 1990. Cervical epidural anaesthesia for carotid artery surgery. *Canadian Journal of Anaesthesia* **37**(3), 353–358.

Bove EL, Fry WJ, Gross WS and Stanley JC. 1979. Hypotension and hypertension as consequences of baroreceptor dysfunction following carotid endarterectomy. *Surgery* **85**(6), 633–637.

Boysen, G., Ladgaard-Petersen, H.J., Hennksen, H. *et al.* 1971. The effects of $PaCO_2$ on regional cerebral blood flow and internal carotid artery pressure during carotid clamping. *Anesthesiology* **35**, 286–300.

Brown, M.M. and Humphrey, P.R.D. 1992. Carotid endarterectomy: recommendations for management of transient ischaemic attack and ischaemic stroke. *British Medical Journal* **305**, 1071–1074.

Browse NL and Mansfield AO 1997. Carotid endarterectomy: operative technique. In Browse, N.L., Mansfield, A.O. and Bishop, C.C.R (eds), *Carotid endarterectomy: a practical guide*. Oxford: Butterworth-Heinemann, 98–105.

Busto, R., Globus, M.Y-T., Dietrich, W.D. *et al.* 1989. The effect of mild hypothermia on ischaemic induced release of neurotransmitters and free fatty acids in rat brain. *Stroke* **20**, 904–910.

Callow, A.D., Caplan, L.R., Correll, J.W. *et al.* 1988. Carotid endarterectomy: What is its current status? *American Journal of Medicine* **85**, 835–838.

Cox, C. and Bannister, J. 1994. Anaesthesia for carotid artery surgery. *British Journal of Anaesthesia* **72**, 252.

Cucchiara, R.F., Benefiel, D.J., Matteo, R.S. *et al.* 1986. Evaluation of esmolol in controlling increases in heart rate and blood pressure during endotracheal intubation in patients undergoing carotid endarterectomy. *Anesthesiology* **65**, 528–531.

Davies, M.J., Murrell, G.C., Cronin, K.D. *et al.* 1990. Carotid endarterectomy under cervical plexus block – a prospective clinical audit. *Anaesthesia and Intensive Care* **18**(2), 219–223.

Duncan, L.A., Ruckley, C.V. and Wildsmith, J.A.W. 1995. Cerebral oximetry; useful monitor during carotid artery surgery. *Anaesthesia* **50**, 1041–1045.

Edwards, W.H., Edwards, W.H., Mulherin, J.L. and Jenkins, J.M. 1985. The role of antiplatelet drugs in carotid reconstructive surgery. *Annals of Surgery* **201**, 765–770.

Endarterectomy for Asymptomatic Carotid Artery Stenosis. 1995. Executive committee for ACAS Study. *Journal of the American Medical Association* **273**(18), 1421–1428.

European Carotid Surgery Trialists' Collaborative Group. 1991. MRC European carotid surgery trial: interim results for symptomatic patients with severe (70–99%) or with mild (0–29%) carotid stenoses. *Lancet* **337**, 1235–1243.

Fisher, M., Jones, S. and Sacco, R.L. 1994. Prophylactic neuroprotection for cerebral ischaemia. *Stroke* **25**, 1075–1080.

Gelb, A.W., Boisvert, D.P., Tang, C. *et al.* 1989. Primate brain tolerance to temporary focal cerebral ischaemia during isoflurane or sodium nitroprusside induced hypotension. *Anesthesiology* **70**, 678–683.

Gelb, A.W., Floyd, P., Lok, P. *et al.* 1986. A prophylactic bolus of thiopentone does not protect against prolonged focal cerebral ischaemia. *Canadian Anaesthetic Society Journal* **33**, 173–177.

Green, R.M., Messick, W.J., Ricotta, J.J. *et al*. 1985. Benefits, shortcomings and costs of EEG monitoring. *Annals of Surgery* **201**, 785–791.

Halsey, J.H., McDowell, H.A., Gelmon, S. and Morawetz, R.B. 1989. Blood velocity in the middle cerebral artery and regional cerebral blood flow during carotid endarterectomy. *Stroke* **20**, 53–59.

Halsey, J.H. 1992. Risks and benefits of shunting in carotid endarterectomy. *Stroke* **23**, 1583–1587.

Haynes, C.D. and Dempsey, R.L. 1979. Carotid endarterectomy: Review of 276 cases in a community hospital. *Annals of Surgery* **189**, 258–261.

Hertzer, N.R. and Lees, C.D. 1981. Fatal myocardial infarction following carotid endarterectomy. *Annals of Surgery* **194**(2), 212–218.

Jenkinson, J.L. 1994. Electrical monitoring of the brain and spinal cord. In Walters, F.J.M., Ingram, G.S. and Jenkinson, J.L. (eds), *Anaesthesia and intensive care for the neurosurgical patient*. Oxford: Blackwell Scientific Publications, 122–140.

Jobsis, F.F. 1977. Noninvasive, infrared monitoring of cerebral and myocardial oxygen sufficiency and circulatory parameters. *Science* **198**, 1264–1266.

Kochs, E., Hoffman, W.E., Werner, C. *et al*. 1992. The effects of propofol on brain electrical activity, neurologic outcome and neuronal damage following incomplete ischaemia in rats. *Anesthesiology* **76**, 245–252.

Kresowik, T.F., Worsey, J., Khoury, M.D. *et al*. 1991. Limitations of electroencephalographic monitoring in the detection of cerebral ischaemia accompanying carotid endarterectomy. *Journal of Vascular Surgery* **13**, 439–443.

Kwaan, J.H., Peterson, G.J. and Connolly, J.E. 1980. Stump pressure: an unreliable guide for shunting during carotid endarterectomy. *Archives of Surgery* **115**, 1083–1086.

Lam, A.M., Manninen, P.H., Ferguson, G.G. and Nantau, W. 1991. Monitoring electrophysiologic function during carotid endarterectomy: A comparison of somatosensory evoked potentials and conventional electroencephalogram. *Anesthesiology* **75**, 15–21.

Landesberg, G., Erel, J., Anner, H. *et al*. 1993. Perioperative myocardial ischaemia in carotid endarterectomy under cervical plexus block and prophylactic nitroglycerin infusion. *Journal of Cardiothoracic and Vascular Anesthesia* **7**(3), 259–265.

Lennard, N., Smith, J., Dumville, J. *et al*. 1997. Role of transcranial doppler ultrasonography in preventing thromboembolic stroke after carotid endarterectomy. *British Journal of Surgery* **84**, 562 (abstract).

Markand, O.N., Dilley, R.S., Moorthy, S.S. and Warren, C. 1984. Monitoring of somatosensory evoked responses during carotid endarterectomy. *Archives of Neurology* **41**, 375–378.

Markowitz, I.P., Adinolfi, M.F. and Kerstein, M.D. 1984. Barbiturate therapy in the postoperative endarterectomy patient with a neurologic deficit. *American Journal of Surgery* **148**, 221–223.

Mason, P.F., Dyson, E.H., Sellars, V. and Beard, J.D. 1994. The assessment of cerebral oxygenation during carotid endarterectomy utilising near infrared spectroscopy. *European Journal of Vascular Surgery* **8**, 590–594.

McCormick, P.W., Stewart, M., Goetting, M.G. *et al*. 1991. Noninvasive cerebral optical spectroscopy for monitoring cerebral oxygen delivery and hemodynamics. *Critical Care Medicine* **19**, 89–97.

McKay, R.D., Sundt, T.M., Michenfelder, J.D. *et al*. 1976. Internal carotid artery stump pressure and cerebral blood flow during carotid endarterectomy: modification by halothane, enflurane and innovar. *Anesthesiology* **45**, 390–400.

Messick, J.M., Casement, B., Sharbrough, F.W. *et al*. 1987. Correlation of regional cerebral blood flow (rCBF) with EEG changes during isoflurane anesthesia for carotid endarterectomy: critical rCBF. *Anesthesiology* **66**, 344–349.

Michenfelder, J.D., Milde, J.H. and Sundt, T.M. 1976. Cerebral protection by barbiturate anesthesia. Use after middle cerebral artery occlusion in java monkeys. *Archives of Neurology* **33**, 345–350.

Michenfelder, J.D., Sundt, T.M., Fode, N. and Sharbrough, F.W. 1987. Isoflurane when compared to enflurane and halothane decreases the frequency of cerebral ischaemia during carotid endarterectomy. *Anesthesiology* **67**, 336–340.

Michenfelder, J.D. 1974. The interdependency of cerebral function and metabolic effects following massive doses of thiopental in the dog. *Anesthesiology* **41**, 231–236.

Moffat, J.A., McDougall, M.J., Brunet, D. *et al*. 1983. Thiopental bolus during carotid endarterectomy – rational drug therapy? *Canadian Anaesthetic Society Journal* **30**, 615–622.

Moore, W.S. and Hall, A.D. 1969. Carotid artery back pressure. A test of cerebral tolerance to temporary carotid occlusion. *Archives of Surgery* **99**, 702–710.

Morawetz, R.B., Zeiger, H.E., McDowall, H.A. *et al*. 1984. Correlation of cerebral blood flow and EEG during carotid occlusion for endarterectomy (without shunting) and neurologic outcome. *Surgery* **96**, 184–189.

Moss, E. 1994. Anaesthesia for vascular surgery. In Walters, F.J.M., Ingram, G.S. and Jenkinson, J.L. (eds), *Anaesthesia and intensive care for the neurosurgical patient*. Oxford: Blackwell Scientific Publications, 239–273.

Muir, K.W. and Lees, K.R. 1995. Clinical experience with excitatory amino acid antagonist drugs. *Stroke* **26**, 503–513.

Murphy, P.G., Myers, D.S., Davies, M.J. *et al*. 1992. The antioxidant potential of propofol (2,6 diisopropylphenol). *British Journal of Anaesthesia* **68**, 613–618.

Naylor, A.R. and Ruckley, C.V. 1996. Complications after carotid surgery. In Campbell, B. (ed.), *Complications in arterial surgery. A practical approach to management*, Oxford: Butterworth-Heinemann, 73–88.

Naylor, A.R., Bell, P.R.F. and Ruckley, C.V. 1992. Monitoring and cerebral protection during carotid endarterectomy. *British Journal of Surgery* **79**(8), 735–741.

Naylor, A.R., Wildsmith, J.A.W., McClure, J. *et al*. 1991. Transcranial doppler monitoring during carotid endarterectomy. *British Journal of Surgery* **78**, 1264–1268.

Nehls, D.G., Major, M.C., Todd, M.M. *et al*. 1987. A comparison of the cerebral protective effects of isoflurane and barbiturates during temporary focal ischaemia in primates. *Anesthesiology* **66**, 453–464.

Nevin, M. 1994. Cerebral metabolism. In Walters, F.J.M., Ingram, G.S. and Jenkinson, J.L. (eds), *Anaesthesia and intensive care for the neurosurgical patient*, Oxford: Blackwell Scientific Publications, 46–69.

Newberg, L.A., Milde, J.H. and Michenfelder, J.D. 1983. The cerebral metabolic effects of isoflurane at and above concentrations that suppress cortical electrical activity. *Anesthesiology* **59**, 23–28.

North American Symptomatic Carotid Endarterectomy Trial Collaborators. 1991. Beneficial effect of carotid endarterectomy in symptomatic patients with high grade carotid stenosis. *New England Journal of Medicine* **325**, 445–453.

Ombrellaro, M.P., Freeman, M.B., Stevens, S.L. and Goldman, M.H. 1996. Effect of anesthetic technique on cardiac morbidity following carotid artery surgery. *American Journal of Surgery* **171**, 387–390.

Paydachee, T.S., Gosling, R.G., Bishop, C.C. *et al*. 1986. Monitoring middle cerebral artery velocity during carotid endarterectomy. *British Journal of Surgery* **73**, 98–100.

Pine, R., Avellone, J.C., Hoffman, M. *et al*. 1984. Control of post carotid endarterectomy hypertension with baroreceptor blockade. *American Journal of Surgery* **147**, 763–765.

Rampil, I.J., Holzer, J.A., Quest, D.O. *et al*. 1983. Prognostic value of computerized EEG analysis during carotid endarterectomy. *Anesthesia and Analgesia* **62**, 186–192.

Riles, T.S., Kopelman, I. and Imparato, A.M. 1979. Myocardial infarction following carotid endarterectomy: A review of 683 operations. *Surgery* **85**(3), 249–252.

Rosenthal, D., Stanton, P.E. and Lamis, P.A. 1981. Carotid endarterectomy – The unreliability of intraoperative monitoring in patients having had stroke or reversible ischaemic neurologic deficit. *Archives of Surgery* **116**, 1569–1574.

Rothwell, P.M., Slattery, J. and Warlow, C.P. 1997. Clinical and angiographic predictors of stroke and death from carotid endarterectomy; systematic review. *British Medical Journal* **315**, 1571–1577.

Ruckley, C.V. and Wildsmith, J.A.W. 1992. Carotid endarterectomy: future perspectives. *European Journal of Vascular Surgery* **6**, 229–231.

Ruta, T.S., Drummond, J.C. and Cole, D.J. 1991. A comparison of the area of histochemical dysfunction after focal cerebral ischaemia during anaesthesia with isoflurane and halothane in the rat. *Canadian Journal of Anaesthesia* **38**, 129–135.

Samra, S.K., Dorje, P., Zelenock, G.B. and Stanley, J.C. 1996. Cerebral oximetry in patients undergoing carotid endarterectomy under regional anesthesia. *Stroke* **27**, 49–55.

Sano, T., Drummond, J.C., Patel, P.M. *et al*. 1992. A comparison of the cerebral protective effects of isoflurane and mild hypothermia in a model of incomplete forebrain ischaemia in the rat. *Anesthesiology* **76**, 221–228.

Shapiro, H.M. 1985. Barbiturates in brain ischaemia. *British Journal of Anaesthesia* **57**, 82–95.

Skydell, J.L., Machleder, H.I. and Baker, J.D. 1987. Incidence and mechanism of post-carotid endarterectomy hypertension. *Archives of Surgery* **122**, 1153–1155.

Smith, J.S., Roizen, M.F., Cahalan, M.K. *et al*. 1988. Does anesthetic technique make a difference? Augmentation of systolic blood pressure during carotid endarterectomy: Effects of phenylephrine versus light anesthesia and of isoflurane versus halothane on the incidence of myocardial ischaemia. *Anesthesiology* **69**, 846–853.

Steed, D.L., Peitzman, A.B., Grundy, B.L. and Webster, M.W. 1982. Causes of stroke in carotid endarterectomy. *Surgery* **92**(4), 634–639.

Steen, P.A., Newberg, L., Milde, J.H. and Michenfelder, J.D. 1983. Hypothermia and barbiturates: individual and combined effects on canine cerebral oxygen consumption. *Anesthesiology* **58**, 527–532.

Stoneham, M.D. and Knighton, J.D. 1999. Regional anaesthesia for carotid endarterectomy. *British Journal of Anaesthesia* **83**, 910–919.

Sundt, T.M., Sandok, B.A. and Whisnant, J.P. 1975. Carotid endarterectomy: Complications and preoperative assessment of risk. *Mayo Clinic Proceedings* **50**, 301–306.

Sundt, T.M., Sharbrough, F.W., Anderson, R.E. and Michenfelder, J.D. 1974. Cerebral blood flow measurements during carotid endarterectomy. *Journal of Neurosurgery* **41**, 310–320.

Tangkanakul, C., Counsell, C. and Warlow, C. 1996. Carotid endarterectomy performed under local anaesthetic compared to general anaesthetic: a systematic review of the evidence. In Warlow, C., Van Gijn, J. and Sandercock, P. (eds), *Stroke module of The Cochrane Database of Systematic Reviews*.

Todd, M.M. and Warner, D.S. 1992. A comfortable hypothesis re-evaluated. *Anesthesiology* **76**, 161–164.

Toner, C.C. and Stamford, J.A. 1996. General anaesthetics as neuroprotective agents. *Ballieres Clinical Anesthesiology* **10**(3), 515–533.

Towne, J.B. and Bernhard, V.M. 1980. The relationship of postoperative hypertension to complications following carotid endarterectomy. *Surgery* **88**(4), 575–579.

Watt, I. and Ledingham, I.M. 1984. Mortality amongst multiple trauma patients admitted to an ITU. *Anaesthesia* **39**, 973–981.

Williams, I.M., Vohra, R., Farrell, A. *et al.* 1994. Cerebral oxygen saturation, transcranial Doppler ultrasonography and stump pressure in carotid surgery. *British Journal of Surgery* **81**, 960–964.

Wong, D.H.W. 1991. Perioperative stroke Part 1: General surgery, carotid artery disease and carotid endarterectomy. *Canadian Journal of Anaesthesia* **38**(3), 347–373.

15

Anaesthesia for vascular surgery on the lower limb

JONATHAN P THOMPSON AND GRAHAM SMITH

INTRODUCTION

The incidence of peripheral vascular disease (PVD) increases with age, and the condition affects 5–7 per cent of the middle-aged and elderly populations. The early symptoms of cold extremities, intermittent claudication and paraesthesiae may progress in 25 per cent of cases to rest pain and gangrene without treatment. Several studies have established an association between smoking, peripheral arterial and coronary artery disease, and patients with PVD are at high risk of developing complications after anaesthesia and surgery.

Indications for intervention

Although symptomatic improvement may be achieved by medical therapy, active intervention may be required for severe, disabling symptoms. Patients should stop smoking, and cardiac failure and polycythaemia may require treatment. There is little evidence of benefit from vasodilators or antiplatelet drugs, although these may be prescribed

for associated cardiovascular or cerebrovascular disease. If such general measures are ineffective or unsuccessful, minimally invasive surgical or interventional radiological techniques are often attempted. At the Leicester Royal Infirmary, approximately 70 per cent of patients referred with disabling symptoms of PVD are treated currently by angioplasty or endovascular techniques, with no involvement of the anaesthetist.

PERCUTANEOUS TRANSLUMINAL ANGIOPLASTY

Percutaneous transluminal angioplasty (PTA) is an established treatment for intermittent claudication, rest pain or lower limb ischaemia caused by stenoses or occlusions of the iliac, femoral and popliteal vessels, and good success rates have been reported with infrapopliteal angioplasty (Varty et al., 1995). In general, treatment of discrete isolated lesions of the iliac, or femoropopliteal vessels is the most successful with overall patency rates of 50–70 per cent at five years. The rate of complications which require subsequent bypass surgery (i.e. acute occlusion at the site of the lesion caused by thrombosis or dissection, and distal embolism) should be around 0.5 per cent; the morbidity and mortality rate associated with PTA is low. Factors historically associated with poor results are a disease segment length > 10 cm, distal disease, poor distal run-off and diabetes mellitus. Although recurrent disease may be amenable to repeated angioplasty, or the addition of fibrinolytic therapy, patients who present for conventional surgery have more extensive, diffuse or advanced disease, recurrent disease, or rarely an acute complication of PTA. These patients are likely to have more extensive coronary and cerebrovascular disease, to have continued to smoke and may be at even greater risk of developing cardiovascular complications.

PERIPHERAL VASCULAR RECONSTRUCTION

The indications for reconstructive surgery are ischaemic rest pain, tissue loss (ulceration or gangrene), severe claudication with disease at certain anatomical sites (femoropopliteal, popliteal or distal), or failure of non-surgical procedures (Table 15.1). The operation may be classified as either an inflow or outflow procedure. Inflow procedures are performed to bypass obstruction in the aorto-iliac segment; outflow procedures bypass obstruction distal to the inguinal ligament. There is an increasing trend for distal reconstructions, as far as the ankle or the foot, although the risk of failure and limb loss implies that these should be reserved for critical ischaemia rather than intermittent claudication. Up to 30 per cent of patients with symptoms of claudication may be suitable for aorto-iliac reconstruction, usually by percutaneous transluminal angioplasty, although an open procedure involving a transperitoneal or oblique retroperitoneal abdominal incision may be required (Davies *et al.*, 1990). In occasional cases, usually where the patient is particularly frail, axillobifemoral, unilateral axillopopliteal or crossover femorofemoral grafts may be performed. Operations involving the axilla are not suitable in

Table 15.1 *Indications for peripheral vascular reconstructive surgery*

- Ischaemic rest pain
- Tissue loss (ulceration or gangrene)
- Severe intermittent claudication with disease at certain anatomical sites (femoropopliteal, popliteal or distal)
- Failure of non-surgical treatment

these circumstances for regional anaesthesia (though judiciously supplemented local anaesthetic is often used), but the anaesthetic considerations are essentially similar to those for the commoner outflow procedures of femoral, popliteal and distal bypass grafting. Outflow procedures vary widely in their complexity, but commonly involve a bypass from femoral artery to popliteal, or crural vessels (anterior or posterior tibial, or tibioperoneal artery).

The graft material used is either synthetic usually PTFE (polytetrafluoroethylene) or autogenous saphenous vein (ASV). ASV bypass procedures can be performed *in situ*, or reversed. Synthetic PTFE grafts may be used for femoropopliteal reconstruction. Early reports of comparable patency rates to ASV have not been confirmed, particularly for operations below the knee (Sayers *et al.*, 1993). Synthetic grafts may, however, be preferred if the saphenous vein is too small, is missing or has been damaged by thrombophlebitis. The advantages over ASV include a shorter operative time because there is no venous dissection, which is especially important in the poorer risk patient.

In situ ipsilateral long saphenous grafts involve exposure of the saphenous vein along its length, ligation of side branches, and anastomosis of the proximal end to the common femoral artery. As venous valves impair distal flow, they are destroyed using a valvulotome, and the vein attached to the distal artery. The advantages of this technique are that the larger proximal saphenous vein matches the size of the larger proximal femoral artery (and the smaller distal ends also match), and that the vein is not removed from its bed, thereby obviating twisting or kinking of the vessel. The graft may be checked by angiography, angioscopy, or Doppler flow measurements (Davies *et al.*, 1993a) in addition to palpation. Early reports of improved patency rates with this technique (Buchbinder *et al.*, 1981; Leather *et al.*, 1981) compared with reversed vein grafting have not been confirmed by subsequent studies (Varty *et al.*, 1993).

Reversed saphenous vein grafts may be performed to avoid the problems associated with venous valves. The whole length of vein is detached, the branches ligated, the vein flushed, its alignment reversed and the vein tunnelled subcutaneously before attachment to the artery. Venous spasm may be decreased by flushing with warm heparinized blood rather than cold fluids, and minimizing handling of the vein. It is important to avoid trauma, kinking or twisting. The duration of surgery with both reversed and *in situ* ASV operations is prolonged, but for distal reconstruction these techniques have a higher patency rate than the use of prosthetic grafts. Successful surgical outcome depends on many factors, but up to 30 per cent of all infragenicular grafts require revision surgery or angioplasty (Taylor *et al.*, 1990; London *et al.*, 1993). The contribution of anaesthesia to surgical outcome is discussed below.

Early graft occlusion may occur in 20 per cent of cases (Dunlop *et al.*, 1995) and is caused usually by technical problems related to graft size, twisting or kinking; other factors include hypotension, hypothermia or peripheral vasoconstriction. As the limb is ischaemic, re-exploration is a matter of urgency. Embolectomy may be sufficient, but graft replacement may be required, especially of prosthetic grafts. Late graft failure (more than 30 days after operation) is commonly caused by intrinsic factors and occurs in approximately 15–20 per cent of all grafts; 80 per cent in the first year after surgery. The usual causes of late graft stenosis are atherosclerosis or intimal hyperplasia, the aetiology of which involves surgical trauma, inflammatory mediators, pre-existing venous pathology and haemodynamic stresses caused by pulsatile arterial pressures acting on the venous graft wall (Varty *et al.*, 1993).

PRE-OPERATIVE ASSESSMENT

Pre-operative assessment of the patient presenting for arterial reconstructive surgery of the lower limb is essentially similar to that of patients undergoing other vascular procedures. However, whilst patients presenting for aortic surgery are investigated extensively, because of the semi-urgent nature of many peripheral vascular surgical procedures, time may not permit complicated invasive diagnostic tests of cardiovascular function. Furthermore, less senior anaesthetists may be involved because surgery often takes place outside normal working hours.

Patients with peripheral vascular disease usually have widespread vascular disease (Hertzer *et al.*, 1984), with a high incidence of hypertension, ischaemic heart and cerebrovascular disease, diabetes mellitus and renal disease; they are usually smokers and have associated respiratory disease. Consequently, long-term survival after peripheral

revascularization may be less than 65 per cent at twelve months (Thompson *et al.*, 1993). The commonest causes of morbidity and mortality amongst patients undergoing peripheral vascular surgery are myocardial ischaemia and infarction (Mangano, 1990). Hertzer and colleagues (1987) found that 50 per cent of deaths after peripheral vascular surgery were related to cardiac causes. Peri-operative myocardial ischaemia occurs in approximately 38 per cent of vascular surgical patients (McCann and Clements, 1989; Mangano, 1990). Ischaemia in the peri-operative period is associated with subsequent myocardial infarction (Slogoff and Keats, 1985; Pasternack *et al.*, 1989; Raby *et al.*, 1989; Mangano, 1990; Fleisher *et al.*, 1991; Christopherson *et al.*, 1993) with an incidence in the range 2.8–4.5 per cent (Hertzer *et al.*, 1987; Taylor *et al.*, 1991; Yeager *et al.*, 1994; Bode *et al.*, 1996). Frequently, peri-operative myocardial infarctions are silent (Yeager *et al.*, 1987) with a mortality of up to 50 per cent. In a recent study of 423 patients undergoing femoral to distal arterial bypass surgery, 13 of the 19 peri-operative myocardial infarctions (4.5 per cent overall) were silent (Bode *et al.*, 1996).

Over the last two decades several investigators have attempted to assess the risks associated with particular conditions in relation to peri-operative myocardial ischaemia, but these attempts have produced conflicting results. Moreover, the answers to apparently simple issues including the extent of peri-operative risk associated with hypertension have proved elusive. Unfortunately, different surgical populations have been examined in many previous studies, even though general surgical patients are likely to possess a pattern of concomitant medical disease different from that in patients with widespread vascular disease. For example, the widely-quoted Goldman cardiac risk index probably underestimates the risks of vascular surgery (Gersh *et al.*, 1991; Fleisher, 1996). Furthermore, in many studies of peri-operative cardiac risk, several operative procedures, including abdominal aortic aneurysm repair, carotid endarterectomy, and lower limb peripheral vascular reconstruction have been grouped under the classification 'peripheral vascular surgery'. Although not subject to the sudden haemodynamic changes and fluid shifts associated with aortic cross-clamping, and the respiratory effects of a large abdominal incision, lower-limb vascular reconstruction may be prolonged, and accompanied by hypothermia and hypovolaemia. Hypothermia *per se* may be associated with myocardial ischaemia (Frank *et al.*, 1993).

However, suggestions that there are large differences in cardiac morbidity and mortality between patients undergoing different major vascular procedures are not confirmed by the available data. In a prospective study of more than 1500 patients undergoing vascular surgical procedures, the incidence of myocardial infarction was similar after both infrainguinal (3.5 per cent) and aortic surgery (4.0 per cent) (Yeager, 1994). Clinical evidence of coronary artery disease seems to be a better predictor of the occurrence of peri-operative cardiac events than the type of surgery performed. (Krupski *et al.*, 1993; L'Italien *et al.*, 1995). In a review of several studies involving several thousand vascular surgical patients clinical suspicion of coronary artery disease was associated with a doubling in late mortality rates (Hertzer *et al.*, 1987; ACC, 1996).

The influence of factors noted to increase peri-operative risk in the 1970s and 1980s (Goldman *et al.*, 1977; Detsky *et al.*, 1986) probably diminished in the late 1990s as a consequence of advances in cardiology. For example, the widespread use of thrombolysis and percutaneous coronary angioplasty after myocardial infarction has decreased the incidence of re-infarction within six months. The American College of Cardiology has therefore abandoned the absolute time interval since infarction as an independent factor in peri-operative cardiac risk (ACC, 1996; Fleisher, 1996).

Incidence of peri-operative myocardial ischaemia

Ischaemic heart disease is present in 36 per cent or more patients with peripheral vascular disease (Bode *et al.*, 1996). In a review of six studies of 4642 patients undergoing a variety of vascular procedures, peri-operative cardiac events (myocardial infarction, ischaemia, arrhythmia or congestive cardiac failure) occurred in 16 per cent of patients with clinical evidence of coronary artery disease compared with 1.7 per cent without (Hertzer *et al.*, 1987).

Why is risk assessment important?

Many of the factors which contribute to the pathogenesis of peripheral vascular disease, (smoking, diabetes, hyperlipidaemia) are also risk factors for coronary artery disease. In the widely quoted Cleveland Clinic series of 1000 patients presenting for peripheral vascular surgery who underwent routine pre-operative coronary angiography, only 8 per cent had normal coronary vessels, and 32 per cent had 'mild' to 'moderate' coronary artery disease . Clinical indicators of coronary artery disease correlated well with the findings on angiography (Hertzer *et al.*, 1984).

Unfortunately, the usual presenting symptoms of coronary artery disease are frequently masked in the patient with peripheral vascular disease. Exercise tolerance is a useful clinical indicator of the severity of ischaemic heart disease (McPhail *et al.*, 1988), but in this section of the population, it is almost invariably limited by intermittent claudication, previous amputation, or old age. Such patients may have adapted to a lifestyle with little exercise, have few symptoms and a normal ECG at rest even though they may have severe coronary artery disease. In addition, myocardial ischaemia when present may be asymptomatic. In the Cleveland series, 15 per cent of patients without suspected disease had severe coronary artery disease requiring surgical correction. Major peripheral vascular surgery may be prolonged, leading to hypothermia, and shifts in intra- and extravascular fluid volumes. These factors combine with the effects of co-existing disease to produce a high morbidity and mortality from peripheral vascular surgery (Mangano *et al.*, 1990; Ashton *et al.*, 1993). It is therefore imperative to carefully assess the presence of cardiovascular risk factors in patients who may not have overt symptoms.

SCREENING

Screening tests have an associated morbidity and even mortality. They may be expensive, and unnecessary for many patients, and consequently many attempts have been made to target screening more effectively. A particular test can only be justified if the results affect treatment and outcome (ACC, 1996). Whilst the pre-operative investigation of the very high- or very low-risk patient is more straightforward there has, until recently, been little consensus on the optimum strategy for the patient of intermediate risk. The major problem which has so far proved elusive is to define which patients with symptoms or a history suggestive of ischaemic heart disease benefit from invasive pre-operative assessment.

The evidence regarding hypertension illustrates these difficulties. Standard teaching states that hypertension increases the risks of anaesthesia. However, whilst untreated hypertension is well known to be associated with increased haemodynamic lability, in multivariate risk analyses (Detsky et al., 1986; Goldman et al., 1977), controlled hypertension has not proved a consistent predictor of peri-operative cardiac events. Nonetheless, patients presenting to hospital with a high systemic arterial pressure on admission may demonstrate increased haemodynamic instability on laryngoscopy and intubation, and may be more at risk for development of myocardial ischaemia (Bedford and Fenstein, 1980; Stone et al., 1988a, b). Clearly, if there is untreated hypertension, elective surgery should be postponed until arterial pressure is under adequate control, although 'adequate control' has not been defined and in a patient with critical ischaemia, postponement of surgery may risk loss of the limb. Three small studies suggested that pre-operative beta-blockade may be beneficial in reducing the incidence of peri-operative myocardial ischaemia (Stone et al., 1988a, b; Pasternak et al., 1989), although there is limited evidence for beneficial effects of other antihypertensive therapy.

In an attempt to clarify peri-operative cardiac risk assessment, the American College of Cardiologists and American Heart Association recently evaluated the literature of the last two decades in order to produce some guidelines for the cardiovascular evaluation of patients presenting for non-cardiac surgery (ACC, 1996). Whilst these are influenced inevitably by United States practice, some of the conclusions may be applied universally. In spite of – or perhaps as a consequence of – all the extensive laboratory tests and invasive investigations available, the starting point for pre-operative assessment remains a thorough history and clinical examination; the objective is to identify and assess potentially serious or correctable disorders. Emphasis should be placed not only on the presence, but the severity of cardiac symptoms in order that some assessment of functional capacity be made. Which tests should be performed is discussed below.

SYMPTOMS

Symptoms of cardiac disease may be absent in a large proportion of patients with significant coronary disease. Hertzer and colleagues (1984) investigated 1000 consecutive patients scheduled for peripheral vascular surgery with coronary angiography. Thirty-seven per cent of those without symptoms had coronary stenoses > 70 per cent compared with 78 per cent of those with symptoms; of these, the majority had multivessel disease. The presence of symptoms is therefore indicative of coronary pathology *to some degree.*

Pre-operative history and examination should therefore focus on assessment of the cardiovascular and respiratory systems. In particular, symptoms and signs relating to congestive cardiac failure and angina should be sought. Existing cardiac failure has been shown consistently to correlate with peri-operative cardiac morbidity (Goldman et al., 1977; Detsky et al., 1986; Mangano, 1990) and its detection is paramount. However, the detection of clinical signs of cardiac failure varies widely between observers, clinical signs correlate poorly with ejection fraction, and are insensitive for increased elevated pulmonary capillary wedge pressure, although highly specific (Gersh et al., 1991). Recent myocardial infarction or the presence of stable or unstable angina increases the risk of peri-operative myocardial infarction (Detsky et al., 1986; Shah et al., 1990), although because of improvements in medical therapy, the ACC has now abandoned as a risk factor the absolute time post 30 days after infarction. If angina is associated with symptoms of left ventricular dysfunction (dyspnoea, syncope), it is suggested that peri-operative myocardial ischaemia is associated with left ventricular dysfunction. Such symptoms are therefore particularly relevant. In addition, cardiac outcome after surgery is affected by co-existing medical conditions including diabetes, renal dysfunction, and cerebrovascular disease, in addition to old age. Hypertension and diabetes mellitus are not

Table 15.2 *Why is peripheral vascular surgery 'high risk'?*

- Many risk factors for peripheral vascular disease are also risk factors for coronary artery disease
- The usual symptoms of coronary artery disease may be masked by intermittent claudication, old age, amputation or arthritis.
- Procedures are often lengthy, with the risk of hypothermia, blood loss, changes in vascular volumes, blood pressure and heart rate.
- Myocardial ischaemia is common, commonly silent, and associated with myocardial infarction.

Table 15.3   *Clinical stratification of pre-operative cardiac risk factors before functional assessment (ACC, 1996)*

Major	Intermediate	Minor
A recent myocardial infarct (within 7–30 days)	Mild angina	Age > 70 years
Unstable or severe angina	A previous myocardial infarct	Abnormal ECG findings
Severe valvular disease	(> 30 days)	Heart rhythm other than sinus
Uncontrolled congestive cardiac failure	Diabetes mellitus	Uncontrolled hypertension
Atrioventricular block	Treated congestive cardiac failure	Previous stroke

proven *independent* predictors of morbidity but *are* important correlates of coronary artery disease (CAD). Peripheral vascular surgery is rated as high risk (Table 15.2), so that the assessment of all these conditions must be thorough, and their presence should lower the threshold for further testing.

Risk classification and further investigation

The joint American College of Cardiology and American Heart Association Task Force allocated patients to one of three groups (Table 15.3). It is suggested that high-risk patients should undergo further invasive assessment almost regardless of the surgical procedure (Table 15.4). For low-risk patients (i.e. age <70 years with no risk factors), no special tests are required (ACC, 1996). For medium or minor risk patients, some assessment of functional capacity is required. Activity scales such as the Duke Activity Status Index (Hlatky *et al.*, 1989) provide a framework for this. Briefly, peri-operative cardiac risk is increased in patients unable to sustain moderate physical activity as rated by four metabolic equivalents, e.g. walking on the flat at 4 mph, walking up a hill, climbing a flight of stairs, scrubbing floors or playing golf. For patients of medium clinical risk with good functional capacity

undergoing peripheral vascular surgery, further non-invasive tests are recommended, and are mandatory if functional capacity is poor (Table 15.4). The precise tests depend on the symptoms and are detailed below, but exercise ECG, 24-hour ECG, echocardiography, radionuclide angiography, or dipyridamole–thallium scanning are among the possibilities. It is recommended that high-risk patients, and those with intermediate risk, but poor functional capacity and abnormalities or equivocal results on non-invasive testing, undergo coronary angiography and cardiological referral. If angina is associated with symptoms of left ventricular dysfunction such as dyspnoea or syncope, it is suggested that peri-operative myocardial ischaemia will produce left ventricular dysfunction. No further non-invasive tests are indicated and the patient should undergo coronary angiography. The question of possible coronary revascularization is discussed below.

INVESTIGATIONS

In the evaluation of a screening test for its ability to correctly identify patients who are, and who are not, at risk of peri-operative myocardial ischaemia, the terms 'positive' and 'negative predictive value' are often used. The positive predictive value of a test is the probability of disease in a patient with a positive

Table 15.4   *Suggested strategy for peri-operative cardiac assessment before peripheral vascular surgery*

Situation	Action*
No clinical risk factors, good functional capacity *or* Minor clinical risk factors, good functional capacity	Proceed to surgery
Minor clinical risk factors, poor functional capacity *or* Intermediate clinical risk, good functional capacity	Further assessment by exercise ECG, ambulatory ECG, DPTA, radionuclide angiography or DSE. Proceed to coronary angiography if results positive or equivocal
Intermediate clinical risk, poor functional capacity, *or* High clinical risk	Cardiological referral and coronary angiography

*DPTA, dipyridamole–thallium angiography; DSE, dobutamine stress echocardiography.

test result, and the negative predictive value refers to the probability of no disease in a patient with a negative test result. In contrast to specificity and sensitivity, the predictive value of a test depends on the prior probability of the outcome in question, as well as the specificity and sensitivity of the test. The value of a particular screening test therefore depends on the tested population (Goldman, 1995) which varies between studies.

Electrocardiography

Despite its limitations in sensitivity (it may be normal in up to 50 per cent of patients with single vessel coronary artery disease) (Chaitman, 1986), resting 12-lead electrocardiography is mandatory for all peripheral vascular surgical patients. It is non-invasive, gives valuable information about previous myocardial infarction, ventricular hypertrophy, arrhythmias, electrolyte or conduction disturbances and is generally considered part of the physical examination (ACC, 1996).

Exercise electrocardiography

The widespread use of exercise electrocardiography in vascular patients is limited by technical difficulties and the effect of intermittent claudication on the ability to exercise, though supplemental arm ergometry can be performed if claudication becomes limiting (Cutler et al., 1981). Up to 25 per cent of patients with no clinical history of coronary artery disease and a normal resting ECG have an abnormal exercise ECG. If the resting ECG is abnormal or there is a history of myocardial infarction, the frequency of such abnormalites is 35–50 per cent (ACC, 1996). Only 50 per cent of the vascular surgical population will be able to reach a heart rate >75 per cent of age-predicted maximum. Inability to reach 85 per cent of maximal heart rate is predictive of adverse cardiac events (Cutler et al., 1981; McPhail et al., 1988), and ECG abnormalities at low workloads are associated with increased peri-operative cardiac risk. The overall positive predictive value of exercise electrocardiography in vascular patients is around 16–20 per cent with a negative predictive value of 93–99 per cent, and it is recommended as the test of choice for assessment of functional capacity in patients with potential myocardial ischaemia (ACC, 1996). In patients with abnormalities on resting ECG which preclude interpretation of ST changes (left bundle branch block, left ventricular hypertrophy with strain, digoxin effect), other tests are recommended.

Ambulatory electrocardiography

Several authors have investigated the relationship between ambulatory electrocardiography and peri-operative cardiac outcome. In vascular surgical patients, the incidence of pre-operative myocardial ischaemia is 12–24 per cent (McPhail et al., 1988; Ouyang et al., 1989; Pasternack et al., 1989; Raby et al., 1989; Mangano et al., 1990; Fleisher et al., 1991; Muir et al., 1991; Landesberg et al., 1993). In the majority of patients these episodes of myocardial ischaemia were silent (Knight et al., 1989). Silent myocardial ischaemia was even more common after operation, occurring in 39–61 per cent of patients (Ouyang et al., 1989; Mangano et al., 1990; Landesberg et al., 1993). Several of these studies demonstrated an increased incidence of adverse peri-operative cardiac events (myocardial infarction, arrhythmia, cardiac failure or unstable angina) in patients with episodes of ischaemia before operation, with a positive predictive value of 35–40 per cent (Raby et al., 1989; Fleisher et al., 1991). The negative predictive value of a normal ambulatory ECG for an uneventful outcome is 86–99 per cent, though this depends on the study population (Goldman, 1995).

Some have suggested that ambulatory electrocardiography should be used routinely before operation in vascular surgical patients, recognizing that 10 per cent or more (Mangano et al., 1990) may have underlying ECG abnormalities which preclude interpretation of ST-segment abnormalities (Cunningham, 1994). Many of the studies performed so far have not been standardized, with variations in study design including performance in hospital or at home, interpretation of individual abnormalities, and description of results from ambulatory electrocardiography as either positive or negative, with no attempt at stratification of risk (ACC, 1996; Fleisher, 1996). Landesberg and colleagues (1993) found that only prolonged (>2 hours) pre-operative ischaemic episodes were predictive of post-operative cardiac morbidity. Whilst ambulatory electrocardiography has proved useful in demonstrating the incidence of myocardial ischaemia in the peri-operative period, it cannot be recommended for routine use and is no more useful than dipyridamole–thallium imaging for the prediction of peri-operative cardiac events or the need for coronary angiography (Fleisher et al., 1995a). However, it may prove useful in the assessment of selected patients who are unable to exercise.

Dipyridamole–thallium angiography

Over the last decade several studies have attempted to define the role of dipyridamole–thallium angiography (DPTA) in predicting peri-operative cardiac risk. In one of the early reports, Eagle *et al.* (1989) retrospectively studied 200 patients undergoing vascular surgery. Thirty per cent of the patients with a positive scan had a peri-operative cardiac event, 7 per cent of them fatal. The positive predictive value of a positive scan was only 16 per cent, but the negative predictive value of a normal scan was 99 per cent. When taken with clinical indicators (age, angina, diabetes, ECG evidence of Q waves or ventricular ectopic activity), a positive scan (redistribution defect or ischaemic changes during DPTA) correlated with the occurrence of cardiac events. It was therefore suggested as being useful in the assessment of the patient of intermediate risk. However, Mangano and colleagues (1991) suggested that routine pre-operative DPTA was not warranted because the positive predictive value decreased to 5 per cent when clinicians were blinded to the scan results, and 54 per cent of the adverse cardiac outcomes occurred in patients without redistribution defects. It may be less useful in diabetic patients (Lane *et al.*, 1989). In the largest study so far, DPTA was found to be of less value than clinical suspicion or an age > 65 years in 457 patients undergoing aortic surgery (Baron *et al.*, 1994). In 17 studies performed on 2679 patients between 1985 and 1994, the overall positive predictive value was 4–20 per cent, and a normal scan had a negative predictive value of 99–100 per cent. It has been suggested that risk assessment may be improved by scoring or quantifying abnormalities on DPTA (ACC, 1996), though its role in pre-operative cardiac evaluation is likely to be limited to patients with moderate symptoms of coronary artery disease and in whom exercise or ambulatory electrocardiography is unsuitable.

Radionuclide angiography

Radionuclide angiography may be used to assess left ventricular function and is particularly useful in patients with symptoms of cardiac failure. However, the value of this technique for screening is doubtful; several prospective and retrospective studies have produced conflicting results. Initial studies suggested that radionuclide angiography could be used at rest to stratify the risk of peri-operative myocardial infarction in patients undergoing peripheral vascular surgery (Jain *et al.*, 1985; Pasternack *et al.*, 1985).

Risk was increased particularly if resting ejection fraction was less than 35 per cent (Pasternack *et al.*, 1985; Kazmers *et al.*, 1988). However, more recent studies have failed to confirm these findings (Franco *et al.*, 1989), and the role of resting left ventricular function as a predictor of adverse peri-operative cardiac events is doubtful (Cunningham, 1994; ACC, 1996).

Dobutamine stress echocardiography

Dobutamine stress echocardiography (DSE) has potential advantages over other tests because it may allow dynamic assessment of ventricular function, although experience is limited. In two studies where physicians were blinded to the results, the positive predictive values for adverse cardiac outcome were 7 and 14 per cent respectively, with a negative predictive value of 100 per cent (Eichelberger *et al.*, 1993; Poldermans *et al.*, 1993).

Interpretation of the investigations mentioned above requires special expertise, and is subjective to some degree. Meta-analysis of trials involving the efficacy of DPTE, radionuclide angiography, DSE and ambulatory electrocardiography in risk assessment suggested that all four tests were similarly predictive of myocardial ischaemia with overlapping confidence intervals. Therefore the choice of test should account for local expertise (Mantha *et al.*, 1994).

Coronary angiography

Coronary angiography is the definitive investigation of coronary artery disease and the need for revascularization. The indications are similar to those applied in other circumstances and include angina unresponsive to medical therapy, unstable angina, other test results indicative of high cardiac risk, or equivocal results in a clinically high-risk patient. For patients with unstable or unresponsive angina, non-invasive testing is therefore not required and the patient should be scheduled immediately for coronary angiography (Table 15.4) (Fleisher, 1996).

SHOULD PATIENTS HAVE CORONARY REVASCULARIZATION BEFORE PERIPHERAL VASCULAR SURGERY?

Several retrospective studies have assessed the place of coronary revascularization by conventional bypass surgery (Hertzer *et al.*, 1984; Reul *et al.*, 1986) or angioplasty (Elmore *et al.*, 1993; Gottlieb *et al.*, 1998) before subsequent peripheral vascular surgery, but there are few prospective data. The risks of peripheral vascular surgery in patients with documented severe coronary artery disease were decreased in those who had prior coronary revascularization (Hertzer *et al.*, 1984) and furthermore, the long-term risks of coronary artery disease were diminished (Hertzer *et al.*, 1986; 1987; Rihal *et al.*, 1995). In a prospective study of 1546 patients with known coronary artery disease who underwent high-risk noncardiac surgery, the combined risk of death or myocardial infarction was less than 2% in those who had undergone coronary revascularization compared with over 4% in medically treated patients, though there was no difference between groups in patients with single vessel coronary disease. The benefit from coronary artery bypass grafting persisted for up to six years (Eagle *et al.*, 1997). Small observational studies have suggested that the risks of perioperative cardiac death are low in patients who have undergone prior coronary angioplasty (Elmore *et al.*, 1993; Gottlieb *et al.*, 1998). However, the peri-operative morbidity and mortality of cardiac surgery in vascular patients is appreciable; and angioplasty with or without intracoronary stenting is not without risks, including the need for emergency coronary artery bypass grafting. The risks of angioplasty are greater in the elderly, those with systemic atherosclerosis and diabetes (Rihal, 1998). Moreover, the optimal timing of peripheral vascular surgery after coronary angioplasty is not known. In the first few days, the angioplasty site remains at risk of acute vessel closure or thrombosis, whilst the risk of restenosis increases in the first few months; operation after 'at least several days' (ACC, 1996) or 'thirty to forty days' (Rihal, 1998) has been recommended.

The risks of coronary revascularization should also be considered. It is only indicated before peripheral vascular reconstruction if the combined morbidity and mortality is likely to be lower than from vascular surgery alone, and the long-term outcome significantly improved (ACC, 1996). The precise risk/benefit ratio for an individual patient depends on many factors, including local expertise in vascular and coronary revascularization surgery (Fleisher, 1996). However, overall benefits are only likely if the mortality from coronary revascularization is low (2–3 per cent) and the estimated mortality from the vascular surgery is more than 5 per cent (Mason *et al.*, 1995).

Therefore, the indications for coronary angioplasty or surgery are the same as conventional indications for these procedures when peripheral vascular surgery is not being considered (de Bono, 1991; ACC, 1996). For coronary artery bypass grafting these are severe left main stem disease, severe proximal triple vessel disease with left ventricular dysfunction, and intractable ischaemia despite maximal medical therapy in a patient with an acceptable risk for coronary artery revascularization (ACC, 1991). Unfortunately in the absence of prospective controlled clinical trials, the benefits of prior angioplasty or CABG in terms of overall morbidity and mortality in patients scheduled for peripheral vascular surgery remain unproven.

Much of the literature on pre-operative evaluation and peri-operative management of a patient with cardiovascular disease has emanated from the United States, where cardiological referral and investigation may differ from practice in the United Kingdom. In the multifactorial context of peri-operative myocardial ischaemia and infarction, which depends on the balance of coronary oxygen supply and demand, coronary thrombosis, and factors relating to coronary tone, it is recognized that in a situation of changing pathophysiology, the value of pre-operative testing is inevitably limited (Mangano, 1995). In particular, no single pre-operative test is likely to prove discriminating for pre-operative cardiac risk assessment (Fleisher, 1996).

Other pre-operative factors

DIABETES MELLITUS

Diabetes mellitus is common in patients presenting for peripheral vascular reconstruction (Thompson *et al.*, 1993). These patients have a high incidence of associated coronary artery disease (Nesto *et al.*, 1990) and a higher cardiovascular risk from peripheral vascular surgery. In addition, the late results of surgery that are often worse than those for the non-diabetic, partly because of the associated cardiovascular and renal disease, but also the advanced stage of local disease when surgery is considered (Burden, 1992).

The presence of autonomic neuropathy should be specifically sought. This may not only predispose to peri-operative cardiovascular instability, but has also been suggested as the best predictor of silent coronary disease (Fleisher, 1996); the threshold for pre-operative testing therefore should be lower in the diabetic patient. Peri-operative considerations regarding the management of diabetes are similar to those for non-vascular surgery, although the prolonged nature, and possible metabolic disruption from the surgery, make an intravenous insulin regime with frequent monitoring of blood glucose concentration mandatory for all but the briefest of procedures.

ADVANCED AGE

Most patients presenting for peripheral vascular surgery are elderly. Although chronological age does not always correlate with physiological reserve, decreased exercise levels in the elderly may mask cardiorespiratory symptoms and age has often proved an independent risk factor for cardiac complications (Goldman *et al.*, 1977; Shah *et al.*, 1990; Goldman, 1995).

LIPID DISEASES

Hyperlipidaemia, particularly elevated low-density lipoprotein (LDL), is associated with coronary artery disease. Type IV hyperlipidaemia (elevated very low-density lipoprotein, VLDL) is particularly associated with peripheral vascular disease (Greenhalgh *et al.*, 1975). Although hyperlipidaemia has not proved to be an independent risk factor for peri-operative cardiac morbidity (Goldman, 1995; Goldman *et al.*, 1977), it is associated with smoking, lack of exercise and coronary artery disease.

COLLAGEN VASCULAR DISORDERS

Vascular disease may exist in several diseases which occur in younger patients. Patients with systemic lupus erythematosus and lupus anticoagulant may present for peripheral reconstructive surgery. The arteritides of polyarteritis nodosa and rheumatoid arthritis generally respond to steroids, but infective arteritis is rare and therefore it is unusual to encounter such patients presenting at a young age for vascular surgery.

BUERGER'S DISEASE

Buerger's disease, characteristically occurring in male smokers aged 20–45 years, is an obliterative thromboangiitis which usually affects distal vasculature. There is no association with diabetes or hyperlipidaemia, and ECG findings are often normal. Although sympathectomy, anticoagulation or prostaglandin infusion may be successful in terms of symptom relief, arterial bypass may be required in cases of severe skin ulceration or gangrene. As cessation of smoking almost always leads to improvement, patients presenting for surgery (reconstruction or amputation) are usually inveterate smokers with associated cardiorespiratory pathology, with a physiological age exceeding their chronological age.

POPLITEAL AND FEMORAL ANEURYSMS

Aneurysms of the popliteal artery have been compared with abdominal aortic aneurysms in that both occur in the same population, often co-exist in the same patient, and are commonly asymptomatic. Consequently they may be associated with complications by the time patients present clinically, with symptoms of tissue necrosis, rest pain, intermittent claudication or a tender popliteal swelling. Complications include thrombosis, embolization, and vein or nerve compression. Gangrene occurs in 20 per cent of patients at some stage. Treatment commonly comprises autogenous saphenous vein grafting, which occasionally requires the patient to be supine for groin exploration and prone for popliteal dissection. Distal grafting may be required for ischaemic symptoms.

Femoral aneurysms are most commonly iatrogenic, following aortofemoral bypass grafting or femoral catherization, but they may occur in the elderly arteriopath in association with other aneurysms.

Popliteal entrapment syndrome and cystic adventitial disease

Two rare causes of popliteal obstruction in otherwise healthy young adults are popliteal entrapment syndrome and cystic adventitial disease. Both cause symptoms of intermittent calf claudication, and the patients are often non-smokers.

Popliteal entrapment syndrome Popliteal entrapment syndrome is caused by muscular compression of the popliteal artery and characteristically affects physically active young adult males with strong muscular development. Two of the larger series have been described in soldiers, and the syndrome is caused by anomalies of popliteal anatomy (Eastcott *et al.*, 1992). Pulses are typically normal, but the posterior tibial pulse may disappear when the foot is plantar-flexed with the knee extended. Although intermittent claudication is the commonest symptom, local arterial damage may result in popliteal stenosis, aneurysm and thromboembolic ischaemia. Treatment comprises surgical decompression and, if necessary, resection of the diseased vessel.

Cystic adventitial disease Cystic adventitial disease is caused by ganglion-like hypertrophy of the investing tissues of the popliteal artery and causes unilateral claudication with a localized popliteal bruit. Flexion of the knee increases the obstruction (in contrast with popliteal entrapment syndrome) and ischaemic complications are rare. Symptoms may be relieved by aspiration of the cyst, though it tends to recur and operative reconstruction with reversed vein grafting may be required.

Some surgeons prefer to operate with these patients in the prone position. They rarely require any special anaesthetic precaution.

ANAESTHETIC MANAGEMENT

There has been enormous effort expended in attempting to identify risk factors in individual patients. Although there are guidelines (Gersh *et al.*, 1991; ACC, 1996), there is no accord on the best management for individual patients. This may not be surprising because the choice of premedication, pre-operative therapy, anaesthetic technique and monitoring is influenced by many factors. However, several studies on various aspects of *peri-operative* management show that anaesthetic technique and management *is* important in overall outcome (Frank *et al.*, 1993; Mangano, 1995).

Pre-operative evaluation and preparation

Pre-operative evaluation and investigations may reveal treatable medical conditions which should be optimized before surgery. For the elective procedure this should be straightforward, but for patients presenting with a critically ischaemic limb, the benefits

of prolonged pre-operative evaluation and therapy must be balanced against the risks of progressive limb ischaemia.

Patients for peripheral vascular reconstruction have commonly undergone recent angiography to define the nature and severity of their pathology. The patient with a critically ischaemic limb may also be receiving anticoagulant medication. Full anticoagulation is a near total contraindication to regional anaesthesia and the relevance of low-dose heparin and prophylactic aspirin regimes is discussed below.

Concurrent diseases including diabetes, hypertension and ischaemic heart disease should be managed conventionally. For diabetic patients, the prolonged nature of peripheral vascular surgery requires the use of a glucose/insulin regimen. Regional techniques may be associated with less nausea, vomiting, and constitutional upset and may be preferable in the diabetic patient.

Hypertensive patients should be assessed thoroughly for the presence of end-organ damage and should continue their antihypertensive medication until the morning of surgery. There is evidence that pre-operative beta-blockade may diminish perioperative tachycardia, hypertension and ischaemic episodes (Stone *et al.*, 1988a, b). It may also be considered appropriate for the patient with ischaemic heart disease in the absence of contraindications. The threshold for invasive monitoring in the patient with hypertension or overt ischaemic heart disease is lowered, and specific monitoring for myocardial ischaemia should be considered, though this has limitations (Ansley *et al.*, 1996; Yang, 1996). Measures to prevent the pressor responses to tracheal intubation and intra-operative stimuli should be taken, for example the use of short-acting opioids or beta-blockers (Crawford *et al.*, 1987; Korpinen *et al.*, 1995; Miller *et al.*, 1991, 1993).

The presence of overt symptoms of systemic sepsis is a relative contraindication to regional anaesthesia. Such patients may require resuscitation with intravenous fluids guided by invasive monitoring where appropriate, and intravenous antibiotics.

Quality of life is better after limb salvage than after amputation (Pell *et al.*, 1993; Thompson *et al.*, 1995) and patients requiring amputation of part or all of the lower limb have usually undergone previous surgery in an attempt to preserve the limb. The decision to amputate is usually protracted and therefore the patient has time to come to terms with the surgery. They also may have some preference regarding anaesthetic technique (see below). However, psychological preparation and occupational therapy are important parts of pre-operative preparation.

Premedication

Several considerations affect the choice of premedication. The effects of concurrent disease may be prominent, and excessive sedation or associated respiratory depression should be avoided (Knight *et al.*, 1989). Anxiolysis is often desirable for some patients. Many patients presenting for vascular reconstruction or amputation may be dependent on opioid analgesics so the effects of opioid tolerance may be a problem. Other elderly patients may be susceptible to the depressant effects of opioids, or receiving many other drugs, so that individual assessment is required and premedication prescribed cautiously. Concurrent antihypertensive or anti-anginal drugs, or bronchodilators should be continued up to the morning of surgery. Prescribed premedication commonly comprises a benzodiazepine, combined with other specific therapy depending on the patient's condition, but is often omitted according to the patient's and the anaesthetist's preference.

General anaesthetic techniques

INDUCTION

Anaesthesia should be induced as smoothly as possible, with appropriate monitoring in place (see below). Cardiovascular stability and histamine release may be determinants of the choice of intravenous anaesthetic agent, although the rate of administration and total mass of drug used are probably more important in terms of cardiovascular stability. A commonly used technique is balanced anaesthesia with nitrous oxide, opioids and inhalational agents. Intermittent positive ventilation is commonly used with neuromuscular block produced by one of the shorter acting non-depolarizing agents, balancing cardiovascular stability with the possibility of accumulation on repeated dosing in the elderly or those with impaired hepatic or renal function.

AIRWAY MANAGEMENT

The duration of surgery has traditionally dictated airway maintenance with a tracheal tube. Specific manoeuvres to diminish the pressor responses to intubation are advisable. The most commonly used methods are boluses of short-acting intravenous opioids such as fentanyl or alfentanil (Crawford *et al.*, 1987), beta-blockers such as esmolol (Miller *et al.*, 1991) or a combination (Korpinen *et al.*, 1995) to decrease pressor responses. The laryngeal mask airway is associated with less pressor effect (Wilson *et al.*, 1992) and may be suitable for some procedures.

MAINTENANCE

There is no evidence for the superiority of any specific general anaesthetic technique (Forrest *et al.*, 1990) although some authors debate the disadvantages of nitrous oxide or any volatile agent (myocardial depression) or specifically isoflurane (coronary steal) in the high-risk patient. The prolonged nature of peripheral vascular reconstruction and the possibility of poor respiratory function imply that a balanced technique with controlled ventilation is probably preferable. A total intravenous technique could be used, although there is no evidence for any benefit in outcome.

Whatever technique is used, the most important principle is meticulous attention to detail particularly regarding the cardiovascular and respiratory systems and maintenance of temperature. It is essential to maintain haemodynamic stability because tachycardia with hypotension and hypertension have been associated with myocardial ischaemia per- and post-operatively (Slogoff and Keats, 1985; McCann and Clements, 1989). Analgesic requirements for femoropopliteal or distal reconstruction are generally moderate, though opioids are required. Intravenous glyceryl trinitrate is useful in the intra-operative management of myocardial ischaemia, particularly when associated with hypertension. It has theoretical attractions as prophylactic use against intra-operative ischaemia, but the evidence for this is limited, more recent studies suggesting no benefit (Dodds *et al.*, 1993). It also carries the risk of inducing hypotension.

Methods to conserve heat should always be used. Hypothermia leads to vasoconstriction and shivering with adverse effects on myocardial oxygen demand. Hypothermia usually persists for several hours post-operatively, because thermoregulation is impaired by the effects of general anesthesia and opioids. It may be associated with myocardial ischaemia (Frank *et al.*, 1993) and post-operative discomfort (Kurz *et al.*, 1995). For prolonged vascular reconstructive surgery, vasoconstriction associated with hypothermia may impair peripheral perfusion in the initial post-operative period. This may confuse the diagnosis of hypoperfusion caused by graft failure and may possibly predispose to graft thrombosis.

Active measures to prevent heat loss should be undertaken during prolonged vascular reconstructive surgery, including the use of a thermal mattress, topical warming blankets and insulation for exposed areas, and the use of warmed intravenous fluids. The use of a circle breathing system with soda lime absorber helps to diminish heat loss. All potential pressure areas should be protected by the use of padding.

FLUIDS AND MONITORING

Good per-operative hydration is required with judicious replacement of blood loss. If cardiac function is poor, fluids should be administered with caution and be guided by invasive monitoring. In the absence of blood loss, intravenous fluid requirements are often modest, as the 'third space' fluid losses are small because of the peripheral nature of this type of surgery.

A urinary catheter may be needed, because of the prolonged nature of most arterial reconstructions. Temperature monitoring is mandatory for all but the briefest of procedures, and neuromuscular transmission should always be monitored when muscle relaxants are used. The patients are usually elderly, with potentially impaired renal and hepatic function, and cumulation is possible during the course of a prolonged procedure. Routine monitoring of the ECG is limited in the detection of myocardial ischaemia and multilead or ST-segment monitoring is more sensitive. The AHA/ACC Working Party suggested that ST-segment monitoring should be used routinely (ACC, 1996; Fleisher, 1996) although it has limitations (Yang, 1996). Because myocardial ischaemia is common in the post-operative period (Mangano, 1990) and is often silent (Ouyang *et al.*, 1989; Fleisher *et al.*, 1991) continued specific monitoring for myocardial ischaemia should be considered in the high-risk patient.

Transoesophageal echocardiography may be useful for assessing ventricular function and early detection of myocardial ischaemia. However, there are few anaesthestists in the United Kingdom skilled in its use.

Invasive arterial pressure monitoring is necessary during prolonged procedures. It is not without morbidity and the use of Allen's test is unreliable in this context.

Invasive monitoring of central venous pressure or pulmonary artery pressure may be indicated in some patients presenting for peripheral vascular reconstruction. Berlauk and colleagues (1991) compared the use of a pulmonary artery flotation catheter on the pre-operative night (more than 12 hours) with conventional monitoring for 3 hours, before peripheral vein grafting for occlusive vascular disease. An algorithm was used to attain stated haemodynamic end-points pre-operatively. The use of a pulmonary artery catheter was associated with more haemodynamic stability and fewer intra-operative adverse events. The authors reported less post-operative cardiac morbidity and decreased graft thrombosis, but there was no significant effect on the incidence of myocardial infarction or cardiac death. There was a 4.4 per cent incidence of catheter-related morbidity. The study excluded patients with a history of recent myocardial infarction, congestive cardiac failure, symptomatic valvular disease or unstable angina (i.e. all the conventional indications for invasive central monitoring) and some of the conclusions were not supported by the data presented.

Routine use of a pulmonary artery catheter is therefore not justified, though it clearly has a role for selected patients, in particular those with cardiac failure pre-operatively. Its use should be based on the patient's clinical condition, the surgical procedure and the clinical setting within which the practice is based (ASA, 1993). In addition, the successful use of a pulmonary artery catheter depends on correct interpretation of measured and derived variables and therapeutic interventions should reflect the appropriate physiology and pharmacology (Beattie, 1996). A central venous catheter is therefore more commonly used, and allows the administration of inotropes and vasoactive drugs, as well as monitoring of central venous pressure.

RECOVERY FROM ANAESTHESIA

During tracheal extubation and emergence from anaesthesia, there is increased risk of the patient developing tachycardia, hypertension and myocardial ischaemia (Edwards *et al.*, 1994). Before tracheal extubation, patients should be normothermic, normovolaemic, have a haematocrit >30 per cent and be pain-free in order to minimize this risk. If these criteria are not met, post-operative ventilation should be considered. Specific measures such as intravenous glyceryl trinitrate or esmolol may be used to diminish the pressor response to tracheal extubation (Dyson *et al.*, 1990).

Regional anaesthetic techniques

Many peripheral vascular operations may be managed with regional techniques, using them alone or combined with sedation or light general anaesthesia. Because of the prolonged nature of some reconstructive procedures, continuous techniques are often preferred to single-injection methods to ensure sufficient duration of block. A catheter technique also has the advantage that it may be used for post-operative analgesia. Combined spinal epidural anaesthesia techniques may be used increasingly for peripheral vascular surgery.

EFFECTS ON OUTCOME

Regional anaesthesia has several theoretical advantages over general anaesthesia. These include modification of the cardiovascular and metabolic responses to stress (Kehlet, 1984), and effects on blood coagulation (Tuman *et al.*, 1991; Christopherson *et al.*, 1993; Rosenfeld *et al.*, 1993) and respiratory function (Raggi *et al.*, 1987). However, several studies performed to see if these potential benefits are accompanied by a decrease in cardiovascular morbidity and mortality have produced conflicting results. In a mixed population of patients undergoing a variety of vascular procedures (abdominal aortic, carotid and peripheral vascular reconstruction), Yeager and colleagues (1987) found a decrease in morbidity and mortality amongst patients receiving epidural block. However, others have found no effect of anaesthetic technique on cardiovascular outcome in either mixed surgical (Baron *et al.*, 1991; Davies *et al.*, 1993b; Jayr *et al.*, 1993) or vascular patients (Cook *et al.*, 1986; Christopherson *et al.*, 1993; Bode *et al.*, 1996). A review of outcome studies concluded that the only studies showing a significant benefit on cardiovascular outcome had been small with little control of the extent of surgery (Blake, 1995).

The largest and most recent prospective randomized study to compare epidural, subarachnoid and general anaesthesia in patients undergoing peripheral vascular surgery was undertaken in 423 patients scheduled for femorodistal reconstruction (Bode *et al.*, 1996). The patients were of a high risk for perioperative myocardial complications: 86 per cent had diabetes mellitus, 69 per cent were hypertensive, 41 per cent smoked and 36 per cent had a history of previous myocardial infarction. The incidence of myocardial events (myocardial infarction, angina, congestive cardiac failure) or death was 2–6 per cent (with no significant differences between the three groups), and the study was abandoned because the incidence of significant events was so low that unfeasible numbers of patients would have been required to demonstrate any difference in outcome. All patients were monitored using a pulmonary artery catheter for 48 hours post-operatively and they received prophylactic glyceryl trinitrate infusions, albeit without predetermined end-points.

This degree of peri-operative care may have contributed to the low overall morbidity and mortality, even in a high-risk diabetic population. In addition, a particular feature of the study was that surgical variables were well controlled, in contrast with some previous studies. Also of note, although without obvious explanation, were the higher death rate and trend towards increased morbidity in a subgroup which had inadequate regional anaesthesia. In an accompanying editorial Go and Browner (1996) combined the results of all previous studies and found no difference in peri-operative or short-term cardiac mortality between epidural and general anaesthesia (95 per cent confidence intervals of +3 to –3 per cent). Combining the outcomes of any cardiac event or death, there was a possible benefit of general anaesthesia of up to 1.5 per cent (95 per cent confidence intervals –4 to +7 per cent). It was concluded that a larger sample size might find a statistically, but not a clinically, significant difference in outcome between regional and general anaesthesia, suggesting that further research in this area is unlikely to be required.

SURGICAL STRESS

One of the cited advantages of regional compared with general anaesthesia is that it may diminish the stress response to surgery. Attenuation of stress-mediated tachycardia and hypertension, and decreases in preload and afterload, all produced by sympathetic block and contributing to decreases in myocardial oxygen consumption are attractive concepts in the patient with cardiovascular disease. Conversely, decreased coronary perfusion pressure due to hypotension may be catastrophic in some patients with severe coronary artery disease (Caplan et al., 1988), although good blood pressure management may diminish this risk. Therefore, any possible beneficial effect of regional anaesthesia on cardiovascular variables depends on the level of sympathetic blockade, baseline blood volume, cardiovascular function and technique used; it may be harmful if performed injudiciously (Gelman, 1996).

Epidural analgesia has been used to diminish the neuroendocrine response to major surgery (Gelman, 1996). Lower-limb vascular reconstructive surgery causes less pain and surgical stress than major intra-abdominal or orthopaedic surgery, so the potential benefits are less. However, epidural anaesthesia prolonged into the post-operative period has been associated with a smaller increase in plasma catecholamines after peripheral vascular reconstruction, but with no effect on urinary cortisol (Breslow et al., 1993). The effect on catecholamines probably resulted from improved analgesia (Parker et al., 1995) . Although the concept of decreasing the potentially harmful effects of the stress response to surgery is attractive, there is little evidence to show that this is associated with improved outcome.

EFFECTS ON PERIPHERAL BLOOD FLOW AND COAGULATION

Blood flow through a graft is a major determinant of immediate graft patency in peripheral arterial reconstructive surgery (Bandyk et al., 1985; Davies et al., 1993a; Atassanoff, 1996). Limb blood flow depends on cardiac output, peripheral vascular resistance and circulating blood volume, and may be decreased by hypothermia, hypovolaemia and pain. The effect of an epidural on graft blood flow was first demonstrated about thirty years ago, graft flow increasing by over 50 per cent (Cousins and Wright, 1971). The arterial pressure remained unchanged, so the increase was attributed to a reduction in peripheral vascular resistance. These findings have since been confirmed (Hickey et al., 1995). Surgical sympathectomy has a similar effect and is used therapeutically for vasospastic disease (Tracy and Reid, 1992).

The stress response to surgical trauma includes a tendency to increased blood coagulation mediated by several pathways, including an increase in circulating procoagulant factors, factor VIII, von Willebrand factor and fibrinogen (Gelman, 1993), increased platelet aggregation (McDaniel et al., 1984; Naesh et al., 1994), a decrease in inhibitors of coagulation antithrombin III and protein C (Flinn et al., 1984; McDaniel et al., 1984) and inhibition of fibrinolysis (Gelman, 1993). Epidural block has been shown to attenuate this hypercoagulability by effects on platelets, coagulation factors and the fibrinolytic pathway (Borg and Modig, 1985; Naesh et al., 1994). Regional anaesthesia results in a decrease in the incidence of deep venous thrombosis (Modig et al., 1983) after hip surgery as a result of effects on peripheral blood flow and attenuation of the hypercoagulable post-operative state. Several studies have therefore looked at the relationship between graft function and regional anesthesia.

Tuman and colleagues (1991) used thromboelastography (TEG) to indicate fibrinogen–platelet activity and compare the effects of anaesthetic technique on outcome after major vascular surgery. Patients received epidural analgesia and the attention of the acute pain team for a mean of 2.4 days post-operatively. The general anaesthesia group received intramuscular opioids for pain relief, and another group undergoing non-vascular surgery acted as controls for the TEG variables, there being evidence of accelerated coagulation before surgery in the vascular patients. With general anaesthesia coagulability increased further and graft failure occurred in 20 per cent. Post-operative graft thrombosis was reduced significantly in the vascular patients who received epidural block, and this was associated with a reduction in coagulability towards the level of the non-vascular controls. Similar changes occurred in the non-vascular patients who received an epidural. The incidence of cardiovascular and respiratory morbidity was also reduced in the epidural group.

Christopherson and colleagues (1993) assessed the effects of an epidural on peri-operative cardiac morbidity in 100 patients undergoing infra-inguinal reconstruction. There was an increased rate of re-operation for graft occlusion in the general anaesthesia group (11 vs. 2 patients), but no difference in peri-operative cardiac outcome and the study was terminated early. In a subset of these patients, plasma indicators of fibrinolytic activity were also measured 24 and 72 hours after operation. There was some indication of decreased fibrinolysis in the general anaesthetic group and it was suggested that impaired fibrinolysis renders some patients susceptible to peri-operative thrombosis.

These studies attracted much attention because of the suggestion that general anaesthesia is associated with impaired fibrinolysis (and hence hypercoagulability) that may contribute to graft failure. However, several factors relating to graft thrombosis were not controlled in these studies, which were designed primarily to examine peri-operative cardiac morbidity. These factors included peri-operative administration of heparin, dextran, non-steroidal anti-inflammatory drugs and antiplatelet drugs (Gelman, 1993), and surgical factors, including disease severity, although no difference was reported between the groups. However, the overall incidence of graft failure (13 per cent) was high (Kupelli, 1993).

A retrospective analysis of patients in the same study by the same authors, while re-affirming the apparent association between general anaesthesia, impaired fibrinolysis and graft thrombosis, also found that poor run-off at operation was noted more often in the general anaesthesia group, suggesting that randomization of technical surgical factors may have been 'less than optimal' (Perler et al., 1995). A total of 14 surgeons performed the operations, and individual complication rates were not reported. However, re-operation salvaged several of the grafts in the general anaesthesia group to produce similar secondary patency rates in the groups. The authors suggested that 'it is possible that technical problems at the original operation may have occurred more frequently in the general anaesthesia group'. Conclusions regarding the effect of epidural anaesthesia on graft function after peripheral reconstruction must therefore be viewed with caution.

In an analysis of their work on the effect of anaesthetic technique (regional or general anaesthesia) on cardiac outcome after femorodistal reconstruction, Pierce et al. (1997) found no difference in the rates of graft occlusion, re-operation or amputation. This study was designed to analyse cardiac outcome in a group of high-risk patients (over 80 per cent diabetic). There was a low rate of graft complication (>97 per cent patent at 30 days) and low statistical power, possibly attributable to close post-operative monitoring for 48–72 h and administration of heparin and aspirin to all patients. However, this study uniquely recorded surgical variables including indication for surgery, type and site of graft, and grade of surgeon, in accordance with accepted reporting standards

(Rutherford, 1991). Another recent retrospective study of 294 patients undergoing infra-inguinal revascularization with general or epidural anaesthesia found no difference in mortality or early graft thrombosis (14 per cent epidural, 9.4 per cent general) (Schunn et al., 1998). Although the factors involved in early and late graft failure may differ, it is clear that several influences alter graft patency. Late graft failure (more than 30 days after operation) is caused more commonly by intrinsic factors such as anastomotic stenosis, vein stricture and kinking, rather than compromised distal outflow, hypotension or hypercoagulability (Donaldson et al., 1992). These data suggest therefore that any potential benefits of epidural anaesthesia (continued into the post-operative period) are minor and insignificant in the overall context of graft survival. Clearly, more well-controlled prospective randomized trials are required.

EPIDURAL ANAESTHESIA, ANTICOAGULANTS AND ASPIRIN

The subject of epidural or subarachnoid anaesthesia in patients taking antiplatelet medication or thromboprophylaxis with heparin has been much debated during the last decade. Several retrospective reviews of peri-operative anticoagulant use have suggested that low dose (5000 IU) prophylactic or intra-operative heparin is safe (Berqvist et al., 1992), provided that the heparin is not administered within 4 hours before, or 1 hour after, institution of the block (Wildsmith and McClure, 1991). In the widely-quoted prospective study of Rao and El-Etr (1981), 4000 patients underwent peripheral vascular surgery with epidural or continuous subarachnoid anaesthetic and peri-operative heparin without neurological complications. Particular precautions were taken, including close attention to the timing of anticoagulant administration, titration of heparin according to measured activated clotting times and postponement of surgery if blood was encountered at any stage during insertion of the epidural catheter.

The recent introduction of low-molecular-weight heparins (LMWHs) into clinical practice has led to a resurgence of awareness of the problem of undertaking spinal and epidural anaesthesia in patients receiving thromboprophylaxis with these drugs. Enoxaparin was the first LMWH introduced in 1993 into the United States. Shortly afterwards, sporadic case reports of epidural haematoma led the Food and Drug Administration to issue a warning in 1997 on the problems associated with LMWHs. The frequency of spinal haematoma in this population was assessed as between 1/1000 and 1/10 000 central blocks (Horlocker and Heit, 1997). However, in Europe LMWHs were introduced in 1987 and Bergqvist *et al.* (1992) estimated that more than 1 000 000 patients received LMWHs safely in association with regional anaesthesia. An important difference between the North American and European experience was that much higher doses of LMWHs were used in North America. The issue is also discussed in Chapter 10.

If cancellation of surgery is deemed necessary in these circumstances, the risk:benefit ratio of regional anaesthesia is altered markedly, and the question of what to do if blood is encountered on insertion of the catheter has not been fully resolved. It has been suggested that all patients taking aspirin should have the bleeding time assessed before epidural anaesthesia (Macdonald, 1991), but the variability of this test in the clinical setting precludes its routine use at present. In a retrospective study of 1000 patients who had regional techniques, 39 per cent of whom were taking non-steroidal anti-inflammatory drugs, there were no neurological complications (Horlocker *et al.*, 1990) and data from the CLASP (1994) trial confirmed epidural anaesthesia was safe in the patient taking aspirin.

In summary, there is no convincing evidence at present that either general or regional anaesthesia *per se* is superior in terms of cardiovascular or respiratory function for peripheral vascular surgery. This is perhaps not surprising in view of the large number of dynamic variables in any clinical situation. The evidence to suggest that graft survival is improved when a regional technique is used is flawed, and further studies are necessary. At present, the choice of technique should be determined by other factors such as the duration of operation, pre-operative status and patient preference.

POST-OPERATIVE MANAGEMENT

Over the last few years, there has been increasing interest in the importance of careful management in the post-operative period. The benefits of good pain management, respiratory care, oxygen therapy and cardiovascular monitoring have been recognized. There are specific problems for the vascular surgical patient, including hypothermia, hypoxaemia and myocardial ischaemia.

Hypothermia

Elderly patients undergoing prolonged surgical procedures, including peripheral vascular reconstruction, are at particular risk of hypothermia. This is associated with shivering, thermal discomfort (Kurz *et al.*, 1995), increased sympathetic nervous activity and oxygen consumption, and may increase the risk of post-operative morbidity (Slotman *et al.*, 1985). Using Holter monitoring for 24 hours after lower-limb revascularization, Frank and colleagues (1993) studied 100 consecutive patients, and found that hypothermia (core temperature < 35°C) was associated with hypoxaemia, angina and myocardial ischaemia. There was no association between type of anaesthesia (regional or general) and the occurrence of hypothermia or myocardial ischaemia. Close attention to temperature monitoring and intra-operatively conservation of heat is therefore required.

Post-operative hypoxaemia

The aetiology of post-operative hypoxaemia is multifactorial, but predisposing conditions include age, pre-operative status, site and duration of surgery, and administration of opioids. Lung volumes, including forced vital capacity and functional residual capacity, decrease for several days after surgery and this leads to ventilation–perfusion mismatch and hypoxaemia (Craig, 1981). These changes are less marked than after upper abdominal surgery, but they are still important after peripheral vascular surgery because the patient population is at high risk of developing myocardial ischaemia.

Post-operative nocturnal hypoxaemia is common after surgery, and is undetectable clinically in 95 per cent of cases (Moller *et al.*, 1990). It may be associated with myocardial ischaemia (Pateman and Hanning, 1989; Rosenberg *et al.*, 1990; Reeder *et al.*, 1991), particularly if prolonged (> 5 min) and severe (SpO_2 < 85 per cent) (Gill *et al.*, 1992). Supplementary oxygen improves the mean saturation, but episodic hypoxaemia may still occur (Rosenberg *et al.*, 1992). The associated myocardial ischaemia may also be reversed by oxygen administration, but may occur during the first two post-operative nights in some patients even when oxygen saturation is within the normal range (Reeder *et al.*, 1992).

It has been suggested that oxygen should be administered to all patients after operation for 24 hours and to 'at-risk' patients for at least another 3–4 days, and be accompanied by monitoring by pulse oximetry or blood gas analysis (Oh, 1992). Most of the data on post-operative hypoxaemia refer to abdominal surgical patients and it may be less severe after peripheral vascular surgery, but data are lacking. At present, it seems sensible that supplementary oxygen is given to all vascular patients for at least 24 hours after operation, and that 'high-risk' patients should be monitored with pulse oximetry and receive supplementary oxygen for a further 2–3 days. There is no consensus on the dose or duration of oxygen, and no evidence at present that outcome is affected.

Myocardial ischaemia

Adverse cardiac events occur more commonly after, rather than before or during, operation (Mangano *et al.*, 1990). The risk of post-operative ischaemia is increased if there is intra-operative ischaemia (Dodds *et al.*, 1993): post-operative ST-segment changes are a strong predictor of adverse peri-operative cardiac events (Fleisher *et al.*, 1995b). Furthermore, if the patient does suffer a peri-operative myocardial infarction, the incidence of subsequent post-operative myocardial infarction is greatly increased (Fleisher, 1996; ACC, 1996), and long-term survival is shortened (Mangano *et al.*, 1992).

Mangano and colleagues (1990) used continuous ECG monitoring in 474 patients at high risk of coronary artery disease, but undergoing non-cardiac surgery, from 2 days before to 2 days after operation. They found that 41 per cent of ischaemic episodes occurred post-operatively compared with 20 per cent pre- and 25 per cent intra-operatively, and that 47 per cent of ischaemic events occurred after the third post-operative day. Post-operative ischaemia was often precipitated by tachycardia, and ischaemia in the early post-operative period was associated with a ninefold increase in the incidence of major cardiac complications. Several episodes of ischaemia were not accompanied by haemodynamic aberrations, and were commonly asymptomatic, as others have found (Knight *et al.*, 1989; Muir *et al.*, 1991; Landesberg *et al.*, 1993; Gill *et al.*, 1996).

McCann and Clements (1989) used continuous Holter monitoring from the night before, until the third night after, surgery in 50 patients undergoing lower-extremity revascularization. Thirty-eight per cent of patients had evidence of myocardial ischaemia which was associated with cardiac morbidity. All except one of these episodes were painless and undetectable clinically; an association with tachycardia was noted. There were no differences in clinical characteristics between those with and those without ischaemia, and it was suggested that prolonged post-operative monitoring was worthwhile.

Although it may have limitations (Yang, 1996), prolonged cardiac monitoring with multiple lead ECG and ST-segment monitoring is probably worthwhile in the higher risk patient, particularly if there has been intra-operative hypotension or evidence of myocardial ischaemia. Optimization of cardiovascular status, fluid balance, haematocrit, oxygenation and analgesia are essential before and during surgery to minimize the risks of cardiovascular morbidity (and may contribute to surgical outcome), but any benefit is unlikely to be realized without similar attention after operation. This implies high dependency-type care, with its attendant resource implications.

Post-operative analgesia

The extent of post-operative pain after peripheral vascular surgery is considerably less than that after more proximal intra-abdominal surgery. Occasionally, surgery itself relieves ischaemia-induced rest pain. Unless the patient has received an intra-operative extradural as part of the anaesthetic technique therefore, it is not usually necessary to use advanced analgesic techniques and, because ileus is not a problem, the change from parenteral to oral opioid administration may occur early in the post-operative period.

LOWER LIMB AMPUTATION

The indications for amputation of a varying part of the lower limb have changed with developments in vascular surgery. Absolute indications include failed vascular reconstruction, the presence of severe infection with loss of function, infected gangrene with the risk of systemic septicaemia (particularly in the diabetic), and severe, intractable rest pain in a patient unfit for more prolonged surgery. Relative indications include intractable ischaemic ulceration and combined arterial ischaemic and venous occlusive disease (Robinson, 1992). In 1989, of the referrals for limb fitting in the United Kingdom, 67 per cent of patients had amputation for vascular insufficiency, and 24 per cent were diabetic (Eastcott and Redhead, 1992). Vascular reconstructive surgery is more likely to fail if the patient continues to smoke cigarettes, is diabetic or has severe or multilevel disease (Eastcott et al., 1992).

Apart from those related to trauma, patients presenting for amputation are likely to have severe widespread vascular disease, have had recent previous anaesthetics, and may have been bed-bound, resulting in debilitation and poor nutritional state. The administration of large doses of opioid analgesics may result in tolerance and the overall condition of the patient is thus likely to be worse than when the individual presented for elective vascular reconstruction. It is vital to consider the specific treatment of concomitant medical conditions, and physiotherapy, antibiotics and treatment of cardiovascular disease may be required before surgery. The overall mortality rate is 7–10 per cent.

Amputation may be performed at a number of levels: toes, transmetatarsal, ankle or Syme's operation, below, through or above knee. The risks are greater with more proximal surgery, if only because the patient's general condition may be worse. Between 15 and 20 per cent of patients undergoing below-knee amputation subsequently require above-knee amputation. The long-term survival at two years after above-knee amputation is 33–66 per cent, with 12–24 per cent having also lost the opposite limb by this time (Eastcott and Redhead, 1992).

Patients presenting for amputation therefore have risk factors additional to those present in patients presenting for vascular reconstructive surgery, and a careful anaesthetic technique is important. Stump survival is influenced by several factors, particularly blood flow, and a careful anaesthetic technique avoiding hypotension, hypothermia and hypovolaemia is paramount. Regional anaesthesia by subarachnoid or epidural routes is known to improve peripheral blood flow, decrease platelet hyperaggregability, and is associated with improvement in thromboelastographic markers of fibrinogen–platelet activity in vascular surgical patients (see above). There may be less disturbance of respiratory function or disruption of diabetic control regimens, decreased blood loss (Mann and Bissett, 1983; Cook et al., 1986), and there is some evidence that regional techniques may also decrease the incidence of phantom-limb pain (see below).

A controlled spinal or epidural anaesthetic therefore has several potential advantages, provided that intravenous fluids are used judiciously and undue hypotension is avoided, although in a small study comparing the effects of spinal anaesthesia with sedation and general anaesthesia, there were no differences in cardiovascular or respiratory morbidity (Mann and Bissett, 1983). The main disadvantages of regional techniques are concerns over systemic anticoagulation and patient objection, as many patients would prefer to be unconscious. An alternative is the combination of sciatic and 'triple' (femoral, obturator and lateral cutaneous nerve of the thigh) nerve blocks with a light general anaesthetic. When prolonged post-operatively, nerve blockade may contribute to diminished phantom pain (Fisher and Meller, 1991), although the evidence is conflicting (Elizaga et al., 1994).

Phantom limb pain

Phantom limb pain can be defined as pain felt in the absent part of the limb. Two types of pain predominate. One type is a burning or throbbing pain, while the other presents as an abnormal ischaemic discomfort ranging from mild to excrutiating. This is separate from phantom-limb sensation, which does not include pain, but usually includes paraesthesiae, and a feeling of limb distortion and is present in almost all amputees, and usually disappears in the first year after amputation. Stump pain, distinct from phantom pain, is the painful sensory phenomenon perceived in the region of amputation that may be localized to one small area or occur diffusely throughout the amputated region (Wesoleski and Lema, 1993).

The prevalence of some degree of phantom pain has been reported at up to 80 per cent one year after traumatic amputation (Sherman, 1994), although it is less after amputation for peripheral vascular disease. It tends to diminish in severity and frequency with time (Jensen and Rasmussen, 1994), but persistent, severe pain may still occur in 5–10 per cent of patients two years after amputation. Phantom pain is very difficult to treat, and the number of differing medical, psychological and surgical treatments available attest to this. A survey in the United States in 1980 showed that 68 unrelated treatments were in use at that time, each with its enthusiasts, but none had been shown to be universally successful (Sherman et al., 1980). The majority of surgical treatments, including rhizotomy, cordotomy or thalamotomy have proven ineffectual. Dorsal-root entry-zone lesions may be more effective in the treatment of phantom pain except when amputation has been performed for cancer or vascular insufficiency. Dorsal-column stimulation has also been unsuccessful.

One theory of phantom pain suggests that the pain is a 'memory' of pre-existing pain. Phantom pain closely resembles pre-existing pain in location and character in 36 per cent of amputees (Loeser, 1990; Jensen and Rasmussen, 1994), and it occurs much more commonly in those with pain before amputation and on the day of amputation compared with those without pain. Furthermore, in patients with established phantom pain, subsequent subarachnoid anaesthesia may cause re-appearance of phantom pain, or the appearance of phantom pain in others. Prolonged post-operative femoral or sciatic nerve blockade has been used to provide post-operative stump analgesia, and diminish opioid requirements (Pavy and Doyle, 1996) and one report suggested that phantom pain in a group of vascular patients at one year might be decreased in this way, compared with historical controls (Fisher and Meller, 1991). In contrast, however, no benefit in terms of analgesia, opioid requirements or phantom limb pain at six months was found from prolonged sciatic nerve blockade (mean 4.1 days) in a heterogeneous group of amputees (Elizaga et al., 1994). Cousins (1979) demonstrated that pre-operative chemical lumbar sympathectomy produced a significant relief of rest pain for a mean duration of almost six months in 386 patients with vascular insufficiency of the lower limbs. Notably, of those patients who subsequently required amputation, no patient experienced phantom pain.

Perhaps the most well-known preventative strategy involves pre-operative epidural anaesthesia. Bach and colleagues (1988) used pre-operative epidural anaesthesia with morphine and/or bupivacaine to abolish pain for 72 hours before operation, in 11 patients scheduled for lower limb amputation and in whom there was no contraindication to the epidural. The block was continued through the operation and for three days afterwards, control patients receiving general anaesthesia and systemic opioid analgesics post-operatively. The patients who received epidurals experienced less phantom pain (defined as any painful sensation referred to the amputated limb), at seven days, and were all pain free at six months and one year later. However, patients whose pain was not abolished by the epidural were excluded from further analysis, and the differences between groups were not statistically significant at seven days or one year.

Jahangiri and colleagues (1994) found a significant decrease in the incidence of phantom pain and phantom limb sensation 7 days, 6 months and one year after amputation in patients who received epidural diamorphine, clonidine and bupivacaine pre- and post-operatively compared with those receiving on-demand opioids, in a prospective, open study. However, in the largest and best-designed study to date, patients were randomized to receive either epidural bupivacaine and morphine, or epidural saline with oral and intramuscular morphine, for 18 hours before lower limb amputation (Nikolajsen et al., 1997). Following surgery under standard general anaesthesia, epidural morphine and bupivacaine was continued in all patients for approximately one week. The incidence of phantom and stump pain was high (75 per cent compared with 69 per cent after 12 months in the pre-operative epidural and control groups respectively), with no differences in opioid requirements or pain intensity at any point during the study. The effect of epidural analgesia on the subsequent development of phantom or stump pain following limb amputation is therefore uncertain. In view of the high incidence and refractory nature of phantom pain, further research is required.

NEWER THERAPEUTIC TECHNIQUES

Angioplasty

Non-invasive techniques have increased in popularity over the last two decades. At the Leicester Royal Infirmary, approximately 70 per cent of patients referred with symptoms of peripheral vascular disease are treated by angioplasty, local fibrinolysis or endovascular techniques. Angioplasty is ideal for discrete iliac or femoropopliteal occlusions, although its place is expanding rapidly, and it is usually performed in the radiology department, with no involvement of the anaesthetist. The risks of sedation in the radiology department are well recognized, and it may be that anaesthetic input is required for angioplasty in the ill patient. In this case, the problems of sedation or a general anaesthetic technique in a darkened, distant environment may be compounded by the poor condition of the patient, and regional techniques may be a useful alternative. A recognized complication of angioplasty is distal embolization or occasionally perforation, and surgery may be required as an emergency in these circumstances, when pre-operative preparation may be minimal. Re-stenosis may occur in around 30 per cent of cases.

Endovascular techniques

Endovascular stenting involves the insertion of a self-expandable or balloon-expandable endoprosthesis, and is well established in the treatment of aorto-iliac occlusive disease where anaesthesia is required (Dietrich, 1996). Its use in femoral or popliteal arterial disease is less well established (Henry and Amor, 1996). Indications at present are residual stenosis after angioplasty, undilatable stenosis after angioplasty, dissection after angioplasty, or re-stenosis (Table 15.5). As with angioplasty, anaesthetic involvement is limited because these procedures are commonly performed under local anaesthesia with sedation, but they may present a real challenge when anaesthetic assistance is required. The judicious use of a regional technique might have advantages under these circumstances. The subsequent use of small doses of intravenous heparin (5000 IU) after an appropriate interval in this situation should not be regarded as a contraindication to regional anaesthesia.

Future developments

It is likely that the use of non-invasive treatment of peripheral vascular disease will continue to increase. In addition, the recognition that improvements in medical conditions, particularly cardiac failure, can lead to improvements in symptoms and signs of peripheral vascular disease (Eastcott *et al.*, 1992), may influence the numbers of patients presenting for vascular reconstruction. However, with an ageing population, and a recognition of the benefits of treatment for the elderly, it may be that the patients presenting for surgery and anaesthesia are those in whom medical therapy or non-invasive techniques

Table 15.5 *Indications for endovascular procedures in the lower limb*

- Residual stenosis after angioplasty
- Undilatable stenosis after angioplasty
- Dissection after angioplasty
- Re-stenosis

have failed. The contribution of good anaesthetic management becomes even more important for a successful outcome.

REFERENCES

ACC, 1991. Guidelines and indications for coronary artery bypass graft surgery: a report of the American College of Cardiology/American Heart Association Task Force on Assessment of Diagnostic and therapeutic cardiovascular procedures (Subcommittee on coronary artery bypass surgery). *Journal of American College of Cardiology* **17**, 543–589.

ACC, 1996. Guidelines for Perioperative Cardiovascular Evaluation for Noncardiac Surgery: Report of the American College of Cardiology/American Heart Association Task Force on Practice Guidelines (Committee on Perioperative Cardiovascular Evaluation for Noncardiac Surgery). *Journal of American College of Cardiology* **27**, 910–948.

Ansley, D.M., O'Connor, P., Merrick, P.M. *et al.* 1996. On line ST-Segment analysis for detection of myocardial ischaemia during and after coronary revascularization. *Canadian Journal of Anaesthesia* **43**, 995–1000.

ASA, 1993. Practice Guidelines for Pulmonary Artery Catheterization. A Report by the American Society of Anesthesiologists Task Force on Pulmonary Artery Catherization. *Anesthesiology* **78**, 380–394.

Ashton, C.M., Petersen, N.J., Wray, N.P. *et al.* 1993. The incidence of perioperative myocardial infarction in men undergoing noncardiac surgery. *Annals of Internal Medicine* **118**, 504–510.

Atanassoff, P.G. 1996. Effects of regional anesthesia on perioperative outcome. *Journal of Clinical Anesthesia* **8**, 446–455.

Bach, S., Noreng, M.F. and Tjellden, N.U. 1988. Phantom limb pain in amputees during the first 12 months following limb amputation, after preoperative lumbar epidural blockade. *Pain* **33**, 297–301.

Bandyk, D.F., Cato, R.F. and Towne, J.B. 1985. A low flow velocity predicts failure of femoropopliteal and femorotibial bypass grafts. *Surgery* **98**(4), 799–809.

Baron, J-F., Bertrand, M., Barre, E. *et al.* 1991. Combined epidural and general anesthesia versus general anesthesia for abdominal aortic surgery. *Anesthesiology* **75**, 611–618.

Baron, J-F., Mundler, O., Bertrand, M. *et al*. 1994. Dipyridamole-thallium scintigraphy and gated radionuclide angiography to assess cardiac risk before abdominal aortic surgery. *New England Journal of Medicine* **330**, 663–669.

Beattie, C. 1996. Anaesthesia for major vascular surgery. *Canadian Journal of Anaesthesia* **43**, R3–R7

Bedford R.F. and Fenstein, B. 1980. Hospital admission blood pressure: a predictor for hypertension following endotracheal intubation. *Anesthesia and Analgesia* **59**, 367–370.

Berlauk, J.F., Abrams, J.H., Gilmour, I.J. *et al*. 1991. Preoperative optimization of cardiovascular hemodynamics improves outcome in peripheral vascular surgery. *Annals of Surgery* **214**, 289–297.

Bergqvist, D., Lindblad, B. and Matzsch, T. 1992. Low molecular weight heparin for thromboprophylaxis and epidural/spinal anaesthesia – is there a risk? *Acta Anesthesiologica Scandinavica* **36**, 605–609.

Blake, D.W. 1995. The general versus regional anaesthesia debate: time to re-examine the goals. *Australia and New Zealand Journal of Surgery* **65**, 51–56.

de Bono, D.P. and Rose, E.L. 1991. Silent myocardial ischaemia in preoperative patients: What does it mean, and what should be done about it? *British Journal of Anaesthesia* **67**, 367–368.

Borg, T. and Modig, J. 1985. Potential antithrombotic effects of local anaesthetics due to their inhibition of platelet aggregation. *Acta Anesthesiologica Scandinavica* **29**, 739–742.

Bode, R.H., Lewis, K.P., Zarich, S.W. *et al*. 1996. Cardiac outcome after peripheral vascular surgery: Comparison of general and regional anesthesia. *Anesthesiology* **84**, 3–13.

Breslow, M.J., Parker, S.D., Frank S.M. *et al*. 1993. Determinants of catecholamine and cortisol responses to lower extremity revascularization. *Anesthesiology* **79**, 1202–1209.

Buchbinder, D., Singh, J.K., Karmody, A.M. *et al*. 1981. Comparison of patency rate and structural change of 'in-situ' and reversed vein arterial bypass. *Journal of Surgical Research* **30**, 213–222.

Burden, A.C. 1992. Diabetes and vascular disease. In Bell, P.F.R., Jamieson, C.W. and Vaughan Ruckley, C. (eds), *Surgical management of vascular disease*. London: W.B. Saunders.

Caplan, R.A., Ward, R.J., Posner, K. and Cheney, F.W. 1988. Unexpected cardiac arrest during spinal anesthesia: A closed claims analysis of predisposing factors. *Anesthesiology* **68**, 5–11.

Chaitman, B.R. 1986. The changing role of the exercise electrocardiogram as a diagnostic and prognostic test for chronic ischemic heart disease. *Journal of the American College of Cardiology* **8**, 1195–1210.

Christopherson, R., Beattie, S., Frank. *et al*. 1993. Perioperative morbidity in patients randomized to epidural or general anesthesia for lower extremity vascular surgery. *Anesthesiology* **79**, 422–434.

CLASP Collaborative Group 1994. CLASP: a randomised trial of low-dose aspirin for the prevention and treatment of pre-eclampsia among 9364 pregnant women. *Lancet* **343**(8898), 619–629.

Cook, P.T., Davies, M.J., Cronin, K.D. and Moran, P. 1986. A prospective randomised trial comparing spinal anaesthesia using hyperbaric cinchocaine with general anaesthesia for lower limb vascular surgery. *Anaesthesia and Intensive Care* **14**, 373–380.

Cousins, M.J. and Wright, C.J. 1971. Graft, muscle, skin blood flow after epidural block in vascular surgical procedures. *Surgery, Gynecology and Obstetrics* July, 59–64.

Cousins, M.J. 1979. Neurolytic lumbar sympathetic blockade: duration of denervation and relief of rest pain. *Anaesthesia and Intensive Care* **7**, 271– 235.

Craig, D.B. 1981. Postoperative recovery of pulmonary function. *Anesthesia and Analgesia* **60**, 46–52.

Crawford, D.C., Fell, D., Achola, K.J. and Smith, G. 1987. Effects of alfentanil on the pressor and catecholamine responses to tracheal intubation. *British Journal of Anaesthesia* **59**, 707–712.

Cunningham, A.J. 1994. Anaesthesia for abdominal and major vascular surgery. In Nimmo, W.S., Rowbotham, D.J. and Smith, G. (eds), *Anaesthesia*. London: Blackwell.

Cutler, B.S., Wheeler, H.B., Paraskos, J.A. and Cardullo, P.A. 1981. Applicability and interpretation of electrocardiographic stress testing in patients with peripheral vascular disease. *American Journal of Surgery* **141**, 501–506.

Davies, A.H., Ramarakha, P., Collin, J. and Morris, P.J. 1990. Recent changes in the treatment of aortoiliac occlusive disease by the Oxford Regional Vascular Service. *British Journal of Surgery* **77**, 1129–1131.

Davies, A.H., Magee, T.R., Baird, R.N. and Horrocks, M. 1993a. Intraoperative measurement of graft resistance as a predictor of early outcome. *British Journal of Surgery* **80**, 854–857.

Davies, M.J., Silbert, B.S., Mooney, P.J. *et al*. 1993b. Combined epidural and general anaesthesia versus general anaesthesia for abdominal aortic surgery: A prospective randomised trial. *Anaesthesia and Intensive Care* **21**, 790–794.

Detsky, A.S., Abrams, H.B., Forbath, N. *et al*. 1986. Cardiac assessment for patients undergoing noncardiac surgery: a multifactorial risk index. *Archives of Internal Medicine* **146**, 2131–2134.

Dietrich, E.B. 1996. Stenting of iliac arteries. In Sigwart U. (ed.), *Endoluminal stenting*. London: W.B. Saunders, 468–475.

Dodds, T.M., Stone, J.G., Coromilas, J. *et al*. 1993. Prophylactic nitroglycerin infusion during noncardiac surgery does not reduce perioperative ischemia. *Anesthesia and Analgesia* **76**, 705–713.

Donaldson C., Mannick, J.A. and Whittemore, A.D. 1992. Causes of primary graft failure after in situ saphenous vein bypass grafting. *Journal of Vascular Surgery* **15**(1), 113–120.

Dunlop, P., Hartshorne, T., Bolia A. *et al*. 1995. The long-term outcome of infrainguinal graft surveillance. *European Journal of Vascular and Endovascular Surgery* **10**, 352–355.

Dyson, A., Isaac, P.A., Pennant, J.H. *et al*. 1990. Esmolol attenuates cardiovascular responses to extubation. *Anesthesia and Analgesia* **71**, 675–678.

Eagle, K.A., Rihal, C.S., Mickel, M.C. *et al*. 1997. Cardiac risk of noncardiac surgery – Influence of coronary disease and type of surgery in 3368 operations. *Circulation* **96**, 1882–1887.

Eagle, K.A., Coley, C.M., Newell, J.B. *et al*. 1989. Combining clinical and thallium data optimizes preoperative assessment of cardiac risk before major vascular surgery. *Annals of Internal Medicine* **110**, 859–866.

Eastcott, H.H.G. and Redhead, R.G. 1992. Amputations. In Eastcott, H.H.G. (ed.), *Arterial surgery*. Edinburgh: Churchill Livingstone.

Eastcott, H.H.G., Veith, F.J. and Bergan, J. 1992. Chronic ischaemia. In Eastcott, H.H.G. (ed.), *Arterial surgery*. Edinburgh: Churchill Livingstone.

Edwards, N.D., Alford, A.M., Dobson, P.M.S. *et al*. 1994. Myocardial ischaemia during tracheal intubation and extubation. *British Journal of Anaesthesia* **73**, 537–539.

Eichelberger, J.P., Schwarz, K.Q., Black, E.R. *et al*. 1993. Predictive value of dobutamine echocardiography just before noncardiac vascular surgery. *American College of Cardiology* **72**, 602–607.

Elizaga, A.M., Smith, D.G., Sharar, S.R. *et al*. 1994. Continuous regional analgesia by intraneural block: Effect on postoperative opioid requirements and phantom limb pain. *Journal of Rehabilitation Research and Development* **31**, 179–187.

Elmore, J.R., Hallett, J.W.Jr., Gibbons, R.J. *et al*. 1993. Myocardial revascularization before abdominal aortic aneurysmorraphy: effect of coronary angioplasty. *Mayo Clinic Procedures* **68**, 637–641.

Fisher, A. and Meller, Y. 1991. Continuous postoperative regional analgesia by nerve sheath block for amputation surgery – a pilot study. *Anesthesia and Analgesia* **72**, 300–303.

Fleisher, L.A., Rosenbaum, S.H., Nelson. *et al*. 1991. The predictive value of preoperative silent ischemia for postoperative ischemic cardiac events in vascular and nonvascular surgery patients. *American Heart Journal* **122**, 980–986.

Fleisher, L.A. 1996. Perioperative management of the cardiac patient undergoing noncardiac surgery. In Barash, P.G. (ed.), *American Society of Anesthesiologists Refresher Course* **24**, 70–84.

Fleisher, L.A., Rosenbaum, S.H., Nelson, A.H. *et al*. 1995a. Preoperative dipyridamole thallium imaging and ambulatory electrocardiographic monitoring as a predictor of perioperative cardiac events and long-term outcome. *Anesthesiology* **83**, 906–917.

Fleisher, L.A., Nelson, A.H. and Rosenbaum, S.H. 1995b. Postoperative myocardial ischemia: Etiology of cardiac morbidity or manifestation of underlying disease? *Journal of Clinical Anesthesia* **7**, 97–102.

Flinn, W.R., McDaniel M.D., Yao, J.S.T. *et al*. 1984. Antithrombin III deficiency as a reflection of dynamic protein metabolism in patients undergoing vascular reconstruction. *Journal of Vascular Surgery* **1**, 888–895.

Forrest, J. B., Cahalan, M.K., Rehder K. *et al*. 1990. Multicenter study of general anesthesia II: results. *Anesthesiology* **72**, 262–268.

Franco, C.D., Goldsmith, J., Veith, F.J. *et al*. 1989. Resting gated pool ejection fraction: a poor predictor of perioperative myocardial infarction in patients undergoing vascular surgery for infrainguinal bypass grafting. *Journal of Vascular Surgery* **10**, 656–661.

Frank, S.M., Beattie, C., Christopherson, R. *et al*. 1993. Unintentional hypothermia is associated with postoperative myocardial ischaemia. *Anesthesiology* **78**, 468–476.

Gelman, S. 1993. General versus regional anesthesia for peripheral vascular surgery. *Anesthesiology* **79**, 415–418.

Gelman, S. 1996. Regional vs. General anesthesia for lower extremity vascular surgery. International Anaesthetic Research Society Review Course Lectures 52–55 (supplement to *Anesthesia and Analgesia*, March 1996).

Gersh, B.J., Rihal, C.S., Rooke, T.W. and Ballard, DJ. 1991. Evaluation and management of patients with both peripheral vascular and coronary artery disease. *Journal of the American College of Cardiology* **18**, 203–214.

Gill, N.P., Wright, B. and Reilly, C.S. 1992. Relationship between hypoxaemia and cardiac ischaemic events in the perioperative period. *British Journal of Anaesthesia* **68**, 471–473.

Gill, J.B., Carins, J.A., Roberts, R.S. *et al.* 1996. Prognostic importance of myocardial ischemia detected by ambulatory monitoring early after acute myocardial infarction. *New England Journal of Medicine* **334**, 65–70.

Go, A.S. and Browner, W.S. 1996. Cardiac outcomes after regional or general anesthesia. Do we have the answer? *Anesthesiology* **84**, 1–2.

Goldman, L. 1995. Cardiac risk in noncardiac surgery: an update. *Anesthesia and Analgesia* **80**, 810–820.

Goldman, L., Caldera, D.L. and Nussbaum, S.R. 1977. Multifactorial index of cardiac risk in noncardiac surgical procedures. *New England Journal of Medicine* **297**, 845–850.

Gottlieb, A., Banoub, M., Sprung, J. *et al.* 1998. Perioperative cardiovascular morbidity in patients with coronary artery disease undergoing vascular surgery after percutaneous transluminal coronary angioplasty. *Journal of Cardiothoracic and Vascular Anesthesia* **12**, 501–506.

Greenhalgh, R.M., Taylor, G.W., Lewis, B. and Kaye, J. 1975. Serum lipids in stenosing and dilating forms of peripheral arterial disease. *Journal of Cardiovascular Surgery* **16**, 150–151.

Henry, M. and Amor, M. 1996. Stenting of femoral and popliteal arteries. In Sigwart, U. (ed.), *Endoluminal stenting*. London: W.B. Saunders, 468–475.

Hertzer, N.R., Young, J.R., Beven, E.G. *et al.* 1984. Coronary artery disease in peripheral vascular patients: a classification of 1000 coronary angiograms and results of surgical management. *Annals of Surgery* **199**, 223–233.

Hertzer, N.R., Young, J.R., Beven, E.G. *et al.* 1986. Late results of coronary bypass in patients with peripheral vascular disease, I: five-year survival according to age and clinical cardiac status. *Cleveland Clinic Quarterly* **53**, 133–143.

Hertzer N.R., Young, J.R., Beven, E.G. *et al.* 1987. Late results of coronary bypass in patients with peripheral vascular disease, II: five-year survival according to sex, hypertension and diabetes. *Cleveland Clinic Journal of Medicine* **54**, 15–23.

Hickey, N.C., Wilkes, M.P., Howes, D. *et al.* 1995. The effect of epidural anaesthesia on peripheral resistance and graft flow following femorodistal reconstruction. *European Journal of Endovascular Surgery* **9**, 93–96.

Hlatky,. M.A., Boineau, R.E., Higginbotham, M.B. *et al.* 1989. A brief self-admistered questionnaire to determine functional capacity (the Duke Activity Status Index). *American Journal of Cardiology* **64**, 651–654.

Horlocker, T.T. and Heit, J.A. 1997. Low molecular weight heparin: biochemistry, pharmacology, perioperative prophylaxis regimens, and guidelines for regional anaesthetic management. *Anesthesia and Analgesia* **85**, 874–885.

Horlocker T.T., Wedel, D.J. and Offord, K.P. 1990. Does preoperative antiplatelet therapy increase the risk of hemorrhagic complications associated with regional anesthesia? *Anesthesia and Analgesia* **70**, 631–634.

Jahangiri, M., Bradley, J.W.P., Jayatunga, A.P. and Dark, C.H. 1994. Prevention of phantom pain after major lower limb amputation by epidural infusion of diamorphine, clonidine and bupivacaine. *Annals of the Royal College of Surgeons of England* **76**, 324–326.

Jain, K.M., Patil, K.D., Doctor, U.S. and Peck, S.L. 1985. Preoperative cardiac screening before peripheral vascular operation. *American Surgeon* **51**, 77–81.

Jayr, C., Thomas, H., Rey, A. *et al.* 1993. Postoperative pulmonary complications: Epidural analgesia using bupivacaine and opioids versus parenteral opioids. *Anesthesiology* **78**, 666–676.

Jensen, T.S. and Rasmussen, P. (1994) Phantom pain and other phenomena after amputation. In Wall, P.D. and Melzack, R. (eds.), *Textbook of pain*, Edinburgh: Churchill Livingstone, 651–665.

Kazmers, A., Cerquiera, M.D. and Zierler, R.E. 1988. The role of preoperative radionuclide ejection fraction in direct abdominal aortic aneurysm repair. *Journal of Vascular Surgery* **8**, 128–136.

Knight A.A., Hollenberg, M., London, M.J. and Mangano, D.T. 1989. Myocardial ischaemia in patients awaiting coronary artery bypass grafting. *American Heart Journal* **117**, 1189–1195.

Korpinen, R, Saarnivaara, L, Siren, K. and Sarna, S. 1995. Modification of the haemodynamic responses to induction of anaesthesia and tracheal intubation with alfentanil, esmolol, and their combination. *Canadian Journal of Anaesthesia* **42**(4), 298–304.

Krupski, W.C., Layug, E.L., Reilly, L.M. *et al.* 1993. Comparison of cardiac morbidity rates between aortic and infrainguinal operations: two-year follow up. Study of perioperative ischemia research group. *Journal of Vascular Surgery* **18**, 609–615.

Kupelli, I.A. 1994. Factors affecting outcome in patients undergoing peripheral vascular surgery: 1. *Anesthesiology* **80**, 484.

Kurz, A., Sessler, D.I., Narzt, E. *et al.* 1995. Postoperative hemodynamic and thermoregulatory consequences of intraoperative core hypothermia. *Journal of Clinical Anesthesia* **7**, 359–366.

Landesberg, G., Luria, M.H., Cotev, S. *et al.* 1993. Importance of long-duration postoperative ST-segment depression in cardiac morbidity after vascular surgery. *Lancet* **341**, 715–719.

Lane, S.E., Lewis, S.M., Pippin, J.J. *et al.* 1989. Predictive value of quantitative dipyridamole-thallium scintigraphy in assessing cardiovascular risk after vascular surgery in diabetes mellitus. *American Journal of Cardiology* **64**, 1275–1279

Leather, R.P., Shah, D.M. and Karmody, A.M. 1981. Infrapopliteal arterial bypass for limb salvage: Increased patency and utilization of the saphenous vein used 'in situ'. *Surgery* **90**, 1000–1008.

L'Italien, G.J., Cambria, R.P., Cutler, B.S. *et al.* 1995. Comparative early and late cardiac morbidity rates between aortic and infrainguinal operations: two-year follow-up. Study of Perioperative Ischemia research group. *Journal of Vascular Surgery* **21**, 935–944.

London, N.J.M., Sayers, R.D., Thompson, M.M. *et al.* 1993. Interventional radiology in the maintenance of infrainguinal vein graft patency. *British Journal of Surgery* **80**, 187–193.

Loeser, J.D. 1990. Pain after amputation: Phantom limb and stump pain. In Bonica, J.J. (ed.), *The management of pain*. Philadelphia: Lea & Febiger, 244–256.

Mangano, D.T. 1990. Perioperative cardiac morbidity. *Anesthesiology* **72**, 153–184.

Mangano, D.T. 1995. Preoperative risk assessment: Many studies, few solutions. Is a cardiac risk assessment paradigm possible? *Anesthesiology* **83**, 897–901.

Mangano, D.T., Browner, W.S., Hollenberg, M. *et al.* 1990. Association of perioperative myocardial ischaemia with cardiac morbidity and mortality in men undergoing noncardiac surgery: The study of the perioperative ischemia research group. *New England Journal of Medicine* **323**, 1781–1788.

Mangano, D.T., Browner, W.S., Hollenberg, M. *et al.* 1992. Long-term cardiac prognosis following noncardiac surgery. The study of perioperative ischemia research group. *Journal of the American Medical Association* **268**, 233–239.

Mangano, D.T., London, M.J., Tubau, J.F. *et al.* 1991. Dipyridamole thallium-201 scintigraphy as a preoperative screening test: A reexamination of its predictive potential. *Circulation* **84**, 493–502.

Mangat, P.S. and Jones, J.G. 1993. Perioperative hypoxaemia. In Kaufman, L. (ed.), *Anaesthesia review 10*. Edinburgh, Churchill Livingstone, 83–105.

Mann, R.A.M. and Bisset, W.I.K. 1983. Anaesthesia for lower limb amputation: A comparison of spinal analgesia and general anaesthesia in the elderly. *Anaesthesia* **38**, 1185–1191.

Mantha, S., Roizen, M.F., Barnard, J. *et al.* 1994. Relative effectiveness of four preoperative tests for predicting adverse cardiac outcomes after vascular surgery: A meta-analysis. *Anesthesia and Analgesia* **79**, 422–433.

Mason, J.J., Owens, D.K., Harris, R.A., Cooke, J.P. and Hlatky, M.A. 1995. The role of coronary angiography and coronary revascularisation before noncardiac vascular surgery. *Journal of the American Medical Association* **273**, 1919–1925.

McCann, R.L. and Clements, F.M. 1989. Silent myocardial ischaemia in patients undergoing peripheral vascular surgery. *Journal of Vascular Surgery.* **9**, 583–587.

McDaniel, M.D., Pearce W.H., Yao, J.S.T. *et al.* 1984. Sequential changes in coagulation and platelet function following femorotibial bypass. *Journal of Vascular Surgery* **1** (**2**), 261–268.

MacDonald, R. 1991. Aspirin and extradural blocks. *British Journal of Anaesthesia* **66**, 1–3.

McPhail, N., Calvin, J.E., Shariatmadar, A. *et al.* 1988. The use of preoperative exercise testing to predict cardiac complications following arterial reconstruction. *Journal of Vascular Surgery* **7**, 60–68.

Michaels, J.A., Payne, S.P.K. and Galland, R.B. 1996. A survey of methods used for cardiac risk assessment prior to major vascular surgery. *European Journal of Vascular and Endovascular Surgery* **11**, 221–224.

Miller, D.R., Martineau, R.J., O'Brien, H. *et al.* 1993. Effects of alfentanil on the hemodynamic and catecholamine response to tracheal intubation. *Anesthesia and Analgesia* **76**, 1040–1046.

Miller, D.R., Martineau, R.J., Wynands, J.E. and Hill, J. 1991. Bolus administration of esmolol for controlling the haemodynamic response to tracheal intubation: the Canadian multicentre trial. *Canadian Journal of Anaesthesia* **38**, 849–858.

Modig, J., Borg, T., Bagge, L. and Saldeen, T., 1983. Role of extradural and of general anaesthesia in fibrinolysis and coagulation after total hip replacement. *British Journal of Anaesthesia* **55**, 625–628.

Moller, J.T., Wittrup, M. and Johansen, S.H. 1990. Hypoxemia in the postanesthesia care unit: An observer study. *Anesthesiology* **73**, 890–895.

Muir, A.D., Reeder, M.K., Foex, P. *et al.* 1991. Preoperative silent myocardial ischaemia: Incidence and predictors in a general surgical population. *British Journal of Anaesthesia* **67**, 373–377.

Naesh, O., Haljamae, H.J., Hindberg, I. *et al.* 1994. Epidural anaesthesia prolonged into the postoperative period prevents stress response and platelet hyperaggregability after peripheral vascular surgery. *European Journal of Vascular Surgery* **8**, 395–400.

Nesto, R.W., Watson, F.S., Kowalchuk, G.J. *et al.* 1990. Silent myocardial ischemia and infarction in diabetics with peripheral vascular disease: Assessment by dipyridamole thallium-201 scintigraphy. *American Heart Journal* **120**, 1073–1077.

Nikolajsen, L., Ilkjaer, S., Christensen, J.H., Kroner, K and Jensen, T.S. 1997. Randomised trial of epidural bupivacaine and morphine in prevention of stump and phantom pain in lower-limb amputation. *Lancet* **350**, 1353–1357.

Oh, T.E. 1992. Postoperative hypoxaemia. In Atkinson, R.S., Adams, A.P. (eds), *Recent advances in anaesthesia and analgesia 17*. Edinburgh, Churchill Livingstone, 103–117.

Ouyang, P., Gerstenblith, G., Furman, W.R. *et al.* 1989. Frequency and significance of early postoperative silent myocardial ischaemia in patients having peripheral vascular surgery. *American Journal of Cardiology* **64**, 1113–1116.

Parker, S.D, Breslow, M.J., Frank, S.M. *et al.* 1995. Catecholamine and cortisol responses to lower extremity revascularisation: Correlation with outcome variables. *Critical Care Medicine* **23**, 1954–1961.

Pasternack, P.F., Imparato, A.M., Riles, T.S. *et al.* 1985. The value of the radionuclide angiogram in the prediction of perioperative myocardial infarction in patients undergoing lower extremity revascularisation procedures. *Circulation* **72** (Suppl. 2, Part 2), 13–17.

Pasternack, P.F., Grossi, E.A., Baumann, F.G. *et al.* 1989. Beta blockade to decrease silent myocardial ischaemia during peripheral vascular surgery. *American Journal of Surgery* **158**, 113–116.

Pateman, J.A. and Hanning, C.D. 1989. Postoperative myocardial infarction and episodic hypoxaemia. *British Journal of Anaesthesia* **63**, 648–650.

Pavy, T.-J.G. and Doyle, D.L. 1996. Prevention of phantom limb pain by infusion of local anaesthetic into the sciatic nerve. *Anaesthesia and Intensive Care* **24**, 599–600.

Pell, J.P., Donnan, P.T., Fowkes, F.G.R. and Ruckley, C.V. 1993. Quality of life following lower limb amputation for peripheral vascular disease. *European Journal of Vascular and Endovascular Surgery* **7**, 448–451.

Perler, B.A., Christopherson, R., Rosenfeld, B.A. *et al.* 1995. The influence of anesthetic method on infrainguinal bypass graft patency: A closer look. *American Surgeon* **9**, 784–789.

Pierce, E.T., Pomposelli, F.B., Stanley, G.D. *et al.* 1997. Anesthesia type does not influence early graft patency or limb salvage of lower extremity arterial bypass. *Journal of Vascular Surgery* **25**, 226–232.

Poldermans, D., Fioretti, P.M., Forster, T. *et al.* 1993. Dobutamine stress echocardiography for assessment of perioperative cardiac risk in patients undergoing major vascular surgery. *Circulation.* **87**, 1506–1512.

Raby, K.E., Goldman, L., Creager, M.A. *et al.* 1989. Correlation between preoperative ischemia and major cardiac events after peripheral vascular surgery. *New England Journal of Medicine* **321**, 1296–1300.

Raggi, R., Dardik, H. and Mauro, A.L. 1987. Continuous epidural anesthesia and postoperative epidural narcotics in vascular surgery. *American Journal of Surgery* **154**, 192–197.

Rao, T.L.K. and El-Etr, A.A. 1981. Anticoagulation following placement of epidural and subarachnoid catheters: An evaluation of neurologic sequelae. *Anesthesiology* **55**, 618–620.

Reeder, M.K., Muir, A.D., Foex, P. *et al.* 1991. Postoperative myocardial ischaemia: temporal association with nocturnal hypoxaemia. *British Journal of Anaesthesia* **67**, 626–631.

Reeder, M.K., Goldman, M.D., Loh, L. *et al.* 1992. Postoperative hypoxaemia after major abdominal vascular surgery. *British Journal of Anaesthesia* **68**, 23–26.

Reul G.J. Jr, Cooley D.A., Duncan J.M. *et al.* 1986. The effect of coronary bypass on the outcome of peripheral vascular operations in 1093 patients. *Journal of Vascular Surgery* **3**, 788–798.

Rihal, C.S. 1998. The role of myocardial revascularisation preceding noncardiac surgery. *Progress in Cardiovascular Diseases* **40**, 383–404.

Rihal, C.S., Eagle, K.A., Mickel, M.C. *et al.* 1995. Surgical therapy for coronary artery disease among patients with combined coronary artery and peripheral vascular disease. *Circulation* **91**, 46–53.

Robinson, K.P. 1992. Amputations in vascular patients. In Bell, P.F.R., Jamieson, C.W. and Vaughan Ruckley, C. (eds), *Surgical management of vascular disease.* London: W.B. Saunders.

Rosenberg, J., Rasmussen V., Jessen, F.V. *et al.* 1990. Late postoperative episodic and constant hypoxaemia and associated ECG abnormalities. *British Journal of Anaesthesia* **65**, 684–691.

Rosenberg, J., Pedersen M.H., Gebuhr, P. and Kehlet, H. 1992. Effect of oxygen therapy on late postoperative episodic and constant hypoxaemia. *British Journal of Anaesthesia* **68**, 18–22.

Rosenfeld, B.A, Beattie, C., Christopherson, R. *et al.* 1993. The effects of different anesthetic regimens on fibrinolysis and the development of postoperative arterial thrombosis. *Anesthesiology* **79**, 435–443.

Rutherford, R.B. 1991. Standards for evaluating results of interventional therapy for peripheral vascular disease. *Circulation* **83**(Suppl. 2), I 6–I 11.

Sayers, R.D., Thompson, M. M., London, N.J.M. *et al.* 1990. Selection of patients with critical limb ischaemia for femorodistal vein bypass. *European Journal of Vascular and Endovascular Surgery* **7**, 291–297.

Shah, K.B., Kleinman, B.S., Rao, T.L.K. *et al.* 1990. Angina and other risk factors in patients with cardiac diseases undergoing non-cardiac operations. *Anesthesia and Analgesia* **70**, 240–247.

Sherman, R.A. 1994. Phantom limb pain: Mechanism-based management. *Clinics in Podiatric Medicine and Surgery* **11**, 85–106.

Sherman,R.A., Sherman, C.J. and Gall, N.G. 1980. A survey of current phantom limb pain treatment in the United States. *Pain* **8**, 85–99.

Slogoff, S. and Keats, A.S. 1985. Does perioperative myocardial ischemia lead to postoperative myocardial infarction? *Anesthesiology* **62**, 107–114.

Slotman, G.J., Jed, E.H. and Burchard, K.W. 1985. Adverse effects of hypothermia in postoperative patients. *American Journal of Surgery* **149**, 495–501.

Stone, J.G., Foex, P., Sear, J.W. *et al.* 1988. Myocardial ischaemia in untreated hypertensive patients: effect of a single small oral dose of a beta-adrenergic blocking agent. *Anestheseiology* **68**, 495–500.

Stone, J.G., Foex, P., Sear, J.W. *et al.* 1988. Risk of myocardial ischaemia during anaesthesia in treated and untreated hypertensive patients. *British Journal of Anaesthesia* **61**, 675–679.

Taylor, L.M., Yeager, R.A., Moneta, G.L. *et al.* 1991. The incidence of perioperative myocardial infarction in general vascular surgery. *Journal of Vascular Surgery* **15**(1), 52–61.

Taylor, P.R., Wolfe, J.H.N., Tyrell, M.R. *et al.* 1990. Graft stenosis: justification for 1–year surveillance. *British Journal of Surgery* **77**, 1125–1128.

Thompson, M.M., Sayers, R.D., Varty, K. *et al.* 1993. Chronic critical leg ischaemia must be redefined. *European Journal of Vascular and Endovascular Surgery* **7**, 420–426.

Thompson, M.M., Sayers, R.D., Reid, A. *et al.* 1995. Quality of life following infragenicular bypass and lower limb amputation. *European Journal of Vascular and Endovascular Surgery* **9**, 310–313.

Tracy, G.D. and Reid, W. 1992. Sympathectomy. In Eastcott, H.H.G. (ed.), *Arterial surgery*. Edinburgh: Churchill Livingstone.

Tuman, K.J., McCarthy, R.J., March, R.J. *et al.* 1991. Effects of epidural anesthesia and analgesia on coagulation and outcome after major vascular surgery. *Anesthesia and Analgesia* **73**, 696–704.

Varty, K., Allen, K.E., Bell, P.R.F. and London, N.J.M. 1993. Infrainguinal vein graft stenosis. *British Journal of Surgery* **80**, 825–833.

Varty, K., Bolia, A., Naylor, A.R., Bell, P.R.F. and London, N.J.M. 1995. Infrapopliteal percutaneous transluminal angioplasty: A safe and successful procedure. *European Journal of Vascular and Endovascular Surgery* **9**, 341–345.

Wesolowski, J.A. and Lema, M.J. 1993. Phantom limb pain. *Regional Anaesthesia* **18**, 121–127.

Wildsmith, J.A.W. and McLure, J.H. 1991. Anticoagulant drugs and central nerve blockade. *Anaesthesia* **46**, 613–614.

Wilson, I.G., Fell, D., Robinson, S.L. and Smith, G. 1992. Cardiovascular responses to insertion of the laryngeal mask. *Anaesthesia* **47**, 300–302.

Yang, H. 1996. Intraoperative automated ST segment analysis: a reliable 'Black Box'? *Canadian Journal of Anaesthesia* **43**, 1041–1051.

Yeager, M.P., Glass, D., Neff, R.K. and Brinck-Johnsen, T. 1987. Epidural anesthesia and analgesia in high-risk surgical patients. *Anesthesiology* **66**, 729–736.

Yeager, R.A., Moneta, G.L., Edwards, J.M. *et al.* 1994. Late survival after perioperative myocardial infarction complicating vascular surgery. *Journal of Vascular Surgery* **20**, 598–606.

16

Anaesthesia for upper limb procedures

DAVID M COVENTRY

INTRODUCTION

Even a specialist vascular anaesthetist is unlikely to be presented with upper limb vascular pathology on more than an occasional basis. With the exception of fistula formation for chronic haemodialysis, this diverse group is small in comparison to the numbers presenting for lower limb vascular reconstruction. With advances in techniques of subclavian angioplasty and stenting, it is likely that the number of patients presenting for conventional reconstructive surgery will decline still further.

Chronic ischaemia of the upper limb may reflect widespread atherosclerotic disease or may result from thoracic outlet obstruction in an otherwise healthy individual. In addition, peripheral ischaemia can, on occasion, result from small vessel occlusion from a variety of less common medical conditions such as Buerger's disease or connective tissue disorders. Although most are not amenable to surgical reconstruction, the development of video-assisted thoracoscopic sympathectomy offers a much less invasive technique for palliation than was previously possible. Despite this, its value for vasospastic or obliterative disease remains contentious in all but a few specific situations. Acute ischaemia of the upper limb usually results from trauma, iatrogenic injury or embolism, but is increasingly being seen as a result of recreational drug abuse and inadvertent intra-arterial injection. The anaesthetist has a role here not only in the provision of anaesthesia for reconstruction and fasciotomy, but also in the provision of regional analgesia for pain relief and vasodilatation in the post-operative or post-injury period.

This group of patients therefore provide the anaesthetist with a formidable variety of clinical challenges in assessment, monitoring, general and regional anaesthetic technique, and pain relief.

ANAESTHESIA FOR VASCULAR ACCESS PROCEDURES

The most commonly encountered vascular procedures performed on the upper limb are those involving the establishment of vascular access to allow chronic haemodialysis. These patients often present with recurrent problems, with renal transplantation where appropriate, as the only permanent solution. When it is possible, a direct arteriovenous fistula provides the most satisfactory dialysis access, with the more peripheral sites, such as the anatomical 'snuff box' or classic Brescia–Cimino radiocephalic fistula at the wrist, being considered the most generally suitable. If patency subsequently becomes a problem, more proximal sites such as the brachiocephalic

(Dunlop *et al.*, 1986) or brachioaxillary fistula may be considered, with polytetrafluoroethylene (PTFE) graft fistulae reserved for the patient for whom all other autologous possibilities have been utilized (Coburn and Carney, 1994). Because the majority of patients are already receiving haemodialysis via a central vein, most vascular access procedures are carried out on an elective basis and the fistula is not utilized until it 'matures' some weeks later. Occasionally, patients may present more urgently with early complications such as bleeding or thrombosis of the fistula, when surgical thrombectomy or transluminal angioplasty may be required to restore blood flow.

Pre-operative assessment

Assessment of the patient with renal failure should begin by ascertaining its aetiology where possible, because this may provide valuable information regarding other potential end-organ pathology. Common causes include hypertension, diabetes mellitus and chronic glomerulonephritis, while diseases such as polycystic kidney, chronic pyelonephritis, systemic lupus or vasculitis affecting the kidney are less common (Brenner and Rector, 1996). As well as being a common cause, hypertension is also one of the common presenting complications of chronic renal failure and is almost always present at some stage (Marsland and Bradley, 1983; Heino *et al.*, 1986). In most patients, this is a result of fluid overload as a consequence of sodium and water retention, but in a few it may be a result of excessive plasma renin activity despite an apparently euvolaemic state (Weir and Chung, 1984; Galla and Luke, 1996). In the former group, adequate dialysis with removal of excess fluid, along with improvements in dialysis technology, have resulted in a significant reduction in those requiring antihypertensive medication, but a few of the latter group of patients may require one of the potent antihypertensive agents such as beta-blockers, calcium antagonists and angiotensin-converting enzyme inhibitors. However, it would appear that the use of recombinant erythropoietin and the subsequent increase in haematocrit may have increased the prevalence of hypertension by up to one-third (Galla and Luke, 1996). Care should therefore be taken to ensure that hypertension is well controlled (Goldman and Calders, 1979) and that the appropriate medication is prescribed on the day of surgery. A history of

ischaemic heart disease should be sought, especially in the more elderly patient (Weir and Chung, 1984).

Particular attention should be paid to assessing symptoms and signs of fluid overload and congestive cardiac failure. This may be further exacerbated by anaemia, pericardial effusion (May and Mitch, 1996) or a previous large atrioventricular fistula. A unique form of pulmonary oedema may occur even in the absence of volume overload and is associated with normal or mildly elevated intracardiac and pulmonary wedge pressures. This is thought due to increased permeability of the alveolar capillary membrane and usually responds to vigorous dialysis. The dialysis schedule should be examined for wet and dry weights and for any problems such as cardiovascular instability occurring during dialysis. Where possible, haemodialysis should be performed during the afternoon of the day prior to surgery to permit equilibration of fluid and electrolytes and to avoid persistent heparinization which may occur up to 10 hours after dialysis. Bleeding time may be further prolonged by platelet dysfunction or a reduction in certain coagulation factors, primarily the vitamin K-dependent factors (II, VII, IX, X) and factor V. Stewart and Castaldi (1967) observed that platelet function should return to normal with frequent and adequate dialysis. With the introduction of biosynthetic erythropoietin (Winearls *et al.*, 1986) anaemia should be less of a problem, although haematocrit is best kept below 35 per cent to prevent problems with fistula thrombosis (Winearls, 1992). Diabetes, when present, should be well controlled and plans made for its peri-operative management.

Because the vast majority of patients will be best managed with a regional anaesthetic technique, any existing peripheral neuropathy or proximal myopathy, not uncommon in patients with chronic renal failure, should be sought and documented (Maddern, 1983). The patient's mental state should be sympathetically assessed as many will be anxious or depressed from frequent hospitalization or previous fistula failure, whereas others may be somnolent or frankly confused from biochemical derangement or relative hypoxaemia. Other factors which may complicate intra-operative management should be sought, such as orthopnoea or skeletal discomfort from pseudogout, uraemic osteodystrophy (May and Mitch, 1996) or concomitant osteoporosis, all of which may be further aggravated by poor nutritional status. It should be clear from this discussion that a settled co-operative patient is best obtained by careful patient positioning and attention to these details rather than the injudicious use of sedative agents.

Pre-operative work up should include a full blood count, electrolyte estimations, blood glucose concentration where appropriate, and a recent chest X-ray to assess cardiomegaly, fluid overload, pleural or pericardial effusion or signs of pulmonary infection. An electrocardiogram is useful to detect or confirm abnormalities of rate and rhythm, ischaemia, ventricular hypertrophy or biochemical disturbance. Because digoxin is excreted in the urine, blood concentrations should be determined in patients receiving this particular medication prior to surgery (Weir and Chung, 1984). Coagulation studies may be necessary and, if significant respiratory dysfunction exists, arterial blood gas estimation is useful as a baseline and to determine acid–base status. Medical staff should appreciate that, in addition to many of these patients having impaired immunity and therefore being susceptible to infection, many receiving chronic haemodialysis may also be carriers of hepatitis B or C and cytomegalovirus infection. The appropriate precautions should therefore be taken (Strom, 1982).

Regional anaesthesia

RENAL FAILURE

It follows from the initial discussion that the use of regional anaesthesia may greatly simplify the management of the renal failure patient, given the complexity of pre-existing disease and the effects it may have on drug distribution and excretion. The pharmacokinetics of many drugs may be altered by changes in compartment volume, electrolytes, pH and total protein or by alterations in cardiac output or rates of excretion. Uraemia potentiates the effect of most sedative drugs, reducing requirements by up to 50 per cent (Kovatis, 1993). When sedative premedication is felt appropriate, a small dose of an orally administered benzodiazepine such as temazepam should suffice (Breimer et al., 1980). It has a short duration of action and is biotransformed to inactive compounds, unlike diazepam and lorazepam. Sedation may be cautiously supplemented later with increments of midazolam or a low-dose propofol infusion if necessary.

When it comes to the choice of local anaesthetic agent, lidocaine is the most commonly used. Although acidosis may reduce the threshold for CNS toxicity in the patient with renal failure, an increased

binding to α_1-acid glycoprotein may lower the unbound plasma fraction and therefore return its therapeutic ratio towards normal (Tucker, 1986). Bupivacaine is inherently more cardiotoxic and the associated prolonged motor block is neither desirable nor appreciated by most patients. Gould and Aldrete (1983), have described a case of bupivacaine cardiotoxicity occurring with a dosage within conventional guidelines in a patient with renal failure.

TECHNIQUE

Although simple distal fistulae can be created using local infiltration alone, regional blockade provides superior analgesia particularly when tunnelling is anticipated. Operating conditions are also improved by the accompanying motor block, and the sympathetic block produces vasodilatation and improved flow characteristics well into the early post-operative period. Despite the absence of definitive morbidity and mortality studies, brachial plexus block using the axillary approach appears to have few potential problems, with the possible exception of intravenous toxicity, and should therefore be the technique of choice. Unlike central neuronal block of the lower limbs, there is little risk of cardiovascular instability nor as great a concern related to minor degrees of coagulation abnormality. The axillary approach also avoids the potential for pneumothorax with supraclavicular techniques, or the increased orthopnoea possible with the interscalene approach and consequent phrenic nerve blockade.

Until recently, it was generally accepted that the duration of brachial plexus block was shorter in patients with chronic renal failure. Bromage and Gertel (1972) reported a reduction in duration of 38 per cent using the supraclavicular approach. However, more recent work with the axillary (Beauregard et al., 1987) and interscalene approaches (McEllistrem et al., 1989) failed to demonstrate any difference in either latency or duration using lidocaine 1 per cent with epinephrine or lidocaine 1 per cent plain, respectively. These studies also demonstrated that using plain lignocaine by the interscalene approach was unlikely to produce analgesia lasting over 1 hour whereas lidocaine with epinephrine 1 : 200 000 by the axillary approach provided analgesia of over 3 hours duration. This technique should therefore suffice for the vast majority of upper limb vascular surgery. Although bupivacaine has also been recommended for this purpose, the vast majority of patients do not appreciate the long duration of motor block produced with this agent despite theoretical advantages of a prolonged sympathetic block.

Technique of axillary block

Prior to performing the plexus block, venous access should be secured avoiding possible future fistula sites, such as the forearm. Strict aseptic precautions should be adhered to at all times and particular care given to patient positioning and comfort as previously described. A multiple-injection technique of axillary block utilizing a peripheral nerve stimulator has been shown to produce a rapid and complete block of the plexus in up to 97 per cent of patients (Fig. 16.1). In addition almost 50 per cent of blocks are complete within 10 min of injection. However, when the radial nerve is not specifically located, it is inadequately blocked in 40 per cent of patients. The ulnar nerve does not need specific location, appearing to be blocked by spread from other injection sites. To achieve a reliable, complete and rapid block, local anaesthetic is therefore deposited in three areas from a single injection site (Coventry *et al.*, 1996). Similar success has also been reported recently with a multiple-injection mid-humoral approach (Macchi *et al.*, 1996; Narchi and Dupre, 1996).

Following aseptic preparation, the skin overlying the axillary artery is infiltrated with local anaesthetic

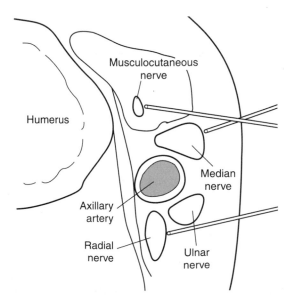

approximately 2 cm lateral to the border of pectoralis major. The musculocutaneous nerve is first located by eliciting biceps contraction with a stimulation current of 2 mA, and then the optimum needle position is established at 0.5 mA. This nerve is easily blocked with an injection of 5 mL lidocaine 1.5 per cent with epinephrine 1 : 200 000 avoiding the need for a subsequent large-volume injection around the plexus. The median nerve is similarly located by eliciting flexion of fingers and thumb and blocked with a further 15 mL of solution. The insulated needle is then withdrawn subcutaneously and passed inferior to the artery to locate the radial nerve by eliciting finger extension and or triceps contraction. The radial block is accomplished with a further 10 mL of solution, making a total injection volume of 30 mL. Where surgery in the upper arm is anticipated, a larger subcutaneous injection below the artery at the time of initial infiltration should guarantee blockade of the intercostobrachial and medial brachial cutaneous nerves.

This technique provides a dense sensory and motor block, but where there are constraints on dosage, such as a particularly cachexic and acidotic patient, lignocaine 1 per cent with adrenaline 1 : 200 000 can be substituted, the total volume of injection reduced (musculocutaneous 4 mL, median 10 mL, radial 6 mL) or more selective blockade performed.

In the post-operative period, supplementary oxygen should be continued until residual sedation has regressed or while clinically indicated. Simple oral analgesic preparations usually suffice for post-operative pain relief. Non-steroidal anti-inflammatory agents are best avoided due to their effects on bleeding and residual renal function. If parenteral analgesia is required in the early post-operative period, 1 mg increments of intravenous diamorphine are administered until pain is controlled.

CHRONIC UPPER LIMB ISCHAEMIA

Symptomatic upper limb ischaemia is much less commonly encountered than the corresponding disease of the lower limb, mainly because of the rich collateral circulation around the shoulder and the lower metabolic requirements of the limb under normal circumstances. Chronic ischaemia is most frequently caused by atheromatous disease in the aortic arch or proximal aortic branches, but may on occasion be related

Figure 16.1 *Relationship of the major brachial plexus nerves to the axillary artery in the upper arm. Redrawn with permission from Baxter and Coventry, 1999.*

to previous trauma, iatrogenic injury, radiation injury or thoracic outlet syndrome. A further group of patients may present with digital ischaemia as a result of vasospastic disease, vasculitis or connective tissue disorder. In the case of patients with unilateral digital ischaemia not falling into one of these categories, a proximal source of embolism such as the left atrium or a subclavian artery aneurysm should be considered (Hight *et al.*, 1976). When symptoms develop, the patient usually complains of weakness and paraesthesia which may on occasion be accompanied by symptoms and signs of vertebrobasilar ischaemia resulting from subclavian steal syndrome (Killen *et al.*, 1966).

Subclavian steal syndrome

The subclavian steal syndrome occurs when there is occlusion of the subclavian or innominate artery proximal to the origin of the ipsilateral vertebral artery (Fig. 16.2). Exercise of the affected arm and the increase in blood flow required is provided by retrograde flow from the ipsilateral vertebral artery, diverting blood flow from the circle of Willis and resulting in symptoms and signs of cerebral ischaemia. The

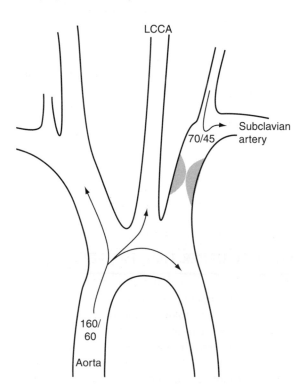

Figure 16.2 *Subclavian steal, resulting from retrograde flow from the ipsilateral vertebral artery.*

resulting vertebrobasilar ischaemia induces symptoms such as vertigo, diplopia or ataxia and may lead to syncopal episodes. Symptoms of arm ischaemia, more commonly the left, are frequently present and occasionally the elderly may develop ischaemic necrosis of the corresponding fingertips. A stroke resulting from subclavian artery disease is extremely uncommon (Holleman *et al.*, 1980). There is often a diminished or absent pulse in the affected arm and the systolic pressure is likely to be at least 20 mmHg lower (Killen *et al.*, 1966). Diagnosis is confirmed by duplex scanning and arch aortography. Nicholls and colleagues (1991) have pointed out that retrograde flow *per se* is not an indication for surgery as many individuals exhibiting this phenomenon are asymptomatic whilst others remain symptomatic despite surgical restoration of the posterior cerebral circulation. Accurate selection of patients who may benefit from surgery therefore remains imprecise and is best made on an individual clinical basis until such times as more informative investigations are available.

CORONARY–SUBCLAVIAN STEAL SYNDROME

A rare late complication of coronary revascularization using the left internal mammary artery (LIMA) is coronary–subclavian steal syndrome. First described by Harjola and Valle (1974), the steal of myocardial perfusion occurs when development of a subtotal stenosis in the left subclavian artery produces reversal of blood flow through the patent LIMA graft (Fig. 16.3). The patient often presents with dizziness or other cerebral vascular symptoms in association with angina pectoris and usually has a systolic blood pressure at least 20 mmHg lower in the ipsilateral arm. Diagnosis is confirmed by aortic arch and carotid angiography. With increasing numbers of LIMA bypass procedures being carried out and patient survival increasing, it can be anticipated that the incidence of angiographically demonstrated steal, currently 0.44 per cent, may increase in the future (Martin and Rock, 1988).

ANAESTHETIC MANAGEMENT OF SUBCLAVIAN PROCEDURES

Many patients, including those with coronary–subclavian steal, can now be offered subclavian artery angioplasty and stenting techniques (Levitt *et al.*, 1992) and will not therefore be presented to the anaesthetist. For those requiring definitive surgery for a discrete lesion, arterial reconstruction offers an

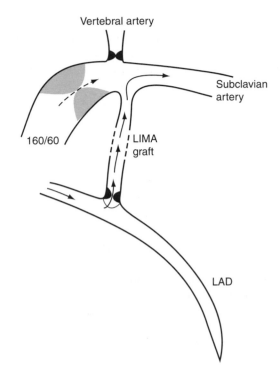

Vertebral artery

Subclavian
artery

160/60

LIMA
graft

LAD

Figure 16.3 *The steal of myocardial perfusion occurs when development of a proximal subtotal stenosis in the left subclavian artery produces reversal of blood flow through the patient IMA graft. LAD = left anterior descending artery; LIMA = left internal mammary artery.*

excellent chance of success (Holleman *et al.*, 1980; Welling *et al.*, 1981).

In patients with widespread atherosclerotic disease, the physiological insult of a thoracotomy necessary for a prosthetic graft to the aortic arch is best avoided as mortality rates of 6–10 per cent were reported at an early stage (Fields, 1972). Even after allowing for improvements in anaesthetic management and surgical technique since that time, it remains safer and as effective to employ an extrathoracic approach such as carotid–subclavian bypass. Axillo-axillary bypass is an alternative in patients with ipsilateral carotid disease and a prosthetic graft to the aortic arch is considered only when there are other complicating circumstances. Early concern that the carotid–subclavian bypass would cause carotid steal with neurological symptoms has been allayed by extensive clinical and laboratory experience (Cook *et al.*, 1972; Williams *et al.*, 1973).

Pre-operative assessment of the arteriopathic patient should be along the lines described earlier in this volume and anaesthesia should be conducted using similar principles of management as carotid endarterectomy (Chapter 14). The two main objectives in the anaesthetic management of carotid–subclavian bypass should be myocardial protection and a technique designed to facilitate early neurological evaluation. Neurological dysfunction may occur as a result of plaque embolization or intolerance of carotid cross-clamping secondary to inadequate collateral perfusion.

The anaesthetic technique and invasive monitoring requirements depend on the particular patient and degree of myocardial dysfunction. All patients should have invasive arterial pressure monitoring in the contralateral arm and if central venous pressure monitoring is indicated, an antecubital long line will avoid vascular puncture and lines in the area of the surgical field.

Due to the demands of surgery, most vascular surgeons prefer the optimal operating conditions provided by general anaesthesia, and regional anaesthesia in this area is difficult. Maintenance of arterial pressure is essential to maintain adequate coronary and cerebral perfusion. Hyperventilation and significant hypocapnia should be avoided because Thompson (1986) described increased retrograde vertebral artery flow and increased subclavian steal under these circumstances. In addition Cone (1994) reported an exercise-induced transient global amnesia in a patient with subclavian steal and carotid artery disease by merely exercising the hand to facilitate venous cannulation. This indicates the possibility of a more significant cerebral ischaemic deficit in those with widespread vascular disease and highlights the importance of carotid duplex scanning pre-operatively. For methods of assessing cerebral perfusion during anaesthesia and carotid cross-clamping, the reader is referred to Chapter 14.

In order to monitor neurological function continuously, Ponzio and colleagues (1992) have recommended carrying out carotid–subclavian bypass using cervicobrachial plexus anaesthesia. This technique can be performed as a high volume (30–40 mL) interscalene approach and allows monitoring of neurological status during carotid occlusion and may minimize interference with cardiovascular and respiratory function. However, the inferior operating conditions, length of procedure and the potential problems of bradycardia, hypotension, syncopal episodes and phrenic nerve paralysis do not merit the routine use of this technique. The addition of a superficial cervical plexus block to general anaesthesia does, however, provide extra cardiovascular stability and useful postoperative analgesia and is easily performed with few potential adverse effects.

In the post-operative period, all patients should be monitored in a high-dependency unit with facilities for invasive pressure monitoring and regular assessment of neurological function for the first 24 hours. Analgesia can often be managed with simple preparations following block regression and anti-emesis provided with ondansetron as it lacks the sedative potential of alternative agents.

Thoracic outlet compression syndrome

The thoracic outlet syndrome is caused by compression of the subclavian artery or brachial plexus at a number of sites in the neck or shoulder girdle including the costoclavicular space, interscalene triangle or insertion of pectoralis minor at the coracoid process. More than 50 per cent of these patients will present with neurological symptoms of pain, paraesthesia or weakness of the arm or hand with the remainder presenting with additional vascular problems. These may range from claudication to acute ischaemia as a result of axillary artery thrombosis or peripheral embolization.

In most cases, the syndrome occurs as a result of neurovascular compression from a well-developed cervical rib or by a congenital anomaly of the first rib or fibrous band arising from it. The variety of presentations ensure that diagnosis is rarely straightforward and usually requires confirmation by chest radiography and subsequent ultrasonography or arteriography. Davies and colleagues (1991) recommended managing the majority of patients presenting with arterial stenosis by cervical rib resection using a supraclavicular approach. Cases may be further complicated by intrinsic arterial damage, subclavian aneurysm formation or distal thromboembolic complications (Scher et al., 1984) which may require arterial reconstruction, thrombectomy or embolectomy in addition to the thoracic outlet decompression. Transaxillary first-rib resection and scalenectomy are now less commonly advocated unless there is a particular indication such as complicated vascular reconstruction or symptomatology in the distribution of the lower brachial plexus.

Patients should be assessed along conventional lines. The majority are likely to fall into the American Society of Anesthesiology (ASA) I and II categories and younger age groups, in sharp contrast to the typical arteriopathic vascular patient. For this reason, anaesthesia and surgery are rarely problematic. The surgical dissection should be extrapleural

and therefore unlikely to cause any ventilatory difficulty. Most anaesthetists would advocate a straightforward balanced general anaesthetic technique with single-lumen endotracheal ventilation and intermittent positive-pressure ventilation (IPPV). If the pleura is damaged during dissection care should be taken to fully re-expand the lung prior to closure. Thoracocentesis is not required unless there is damage to the lung, although a chest radiograph should be performed early in the post-operative period or if the patient becomes symptomatic. Analgesia is best managed with a patient-controlled analgesia (PCA) system for the first 24 hours.

THORACOSCOPIC SYMPATHECTOMY

Arterial reconstructive techniques remain the optimal surgical therapy for chronic ischaemic disease of the upper extremity. Advances in angioplasty and stenting techniques have further reduced the number of patients for whom palliative sympathectomy was the only possible hope for alleviation of symptoms. However, with advances in video-assisted thoracoscopic techniques, sympathectomy is again being considered for palliation or as an adjunct to reconstruction in those patients with rest pain, paraesthesia or peripheral ulceration and gangrene.

A thoracoscopic sympathectomy (T2–4) can be carried out with less pain and scarring than traditional open procedures, as well as improving access and reducing risk to adjacent structures. There is now a large body of evidence regarding the general safety of the technique when employed for healthy patients with hyperhidrosis (Drott et al., 1994; Lin et al., 1994), but few controlled trials for peripheral ischaemic complications. The results in Raynaud's disease are uniformly disappointing in the longer term, but some authors describe benefit in the healing of peripheral ulceration resulting from chronic occlusive disease and in the treatment of Buerger's disease (Ishibashi, 1995; Komori et al., 1995). Thoracoscopic sympathectomy has also been suggested for severe angina pectoris although Harlid (1994) reported marked haemodynamic instability during these cases!

Anaesthetic management
Pre-operative assessment of these patients should be along conventional lines with special attention paid to cardiorespiratory function. All patients with symptomatic pulmonary disease should have pulmonary function tests performed as well as a chest X-ray to

assess the existence of complicating pathology such as bullae or apical pleural disease suggestive of adhesions. As well as complicating surgery, this may influence the choice of anaesthetic and intubation technique or the need for post-operative thoracocentesis. Arterial blood-gas estimation may be required on the basis of these tests and the overall clinical picture.

The patient should be fully monitored in the anaesthetic room, paying attention to any blood-pressure discrepancy between arms. Although invasive arterial pressure measurement is extremely useful during thoracoscopic surgery, its use in profoundly ischaemic upper limbs would not only be technically difficult, but potentially problematic.

Major debate surrounds the need for endo-bronchial intubation to selectively ventilate each lung (Hartrey et al., 1994) or whether single-lumen endo-tracheal intubation is sufficient for adequate surgical access and patient safety (Harlid, 1994). In the latter situation, the lungs are not collapsed, but a small carbon dioxide pneumothorax created using a pressure of 5–6 mmHg. In the majority of situations this does not cause significant cardiac embarrassment. Ventilation can be continued using smaller tidal volumes or high frequency ventilation employed (Graham et al., 1993). Jedeikin and colleagues (1992) reported a series of 58 patients in which the lungs were alternately collapsed, and ventilation controlled with 100 per cent oxygen. They reported only minimal problems with gas exchange. The experience of the author, and of others (Gilligan et al., 1993; Graham et al., 1993; Quinn et al., 1993) is that significant arterial desaturation can occur during one-lung anaesthesia on the second side, even when the lung is fully inflated under direct vision. It appears that there may be a significant period of time after re-inflation of the first lung when pulmonary physiology remains disturbed and inadequate to sustain oxygenation of blood perfusing that lung. This may on occasion lead to abandonment of the procedure (Graham et al., 1993).

Patients are usually positioned supine, with the arms abducted, in a slight reverse Trendelenberg position or in the prone position. It is claimed that the latter improves access and allows surgery to proceed without selective collapse of the lungs or the requirement for high-frequency jet ventilation or endobronchial intubation.

Patients with impaired myocardial function may be at particular risk of developing significant hypotension from the effects of the increased intrathoracic pressure reducing preload and cardiac output as well as the direct effects of T2–4 sympathectomy on myocardial contractility (Drott et al., 1994). Tachycardia may be particularly troublesome and result in significant increases in myocardial oxygen consumption. Oxygen delivery should therefore be optimal, because significant oxygen desaturation will not be tolerated. Eisenkraft (1990) has shown that propofol does not abolish the pulmonary vasoconstrictor response and may therefore better preserve the ventilation : perfusion ratio. Harlid (1994) has used this as a basis for a propofol-based intravenous technique in his series of 125 patients using single-lumen endotracheal anaesthesia. These were performed without problems of significant hypoxaemia. Inotropic support may however be required during carbon dioxide insufflation in particularly compromised individuals.

In the immediate post-operative period, chest pain can be a significant problem despite local anaesthetic infiltration at the incision sites. Intrapleural bupivacaine instillation has been advocated by Plastow and Weisz (1993), while Gilligan and colleagues (1993) advocated leaving apical intrapleural catheters to allow bupivacaine 'top-ups' and also to facilitate aspiration of any residual pneumothorax. The analgesia can be supplemented initially with increments of intravenous morphine until optimal pain relief is achieved. Subsequent discomfort can then usually be controlled with simple analgesic preparations. A chest radiograph should be obtained early in the post-operative period and repeated at 24 hours or before if the patient becomes symptomatic. Supplementary oxygen should be continued for at least 24 hours in this particular patient population.

ACUTE UPPER LIMB ISCHAEMIA

Acute upper limb ischaemia can occur as a result of direct vascular injury or increasingly as a consequence of accidental intra-arterial injection of drugs of abuse. Even in specialist units, brachial artery injuries only account for between 14 and 25 per cent of all vascular injuries (Lambert et al., 1983). Of those, iatrogenic injury from cardiac catheterization via the brachial artery represents a significant proportion, the incidence varying from 0.3 to 12 per cent. The initial injury may be further complicated by intimal damage, thrombosis and peripheral embolism. Surgical management aims to repair the damaged segment with resection, saphenous vein bypass or a generous vein patch and embolectomy if indicated.

The choice of anaesthetic technique will depend on whether the patient is co-operative, has significant associated injuries or will require a section of vein removed from the lower limb. In cases of isolated vascular trauma, most can be managed under axillary block as described earlier in the chapter, with bupivacaine substituted for lignocaine if a longer duration is required. Alternatively, an axillary catheter can be placed and used as the sole technique for blockade or as a technique to supplement general anaesthesia for more complex cases. The catheter technique has the advantage of allowing 'top-ups' for post-operative pain relief and sympathectomy as well as facilitating subsequent embolectomy or re-exploration in patients in whom systemic heparinization may preclude further regional blocks.

The axillary catheter is placed, with a strict aseptic technique, within the neurovascular sheath, anterior to the axillary artery (Pinnock et al., 1996). The catheter is positioned with or without the aid of a peripheral nerve stimulator depending on individual preference. If a stimulator is used, a cannulated needle with a steel hub or a Seldinger-type intravascular cannula with stimulator attached to guidewire can be used. Custom-made catheters such as Contiplex (Braun Medical) have the potential advantage of utilizing non-cutting needles which may reduce the possibility of further vascular trauma. After positioning the needle, most authors advocate injecting at least 10 mL of solution to create space and facilitate catheter advancement. A short extension can then be attached and the cannula secured to skin before covering the entire site with a transparent occlusive dressing.

Dorothee and Robert (1988) described a technique of continuous axillary block for post-operative pain management and sympathectomy. Bupivacaine 0.25 per cent infused at the rate of 0.1 mL/kg/h is a regime used generally, but more recently Iskandar (1996) has described a PCA technique in which the patient received 0.1 mL/kg of bupivacaine 0.25 per cent with a one-hour lockout period. Using this technique, the overall local anaesthetic consumption and need for supplementary analgesia was reduced and patient satisfaction greater than with the continuous infusion technique. Although not proven, sympathectomy may potentially improve the surgical outcome by improving peripheral blood flow and reducing the thrombogenic responses following surgery.

Accidental intra-arterial injection

Another important cause of acute upper limb ischaemia is the inadvertent intra-arterial injection of drugs. Most anaesthetists are aware of the potential for iatrogenic injury with drugs such as sodium thiopentone, but increasingly the accidental intra-arterial injection of a drug of abuse is responsible. The vascular injury is a result of a complex combination of small-vessel obstruction, vasospasm, thrombosis, chemical endarteritis and direct cytotoxic effects on the endothelium (Tait et al., 1994). It is likely that a major initial role is played by vascular occlusion from embolization of filling agents such as talcum powder or corn starch seen particularly with the abuse of oral preparations (Stonebridge et al., 1990). Vasospasm does not appear to play a major role unless perhaps in the case of specific vasoactive agents such as cocaine or methylphenidate (Corser et al., 1985). The variable delay of many patients in seeking medical advice complicates the clinical picture and the frequency of patients taking early discharge further contributes to the difficulty in fully evaluating therapeutic options.

The basis of medical care still consists of elevation of the affected limb, anticoagulation and pain relief. There may be a case to be made for intra-arterial steroid injection to counter small-vessel arteritis while other workers have suggested the use of intra-arterial vasodilators, low-molecular-weight dextran, stellate ganglion block, intra-arterial urokinase (Corser et al., 1985) or systemic Iloprost (Tait et al., 1994), all with variable success.

The anaesthetist's role is in the provision of continuing pain relief or regional anaesthesia for fasciotomy where required. Both can be achieved by using a continuous axillary plexus block. Berger and colleagues (1988) also reviewed and advocated the early use of continuous axillary block for vasodilatation and reported significant success both in relieving ischaemia and in abolishing pain. The block should be continued for 48 hours and accompanied by systemic heparinization. It is clear at this time that no one approach is uniformly successful and a number of patients may still eventually require the peripheral amputation of digits.

REFERENCES

Baxter, A.G. and Coventry, D.M. 1999. Brachial plexus blockade. *Current Anaesthesia and Critical Care*, **10**.

Beauregard, L., Martin, R. and Tetrault, J.P. 1987. Brachial plexus block and chronic renal failure. *Canadian Journal of Anaesthesia* **34**, S118.

Berger, J.L., Nimier, M. and Desmonts, J.M. 1988. Continuous axillary plexus block in the treatment of accidental intra-arterial injection of cocaine. *New England Journal of Medicine* **318**, 930.

Breimer, D.D., Jochemsen, R. and von Albert, H.H. 1980. Pharmacokinetics of benzodiazepenes. *Drug Research* **30**, 875–881.

Brenner, B.M. and Rector, F.C. (eds) 1996. Pathogenesis of renal disease. In *The kidney*, 5th edn. Philadelphia: W.B. Saunders, 1135.

Bromage, P.R. and Gertel, M. 1972. Brachial plexus anesthesia in chronic renal failure. *Anesthesiology* **36**, 488–493.

Coburn, M.C. and Carney, W.I. Jr. 1994. Comparison of basilic vein and polytetrafluoroethylene for brachial arteriovenous fistula. *Journal of Vascular Surgery* **20**, 896–902.

Cone, A.M. 1994. Exercise-induced transient global amnesia in a patient with subclavian steal. *Anaesthesia and Intensive Care* **22**, 95–96.

Cook, C.H., Stemmer, E.A. and Connolly, J.E. 1972. Effect of peripheral resistance on carotid blood flow after carotid-subclavian bypass. *Archives of Surgery* **105**, 9–13.

Corser, G., Masey, S., Jacob, G. *et al.* 1985. Ischaemia following self administered intra-arterial injection of methylphenidate and diamorphine. *Anaesthesia* **40**, 51–54.

Coventry, D.M., Rae, S. and Thomson, M. 1996. A comparison of two neurostimulation techniques of axillary brachial plexus blockade. *Regional Anesthesia* **21** (Suppl. 2S), 23.

Davies, A.H., Walton, J., Stuart, E. and Morris, P.J. 1991. Surgical management of the thoracic outlet compression syndrome. *British Journal of Surgery* **78**, 1193–1195.

Dorothee, M. and Robert, L. 1988. Continuous axillary block for postoperative pain management. *Regional Anesthesia* **13**, 77–82.

Drott, C., Claes, G., Gothberg, G. and Paszkowski P. 1994. Cardiac effects of endoscopic cautery of the upper thoracic sympathetic chain. *European Journal of Surgery* Suppl. 572, 65–70.

Dunlop, M.G., MacKinlay, J.Y. and Jenkins, A.M. 1986. Vascular access: experience with the brachiocephalic fistula. *Annals of the Royal College of Surgeons of England* **68**, 203–206.

Eisenkraft, J.B. 1990. Effects of anaesthetics on the pulmonary circulation. *British Journal of Anaesthesia* **65**, 63–78.

Fields, W.S. 1972. Joint study of extracranial arterial occlusion: VII. Subclavian steal: A review of 168 cases. *Journal of the American Medical Association* **222**, 1139–1143.

Galla, J.H. and Luke, R.G. 1996. Hypertension in renal parenchymal disease. In Brenner, B.M. and Rector, F.C. (eds), *The kidney*, 5th edn. Philadelphia: W.B. Saunders, 2126–2147.

Gilligan, S., Smith, M.B. and Allen, P.R. 1993. Transthoracic endoscopic sympathectomy. *British Journal of Anaesthesia* **70**, 491.

Goldman, L. and Caldera, D.L. 1979. The risks of general anaesthesia and elective operations in the hypertensive patient. *Anesthesiology* **50**, 285–292.

Gould, D.B. and Aldrete, J.A. 1983. Bupivacaine cardiotoxicity in a patient with renal failure. *Acta Anaesthesiologica Scandanavica* **27**, 18–21.

Graham, A.N.J., Lowry, K.G. and McGuigan, J.A. 1993. Anaesthesia for thoracic sympathectomy (letter). *British Medical Journal* **307**, 326.

Harjola, P.T. and Valle, M. 1974. The importance of aortic arch or subclavian angiography before coronary reconstruction. *Chest* **66**, 436–438.

Harlid, R. 1994. Total intravenous anaesthesia with single lumen endotracheal intubation for thoracoscopic sympathectomy. *European Journal of Surgery* Suppl. 572, 37–39.

Hartrey, R., Poskitt, K.R., Heather, B.P. and Durkin, M.A. 1994. Anaesthetic implications for transthoracic endoscopic sympathectomy. *European Journal of Surgery* Suppl. 572, 33–36.

Heino, A., Orko, R. and Rosenberg, P.H. 1986. Anaesthesiological complications in renal trans-plantation: a retrospective study of 500 transplantations. *Acta Anaesthesiologica Scandinavica* **30**, 574–580.

Hight, D.W., Tilney, N.L. and Couch, N.P. 1976. Changing clinical trends in patients with peripheral arterial emboli. *Surgery* **79**, 172–176.

Holleman, J.H., Hardy, J.D., Williamson, J.W. *et al.* 1980. Arterial surgery for arm ischaemia. *Annals of Surgery* **191**, 727–737.

Ishibashi, H., Hayakawa N., Yamamoto, H. *et al.* 1995. Thoracoscopic sympathectomy for Buerger's disease: a report on the successful treatment of four patients. *Surgery Today* **25**, 180–183.

Jedeikin, R., Olsfanger, D., Shachor, D. and Mansoor, K. 1992. Anaesthesia for transthoracic endoscopic sympathectomy in the treatment of upper limb hyperhidrosis. *British Journal of Anaesthesia* **69**, 349–351.

Killen, D.A., Foster, J.H., Gobbel, W.G. *et al*. 1966. The subclavian steal syndrome. *Journal of Thoracic and Cardiovascular Surgery* **51**, 539–560.

Komori, K., Kawasaki, K., Okazaki, J. *et al*. 1995. Thoracoscopic sympathectomy in Buergers disease of the upper extremities. *Journal of Vascular Surgery* **22**, 344–346.

Kovatis, P.G. 1993. Specific considerations with renal disease. In Davidson, J.K., Eckhardt, W.F. and Perese, D.A. (eds), *Clinical anesthesia procedures of the Massachusetts General Hospital*, 4th edn. Boston: Little, Brown, 51–57.

Lambert, M., Ball, C. and Hancock, B. 1983. Management of acute brachial artery occlusion due to trauma or emboli. *British Journal of Surgery* **70**, 639–640.

Levitt, R.G., Wholey, M.H. and Jarmolowski, C.R. 1992. Subclavian artery angioplasty for treatment of coronary artery steal syndrome. *Journal of Vascular Interventional Radiology* **3**, 73–76.

Lin, G-C., Mo, L-R. and Hwang, M-H. 1994. Intraoperative cardiac arrest: A rare complication of T2,3– sympathicotomy for treatment of hyperhidrosis palmaris. *European Journal of Surgery* Suppl. 572, 43–45.

Macchi, P., Pulcini, A., Duflos, P. *et al*. 1996. Evaluation of feasability and efficacy of brachial plexus nerve block in the humeral tunnel in surgery of the hand and forearm. *International Monitor of Regional Anaesthesia* (Abstracts issue), 86.

Maddern, P.J. 1983. Anaesthesia for the patient with impaired renal function. *Anaesthesia and Intensive Care* **11**, 321–332.

Marsland, A.R. and Bradley, J.P. 1983. Anaesthesia for renal transplantation – 5 years experience. *Anaesthesia and Intensive Care* **11**, 337–344.

Martin, J.L. and Rock, P. 1988. Coronary–subclavian steal syndrome: Anesthetic implications and management in the perioperative period. *Anesthesiology* **68**, 933–936.

May, R.C. and Mitch, W.E. 1996 . The pathophysiology of uraemia. In Brenner B.M. and Rector F.C. (eds), *The kidney*, 5th edn. Philadelphia: W.B. Saunders, 2148–2169.

McEllistrem, R.F., Schell, J., O'Malley, K. *et al*. 1989. Interscalene brachial plexus blockade with lidocaine in chronic renal failure – a pharmacokinetic study. *Canadian Journal of Anaesthesia* **36**, 59–63.

Narchi, P. and Dupre, L. 1996. Brachial plexus block. *Proceedings of the 21st meeting of the American Society of Regional Anesthesia*. 199–204.

Nicholls, S.C., Koutlas, T.C. and Strandness, D.E. 1991. Clinical significance of retrograde flow in the vertebral artery. *Annals of Vascular Surgery* **5**, 331–336.

Pinnock, C.A., Fischer, H.B.J. and Jones, R.P. (eds) 1996. Continuous catheter techniques. In *Peripheral nerve blockade*. Edinburgh: Churchill Livingstone, 162–164.

Plastow, S.E. and Weisz, M.T. 1993. Transthoracic endoscopic sympathectomy (letter). *British Journal of Anaesthesia* **70**, 492.

Ponzio, F., Conforti, M., Merlo, M. *et al*. 1992. Carotid–subclavian bypass. Our experience with locoregional anaesthesia. *Minerva Chirurgica (Torino)* **47**, 1347–1350.

Quinn, A.C., Edwards, R.E., Newman, P.J. and Fawcett, W.J. 1993. Treating hyperhidrosis. *British Medical Journal* **306**, 1752.

Scher, L.A., Veith, F.J., Haimovici, H. *et al*. 1984. Staging of arterial complications of cervical rib: Guidelines for surgical management. *Surgery* **95**, 644–649.

Stewart, J.H. and Castaldi, P.A. 1967. Uraemic bleeding: a reversible platelet defect corrected by dialysis. *Quarterly Journal of Medicine (New Series)* **36**, 409–423.

Stonebridge, P.A., Callam, M.J., Farouk, M. and Murie, J.A. 1990. Intra-arterial injection of oral medication in HIV positive drug addicts. *British Journal of Surgery* **77**, 333–334.

Strom, T.B. 1982. Hepatitis, transfusion and renal transplantation- five years later. *New England Journal of Medicine* **307**, 1141–1142.

Tait, I.S., Holdsworth, R.J., Belch, J.J.F. and McCollum, P.T. 1994. Management of intra-arterial injection injury with Iloprost. *Lancet* **343**, 419.

Thompson, R.R. 1986. Anaesthesia and the subclavian steal syndrome. *Anaesthesia* **41**, 1026–1028.

Tucker, G.T. 1986. Pharmacokinetics of local anaesthetics. *British Journal of Anaesthesia* **58**, 717–731.

Weir, P.H.C. and Chung, F.F. 1984. Anaesthesia for patients with chronic renal disease. *Canadian Anaesthetists' Society Journal* **31**, 468–480.

Welling, R.E., Cranley, J.J., Krause, R.J. and Hafner, C.D. 1981. Obliterative arterial disease of the upper extremity. *Archives of Surgery* **116**, 1593–1596.

Williams, C.L., Woods, L.P. and Clemmons, E.E. 1973. Carotid-subclavian bypass grafts for subclavian artery disease. *American Journal of Surgery* **126**, 807–809.

Winearls, C.G., Oliver, D.O., Pippard, M.J. *et al*. 1986. Effects of human erythropoietin derived from recombinant DNA on the anaemia of patients maintained by chronic haemodialysis. *Lancet* **ii**, 1175–1178.

17

Anaesthesia for vascular emergencies

ALASTAIR F NIMMO

INTRODUCTION

Emergency vascular surgery is usually undertaken to treat arterial bleeding or acute arterial occlusion. Most patients are elderly and they typically have multiple medical problems such as heart, lung and kidney disease and diabetes mellitus. A smaller number of patients require emergency vascular surgery because of trauma, and they often have other major injuries. Therefore patients presenting for emergency vascular procedures require urgent surgery for a condition threatening life or limb and usually have other serious illnesses or injuries. Not surprisingly, death or complications during or after surgery are common, and the anaesthetic management and post-operative care of the patient is often challenging and difficult.

EMERGENCY ABDOMINAL AORTIC ANEURYSM REPAIR

The majority of operations on abdominal aortic aneurysms in the United Kingdom are emergency procedures (Naylor *et al.*, 1988), and are performed either because bleeding has occurred from the aneurysm (ruptured aneurysm) or because the aneurysm has become acutely painful and tender and there is considered to be a high risk of rupture (symptomatic or rapidly expanding aneurysm).

Ruptured aneurysm

PRESENTATION AND DIAGNOSIS

Rupture of an aortic aneurysm usually occurs in patients older than 60 years and in men more commonly than in women. Rupture is usually fatal and only a minority of patients undergo emergency surgery (Ingoldby *et al.*, 1986). Many patients die before reaching hospital. Others arrive in hospital alive, but die without reaching the operating room. Sometimes this is because of a delay in making the correct diagnosis or because the patient is transferred from one hospital to another, but in other cases because surgery has been judged to be inappropriate. The mortality rate among those patients who reach hospital is typically 50 per cent and has not improved in recent years (Brimacombe and Berry, 1993; Bradbury *et al.*, 1997).

The classic presentation of a ruptured aneurysm is of a sudden onset of abdominal or lumbar back pain associated with shock and a pulsatile abdominal mass. However, this combination of symptoms and signs is not always present and diagnostic errors are common. Pain may have been present for days or weeks before presentation, caused by rapid aortic expansion, erosion of the aneurysm wall or a small confined leak (Ruckley, 1990). Blood pressure may be normal or at the other extreme the presentation may be with collapse and coma or cardiac arrest. Palpation of the aneurysm may be difficult in the obese. On the other hand, a patient with a palpable aneurysm, but with another cause of pain or shock such as myocardial infarction, may be incorrectly assumed to have a ruptured aneurysm. Ultrasound examination can be used to confirm the presence of an aneurysm, but is not a reliable guide to whether haemorrhage has occurred.

The large majority of ruptured abdominal aortic aneurysms do not extend above the level of the renal arteries and the rupture is usually into the retroperitoneal tissues (Johansson and Swedenborg, 1986). When rupture occurs into the peritoneal cavity, the likelihood of the patient surviving is much reduced (AbuRahma *et al.*, 1991). Occasionally, an aneurysm ruptures into the inferior vena cava to produce an aortocaval fistula. This may give rise to signs of venous engorgement, high-output cardiac failure and a continuous 'machinery' abdominal murmur or thrill so that the diagnosis is made before surgery, or it may be a surprise finding during emergency aneurysm surgery. A primary aorto-enteric fistula occurs when an aneurysm erodes into the bowel, most commonly into adherent duodenum. (A secondary aorto-enteric fistula occurs as the result of previous aortic surgery – typically, there is erosion of the upper end of the aortic graft into the duodenum.) In both cases, minor episodes of gastrointestinal bleeding may occur initially. If the diagnosis is not made at this stage and no surgery undertaken, massive exsanguinating haemorrhage occurs hours to weeks later (Voorhoeve *et al.*, 1996; Nagy and Marshall, 1993).

PRE-OPERATIVE FLUID RESUSCITATION

The usual response of the anaesthetist confronted by a patient with haemorrhagic shock is to give intravenous fluids rapidly in an attempt to restore blood pressure, cardiac output and vital organ perfusion. In a patient with a ruptured aortic aneurysm, this may not be the right thing to do. Brimacombe and Berry (1993, 1994) have reviewed the arguments for and against fluid resuscitation before the aorta is clamped. After the initial bleeding from the aortic

aneurysm, clot formation, retroperitoneal tamponade and hypotension may be important in limiting further haemorrhage. The arguments against fluid resuscitation to restore blood pressure are that this may dislodge clot and overcome tamponade. It may result in further haemorrhage, dilutional coagulopathy and massive blood transfusion. Increased haemorrhage may make the operation technically more difficult for the surgeon. There have been no prospective studies of fluid resuscitation before emergency aortic aneurysm surgery, but some support for a policy of restricting fluid administration before surgery is given by a prospective study of immediate versus delayed fluid resuscitation for hypotensive patients with penetrating torso injuries (Bickell *et al.*, 1994) which concluded that mortality and complication rates were lower when aggressive fluid resuscitation was delayed until the patient reached the operating room. In addition, animal studies of fluid resuscitation after intraperitoneal haemorrhage produced by aortotomy found that very rapid volume resuscitation with either crystalloid or a mixture of hypertonic saline and dextran resulted in more animals dying during the study period (two hours after aortotomy) than when no intravenous fluid was given (Bickell *et al.*, 1991, 1992).

It has been suggested by Crawford (1991) that only sufficient fluid should be given to maintain the systolic blood pressure between 50 and 70 mmHg while Brimacombe and Berry (1993) suggested that a mean blood pressure of 65 mmHg might be a better guide. However, there is no evidence to support any specific figure. A sensible practice is not to give intravenous fluids before the induction of anaesthesia if the patient is conscious and able to obey commands. It would seem more appropriate to give intravenous fluids if severe hypotension is producing symptoms or signs of severe myocardial or cerebral ischaemia. However, in this situation, urgent cross-clamping of the aorta to control bleeding is essential if the patient is to have a chance of survival.

PNEUMATIC ANTISHOCK GARMENT

Sometimes a patient is initially admitted to a hospital where there are no surgeons available who are experienced in emergency abdominal aortic surgery and transfer to another hospital is required. It has been suggested that an inflatable pneumatic antishock garment (PASG), also known as a 'G-suit' or 'military anti-shock trousers' (MAST suit) should be used during transfer. Inflating the garment allows external pressure to be applied to the abdomen and legs and this may both decrease bleeding from the aorta and increase blood pressure. However, the antishock garment makes examination of the patient by the receiving vascular surgeon difficult, and deflation of the garment before surgery may be accompanied by a catastrophic fall in blood pressure. There have been no prospective randomized studies of the use of the PASG in patients with ruptured aneurysms. Studies of the use of the PASG in trauma patients during the transfer from the scene of the accident to hospital have produced conflicting results. A non-randomized observational study (Cayten et al., 1993) found that the use of the PASG in severely hypotensive trauma patients (systolic blood pressure <50 mmHg) was associated with a higher survival rate than when one was not used. On the other hand, a prospective randomized trial in patients with penetrating anterior abdominal injuries and an initial systolic blood pressure ≤90 mmHg showed no benefit (Bickell et al., 1987).

INDICATIONS FOR SURGERY

Occasional cases are reported in which a patient has survived with a small undiagnosed retroperitoneal rupture to undergo surgery weeks or months later. However, for practical purposes it can be assumed that a ruptured abdominal aortic aneurysm is invariably fatal without prompt surgical treatment. Patients who survive surgical repair can be regarded as having had their aneurysm cured. Their long-term survival is little different from that of an age- and sex-matched population and their quality of life is generally good (Rohrer et al., 1988; Stonebridge et al., 1993). A number of factors have been found to be associated with a decreased risk of surviving emergency repair (Table 17.1), but survival may occur in the very elderly or even sometimes following resuscitation from cardiac arrest. It has therefore been argued that emergency surgery is always indicated. However, the present author thinks that most doctors, as well as most patients and their families, would agree that an operation would not be appropriate in the situations defined as relative contraindications by the subcommittee of the Joint Council of the Society for Vascular Surgery and the North American Chapter of the International Society for Cardiovascular Surgery (Hollier et al., 1992):

Table 17.1 *Pre-operative factors associated with a decreased chance of surviving surgery for a ruptured abdominal aortic aneurysm*

- Age > 80 years
- Pre-existing cardiac, pulmonary or renal disease
- Short duration of symptoms before admission
- History of loss of consciousness
- Admission systolic blood pressure < 90 mmHg
- Admission haemoglobin < 80 g/L
- Admission platelet count < 150 × 10⁹/L
- Admission prothrombin time ratio > 1.5
- Cardiac arrest

After AbuRahma et al. (1991), Brimacombe and Berry (1993), Davies et al. (1993), Bradbury et al. (1995).

- Underlying medical condition that would otherwise preclude any significant long-term survival (e.g. terminal cancer).
- Underlying issues relating to quality of life that make repair unreasonable (e.g. demented elderly nursing home patient).

Other situations are less clear-cut. In the very elderly profoundly hypotensive patient who was previously limited by cardiac or respiratory disease, the likelihood of surviving operative repair is low, but the prospect of survival without surgery is zero. Is it better to administer sufficient opioid analgesia to relieve pain and distress and transfer the patient to the ward so that he or she may die there peacefully with their family by their side? Or is it better to transfer the patient to the operating room, knowing that he or she will probably die there or in the intensive-care unit, but hoping that the patient may survive 'against the odds'? Opinions differ. Ideally, such a decision would be made with an accurate knowledge of the patient's medical history and following discussion between the patient, their family, the surgeon and anaesthetist. In practice, information about previous health may not be available, the patient's conscious level may be impaired by hypotension or the effect of opioid analgesics, and the relatives may not yet have arrived in the hospital. However, if an operation is to be undertaken, it is best undertaken at once.

It is sometimes argued that if a decision has been made that the risks of elective repair of an aneurysm in a particular patient outweigh the benefits, and then the patient is subsequently admitted with a ruptured aneurysm, emergency surgery must inevitably be inappropriate. This is illogical. For example, the annual risk of the aneurysm rupturing may have been estimated at less than 5 per cent and the peri-operative mortality associated with elective repair at 10 per cent because of cardiac or respiratory disease, and conservative management was therefore considered appropriate. However, now that the aneurysm has ruptured, the balance of risks and benefits may look very different – for instance, a 100 per cent risk of imminent death without surgery compared to a 50 per cent risk if an operation is undertaken – and surgery may now be appropriate.

THE OPERATION

The operation usually involves a transperitoneal approach with either a midline or transverse abdominal incision, although a few surgeons advocate a retroperitoneal approach to the aorta, and repair of a leaking aneurysm using an aortic stent graft inserted through a common femoral arteriotomy has been described (Yusuf et al., 1994).

The commonest situation is a transperitoneal approach to an aneurysm which has ruptured retroperitoneally. The posterior peritoneum distended with haematoma is exposed. It may be necessary to temporarily clamp the aorta at the level of the diaphragm or to manually compress the aorta against the spine before dissecting and clamping the (usually infrarenal) neck of the aneurysm. There is a risk of tearing the left renal vein or its tributaries during the dissection and the resulting venous bleeding can be impossible to control. (Some surgeons therefore routinely clamp the aorta at the level of the diaphragm rather than clamping the aneurysm neck.) After clamping the aneurysm neck, both common iliac arteries are usually clamped. The aneurysm is opened and its contents evacuated. Bleeding occurs from lumbar vessels in the posterior wall of the aneurysm and these are sutured. The inferior mesenteric artery, if patent, is usually tied off.

A prosthetic tube-shaped graft made of Dacron is anastomosed first to the neck of the aneurysm. The upper part of the Dacron graft itself is then clamped and the upper aortic clamp is removed, testing the upper anastomosis. The lower end of the graft is now sutured to the aortic bifurcation, the graft being thoroughly flushed to remove any clot or atheroma before the lower anastomosis is completed. Then the clamps on the common iliac arteries are released one at a time.

If the common iliac arteries are aneurysmal, it may be necessary to use a Y-shaped aortic graft rather than a tube graft. In this case the internal and external iliac arteries are clamped on each side rather than the common iliac arteries. Two lower anastomoses are fashioned – usually end-to-end anastomoses to the bifurcation of each common iliac artery. The clamps on the iliac vessels are then released one side at a time, with the clamp being taken off the internal iliac artery before the external so that any emboli pass into the internal iliac system where they are less likely to cause ischaemia.

Preparation for surgery

Once the diagnosis of ruptured abdominal aortic aneurysm and the decision to operate have been made, arrangements should be made to transfer the patient without delay directly to the operating room. Prolonged resuscitation in the emergency department is inappropriate, as is the use of an anaesthetic induction room. Anaesthesia should be induced in the operating room. (Occasionally tracheal intubation is required in the emergency department for airway protection or to assist ventilation in the unconscious moribund patient and if surgery is considered appropriate in this situation little or no anaesthesia may be required before aortic clamping.)

Oxygen should be given by face mask. Two large (for example, 14G) peripheral intravenous cannulae should be inserted and at the same time blood samples taken for the cross-matching of 10 units of red cells, fresh frozen plasma and platelets and for the measurement of a full blood count, coagulation screen, urea and electrolytes, and glucose. A brief history of the previous state of health and any drugs being taken (for example, oral anticoagulants!) should be obtained if possible from the patient or the relatives. A brief clinical examination should include assessment of heart rate, blood pressure, peripheral perfusion, conscious level, whether dentures are present and an assessment of whether there are likely to be difficulties with tracheal intubation. In patients having vascular surgery there may be a significant difference in the blood pressure recorded from the two arms – caused by a brachiocephalic or subclavian artery stenosis. If there is such a difference, the higher reading should be regarded as being correct (Frank et al., 1991).

Surgery should not be delayed for the results of blood tests, and the patient should be moved to the operating room while cross-matched blood is being obtained. An electrocardiogram and chest X-ray are useful and in most hospitals can be carried out very quickly when the patient arrives in the emergency department. The electrocardiogram (ECG) may show an acute myocardial infarct or the chest X-ray may suggest that an aneurysm extends to involve the thoracic aorta. However, if a diagnosis of a ruptured aneurysm has been made, one should not wait to obtain these investigations if this will significantly delay transfer to the operating room and on no account should the patient be transferred to the X-ray department.

Analgesia may be required if the patient is in severe pain and anaesthesia is not going to be induced very soon. Small doses of an intravenous opioid may be given in this situation. However, elderly shocked patients are very sensitive to the effects of opioid analgesics which decrease blood pressure by vasodilation, histamine release (morphine and pethidine) and a reduction in sympathetic activity. It has also been suggested that the administration of analgesia can provoke further haemorrhage from a ruptured aneurysm by causing relaxation of tense abdominal muscles with a reduction in tamponade. The administration of opioid analgesics may depress conscious level and result in airway obstruction. Opioids should therefore only be given if the patient has severe pain and should be given in small increments, the aim being only to relieve severe pain rather than to make the patient completely comfortable, unless it has been decided that surgery is inappropriate.

Satisfactory management of anaesthesia and fluid administration requires at least two anaesthetists. In addition to the anaesthetic agents, drugs to treat hypotension or bradycardia (e.g. ephedrine, methoxamine, atropine and adrenaline 10 μg/mL) should be drawn up before the induction of anaesthesia. In the operating room ECG (CM5 modified lead V5, and lead II also if two leads can be displayed simultaneously), non-invasive blood pressure and pulse oximeter monitors and a diathermy electrode should be connected. Ensure that there are two large intravenous cannulae connected to wide-bore intravenous fluid administration sets. 'Y' fluid administration sets should be used so that it is possible to give fluid without interruption when the fluid bags are changed. Blood should be available in the operating room before the induction of anaesthesia. If cross-matched blood is not yet available, group-specific or group O blood should be used. The units of blood should be checked and the first one or two connected to one of the intravenous fluid sets. The blood and intravenous fluid containers should be pressurized and the fluids should pass through a fluid warmer. A urethral catheter is inserted either in the emergency department or in the operating room.

A central venous catheter is not required at this stage unless it has not been possible to insert a large peripheral venous cannula. In that case a large catheter should be inserted into a jugular or subclavian vein. If the patient's condition is stable and there are palpable upper limb pulses, an intra-arterial cannula may be inserted before induction to enable continuous blood pressure monitoring. There may be a significant hypotension on induction and a non-invasive blood pressure monitor may be unable to measure the blood pressure at all. However, prolonged attempts at arterial cannulation should not be allowed to delay surgery. One or both arms should be positioned on arm boards at 90° to the body so that access to intravenous and intra-arterial cannulae is possible during the operation.

Induction of anaesthesia

On induction of anaesthesia a number of factors may combine to produce a decrease in blood pressure which can occasionally be catastrophic and lead to cardiac arrest:

- Reduction in sympathetic drive and endogenous catecholamines.
- Vasodilatation and myocardial depression caused by anaesthetic drugs.
- Decreased venous return caused by positive pressure ventilation.
- Reduction in tamponade may cause further haemorrhage as the abdominal muscles relax.

The surgeons should be scrubbed and the abdomen disinfected and draped before the induction of anaesthesia so that surgery can begin as soon as the patient is unconscious. It must be possible to rapidly infuse fluids during the induction of anaesthesia.

The patient should be assumed to be at risk of aspiration of gastric contents on induction of anaesthesia and a rapid sequence induction technique should be used with pre-oxygenation and cricoid pressure followed by the injection of an intravenous induction agent and suxamethonium. Etomidate produces less of a decrease in blood pressure than thiopentone, propofol or midazolam. Ketamine has been used but, in the hypotensive patient who already has a high sympathetic drive and high endogenous catecholamine production, it may cause a decrease rather than an increase in blood pressure. A retrospective comparison of ketamine and thiopentone for induction in patients with ruptured aneurysms suggested no benefit from the use of ketamine (Beattie et al., 1988).

Not all these patients become hypotensive on induction; in some, laryngoscopy, tracheal intubation and the surgical incision give rise to marked hypertension and tachycardia with a risk of further bleeding and of myocardial ischaemia. To attenuate these responses, an intravenous opioid such as fentanyl or alfentanil may be given before the induction agent unless the patient is moribund with an extremely low or unrecordable blood pressure, or is very drowsy because of the previous administration of an opioid analgesic.

Severe hypotension on induction of anaesthesia should be treated by the rapid infusion of fluids and the injection of vasoconstrictor and sympathometic agents such as methoxamine and ephedrine. The operating table should be tilted head-down. However, the goal at this stage is to avoid hypotension of a severity likely to cause myocardial ischaemia, cardiac arrest or cerebral ischaemia rather than to restore the blood pressure to a normal figure. After intubation of the trachea, the lungs should initially be ventilated gently with oxygen. The tidal volume can be increased and anaesthetic agents added when an acceptable blood pressure is present. If an arterial cannula for continuous monitoring of blood pressure is not in place before the induction of anaesthesia, a rapid guide to whether there has been a marked fall in blood pressure on induction may be provided by an assistant feeling changes in the volume of the pulse, and by looking for changes in the plethysmographic waveform from the pulse oximeter. A decrease in the end-tidal carbon dioxide concentration may provide an indication of a fall in cardiac output.

Maintenance of anaesthesia

A non-depolarizing neuromuscular blocking drug should be given before the effect of suxamethonium has worn off. The surgeon faces a difficult enough task without the patient starting to cough and move! Anaesthesia may be maintained with an intravenous opioid plus nitrous oxide, a volatile anaesthetic such

as isoflurane or a propofol infusion according to the anaesthetist's preference.

Intravenous heparin is not usually given in these patients.

When the surgeon clamps the aorta, afterload increases and so, usually, does the blood pressure. If severe hypertension occurs this may be treated initially by increasing the inspired concentration of volatile anaesthetic or the administration of propofol. However, if this does not readily control the blood pressure it is preferable to infuse glyceryl trinitrate rather than to give a high concentration of an anaesthetic agent with negative inotropic effects. Glyceryl trinitrate should also be infused if ECG signs of myocardial ischaemia develop.

A central venous or pulmonary artery catheter should be inserted once the aorta has been clamped and this is most conveniently introduced through the right internal or external jugular vein. If an arterial cannula is not already in place, one should now be inserted into an upper limb artery. At this stage, a nasogastric tube and nasopharyngeal or oesophageal temperature probe may also be introduced. The haemodynamic goals now are to maintain systemic arterial pressure close to normal and a normal pulmonary capillary wedge pressure or central venous pressure.

Blood and blood product administration

Red cells, fresh frozen plasma (FFP) and platelets should be transfused in addition to the infusion of crystalloid and colloid fluids. The patient should be assumed to have coronary artery disease, and the production of a severe dilutional anaemia by administering far more clear fluid than blood is to be avoided. The aim should be to maintain the haemoglobin concentration above 85 g/L. Intra-operative red cell salvage and retransfusion may be used to decrease the amount of bank blood transfused. However, additional staff are required to set up and operate the autotransfusion system if this is not to delay and distract the anaesthetists managing the patient.

Coagulopathy is usual in patients with a ruptured aneurysm. It is caused not only by dilution of coagulation factors and platelets, but also by disseminated intravascular coagulation. There may not be time to obtain the results of a coagulation screen before surgery and in any case the standard coagulation tests provide limited information about the complex acquired coagulopathy that commonly occurs

(Murphy *et al.*, 1993). FFP and platelets should therefore be ordered as soon as it is decided that surgery is to be undertaken and they should be given after the aorta is clamped. The exact timing of administration of the FFP and platelets should be discussed with the surgeon. For example if brisk bleeding is occurring from a hole in the aorta there is likely to be little benefit in giving them until that bleeding has been controlled. Full blood count and coagulation screen tests should be repeated during and after the operation to help determine the need for further FFP or cryoprecipitate and platelets. At the same time, blood samples should be taken for the measurement of arterial blood-gas tensions and plasma electrolyte concentrations.

Temperature maintenance

The patient is usually hypothermic on arrival in the operating room. Anaesthesia impairs the regulation of body temperature and further heat will be lost from the large abdominal wound if the intravenous fluids and inspired gases are not warmed. Hypothermia during surgical operations is associated with impaired coagulation and increased blood loss (Schmied *et al.*, 1996), post-operative vasoconstriction and myocardial ischaemia (Frank *et al.*, 1993; 1995; 1997) and more frequent wound infections (Kurz *et al.*, 1996). On the other hand, warming ischaemic lower limbs during the period of aortic clamping may be harmful. In an animal study comparing warming and cooling of the lower extremities during the period of aortic clamping, the cardiac output fell more on release of the clamp in the group whose lower limbs had been warmed

Table 17.2 *Methods which can be used to maintain and increase body temperature during emergency abdominal aortic surgery*

- Forced air warming of the upper body
- Warming of intravenous fluids
- Warming of inspired gases
    Low gas flows from a circle system
    Heat and moisture exchanger at the tracheal tube
- Wrapping of upper limbs and head with transparent plastic bags*
- Covering upper limbs and head with towels*
- Warming mattress under the trunk and upper body
- Raising operating room temperature

*If forced air warming is not being used.

(Beebe *et al.*, 1993). A variety of methods can be used to maintain and increase body temperature (Table 17.2). Convective forced-air warming of the chest, upper limbs and head can be very effective in raising the patient's body temperature.

Maintenance of renal function

The patient is at risk of acute renal failure for the following reasons:

- Pre-operative haemorrhagic shock leads to renal tubular ischaemia.
- Suprarenal aortic cross-clamping abolishes renal artery flow producing warm renal ischaemia; infrarenal clamping may cause a reduction in renal blood flow and abnormal intrarenal blood flow distribution.
- Atheromatous emboli or trauma to the renal arteries may occur.
- Post-operative hypotension and low cardiac output may be present, causing further renal hypoperfusion.

General measures to reduce the likelihood of acute renal failure developing include:

- minimizing the duration of any period of suprarenal aortic clamping;
- avoiding hypotension and a low cardiac output during and after surgery by attention to fluid replacement and the use of inotropes; and
- avoiding the use of nephrotoxic drugs.

It has been suggested that giving mannitol, frusemide and dopamine may help preserve renal function. The evidence for a beneficial effect of mannitol and frusemide is conflicting. Other potential beneficial effects of mannitol have been suggested. Paterson and colleagues (1989) found that mannitol given before aortic clamping in elective aortic aneurysm surgery improved post-operative pulmonary function. Dopamine increases renal blood flow by increasing cardiac output and blood pressure, and it has a diuretic action. However, dopamine does not appear to have a specific renal haemodynamic effect in patients undergoing mechanical ventilation (Girbes *et al.*, 1996) and it may cause myocardial ischaemia. If administration of an inotrope is considered appropriate, dopamine may not necessarily be the drug of choice.

Clamp release

Clamp release and reperfusion of the lower limbs results in hypotension and myocardial depression for a number of reasons (Table 17.3). Profound hypotension can on occasion progress to cardiac arrest and death. It is important that the surgeon warns the anaesthetist before releasing the clamps on the aorta or iliac arteries. If glyceryl trinitrate is being infused, this is stopped a few minutes before clamp release. Sufficient fluid should have been administered to raise the pulmonary capillary wedge pressure or central venous pressure up to or slightly above the upper limits of normal (e.g to 16 mmHg and 10 mmHg respectively) before reperfusion. The iliac clamps should be released one at a time and slowly. If an excessive fall in blood pressure occurs then the surgeon should be asked to re-apply the clamp or manually compress the artery. It may be necessary to infuse fluid rapidly to correct hypotension due to hypovolaemia. However, pulmonary capillary wedge (or pulmonary artery diastolic) pressure and/or central venous pressure should be observed closely to avoid excessive administration of fluid when hypotension is due primarily to myocardial depression. The administration of an inotrope may be indicated. Ephedrine (in increments of 3–6 mg) is a useful agent when a mild inotropic and vasoconstrictor effect is desired.

After reperfusion of the lower limbs a metabolic acidosis, systemic hypercapnia with a rise in the measured end-tidal carbon dioxide concentration, and a transient fall in oxygen saturation usually occur. Minute ventilation should be increased provided that severe hypotension is not present and the inspired oxygen concentration may also need to be increased. In the case of profound hypotension, the lungs should be gently ventilated with oxygen alone.

Table 17.3 *Causes of hypotension on clamp release and reperfusion of the lower limbs*

- Hypovolaemia caused by the refilling of empty vasodilated lower-limb vessels
- Blood loss from anastomoses
- Myocardial depression caused by the release of metabolic products from the reperfused ischaemic lower limbs
- Pulmonary micro-embolization leading to pulmonary hypertension and right ventricular dysfunction

After Gelman (1995) and Beebe *et al.* (1993).

If there is little or no hypotension or hypercapnia when the circulation to a leg is restored, this is suggestive of obstruction to blood flow by emboli. If the leg appears ischaemic, an embolectomy catheter may be passed, either through the lower end of the aortic graft or by exploring the femoral artery in the groin. If the leg remains ischaemic the surgeon may need to extend the graft down the leg. Multiple small emboli may lodge in the arteries of the foot resulting in 'trash foot' – typically, the foot is cold and mottled despite the presence of ankle pulses.

POST-OPERATIVE CARE AND COMPLICATIONS

Anaesthesia or sedation and intermittent positive-pressure ventilation should be continued after surgery and patient transfer to the intensive therapy unit. Heat loss should be minimized by keeping the patient well covered during transfer. Haemodynamic instability is common in the early post-operative period and ECG, invasive arterial blood pressure and oxygen saturation should be monitored continuously during the transfer.

Hypertension may occur as a result of peripheral vasoconstriction and inadequate sedation and analgesia, particularly if anaesthesia was maintained with an inhalational agent which has now been discontinued. Hypertension may cause myocardial ischaemia and bleeding and can be treated initially by giving an opioid analgesic and a benzodiazepine or an infusion of propofol. Boluses of all these agents can cause dramatic falls in blood pressure and so should be given cautiously. If the blood pressure remains too high, an antihypertensive agent should be given, for example glyceryl trinitrate by infusion or a beta-blocker.

Equally, hypotension may occur in the early post-operative period as a result of hypovolaemia, cardiac failure or the effects of sedative or analgesic drugs. Hypovolaemia may be the result of continuing bleeding but also commonly accompanies rewarming and peripheral vasodilatation. A further operation is occasionally undertaken in an attempt to control continuing bleeding, but it is more common to find multiple minor bleeding points at re-operation in association with a coagulopathy than to find a discrete bleeding point (Milne *et al.*, 1994). It is therefore important that coagulopathy is corrected as far as possible if continuing haemorrhage is suspected.

Other post-operative complications include lower limb ischaemia, myocardial ischaemia and infarction, cardiac failure, respiratory failure, renal failure, intestinal ischaemia, stroke and paraplegia. However, it should be remembered that typically 50 per cent or more of the patients undergoing surgical repair of a ruptured abdominal aortic aneurysm will be discharged from hospital alive and as already mentioned their long-term survival is little different from that of an age- and sex-matched population and their quality of life is generally good.

Symptomatic non-ruptured aneurysm

Patients presenting with abdominal pain or tenderness without hypotension and who are found to have an abdominal aortic aneurysm may be diagnosed as having a symptomatic but non-ruptured aneurysm. It is presumed that the pain is caused by rapid expansion of the aneurysm and that there is a high likelihood of the aneurysm rupturing within the next few hours or days. Urgent surgery is therefore commonly undertaken. There are, however, two diagnostic pitfalls in this situation. Firstly, a small contained rupture of the aneurysm may already have occurred without producing a haemodynamic disturbance, and a further catastrophic rupture may follow at any moment. Secondly, the pain may be caused by a condition unrelated to the presence of the aneurysm, for example by a myocardial infarct, intra-abdominal malignancy or ischaemic bowel.

The mortality rate associated with the urgent repair of a symptomatic, but unruptured aneurysm is considerably higher than that associated with the elective repair of an asymptomatic aneurysm. One group reported mortality rates of 5 per cent for elective surgery, 26 per cent for urgent surgery for symptomatic unruptured aneurysms and 35 per cent for the repair of ruptured aneurysms (Sullivan et al., 1990). Three factors may contribute to this higher mortality rate. First, patients in whom elective surgery would not be recommended because of advanced age and severe cardiac or respiratory disease may be offered surgery if it appears that rupture of their aneurysm is imminent. Second, when urgent surgery is undertaken shortly after admission to hospital, there is little time for extensive investigation and 'optimization' of the management of co-existing cardiac, respiratory and renal disease. Third, both the abdominal pain with which the patient presents and the patient's death may have a cause other than the aortic aneurysm, for example myocardial or bowel ischaemia.

An urgent computed tomography (CT) scan of the abdomen is often undertaken when a patient is thought to have a symptomatic, but unruptured aneurysm. It may show the presence of retroperitoneal blood if a contained rupture of the aneurysm has occurred, or it may show another unrelated cause of abdominal pain. However, a small retroperitoneal haemorrhage may be difficult to diagnose on a CT scan and both false-negative and false-positive diagnoses of aneurysm rupture occur. If there has been a contained rupture, there is a risk of an extension of the rupture in the X-ray department.

When presented with a patient for urgent repair of a symptomatic aneurysm, the anaesthetist has to decide whether to manage the situation as one would an elective aneurysm repair, establishing invasive haemodynamic monitoring (and perhaps inserting an epidural catheter) before surgery, or whether to manage the patients as if they have a ruptured aneurysm. The first approach is appropriate only if the patient has not been hypotensive at any time and the surgeon feels that it is unlikely that a contained rupture has already occurred. If the aneurysm has not ruptured, intravenous heparin is usually given before the aorta is cross-clamped.

ACUTE LOWER LIMB ISCHAEMIA

Presentation and diagnosis

Acute limb ischaemia typically presents with pain, pallor, pulselessness, paraesthesia and paralysis. It is much commoner in the lower limb than in the upper limb, and may result from arterial occlusion at the level of the aorta, iliac, femoral or popliteal arteries, or of the smaller distal arteries. The main causes are given in Table 17.4. Embolism from the heart was formerly the commonest cause of acute lower limb ischaemia, but this is now a less frequent cause than arterial thrombosis (Giddings and Quraishy, 1994).

Acute lower limb ischaemia is a disease of the elderly. Embolic occlusion usually occurs in patients with heart disease, and arterial thrombosis usually in patients with widespread atheromatous disease. The complications of acute lower limb ischaemia include death, amputation, compartment syndrome, renal failure, deep venous thrombosis and pulmonary

Table 17.4   *Causes of acute lower limb ischaemia*

Embolism
  Cardiac arrhythmias (e.g. atrial fibrillation)
  Mural thrombus
  Valve vegetations
  Atrial myxoma
  Arterial atheroma
Thrombosis
  Atheromatous native vessel
  Arterial graft
  Aneurysm
  Cardiac failure
  Thrombotic states
Dissecting aneurysm
Trauma
  Penetrating
  Blunt
  Iatrogenic
  Traction
Small-vessel disease
  Arteritis

From Giddings and Quraishy (1994) with permission.

embolism (Campbell, 1996). These contribute to a high mortality, 26 per cent of patients presenting to a regional vascular service with acute lower limb ischaemia dying within 30 days of admission (Clason *et al.*, 1989). Most deaths were attributed to cardiovascular or respiratory causes such as myocardial infarct, stroke and bronchopneumonia. Death was more likely in patients with a recent myocardial infarct, those with a history of angina or breathlessness, older patients, and those with a proximal (aorto-iliac) occlusion.

It is sometimes difficult to distinguish between embolism and thrombosis as a cause of acute lower limb ischaemia. Sudden onset of pain, sensory loss and paralysis in a patient without a history of peripheral vascular disease and with atrial fibrillation or a recent myocardial infarction suggests embolism. Thrombosis typically occurs in patients with symptoms or signs of pre-existing peripheral vascular disease. The onset of symptoms may be less sudden and the ischaemia of the limb less complete because of collateral flow.

Treatment

When the diagnosis of acute limb ischaemia is made, heparin is commonly given intravenously as a bolus followed by an infusion. If there is a sensory deficit and paralysis, the arterial obstruction must be relieved urgently or muscle necrosis will occur within approximately six hours. If the ischaemia is thought to be caused by an embolus, embolectomy is undertaken. An incision is made over the femoral or popliteal artery, the artery is exposed and an arteriotomy made. Local clot is removed. To remove remote clot, a Fogarty balloon catheter is advanced into the vessel, the balloon inflated and the catheter withdrawn. After irrigating the vessel with saline, operative arteriography may be carried out. Balloon embolectomy may fail to restore patency of the vessels, particularly if the underlying problem is thrombosis rather than embolism. Further arteriotomies, intra-operative thrombolysis (the instillation of a thrombolytic agent such as streptokinase or urokinase into the occluded artery) or a bypass operation may be required. Fasciotomies may be performed to prevent or treat compartment syndrome.

A saddle embolus is an embolus which impacts at the aortic bifurcation, producing acute ischaemia of both lower limbs. Bilateral common femoral artery embolectomies are performed using Fogarty catheters. Acute aortic obstruction may also be caused by thrombosis of an atherosclerotic aorta or of an aortic aneurysm, and in this situation an aorto-bifemoral or axillo-bifemoral bypass graft may be required.

When acute lower limb ischaemia is thought to be caused by thrombosis rather than embolism, urgent arteriography is usually performed and an interventional radiologist may insert a catheter into the occluded artery for the infusion of a thrombolytic agent. Repeat angiography may reveal that, although the thrombolysis has been successful, there is an underlying atheromatous stenosis. This may be treated by angioplasty, stenting or a bypass graft. Thrombolysis carries a risk of bleeding and fatal stroke may occur.

Anaesthesia

Embolectomy may be performed under local (i.e. infiltration) or general anaesthesia. Even if it is intended that local anaesthesia will be used, an anaesthetist should be present. The patient may be anxious or restless and require sedation. The operator cannot safely manage sedation in addition to concentrating on the operation. The patient may already have been given an opioid analgesic. If sedation is required a small dose of a short-acting benzodiazepine such as midazolam in increments of 0.5 mg intravenously may be used. Alternatively, propofol may be given by intravenous infusion, and has the advantages that fine adjustment of the level of sedation is easier to achieve and that recovery is rapid once the infusion is stopped. Oxygen should be administered by nasal cannulae or face mask and ECG, blood pressure and oxygen saturation monitored. General anaesthesia may be required if embolectomy is unsuccessful and a bypass operation undertaken.

Sometimes spinal or epidural anaesthesia are a suitable alternative to infiltration or general anaesthesia. However, many patients with acute ischaemia will have been receiving intravenous heparin until the time of surgery and most anaesthetists would then consider spinal or epidural anaesthesia to be contraindicated because of concern about the risk of causing an epidural haematoma. Similarly, in patients who have recently received thrombolytic therapy or in whom intra- or post-operative thrombolysis is likely be undertaken, spinal or epidural anaesthesia is probably contraindicated (Onishchuk and Carlsson, 1992).

Although treatment of the ischaemic limb should take place promptly, it is important that the patient's general medical condition should be thoroughly assessed. In addition to a history and physical examination, blood should have been taken for a blood count, urea and electrolytes and glucose and a recent ECG and chest X-ray should be available. Treatment for conditions such as atrial fibrillation with a rapid ventricular response and cardiac failure may need to be given before and during surgery. It may be appropriate to involve a cardiologist in the management of the patient before and/or after surgery and to admit the patient to a high-dependency unit.

Embolectomy or thrombolysis is not appropriate if muscle necrosis has already occurred and the ischaemia of the limb is irreversible. Restoration of circulation to the limb in this situation may cause myocardial depression, cardiac arrhythmia or arrest, and acute renal failure as products of anaerobic metabolism and cell breakdown including potassium and myoglobin return from the limb. If the ischaemia of the limb is irreversible, primary amputation is required. If intravenous heparin is being given, stopping this a few hours before amputation allows a spinal or epidural anaesthetic to be given. Whether spinal or general anaesthesia are given for the amputation, the addition of femoral and sciatic nerve blocks with a long-acting agent such as bupivacaine improves post-operative analgesia. Alternatively an epidural infusion may be used for analgesia after surgery.

Sometimes acute lower limb ischaemia is a preterminal event in a patient about to die of some other condition, for example advanced cardiac or malignant disease. Any intervention other than providing relief of pain is then inappropriate.

ACUTE UPPER LIMB ISCHAEMIA

Acute ischaemia of the upper limb is less common than acute ischaemia of the lower limb. It occurs more often in women than in men and is usually the result of embolism. The patients are less likely to have severe angina or breathlessness than patients with acute lower limb ischaemia and the mortality and amputation rates are lower (Stonebridge et al., 1989). Anaesthetic management of upper limb ischaemia is discussed more fully elsewhere (Chapter 16).

TRAUMA

Presentation and diagnosis

The incidence and pattern of vascular trauma in the United Kingdom and Western Europe differ from that in the United States. Vascular trauma makes up only a small part of the workload of most vascular surgeons in the United Kingdom and penetrating injuries caused by gunshot wounds are much less common than in the United States. The commonest causes of vascular injuries in the United Kingdom are accidents, particularly road-traffic accidents, stabbings and iatrogenic injuries.

Most of the patients injured in accidents and assaults are young. Iatrogenic injuries on the other hand, are more common in elderly patients with pre-existing vascular disease. For example, the femoral artery may be injured during angiography, cardiac catheterization or the insertion of an intra-aortic balloon pump.

Blood vessels are damaged by either blunt or penetrating trauma. The two commonest types of blunt trauma are deceleration injuries to the major vessels and injuries associated with fractured limbs (Mansfield and Wolfe, 1992). Deceleration injuries may cause rupture or avulsion of a vessel when high energies are involved and the resulting severe haemorrhage may be fatal. Partial rupture may occur initially. Blunt trauma in association with orthopaedic injuries sometimes damages only the intima of an artery so that there is no haemorrhage but an intimal flap or thrombus formation may occlude the vessel lumen. Vessel occlusion and signs of ischaemia may first develop some time after the injury. When a penetrating wound completely severs an artery, the ends of the vessel retract and constrict and bleeding may cease. Partially severed arteries on the other hand are more likely to give rise to continuing or recurrent bleeding. Iatrogenic injuries most often involve the common femoral or brachial arteries.

Treatment and anaesthesia

The injured patient with a suspected major vascular injury can appropriately be managed in the emergency department according to the principles taught in the Advanced Trauma Life Support Course for Physicians (Committee on Trauma of the American College of Surgeons, 1993). Very urgent surgery may be required in patients with vascular injuries in the thorax, abdomen or neck. Tracheal intubation may be indicated in the emergency room, or the patient may be transferred to the operating room and anaesthesia induced there. Many of the principles discussed earlier in this chapter in relation to anaesthesia for ruptured abdominal aortic aneurysm repair apply also to anaesthesia for the patient who is shocked as a result of vascular trauma.

When vascular injuries of the limbs cause significant haemorrhage, this is is usually obvious. External haemorrhage may be controlled by applying pressure over the site of bleeding or over the artery proximal to the bleeding point. It is important that vascular injuries causing limb ischaemia are diagnosed promptly and urgent vascular repair undertaken if permanent ischaemic damage to striated muscle is to be avoided.

High-energy limb injuries may result in severe damage affecting bones and muscle as well as artery and vein. If orthopaedic fixation of long-bone fractures precedes vascular repair, an unacceptably long period of ischaemia may result. On the other hand, if

vascular repair is carried out first, subsequent manipulation of the fracture may disrupt the repair. Intraluminal shunts can be used to resolve this dilemma (D'Sa, 1994). Arterial and venous shunts are inserted by the vascular surgeon to bridge the area of vessel injury and restore circulation to the limb distal to the injury. Orthopaedic surgery is then undertaken followed by the definitive vascular repair.

Restoration of blood flow to an ischaemic limb is associated with reperfusion injury, and with the washout of acidic metabolites, potassium and myoglobin from the limb back into the circulation. Therefore, when a venous shunt is inserted to restore venous return it has been recommended that the first few 100 mL of venous blood are discarded. Fasciotomy may be required to prevent the development of compartment syndrome. In the case of an obviously irreparable limb, primary amputation is indicated and the complications of revascularization are then avoided.

Anaesthetic management of the patient with extremity vascular trauma will vary depending on the nature and severity of the associated injuries. A lengthy operation should be anticipated and attention paid to fluid balance and the measurement and maintenance of body temperature.

If myoglobinuria occurs, generation of an alkaline diuresis may prevent renal failure developing. Large volumes of intravenous isotonic saline are given with mannitol and sodium bicarbonate (Slater and Mullins, 1998). In patients at risk of cardiac failure, central venous or pulmonary capillary wedge pressure monitoring may be required.

REFERENCES

AbuRahma, A.F., Woodruff, B.A., Lucente, F.C. et al. 1991. Factors affecting survival of patients with ruptured abdominal aortic aneurysm in a West Virginia community. *Surgery, Gynecology and Obstetrics* **172**, 377–382.

Beattie, W.S., Buckley, D.N., Arciszewski, S.A. et al. 1988. Comparison of ketamine to non-ketamine induction in patients with ruptured aortic aneurysm. *Canadian Journal of Anaesthesia* **35**, S133.

Beebe, D.S., Gauthier, R.L., DeMars, J.J. and Iaizzo, P.A. 1993. Lower extremity hypothermia is beneficial during infra-renal aortic cross-clamping in pigs. *Anesthesia and Analgesia* **77**, 241–249.

Bickell, W.H., Pepe, P.E., Bailey, M.L. *et al*. 1987. Randomized trial of pneumatic antishock garments in the prehospital management of penetrating abdominal injuries. *Annals of Emergency Medicine* **16**, 653–658.

Bickell, W.H., Bruttig, S.P., Millnamow, G.A. *et al*. 1991. The detrimental effects of intravenous crystalloid after aortotomy in swine. *Surgery* **110**, 529–536.

Bickell, W.H., Bruttig, S.P., Millnamow, G.A. *et al*. 1992. Use of hypertonic saline/dextran versus lactated Ringer's solution as a resuscitation fluid after uncontrolled aortic hemorrhage in anesthetized swine. *Annals of Emergency Medicine* **21**, 1077–1085.

Bickell, W.H., Wall, M.J.Jr., Pepe, P.E. *et al*. 1994. Immediate versus delayed fluid resuscitation for hypotensive patients with penetrating torso injuries. *New England Journal of Medicine* **331**, 1105–9.

Bradbury, A.W., Bachoo, P., Milne, A.A. and Duncan, J.L. 1995. Platelet count and the outcome of operation for ruptured abdominal aortic aneurysm. *Journal of Vascular Surgery* **21**, 484–491.

Bradbury, A.W., Makhdoomi, K.R., Adam, D.J. *et al*. 1997. The management of ruptured abdominal aortic aneurysm in the Edinburgh regional Vascular Unit: a 12 year experience 1983–1994. *British Journal of Surgery* (In Press).

Brimacombe, J. and Berry, A. 1993. A review of anaesthesia for ruptured abdominal aortic aneurysm with special emphasis on preclamping fluid resuscitation. *Anaesthesia and Intensive Care* **21**, 311–323.

Brimacombe, J. and Berry, A. 1994. Haemodynamic management in ruptured abdominal aortic aneurysm. *Postgraduate Medical Journal* **70**, 252–256.

Campbell, B. 1996. The acutely ischaemic limb and its treatment. In Campbell, B. (ed.), *Complications in arterial surgery: a practical approach to management*. Oxford: Butterworth-Heinemann, 171–178.

Cayten, C.G., Berendt, B.M., Byrne, D.W. *et al*. 1993. A study of pneumatic antishock garments in severely hypotensive trauma patients. *Journal of Trauma* **34**, 728–735.

Clason, A.E., Stonebridge, P.A., Duncan, A.J. *et al*. 1989. Morbidity and mortality in acute lower limb ischaemia: a 5–year review. *European Journal of Vascular Surgery* **3**, 339–343.

Committee on Trauma of the American ˢ⁻ Surgeons 1993. *Advanced ᵀ⁻* *for Physicians – ˢ⁻* College of Sʳ

Crawford, E.S. 1991. Ruptured abdominal aortic aneurysm: an editorial. *Journal of Vascular Surgery* **13**, 348–350.

D'Sa, A.A.B.B. 1994. Vascular trauma. In Galland, R.B. and Clyne, C.A.C. (eds), *Clinical problems in vascular surgery*. London: Edward Arnold, 166–179.

Davies, M.J., Murphy, W.G., Murie, J.A. *et al*. 1993. Preoperative coagulopathy in ruptured abdominal aortic aneurysm predicts poor outcome. *British Journal of Surgery* **80**, 974–976.

Frank, S.M., Norris, E.J., Christopherson, R. and Beattie, C. 1991. Right- and left-arm blood pressure discrepancies in vascular surgery patients. *Anesthesiology* **75**, 457–463.

Frank, S.M., Beattie, C., Christopherson, R. *et al*. 1993. Unintentional hypothermia is associated with postoperative myocardial ischemia. *Anesthesiology* **78**, 468–476.

Frank, S.M., Higgins, M.S., Breslow, M.J. *et al*. 1995. The catecholamine, cortisol, and hemodynamic responses to mild perioperative hypothermia: A randomized clinical trial. *Anesthesiology* **82**, 83–93.

Frank, S.M., Fleisher, L.A., Breslow, M.J. *et al*. 1997. Perioperative maintenance of normothermia reduces the incidence of morbid cardiac events: A randomized clinical trial. *Journal of the American Medical Association* **277**, 1127–1134.

Gelman, S. 1995. The pathophysiology of aortic cross-clamping and unclamping. *Anesthesiology* **82**, 1026–1060.

Giddings, A.E.B. and Quraishy, M.S. 1994. Management of the acutely ischaemic limb. In Galland, R.B. and Clyne, C.A.C. (eds), *Clinical problems in vascular surgery*. London: Edward Arnold, 19–29.

Girbes, A.R.J., Lieverse, A.G., Smit, A.J. *et al*. 1996. Lack of specific renal haemodynamic effects of different doses of dopamine after infrarenal aortic surgery. *British Journal of Anaesthesia* **77**, 753–757.

Hollier, L.H., Taylor, L.M. and Ochsner, J. 1992. Recommended indications for operative treᵃᵗᵐᵉⁿᵗ of abdominal aortic aneurysms: Rᵉᵖᵒʳᵗ ᵒᶠ subcommittee of the Joiⁿᵗ ᴬᵒⁱ˅ᵃₛᶜᵘˡᵃʳ *Surgery* for Vascular Sᵘʳᵍ⁻ ⁻ᵘⁱⁿᵗᵒ, R. and Mitchell, J.E. 1986. Chaptᵉʳ ⁻ ⁻ᶜᵗ of vascular surgery on community ⁿ⁻ from ruptured aortic aneurysms. *Bᵣ⁻* *Surgery* **73**, 551–553.

Johansson, G. and Swedenborg, J. 1986. Ruptured abdominal aortic aneurysms: a study of incidence and mortality. *British Journal of Surgery* **73**, 101–103.

Kurz, A., Sessler, D.I. and Lenhardt, R. 1996. Perioperative normothermia to reduce the incidence of surgical-wound infection and shorten hospitalization. *New England Journal of Medicine* **334**, 1209–1215.

Mansfield, A.O. and Wolfe, J.H.N. 1992. ABC of vascular diseases – trauma. *British Medical Journal* **304**, 439–442.

Milne, A.A., Murphy, W.G., Bradbury, A.W. and Ruckley, C.V. 1994. Postoperative haemorrhage following aortic aneurysm repair. *European Journal of Vascular Surgery* **8**, 622–626.

Murphy, W.G., Davies, M.J. and Eduardo, A. 1993. The haemostatic response to surgery and trauma. *British Journal of Anaesthesia* **70**, 205–213.

Nagy, S.W. and Marshall, J.B. 1993. Aortoenteric fistulas: Recognizing a potentially catastrophic cause of gastrointestinal bleeding. *Postgraduate Medicine* **93**, 211–221.

Naylor, A.R., Webb, J., Fowkes, F.G.R. and Ruckley, C.V. 1988. Trends in abdominal aortic aneurysm surgery in Scotland (1971–1984). *European Journal of Vascular Surgery* **2**, 217–221.

Onishchuk, J.L. and Carlsson, C. 1992. Epidural hematoma associated with epidural anesthesia: Complications of anticoagulant therapy. *Anesthesiology* **77**, 1221–1223.

Paterson, I.S., Klausner, J.M., Goldman, G. *et al*. 1989. Pulmonary edema after aneurysm surgery is modified by mannitol. *Annals of Surgery* **210**, 796–801.

Rohrer, M.J., Cutler, B.S. and Wheeler, H.B. 1988. Long-term survival and quality of life following ruptured abdominal aortic aneurysm. *Archives of Surgery* **123**, 1213–1217.

Ruckley, C.V. 1990. Ruptured abdominal aortic aneurysm. *Current Practice in Surgery* **2**, 91–96.

Schmied, H., Kurz, A., Sessler, D.I. *et al*. 1996. Mild hypothermia increases blood loss and transfusion requirements during total hip arthroplasty. *Lancet* **347**, 289–292.

Slater, M.S. and Mullins, R.J. 1998. Rhabdomyolosis and myoglobinuric renal failure in trauma and surgical patients: a review. *Journal of the American College of Surgeons* **186**, 693–716.

Stonebridge, P.A., Clason, A.E., Duncan, A.J. *et al*. 1989. Acute ischaemia of the upper limb compared with acute lower limb ischaemia; a 5–year review. *British Journal of Surgery* **76**, 515–516.

Stonebridge, P.A., Callam, M.J., Bradbury, A.W. *et al*. C.V. 1993. Comparison of long-term survival after successful repair of ruptured and non-ruptured abdominal aortic aneurysm. *British Journal of Surgery* **80**, 585–586.

Sullivan, C.A., Rohrer, M.J. and Cutler, B.S. 1990. Clinical management of the symptomatic but unruptured abdominal aortic aneurysm. *Journal of Vascular Surgery* **11**, 799–803.

Voorhoeve, R., Moll, F.L., De Letter, J.A.M. *et al*. 1996. Primary aortoenteric fistula: Report of eight new cases and review of the literature. *Annals of Vascular Surgery* **10**, 40–48.

Yusuf, S.W., Whitaker, S.C., Chuter, T.A.M. *et al*. 1994. Emergency endovascular repair of leaking aortic aneurysm. *Lancet* **344**, 1645.

18

Analysis of costs versus benefit for vascular surgery

MARGARET BOURKE AND ANTHONY J CUNNINGHAM

INTRODUCTION

Cost benefit analysis is the most widely used method of economic evaluation. It entails drawing up a balance sheet of advantages (benefits) and disadvantages (costs) associated with a particular course of action so that choices can be made. Unlike the private sector (where costs, prices, and profits can be used as a guide to decision making for investment) prices to be charged to patients and their health care providers may not reflect the full social benefit of the service. Cost benefit analysis was used to assess flood control programmes in the United States in the 1930s, and was applied in the United Kingdom in the 1960s to transport investment projects, town planning, and more recently, in the 1980s, to education and health care projects (Robinson, 1993a).

ECONOMIC EVALUATION OF HEALTHCARE

Economic evaluation or appraisal is used to describe a number of techniques that may be used to assemble evidence of the expected cost and consequence of different procedures in healthcare. The four main approaches that are currently in use are:

- cost minimization analysis
- cost effectiveness analysis
- cost utility analysis
- cost benefit analysis

Economic evaluation of healthcare is, however, very dependent on whose view point is considered – the patient, the patient's family, the institution, the insurance industry, departments of health, government, or 'society in general'.

Cost minimization analysis

This is an appropriate form of evaluation for use when there is reason to believe that the outcomes of the procedures under consideration are the same. Comparison of daycare surgery with in-patient treatment for varicose veins might be suitable for a cost minimization study. Recent studies indicate that same-day admission and discharge in the first post-operative day after carotid endarterectomy is associated with no difference in clinical outcome

(Kraiss *et al.*, 1995). However, a word of caution is necessary. Cost minimization analysis should be undertaken only when there is evidence to suggest that outcomes are similar. If this evidence is not available, simply concentrating on costs involves the obvious danger of ignoring differences of clinical outcome and providing misleading conclusions.

Cost effectiveness analysis

This is an appropriate technique when the outcome of different investigations or procedures is expected to vary (Robinson, 1993b). The outcome may be expressed in natural units. Measurements may include 'life years gained' after surgical treatment of aneurysmal or occlusive disease of the carotid or abdominal aorta. Information provided by cost effectiveness analysis may be extremely useful in clarifying therapeutic choices for particular disease states.

Cost utility analysis

This is a term used by economists to refer to the satisfaction which consumers derive from goods and services. In the health context, it refers to the subjective level of well-being the patients experience in different states of health. Quality adjusted life-years (QALYs) are calculated by estimating the total life-years gained from a procedure and weighting each year to reflect the quality of life in that year.

To compare outcomes of different programmes, the Rosser index is one measure that is widely used to assign quality of life scores to patients (Mason *et al.*, 1993a). In 1990, United Kingdom cost per quality adjusted year for surgical procedures was given as: £220 for head injury neurosurgical intervention; £490 for subarachnoid haemorrhage neurosurgical intervention; £1180 for hip replacement; £2090 for coronary artery bypass graft; £4718 for renal transplant; £7840 for heart transplant and £107 000 for malignant tumour neurosurgical intervention.

Cost benefit analysis

This is restricted to those forms of evaluation that are used to place a monetary value on benefits or outcomes. This form of analysis may be difficult in some states where healthcare is provided free or substantially above the costs of production. One approach is to seek to establish what price patients would be willing to pay for treatment or services if they were required to pay for them.

CAROTID ENDARTERECTOMY

Carotid endarterectomy (CEA) is the most commonly performed peripheral vascular surgery procedure (Ernst *et al.*, 1987). The number performed in the United States peaked in the mid-1980s at an annual cost of US$1.2 billion. Increasing concerns over the cost of healthcare also surfaced during this time and attempts at cost containment began with the diagnosis-related groups (DRG) hospital reimbursement programme. Increasing concerns about the cost of healthcare coupled with the undetermined efficacy of CEA in preventing stroke were the catalysts for the establishment of two large multicentre trials – the prospective randomized European Carotid Surgery Trialists Collaborative Group (1987) and the North American Symptomatic Carotid Endarterectomy Trial (1991). These studies validated the efficacy of carotid endarterectomy in preventing strokes in symptomatic and asymptomatic patients with significant stenosis (70–99 per cent).

Recent studies have assessed costs versus benefit related to CEA and the utilization of hospital resources. Patient factors contributing significantly to costs include: early pre-operative admission for evaluation and assessment; radiological investigations; anaesthetic technique; post-operative intensive care and high-dependency treatment; and delayed hospital discharge.

Pre-operative evaluation

As in other situations, the objective of evaluation of pre-operative assessment in patients who are to undergo CEA is to determine which diagnostic test yields maximum information, with minimal costs and patient risk. Considering the medical and economic consequences of misdiagnosis, attention has focused on selecting those investigations which identify patients who will potentially benefit from surgery. However, tests such as carotid angiography, the 'gold standard', carry inherent risks and have cost implications. Non-invasive assessment of the carotid artery might reduce the overall cost of the procedure and eliminate the small, but real, procedure related risk of carotid angiography.

Kent and colleagues (1995) assessed the cost effectiveness of four diagnosis strategies employed in the pre-operative investigation of symptomatic patients undergoing evaluation for CEA. These included: (1) duplex sonography (DS); (2) magnetic resonance angiography (MRA); (3) contrast angiography (CA); and (4) combination of duplex sonography and MRA supplemented by carotid angiography for disparate results. In this study, the last noted strategy was associated with the lowest long-term morbidity and mortality in patients with 70–90 per cent stenosis. This combination of techniques had the most favourable cost effectiveness ratio and could potentially replace the current practice of using carotid angiography alone in the pre-operative evaluation of patients with symptomatic carotid stenosis.

Avoiding routine angiography would obviously have a dramatic effect on reducing costs associated with CEA, by an average of US$6500 per patient. Ballard and colleagues (1994a), in a large retrospective review of both symptomatic and asymptomatic patients, compared carotid duplex scan with carotid arteriography to confirm the accuracy of duplex scanning for detecting all grades of disease of the internal carotid arteries. The authors concluded that duplex ultrasonography is a reliable diagnostic tool and can be used as the sole pre-operative investigation for selected patients with extracranial cerebral vascular disease.

Surgeons have relied on the computed tomography (CT) scan to exclude alternative causes of cerebral symptoms and to identify silent infarcts. It was presumed that this information altered the timing of surgical intervention, predicted surgical outcome and helped select patients for non-operative therapy. Routine pre-operative CT scans have been shown to be unnecessary in cost effectivenes studies (Martin *et al.*, 1991). Duplex ultrasound scanning alone, in the majority of incidences, providing adequate anatomical and flow velocity information to allow a safe endarterectomy (Ballard *et al.*, 1994b).

In-patient management

One of the most dramatic consequences of prospective payment has been the gradual reduction in hospital length of stay (LOS) for many surgical procedures.

The appropriate LOS for patients undergoing carotid endarterectomy has been recently re-assessed. Maini and colleagues (1990) reviewed patient outcome and costs of treatment after CEA between 1978 and 1988. They noted a reduction in average LOS from 9.5 days in the first five years of the study to 5.8 days in the second half. The associated constant hospital charge was reduced from US$3113 to US$2620. They concluded that reduction in LOS is the single most important factor responsible for controlling costs of hospitalization with satisfactory early and long-term patient outcome. However, if complications arise during the procedure, significant increases in LOS and hospital costs are to be expected. Appropriate patient selection and choice of anaesthetic technique, surgical expertise, peri-operative patient monitoring and care contributed towards minimizing morbidity and improving patient outcome.

The post-operative management of patients undergoing CEA has changed in recent years with recognition that patients require more high dependency monitoring rather than active intensive care therapy after CEA. A number of recent studies have assessed the outcome of cost effectiveness on intensive-care therapy after CEA. In these studies, less than 20 per cent of patients required intensive care treatment for an average 24 hours (O'Brien and Ricotta, 1991). Current practice is that CEA can be safely performed without routine post-operative intensive care.

Summary

Significant cost savings have been reported, without jeopardy to patients' safety, by comprehensive pre-operative evaluation, avoidance of routine CT scanning, same-day hospital admission, selective intensive-care units and early hospital discharge (Luna and Adyb, 1995).

ABDOMINAL AORTIC ANEURYSM RESECTION

Epidemiological data

Although there is an association between abdominal aortic aneurysm (AAA) and both hypertension and smoking, there is increasing evidence to suggest that biochemical and genetic abnormalities are the primary causes, and that arteriosclerosis is an associated phenomenon (Powell and Greenhalgh, 1989). Further evidence that aneurysmal disease is not simply a variant of occlusive arteriosclerosis comes from epidemiological studies.

Throughout the Western world the mortality from occlusive arteriosclerotic disease is falling. This is probably due to attention to diet, smoking and hypertension. The mortality from AAA, however, appears to be increasing. In England and Wales the age-standardized mortality for AAA rose twentyfold between 1950 and 1984 (Fowkes et al., 1989). In Western Australia, the age-standardized mortality for men over 55 years increased from 34 per 100 000 in 1980 to 46 per 100 000 in 1988 (Norman et al., 1991). These trends have occurred despite several decades of elective surgery undertaken to prevent death from ruptured AAA. The increasing surgical treatment may reflect better diagnostic tests and the elective repair of smaller aneurysms. The increased incidence of ruptured AAA, despite better diagnostic and operative intervention, suggests a rise in the overall prevalence of the disease in the community. In contrast with the poor outcome of AAA rupture, operative mortality for elective repair (Table 18.1) has progressively decreased over the past three decades (Cunningham, 1989).

To prevent the high mortality rate associated with ruptured AAA, population screening was proposed by Mason and colleagues (1993b), with elective operations being performed on patients with the appropriate indications. The survival prospects of the two cohorts were calculated as life expectancies and in terms of life-years. The incremental life-years gained were compared with the incremental costs of the programme. The baseline result and sensitivity analysis indicated that, on the basis of current knowledge, population screening may not be warranted. However, screening programmes might be directed at specific risk groups, in particular men

aged 65–74 years, patients with hypertension, peripheral vascular disease or with a family history of AAA (Darling et al., 1989).

Pre-operative evaluation

Patients who have vascular surgery are considered to have an especially high risk for developing post-operative cardiac complications, the risk of these being reported to range from 5 to 40 per cent. Clinicians have spent a considerable amount of time stratifying these patients into those who may be at higher than average or lower than average risk:

- The first priority is to identify patients for whom the cardiac risks are so high that they outweigh the potential benefits of therapy, thus indicating a more conservative approach.
- The second purpose is to identify patients with clinical problems that might be corrected before surgery.
- The third purpose is to identify those who are most likely to benefit from risk-reducing interventions such as pre-operative percutaneous transcoronary angioplasty (PTCA), bypass surgery or invasive haemodynamic monitoring.

The methods of stratification include clinical risk indexes, exercise stress testing, cardiac imaging, including dipyridamole–thallium scanning (DTS), radionuclide ventriculography (RNV), gated blood-pool ejection-fraction measurement, ambulatory electrocardiographic (AECG) monitoring for silent ischaemia, dobutamine stress echocardiography (DSE) and coronary angiography. Routine coronary angiography before vascular surgery is not feasible because it is invasive and would undoubtedly involve considerable risk and expense if used in all patients. Therefore, the use of non-invasive testing may be the first step in the identification of patients who are at high risk for post-operative cardiac morbidity and mortality, reserving angiography for those patients predicted to be at high risk (Fig. 18.1).

In 1987, Eagle and colleagues developed an algorithm that combined clinical characteristics with dipyridamole-thallium scintigraphy. Unlike most previous studies that included only patients referred by consultant physicians or those considered to be at high risk, these authors studied consecutively enrolled patients, thus reducing referral and selection

Table 18.1 *Elective abdominal aortic aneurysm resection mortality rates*

Period	Mortality (%)
1960–1969	9–18%
1970–1975	4–9%
1976–1986	1–6%

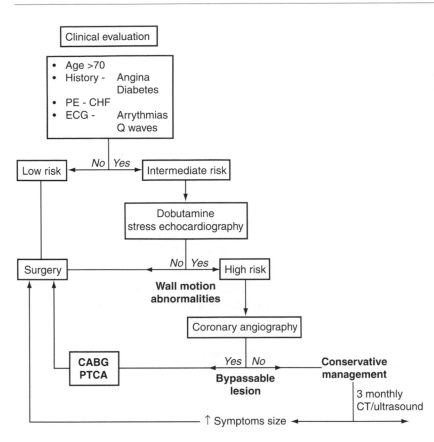

Figure 18.1 *Algorithm for pre-operative assessment.*

bias. Previous knowledge of thallium redistribution may have resulted in altered surgical, anaesthetic and pre-operative medical management.

Which pre-operative test is most effective for predicting adverse peri-operative cardiac outcome? Manta and colleagues (1994) evaluated 56 studies examining one or more of the four tests including DTS, RNV, AECG and DSE. Meta-analysis was performed on 20 studies that met the inclusion criteria. Outcome measures evaluated were cardiac death or myocardial infarction occurring during hospital stay or within one month of surgery. DSE showed good promise for predicting adverse cardiac events after vascular surgery. Incremental dobutamine (10–40 μg/kg/min) was infused, if necessary, to achieve 85 per cent of the age-predicted maximal heart rate in one study (Poldermans *et al.*, 1993). Echocardiographic images were evaluated by two observers blinded to the clinical data of the patients, and results of the test were not used for clinical decision-making. The dobutamine stress test was positive with new or worsened wall-motion abnormality in 35 of 131 patients. All patients with cardiac complications (15 patients) had

a positive dobutamine stress test. No cardiac events occurred in patients with negative tests. Only age >70 years and new wall-motion abnormalities during the dobutamine test were significant predictors of peri-operative cardiac events.

Surgical considerations

Thirty-day mortality after elective AAA repair in the past decade has declined to less than 5 per cent in most centres that manage an adequate volume of cases (Sullivan *et al.*, 1990). The disparity in outcome after AAA rupture and elective repair suggests that early repair should be considered for smaller, lower-risk AAA. The Society for Vascular Surgery/International Society of Cardiovascular Surgery practice guideline now recommends repair of AAA as small as 4 cm in selected patients (Hollier *et al.*, 1992). Once an aneurysm of significant diameter (4–5 cm) is diagnosed, prompt surgical intervention should be considered, unless there are major complications. The only means of improving survival is detection before

Table 18.2 *Incremental cost-effectiveness ratio of early surgery compared with watchful waiting (dollars/QALY)*

Elective operative mortality	Annual rate*		
	0.4%	3.3%	5.4%
2%	WW***	$15 371 ($33 155)**	$8 085 ($18 172)
5%	WW	$17 817 ($39 175)	$8 269 ($19 071)
10%	WW	$23 706 ($67 360)	$8 777 ($21 562)

*Annual rate of abdominal aortic aneurysm rupture or acute expansion.
**The corresponding cost-effectiveness ratios when total charges (hospital plus physician) are substituted for hospital costs are shown in parentheses.
***WW indicates that watchful waiting is the preferred strategy (thus cost effectiveness of early surgery cannot be calculated).
After Katz and Cronenwett, 1994.

Table 18.3 *Comparison of cost-effectiveness ratios for different health care measures*

Early surgery for 4-cm AAA*	$8085–$23 706/QALY
Screening for cervical cancer	$3200–$46 200/QALY
Screening and treating hypertension	$13 600–$69 300/QALY
Beta-blockade after acute myocardial infarction	$5300–$34 200/QALY
Coronary artery bypass	
Single vessel	$51 000/QALY
Left main	$6500/QALY

*Sixty-year-old man with 4-cm abdominal aortic aneurysm with annual rupture rate 3.9–5.4 per cent and elective operative mortality risk 2–10 per cent. After Cronenwett and Katz (1995). Reprinted with permission.

rupture and possibly improved referral rates for elective surgery.

Gilmaker *et al.* (1991) attempted to establish the natural progression of patients with AAA. They found the overall cumulative survival was 51 per cent at five years, with cumulative rupture rate of 12 per cent at five years. The rupture rate was significantly higher (28 per cent at three years) in patients with larger aneurysms (>5 cm). The only reliable predictor of rupture was aneurysm size. Other reports have confirmed that initial AAA size, hypertension (especially diastolic), and chronic obstructive pulmonary disease (COPD) are each independent predictors of AAA rupture. Although not conclusively proven, there is increasing evidence that a positive family history of AAA increases rupture risk, especially when multiple or female relatives are affected (Darling *et al.*, 1989).

The New England Medical Center analysed financial data of 102 patients undergoing elective and emergent abdominal aortic resection over a three-year period from 1986 to 1989 (Breckwoldt *et al.*, 1991). Emergency repairs, although only 12 per cent of the population, accounted for 73 per cent of total losses, with a mean loss of $24 655 per patient. Cronenwett and Katz (1995) found mean hospital costs for ruptured AAA repair were $43 208, nearly double the $24 020 for elective repair. These authors developed a computerized decision analysis model to compare the cost-effectiveness of watchful waiting

with early surgery over a spectrum of clinical scenarios (Cronenwett and Katz, 1995). The variables they considered important were:

• Elective operative mortality.
• Annual rupture rate.
• Patient age.
• Threshold size for elective repair during watchful waiting.
• Patient compliance with follow-up.

The cost-effectiveness ratio for early surgery in a 60-year-old may vary (Table 18.2) from $8085/QALY (at 2 per cent elective operative mortality and 5.4 per cent annual rupture rate) to $23 706/QALY (10 per cent elective operative mortality rate and 3.3 per cent annual rupture rate). The data of Katz and Cronenwett (1994) highlight the additional cost per year of life saved (dollars/QALY) by early surgery versus watchful waiting for a hypothetical cohort of 60-year-old men with a 4-cm AAA at different elective operative mortality rates and different rates of AAA rupture.

In order to put cost-effectiveness of early surgery for 4-cm AAAs into perspective, it is necessary to compare this with the cost effectiveness of generally accepted preventative health measures. In this regard, Table 18.3 shows that the incremental cost effectiveness of a base patient compares favourably with the cost effectiveness of screening for cervical cancer, screening and therapy for hypertension and the use of beta-blockade after acute myocardial infarction. It is also similar to the cost-effectiveness of coronary artery bypass surgery.

Summary

The case for elective aneurysm repair is well established. Despite decreasing mortality rates after elective AAA repair, overall mortality from AAA disease is increasing. Furthermore, emergency aneurysm repair is a financial burden to hospitals. The only means of improving survival is detection before rupture. Targeting at-risk groups may further improve the efficiency of screening programmes.

REFERENCES

Ballard, J.L., Fleig, K., DeLange, M. and Killeen, J.D. 1994. The diagnostic accuracy of duplex ultrasonography for evaluating carotid bifurcation. *American Journal of Surgery* **168**, 123–126.

Breckwoldt, W.L., Mackey, W.C. and O'Donnell, T.F. 1991. The economic implications of high-risk abdominal aortic aneursyms. *Journal of Vascular Surgery* **13**, 798–804.

Cronenwett, J.L. and Katz, D.A. 1995. Cost-effectiveness of operating on small abdominal aortic aneurysms. *Seminars in Vascular Surgery* **8**, 124–134.

Cunningham, A.J. 1989. Anaesthesia for abdominal aortic surgery – a review (Part I). *Canadian Journal of Anaesthesia* **36**, 426–444.

Darling, R.C. III, Brewster, D.C., Darling, R.C. *et al.* 1989. Are familial abdominal aortic aneursyms different? *Journal of Vascular Surgery* **10**, 39–43.

Eagle, K.A., Coley, C.M., Newell, J.B. *et al.* 1989. Combining clinical and thallium data optimizes preoperative assessment of cardiac risk before major vascular surgery. *Annals of Internal Medicine* **110**, 859–866.

Ernst, C.P., Rutklow, I.M., Clevelon, R.J. *et al.* 1987. Vascular surgery in the United States. Report of the Joint Society for Vascular Surgery – International Society for Cardiovascular Surgery, Committee on Vascular Surgery Manpower. *Journal of Vascular Surgery* **6**, 611–621.

European Carotid Surgery Trialists Collaborative Group. 1991. MRC European carotid surgery trial: Interim results for symptomatic patients with severe (70–99%) or with mild (0–29%) carotid stenosis. *Lancet* **333**, 11235–11243.

Fowkes, F.G.R., MacIntyre, C.C.A. and Ruckley, C.V. 1989. Increasive Incidence of aortic aneurysms in England and Wales. *British Medical Journal* **298**, 33–35.

Gilmaker, H., Holmberg, L., Elvin, A. *et al.* 1991. Natural history of patients with abdominal aortic aneurysm. *European Journal of Vascular Surgery* **5**, 125–130.

Hollier, A.H., Taylor, L.M. and Ochsner, J. 1992. Recommended indications for operative treatment of abdominal aortic aneurysms. Report of a subcommittee of the Joint Council of the Society for Vascular Surgery and the International Society for Cardiovascular Surgery. *Journal of Vascular Surgery* **15**, 1046–1056.

Katz, D.A. and Cronenwett, J.L. 1994. The cost-effectiveness of early surgery versus watchful waiting in the management of small abdominal aortic aneurysms. *Journal of Vascular Surgery* **19**, 980–991.

Kent, K.C., Kuntz, K.M., Patel, M.R. *et al.* 1995. Perioperative imaging strategies for carotid endarterectomy. *Journal of the American Medical Association* **274**, 888–893.

Kraiss, L.W., Kilberg, L., Critch, S. and Johansen, K.H. 1995. Short-stay carotid endarterectomy is safe and cost-effective. *American Journal of Surgery* **169**, 512–515.

Luna, G. 1995. Cost effective carotid endarterectomy. *American Journal of Surgery* **169**, 516–518.

Maini, B.S., Mullins, T.F. III, Catlin, J. and O'Mara, P. 1990. Carotid endarterectomy: A ten-year analysis of outcome and cost of treatment. *Journal of Vascular Surgery* **12**, 732–740.

Manta, S., Roizen, M.F., Barnard, J. *et al.* 1994. Relative effectiveness of four preoperative tests for predicting adverse cardiac outcome after vascular surgery: A meta-analysis. *Anesthesia and Analgesia* **79**, 422–433.

Martin, J.D., Valentine, R.J., Stuart, I. *et al.* 1991. Is routine CT scanning necessary in the preoperative evaluation of patients undergoing carotid surgery? *Journal of Vascular Surgery* **14**, 267–270.

Mason, J., Drummond, M. and Torrance, G. 1993. Some guidelines on the use of cost-effectiveness league tables. *British Medical Journal* **306**, 570–572.

Mason, J.M., Wakeman, A.P., Drummond, M.F. and Crumb, B.J. 1993. Population screening for abdominal aortic aneurysm: do the benefits outweigh the costs? *Journal of Public Health Medicine* **15**, 154–160.

Norman, P.E., Castleden, W.M. and Hockey, R.L. 1991. The prevalence of abdominal aortic aneurysms in Western Australia. *British Journal of Surgery* **78**, 1118–1121.

North American Symptomatic Carotid Endarterectomy Trial Collaboration. 1991. Beneficial effects of carotid endarterectomy in symptomatic patients with high-grade carotid stenosis. *New England Journal of Medicine* **325**, 445–453.

O'Brien, M.S. and Ricotta, J.J. 1991. Conserving resources after carotid endarterectomy: selective use of the intensive care unit. *Journal of Vascular Surgery* **14**, 796–802.

Poldermans, D., Fioretti, P.M., Forster, J. *et al*. 1993. Dobutamine stress echocardiography for assessment of perioperative cardiac risk in patients undergoing major vascular surgery. *Circulation* **87**, 1506–1512.

Powell, J. and Greenhalgh, R.M. 1989. Cellular, enzymatic and genetic factors in the pathogenesis of abdominal aortic aneurysms. *Journal of Vascular Surgery* **9**, 297–304.

Robinson, R. 1993. Economic evaluation and health care: cost-effectiveness analysis. *British Medical Journal* **307**, 793–795.

Robinson, R. 1993. Economic evaluation and health care: what does it mean? *British Medical Journal* **307**, 670–673.

Sullivan, C.A., Rohrer, M.J. and Cutler, B.S. 1990. Clinical management of the symptomatic but unruptured abdominal aortic aneurysm. *Journal of Vascular Surgery* **11**, 799–803.

Index

stroke
- after carotid endarterectomy 252
- definition 5
- incidence 5
- lower limb ischaemia and 5
- risk factors 6

stroke volume 67
stump pain 285
stunning 86
subclavian steal syndrome 298–300
sucralfate 195
sudden death syndrome 128
sufentanil 169, 220
superoxide dismutase 182
suxamethonium 223
- effects of renal impairment on 217
- ruptured abdominal aortic aneurysm repair and 309

Swan–Ganz catheter 194
systemic circulation 60, **61**
systemic lupus erythematosus (SLE) 45, 51–2, 239, 276, 295
systemic sclerosis 51
systolic wall motion abnormalities (SWMA) 142

tachycardia 103
Takayasu's arteritis 49, 206
target-controlled infusions of propofol (TCI) 200
telangiectasia, hereditary haemorrhagic 236
temazepam, renal failure and 296
temporal arteritis 49
tetracaine 183
thallium scanning 104
thiazides
- in heart failure 110
- kidney transplantation 223

thiopentone 182
- in carotid arterectomy 259
- effects of renal impairment on 216
- ruptured abdominal aortic aneurysm repair and 310

thoracic epidural anesthesia (TEA) 152, 153, 196
thoracic outlet syndrome (TOS) 27–8, 300–1
thoracoscopic sympathectomy 300–1
thrombin time 236
thromboangiitis obliterans, see Buerger's disease
thromboelastography (TEG), peripheral vascular surgery and 281
thrombolysis 238
thrombophilia in PAOD 44, *44*
thrombophlebitis, malignancy and 240
thrombosis, causes 238–40, *238*
thromboxane A2 (TXA2) 34, 84
- effect of aspirin on 35

thyroid hormones 69
ticlopidine, PAOD and 36, 37
tirilazad in carotid endarterectomy 261
tissue pressure theory of blood flow control 72
total intravenous anaesthesia (TIVA) 199
tPA 238
tranexamic acid 183
transfusion-related lung injury (TRALI) 244
transient ischaemic attack (TIA) 5, 28, 29
- after carotid endarterectomy 252

transient lower limb paralysis 195
transoesophageal Doppler ultrasound, perioperative
- functional principles 143–5
- uses and limitations 145

transoesophageal echocardiography (TOE) 104, 105–6, 133, 168
- limitations 142–3
- monitoring for myocardial ischaemia 142
- monitoring of cardiac function 142
- peri-operative 141–3
- peripheral vascular surgery and 279
- true vs false lumen *168*

trauma, emergency surgery 315
- presentation and diagnosis 315–16
- treatment and anaesthesia 316

treadmill exercise testing 100
triamterene in heart failure 110
tricuspid regurgitation 93
tricuspid stenosis 93
triglyceride
- PAOD and 43
- peripheral arterial disease and 3

troponin 65
trasylol 197

T-wave 139

Ungerleider table 104
unstable (disabling) angina 86
upper limb ischaemia 27–8
- acute 302
- chronic 297–301
- emergency surgery 315

upper-limb procedures
- anaesthesia for vascular access 294–7
- axillary block 297
- pre-operative assessment 295–6
- regional anaesthesia 296–7
- renal failure 296

uraemia in renal transplantation 213
uraemic osteodystrophy 215
urokinase 238

V waves 138
Valsalva manoeuvre 76, 128
valvular heart disease 91–3
- pre-operative assessment 101

varicose veins
- categories *8*
- epidemiology 8
- incidence 31

vascular risk
- antioxidant vitamin E and 45
- modifying 32–4

vascular tone 72
vascular trauma 30
vasculitides 48
vasculitis 48–52, *48*
vasoconstriction 72–4
vasodilatation 73
vasodilators 199